Human Behavior

Human Behavior

An Introduction for Medical Students

Third Edition

Edited by

Alan Stoudemire, M.D.

Professor of Psychiatry
Department of Psychiatry and Behavioral Sciences
Emory University School of Medicine
Atlanta, Georgia

31 Contributors

Lippincott - Raven
P U B L I S H E R S
Philadelphia • New York

Acquisitions Editor: Richard Winters
Developmental Editor: Erin O'Connor
Manufacturing Manager: Dennis Teston
Production Manager: Robert Pancotti
Production Editor: Loretta Cummings
Cover Designer: Karen Quigley
Indexer: Sandi Frank
Compositor: Circle Graphics
Printer: R. R. Donnelley

Printed in the United States of America

9 8 7 6 5 4 3 2 1

Library of Congress Cataloging-in-Publication Data
Human behavior : an introduction for medical students / edited by Alan
    Stoudemire. — 3rd ed.
        p.   cm.
    Includes bibliographical references and index.
    ISBN 0-397-58461-X
    1. Human behavior.   2. Clinical health psychology.   3. Physician and
patient.   4. Psychology.   I. Stoudemire, Alan.
    [DNLM: 1. Behavior.   2. Human Development.   BF 121 H918 1998]
    R726.7.H85   1998
    616'.001'9—dc21
    DNLM/DLC
    for Library of Congress

Care has been taken to confirm the accuracy of the information presented and to describe generally accepted practices. However, the authors, editor, and publisher are not responsible for errors or omissions or for any consequences from application of the information in this book and make no warranty, express or implied, with respect to the contents of the publication.
    The authors, editor, and publisher have exerted every effort to ensure that drug selection and dosage set forth in this text are in accordance with current recommendations and practice at the time of publication. However, in view of ongoing research, changes in government regulations, and the constant flow of information relating to drug therapy and drug reactions, the reader is urged to check the package insert for each drug for any change in indications and dosage and for added warnings and precautions. This is particularly important when the recommended agent is a new or infrequently employed drug.
    Some drugs and medical devices presented in this publication have Food and Drug Administration (FDA) clearance for limited use in restricted research settings. It is the responsibility of the health care provider to ascertain the FDA status of each drug or device planned for use in their clinical practice.

Dedicated to the memory of Boyce Blake and to his family

Contents

Contributing Authors   *xi*

Foreword by Rosalynn Carter   *xvii*

Foreword by Robert O. Pasnau   *xix*

Preface   *xxi*

The Calling of a Physician   *xxv*

Acknowledgments   *xxvi*

Recommended Reference Textbooks   *xxvii*

I   *The Biopsychosocial Model of*
       Understanding Behavior in Health
       and Illness

       1   The Doctor–Patient Relationship   3

            Susan B. Shelton

       2   The Biopsychosocial Model in Medical Practice   36

            Steven A. Cole, Stephen M. Saravay, and
            Richard M. Levinson

       3   Psychological Factors Affecting Medical Conditions
            and Stress Responses   85

            Edward A. Walker and Wayne J. Katon

4   Culture, Ethnicity, and the Practice of Medicine   109

Peter J. Brown, Jessica Gregg, and Bruce L. Ballard

II   *Major Psychological Theories of Human Behavior*

5   Psychoanalytic Psychology   139

Lawrence B. Inderbitzin, Andrew C. Furman, and Mark E. James

6   Behavioral and Social Learning Psychology   182

Pamela G. Dorsett

III   *Human Development through the Lifecycle*

7   Human Sexual Development and Physiology   233

Judith V. Becker, Bradley R. Johnson, and John A. Hunter, Jr.

8   Childhood and Adolescent Development   261

Mary Lynn Dell and Mina K. Dulcan

9   Medicine and the Family   318

Nadine J. Kaslow, Sari Gilman Aronson, and Jennifer P. Wootten

10   Adult and Later-Life Development   340

Thomas Wolman and Troy L. Thompson II

11   The Psychology and Psychobiology of Developmental Trauma   383

Bessel A. van der Kolk

IV   *Biological Basis of Behavior*

12   Neurobiological Aspects of Behavior   403

Cort A. Pedersen, Bradley N. Gaynes, Robert N. Golden, Dwight L. Evans, and John J. Haggerty, Jr.

13   Behavioral Genetics   473

     Miron Baron

V   Clinical Applications

14   Supportive Psychological Care of the
     Medically Ill: A Synthesis of the Biopsychosocial
     Approach in Medical Care   495

     Stephen A. Green

Subject Index   515

Contributing Authors

Sari Gilman Aronson, M.D.

Clinical Assistant Professor
Department of Psychiatry and Internal Medicine
University of Illinois College of Medicine
602 West University Avenue
Urbana, Illinois 61801

Bruce L. Ballard, M.D.

Associate Professor of Clinical Psychiatry
Department of Student Affairs
Cornell University Medical College
445 East 69th Street
New York, New York 10021

Miron Baron, M.D.

Professor of Clinical Psychiatry
Department of Psychiatry
Columbia University College of Physicians and Surgeons
722 West 168th Street
New York, New York 10032

Judith V. Becker, Ph.D.

Associate Dean and Professor of Psychology and Psychiatry
Department of Psychiatry
University of Arizona College of Social and Behavioral Science
1100 University, Douglass Building, 200 West
Tucson, Arizona 85721

Peter J. Brown, Ph.D.

Professor of Anthropology
Departments of Anthropology and Internal Health
Emory University School of Medicine
1440 Clifton Road, Northeast
Atlanta, Georgia 30322

Steven A. Cole, M.D.

Professor of Psychiatry
Hillside Hospital-Long Island Jewish Medical Center
Albert Einstein College of Medicine
1300 Morris Park Avenue
Bronx, New York 10461

Mary Lynn Dell, M.D., Th.M.

Assistant Professor of Psychiatry
The Child Guidance Center of The Children's Hospital of Philadelphia
The University of Pennsylvania
34th Street and Civic Center Boulevard
Philadelphia, Pennsylvania 19104

Pamela G. Dorsett, Ph.D.

Behavioral Institute of Atlanta
6000 Lake Forest Drive, Northwest
Atlanta, Georgia 30328

Mina K. Dulcan, M.D.

Professor of Psychiatry and Behavioral Sciences
Northwestern University Medical School
303 East Chicago Avenue
Chicago, Illinois 60611

Dwight L. Evans, M.D.

Professor and Chair
Departments of Psychiatry, Medicine, and Neuroscience
University of Pennsylvania School of Medicine
36th and Hamilton Walk
Philadelphia, Pennsylvania 19104

Andrew C. Furman, M.D.

Assistant Professor of Psychiatry
Emory University School of Medicine
1440 Clifton Road, Northeast
Atlanta, Georgia 30322

Bradley N. Gaynes, M.D., M.Ph.

Assistant Professor of Psychiatry
University of North Carolina School of Medicine
Campus Box 7160
Chapel Hill, North Carolina 27599

Robert N. Golden, M.D.

Professor and Chair of Psychiatry
University of North Carolina School of Medicine
Campus Box 7160
Chapel Hill, North Carolina 27514

Stephen A. Green, M.D., M.A.

Clinical Professor of Psychiatry
Georgetown University School of Medicine
3800 Reservoir Road, Northwest
Washington, D.C. 20007

Jessica Gregg, M.D.

Department of Anthropology
Emory University School of Medicine
1440 Clifton Road, Northeast
Atlanta, Georgia 30322

John J. Haggerty, Jr., M.D.

Associate Professor of Psychiatry
University of North Carolina School of Medicine
Campus Box 7160
Chapel Hill, North Carolina 27599

John A. Hunter, Jr., Ph.D.

Professor of Psychology
University of Arizona College of Social and Behavioral Science
Douglass Building, 200 West
Tucson, Arizona 85721

Lawrence B. Inderbitzin, M.D.

Professor of Psychiatry and Behavioral Sciences
Emory University School of Medicine
1440 Clifton Road, Northeast
Atlanta, Georgia 30322

Mark E. James, M.D.

Clinical Assistant Professor of Psychiatry and Behavioral Sciences
Emory University School of Medicine
1440 Clifton Road, Northeast
Atlanta, Georgia 30322

Bradley R. Johnson, M.D.

Clinical Assistant Professor of Psychiatry
University of Arizona College of Social and Behavioral Science
Douglass Building, 200 West
Tucson, Arizona 85721

Nadine J. Kaslow, Ph.D.

Associate Professor of Psychiatry
Department of Psychiatry and Behavioral Sciences
Emory University School of Medicine
1440 Clifton Road, Northeast
Atlanta, Georgia 30335

Wayne J. Katon, M.D.

Professor of Psychiatry
Division of Consultation-Liaison Psychiatry
University of Washington School of Medicine
Seattle, Washington 98195

Richard M. Levinson, Ph.D.

Professor of Public Health
Rollins School of Public Health of Emory University
Emory University School of Medicine
1440 Clifton Road, Northeast
Atlanta, Georgia 30322

Cort A. Pedersen, M.D.

Associate Professor of Psychiatry
University of North Carolina School of Medicine
Campus Box 7160
Chapel Hill, North Carolina 27599

Stephen M. Saravay, M.D.

Clinical Professor of Psychiatry
Albert Einstein College of Medicine
1300 Morris Park Avenue
Bronx, New York 10461

Susan B. Shelton, M.D., M.Ed.

Private Practice
27 Lenox Pointe, Northeast
Atlanta, Georgia 30324

Troy L. Thompson II, M.D.

The Daniel Lieberman Professor
Department of Psychiatry and Human Behavior
Jefferson Medical College
1025 Walnut Street, Suite 320
Philadelphia, Pennsylvania 19107

Bessel A. van der Kolk, M.D.

Professor of Psychiatry
Boston University School of Medicine
80 East Concord Street
Boston, Massachusetts 02118

Edward A. Walker, M.D.

Professor
Department of Psychiatry
Division of Consultation-Liaison Psychiatry
University of Washington School of Medicine
Campus Box 356560
Seattle, Washington 98195

Thomas Wolman, M.D.

Clinical Assistant Professor
Department of Psychiatry
University of Pennsylvania School of Medicine
36th and Hamilton Walk
Philadelphia, Pennsylvania 19104

Jennifer P. Wootten, M.D.

Assistant Professor of Psychiatry
Emory University School of Medicine
1440 Clifton Road, Northeast
Atlanta, Georgia 30322

Foreword

We marvel at the clinical, technological, and research advances which have the potential to significantly impact the delivery of health care in America, and we imagine that there may be no limits to scientific progress. However, no technology, no discovery, no pharmacological intervention has transported us beyond the reality that at the essence of health care remains the relationship between a doctor and a patient; and this is most fundamentally true in understanding the emotional and psychological needs of every patient.

Despite our efforts to reduce the stigma of mental illness and emotional problems, millions of Americans are still very fearful about the difficulties that affect their mental, emotional, and social well-being. Patients and their families are afraid to identify these problems, in many instances frightened about what others will think, and often need the help of a physician to understand the nature of their illness and validate the need for help. While we may not be able to overcome this fear and stigma overnight, it is the relationship between doctor and patient which offers an opportunity to be fully responsive to each patient's needs.

The high prevalence of mental and emotional disturbances in the community creates a responsibility for doctors to be sensitive to and cognizant of the mental and emotional needs of their patients and also to develop the readiness to refer them to appropriate specialists when necessary. This requires the study and understanding of human behavior and psychiatry as part of medical education, as well as familiarity with mental disorders that are prevalent in medical settings, such as anxiety disorders, depression, alcoholism, and substance abuse. More than just education, this requires a willingness to clearly hear the mental and emotional concerns of a patient and to make accurate psychiatric diagnoses. The model presented in this text underscores the importance of a carefully cultivated doctor–patient relationship and points to the possibilities for improved quality of care when this framework is conscientiously and consistently applied.

Mrs. Rosalynn Carter

Foreword

It has become increasingly apparent during this era of health care reform that there is a pressing national priority to increase the knowledge of mental disease among all physicians, to implement the understanding of psychiatric treatments and interventions, and to improve the skills of the majority of physicians who will undertake these treatments. The National Institute of Mental Health estimates that sixty percent of the thirty-two million people with mental disease in the United States receive their treatment within the primary care sector entirely. In fact, only one in five with mental illness receives care from the core mental health professionals, with psychiatrists providing only a portion of that care. There is also growing awareness that many nonpsychiatric physicians lack the motivation, the interest, or the conceptual framework that would permit them to provide state-of-the-art treatment to their many patients suffering from mental disorders.

What has been missing in medical education in psychiatry is the excitement and enthusiasm that is so evident in *Human Behavior: An Introduction for Medical Students*, edited by Dr. Stoudemire. The conceptual model that is offered is not peculiar to the behavioral sciences. The biopsychosocial model, in fact, will eventually permeate all of medicine. Beginning with this context and moving through the lifecycle, the biological and psychological factors can be seen as the connecting links that support the scientific application of treatment approaches. This third edition ensures the continued availability of this most needed contribution to medical education and the eventual improvement of the medical care of the citizens of our nation.

Robert O. Pasnau, M.D.
Professor and Assistant Dean
Department of Psychiatry and Biobehavioral Sciences
University of California at Los Angeles
School of Medicine
760 Westwood Plaza
Los Angeles, California 90024

Preface

The essence of being a physician is the ability to integrate excellent medical treatment with compassionate care of the patient. The primary emphasis, however, in medical training is devoted to assimilating a scientific knowledge base and practicing the technical aspects of medical diagnosis and treatment. Relatively little consistent attention is given to acquiring and developing the necessary knowledge and skills to understand and attend to the psychological and emotional needs of patients. With rapid advances in medical science, diagnostic technology, and medical therapeutics over the past 50 years, medical students have been literally crushed by the amount of scientific information they must assimilate. The amount of time and attention devoted to teaching students fundamental principles of human behavior and the psychological aspects of patient care are often given a relatively low priority. The information barrage that students are subjected to, as well as a widespread tendency to determine a specialty choice early in medical school, further contributes to a trend toward narrowness in the training of physicians. In addition, compared to the "hard data" of other scientific disciplines, psychiatry has often appeared diffuse, amorphous, and out of the mainstream of traditional medicine.

There has been an enormous increase in the scientific knowledge base for psychiatry in all of its facets: biological, psychological, and sociological. The biochemical basis for the major mental disorders is gradually being elucidated from studies of aberrant neurotransmitter and receptor activity and molecular genetics. This emerging scientific knowledge has had profound influences on the biological understanding of mental illness. In addition, the field of psychopharmacology has made remarkable advances in providing specific treatments for certain psychiatric illnesses such as psychotic, mood, and anxiety disorders. Advances in neuroradiographic and neuroendocrine probes of the central nervous system have also provided remarkable new ways of measuring biological parameters of normal and abnormal mental functioning. Moreover, while these biological advances may appear to have supplanted the importance of psychoanalytic theories and the perspectives of developmental psychology in psychiatric illness, a growing body of information indicates that certain types of developmental traumas, deprivations, and stresses may have a lasting impact on the central nervous system, leading to altered social behavior, dysfunctional interpersonal relationships, affective instability, and vulnerability to mental disorders. Hence, intriguing scientific evidence is accumulating that may potentially link psychological theories of behavior with neurobiology, enabling a true psychobiologic integration of the behavioral sciences. Where pertinent, this text will point toward trends in this psychobiological body of knowledge.

Throughout this text, the term *biopsychosocial model* will be used. In its essence, this theoretical model emphasizes the importance of understanding behavior and illness from a general systems perspective where multiple biological, psychological, and social systems interact and influence each other. To focus exclusively on one biological, psychosocial, or sociological area while neglecting the others leads to a narrow—and fundamentally mistaken—viewpoint. While in clinical situations necessity and urgency may lead the physician to focus on one given area initially (i.e., attending to a patient's acute myocardial infarction in the emergency room), one must nevertheless not lose sight of the psychological aspects of the illness (the patient's fears and emotional reactions to the heart attack) the effects that the illness might have on other aspects of the patient's life (ability to work and financial affairs), behavioral risk factors that put the patient at risk (i.e., being overweight, smoking cigarettes) or stress that could have actually precipitated the myocardial infarction. Hence, this multidimensional biopsychosocial approach to patient care requires the physician to ultimately assess multiple aspects of the patient's condition in the diagnostic and treatment process.

It is upon the general premise of the biopsychosocial model that this book is based, and it is this viewpoint that forms the predominant theme of the text. The text itself is divided into five sections that address different aspects of a biopsychosocial understanding of human behavior.

The first chapter of the text begins with the cornerstone of the practice of medicine—the doctor–patient relationship. This chapter discusses contractual and psychologic aspects of the doctor–patient relationship framing this relationship within the context of the biopsychosocial model. The basic premises of the biopsychosocial model are discussed in detail in the following chapter, which emphasizes the abundance of scientific evidence to support the validity of the model. While Chapter 2 on the biopsychosocial model discusses at length sociological factors that influence vulnerability for outcome in medical disorders, the next chapter introduces psychological factors that affect medical conditions—with special attention given to the ramifications of stress on the neuroendocrine, immunologic, and cardiovascular systems. The final chapter in this introductory section completes the overview of the biopsychosocial model, examining cultural factors in the practice of medicine.

Section II presents in some detail the basic principles of several major schools of psychology: psychoanalytic and behavioral and social learning theories. The rationale in discussing these several perspectives is addressed in the introduction to the chapter on psychoanalytic psychology and involves a practical decision to cover principles in several major schools of thought in some detail, rather than covering multiple views in a superficial manner, which ultimately would be of little clinical use to medical students. The important principles of psychoanalytic and behavioral theory are presented with emphasis on their practical importance for patient care.

In Section III, fundamentals of normal behavior are dealt with in a comprehensive manner from infancy to later life. This section begins with a discussion of normal human sexual development and provides a basic overview of the normal sexual response cycle. The following chapter on childhood and adolescent development forms a core conceptual framework for the entire text. The section also includes an excellent discussion of *adult* developmental cycles that extends to issues of death and dying. The importance of the family in development and adjusting to illness is also reviewed. This section concludes with an intriguing discussion on one of the most important emerging areas in behavioral science, that is, the neurobiologic effects of developmental stresses and emotional trauma, which as noted above, may serve to integrate psychological and biological perspectives on behavior and mental illness.

Biological aspects of behavior are further discussed in Section IV, addressing two primary areas—neurobiology and behavioral genetics. These chapters present evidence for the biogenetic basis of human behavior, examining data derived from neuroanatomic, neurochemical, and genetic research that should intrigue and interest the most scientifically-oriented student.

The final chapter draws again upon the biopsychosocial model and attempts to integrate the principles discussed in previous chapters to demonstrate how they are useful and important in the care of patients. In this chapter, the specific types of emotional and psychological reactions that patients have to illness are discussed, as well as how they may be managed by physicians using the biopsychosocial model of medical care.

While this text briefly mentions and alludes to the significance of biological, psychological, and social factors in the development of psychiatric illness, specific psychopathological syndromes and the diagnosis and treatment of psychiatric disorders are not specifically addressed. Ideally, this text serves as the basis and entrée to the companion text *Clinical Psychiatry for Medical Students*, which addresses fundamental principles of clinical psychiatry—and also strives for an integrated approach to diagnosis and treatment of the major psychopathological syndromes in psychiatry.

As mentioned earlier in this introduction, the essence of the ideal physician is the ability to practice excellent medicine while attending to the psychological and emotional needs of the patient with compassion. This is certainly not a new concept in medicine and has been the ideal of the profession for centuries. Nowhere has this ethic been more eloquently summarized as in the classic 1927 essay by Dr. Francis Peabody entitled "The Care of the Patient":

> Disease in man is never exactly the same as disease in an experimental animal, for in man the disease at once affects and is affected by what we call the emotional life. Thus, the physician who attempts to take care of patient while he neglects this factor is as unscientific as the investigator who neglects to control all the conditions that may affect his experiment. The good physician knows his patients through and through, and his knowledge is bought dearly. Time, sympathy and understanding must be lavishly dispensed, but the reward is to be found in that personal bond which forms the greatest satisfaction of the practice of medicine. One of the essential qualities of the clinician is interest in humanity, for the secret of the care of the patient is in caring for the patient.

Alan Stoudemire, M.D.

The Calling of a Physician

The thought that I had been granted such a specially happy youth was ever in my mind; I felt it even as something oppressive, and ever more clearly there presented itself to me the question whether this happiness was a thing that I might accept as a matter of course. Here, then, was the second great experience of my life, viz., this question about the right to happiness. As an experience it joined itself to that other one which had accompanied me from my childhood up; I mean my deep sympathy with the pain which prevails in the world around us. These two experiences slowly melted into one another, and thence came definiteness to my interpretation of life as a whole, and a decision as to the future of my own life in particular.

It became steadily clearer to me that I had not the inward right to take as a matter of course my happy youth, my good health, and my power of work. Out of the depths of my feeling of happiness there grew up gradually within me an understanding of the saying of Jesus that we must not treat our lives as being for ourselves alone. Whoever is spared personal pain must feel himself called to help in diminishing the pain of others. We must all carry our share of the misery which lies upon the world. Darkly and confusedly this thought worked in me, and sometimes it left me, so that I breathed freely and fancied once more that I was to become completely the lord of my own life. But the little cloud had risen above the horizon. I could, indeed, sometimes look away and lose sight of it, but it was growing nevertheless; slowly but unceasingly it grew, and at last it hid the whole sky!

"The Right to Happiness" from *Memoirs of Childhood and Youth* by Dr. Albert Schweitzer, translated by C. T. Campion. Used with permission of The Macmillan Company, publishers.

Acknowledgments

The contributors to this textbook are all dedicated clinicians and researchers who represent the very best in academic psychiatry. It has been a pleasure and a privilege to work with them over the years. Their dedication to patient care and medical education will be evident in the quality of the chapters contained herein.

This text could not have been completed without the tireless dedication, loyalty, and effort of my administrative assistant, Ms. Lynda Matthews. Her contribution to this book is greatly appreciated.

Thanks is extended to Dr. Jim Andrews, Clinical Assistant Professor of Psychiatry at Emory University School of Medicine, for his careful and thoughtful review of this text.

Thanks are also extended to the students and faculty of Emory University School of Medicine, as well as to those of other medical schools. Their suggestions regarding the first two editions of this text have, I hope, resulted in a more complete and refined third edition.

Special appreciation is extended to Dr. Steve Rosenberg and his dedicated staff at the National Cancer Institute, National Institutes of Health, who represent the highest ideals of medical science and practice.

Shannon and Dan Amos of Columbus, Georgia provided support, enthusiastic encouragement, and faith in my work that was essential to bringing this third edition to a reality.

Finally, special thanks to Mrs. Rosalynn Carter, Senator Max Cleland, and Mr. Sam Donaldson for their help and advice during difficult times.

Recommended Reference Textbooks

Diagnostic and Statistical Manual of Mental Disorders, 4th ed. Washington, DC. American Psychiatric Association, 1994

> This is the "bible" of descriptive psychiatry. It contains epidemiological and descriptive data of the major psychiatric disorders.

Hales RE, Yudofsky S, Talbott J (eds): Textbook of Psychiatry, 2nd ed. Washington, DC, American Psychiatric Press, 1994

> This is an excellent textbook of clinical psychiatry that is eminently readable and practical. The chapters will provide a somewhat more expanded discussion of the psychopathological syndromes contained in this text.

Kaplan HI, Sadock BJ (eds): Comprehensive Textbook of Psychiatry, 6th ed, Vols 1 and 2. Baltimore, Williams & Wilkins, 1994

> This is an encyclopedic textbook that covers all areas of psychiatry. Detailed and comprehensive, it should be primarily used as a reference source.

Michels R (ed): Psychiatry, Vols I–III. Philadelphia, Lippincott–Raven Publishers, 1996

> This is an excellent and comprehensive textbook of clinical psychiatry. Published in three volumes, the chapters are lucid, well edited, and are kept fresh by a subscription process that periodically updates the material.

Stoudemire A, Fogel BS (eds): Psychiatric Care of the Medical Patient. New York, Oxford University Press, 1993

> This comprehensive textbook is a detailed reference on the psychiatric disorders as encountered in medically ill patients. It contains detailed information regarding diagnosis, psychotherapy, and psychopharmacologic modifications that are required in treating psychiatric disorders in the medically ill.

I

The Biopsychosocial Model of Understanding Behavior in Health and Illness

1

The Doctor–Patient Relationship

Susan B. Shelton

The doctor–patient relationship is often considered the simplest of relationships, but in fact it is one of the most complicated. On the surface, it is the straightforward exchange between a medical expert and a person in need of care. On a deeper level, it is the interaction of two human beings dealing intimately with one another about issues of health, illness, and sometimes death. Unfortunately, this deeper level of interaction is often ignored.

As a medical student or new physician, you may want to maintain emotional distance from patients in order to deal with the enormous pressures of being a physician. Will you know enough to make the diagnosis and offer the right treatment? If the patient dies, will it be your fault? With so much to learn and so many expectations, it is hard to find the time and energy to worry about the nuances of the doctor–patient relationship.

It is tempting to believe that this relationship will automatically happen in a positive way or that it is just a matter of common sense. Most medical students pride themselves on their concern for and commitment to others. However, they also may bring to their profession an idealized if not naïve view of themselves and of their relationships with future patients. This naïveté can lead to frustration and disappointment if it is not tempered with a realistic understanding of the intricate complexities of human personality and the many factors that may influence human behavior in the context of medical illness.

The purpose of both this chapter and this book is to begin to examine the doctor–patient relationship in depth. In many respects, this entire text is devoted to understanding how human behavior is affected by medical illness, which in turn affects the interaction between physician and patient. In this chapter, we will focus on several aspects of the doctor–patient relationship, including:

- Use of the biopsychosocial model
- Empathy
- Styles of relating
- Professional boundaries
- The concepts of transference, countertransference, and the "real" relationship
- Issues of compliance
- Difficult doctor–patient relationships.

The following patient's story introduces many of the major issues to be addressed in this chapter, and it will serve as a reference point throughout this chapter.

A patient with newly diagnosed breast cancer expressed her needs and frustrations in a letter she wrote to her oncologist:

> I am writing this letter as a way to finally be heard by you. . . . At the time of our first meeting, when I told you I was glad to meet you and you countered my honest greeting with a sarcastic remark, "I know you are *not* glad to meet me," you made it perfectly clear that you saw yourself as the "bad guy" and that chemotherapy was going to be a "bad experience." In hindsight, I realize that the relationship you were offering, from the beginning, was never meant to be that of a supportive ally which I so desperately needed during this difficult, stress-filled treatment. Even the setting in which the chemotherapy was administered could never have been conducive to a calm, peaceful reaction. . . .
>
> I am very angry for letting myself be intimidated by you. But I'm also angry and hurt by your impersonal, detached, and at times very rude treatment of me. I came to you anticipating truly professional, innovative, state-of-the-art care. . . . Care does not start and stop with the prescribing of drugs. . . . In addition to your medical opinion, I needed you to support me and encourage me through a very frightening journey. And you were not there for me.
>
> Due to a severe lack of sleep, continuing bladder inflammation problems, poor communication, and other physical and emotional effects of chemo, I gradually became exhausted and unable to cope with life in general, let alone chemo or cancer. You, as my primary physician doing chemotherapy, had a responsibility to remain informed about the results of the various examinations and procedures I was subjected to by doctors you referred me to. You also had a responsibility to communicate to me the impact their findings had on my treatment plan. Instead, I was left with the incredible hassle of trying to get in touch with

them myself and relate their findings to my chemotherapy needs. This
greatly added to the stress I was under.

At our last visit, after talking with me for less than five minutes,
you diagnosed me as severely depressed, referred me to a psychiatrist and suggested that Prozac might help. Then you turned your
back on me while I was crying and walked out the door.

What this patient wanted, and what most patients want from their physicians, is to be heard, understood, and supported. Patients want a physician who
will listen and respond to their individual concerns with empathy and respect.
They want to know that their physician will respond to them when needed and
will not abandon them in the midst of a chronic or terminal illness. As this woman
expressed it, patients want a reliable "ally" who will be emotionally present as
they cope with the uncertainty and pain of their diagnosis and treatment.

To provide this type of support, physicians must understand more than
just the biological and medical aspects of a patient's illness.

BIOPSYCHOSOCIAL MODEL

To know a patient well, one must understand his or her world. As exemplified by the patient letter above, this understanding is not possible through
the use of the biomedical model alone.

The *biomedical* model is defined as an approach to patient care in which
only the biological and medical aspects of a patient's illness are considered
relevant information to be obtained. The model developed out of a prevalent
misconception that one can focus on the disease entity without considering the
person who has the disease (Cassell, 1991). Not included in this model are the
patient's psychological experience and social environment. These omitted
factors can have a major impact on a patient's susceptibility to illness and on
illness outcome.

In contrast, the *biopsychosocial* model is a comprehensive approach to
patient care in which all major aspects of a patient's life are explored (biological, psychological, and social). When used, this approach enables the physician
to provide more effective treatment. This topic will be fully addressed in
Chapter 2 by Drs. Cole, Saravay, and Levinson, as well as in Chapter 14 by Dr.
Green. However, one example may help to illustrate the point.

The oncologist mentioned earlier used the biomedical model in his approach to patient care. He focused on the disease process and pharmacotherapy needed to treat that disease. If he had used the biopsychosocial model,
he would have understood the patient's story that follows.

A CASE STUDY

*JL was a woman in her mid-30s who discovered a lump in her left
breast during a routine breast examination. She was a conscientious*

woman who tried to take care of her health in the same way she took care of her life—through careful planning and control. She saw herself as self-reliant and in charge of what happened to her.

She developed these attributes as a child. She identified with a very controlled and controlling mother and received little emotional support from either parent during times of crisis. When she had a problem or suffered a loss, her mother's advice was always to "get over it."

As an adult, she saw herself as someone who asked for and received little support from others. She was a devoted mother, was active in church and social activities, and had recently made a decision to return to work. Despite a troubled marriage, she felt optimistic about her life.

Her physician assured her that her lump was a cyst, and a mammogram seemed to confirm this. However, attempts to drain the "cyst" were unsuccessful. A difficult biopsy revealed an unsuspected cancer, and the patient underwent a mastectomy. She remained "very strong" throughout these procedures, but felt little support from those around her, including her husband. The patient subsequently went to an oncologist for chemotherapy, and it was in this setting that her "strength" finally gave way.

If the oncologist working with this patient had understood more about her social situation and emotional makeup, he would have realized that she was a woman who was struggling with issues of control and an unspoken need for support. JL had spent her life believing that one could control situations by doing "the right thing" (e.g., doing routine breast examinations) and by being self-sufficient. Overwhelmed by her illness, she found that her attempts at control failed her. A physician who recognized these elements in her life would have been able to give her some sense of control by fully discussing options, assisting her in the decision-making process, and assuring her through action that someone was in charge of her situation and effectively coordinating her care. By recognizing the patient's limited support system, the physician could have provided more personalized care by taking the time to listen to her concerns.

EMPATHY

There is an active component in effective listening, called empathy—the ability to momentarily experience the feelings of another, i.e., to put oneself in another person's place. It is not the same as "feeling sorry" for a patient (sympathy) or offering reassurance (support).

The term has been defined in a variety of ways. A practical definition contains two components. It begins with the ability to experience transiently the feelings of another and to use those feelings to gain an understanding of the other's subjective experience (Zinn, 1993). It ends with the communication of that understanding to the patient. If the understanding is valid, a connection is made that strengthens the doctor–patient relationship.

Empathy is a vital element in establishing a strong therapeutic bond between physician and patient. The patient who feels genuinely understood by the physician is more likely to comply with treatment recommendations and to participate actively in decisions regarding treatment options. He or she is more likely to tell the physician what the physician needs to know to provide optimal care.

Some people believe that empathy cannot be taught and that it is, in fact, an intuitive gift that certain people possess and others lack. They often relegate empathy to the domain of women, and in so doing may subtly denigrate its importance. They see it as the soft side of medicine, what one does when one has nothing else to offer.

If you have had the misfortune to be seriously ill or to have a loved one who was seriously ill, you will empathically understand the true significance of empathy. You have been there. You will be able to recall those physicians who listened to and understood your needs, and those who did not. To you, it will not be a trivial matter. Eventually, it will not be a trivial matter to most of us. Eventually, we will all have a greater understanding of what it means to be a patient than we might wish to have. The development of empathic skills should not have to wait for such an experience.

Ironically, medical students often begin their academic careers with a good deal of empathy. They view their task in humanistic terms, and it is their "education" that changes their views (Spiro, 1993). Students are rarely chosen or rewarded for their empathic abilities and soon learn there are other attributes that will bring them more praise from colleagues. Time pressures and role models often suggest that knowing the right answer is what matters most, and that one can arrive at this with little emotional input from the patient. The patient who insists on telling his or her story in his or her own way may be seen as a nuisance who wastes the physician's valuable and limited time. Lip service may be paid to the issue of empathy: Sure, it's good to be empathic as long as you get the rest of your work done. Fewer people acknowledge that empathy is a critical element of the work and that without understanding the patient, one has understood almost nothing about the patient's illness. This is a radical idea in an era in which science seems to hold the key to accurate diagnoses, and managed care holds the purse strings.

Fortunately, empathy is a skill that can be learned, but only by a person who sees its worth. The mysticism surrounding empathy may stem, in part, from the fact that much of what constitutes an empathic response can occur at a preconscious level. Affective clues are present, but they may resonate on a level at which they are felt before they are understood. For individuals less naturally attuned to the feelings of others, empathy can be taught and, like any skill, becomes easier with practice. Some authors describe it as a trial identification in which one uses one's personal experience and imagination in an attempt to resonate with the experience of another (Zinn, 1993). A physician may ask, "How would I feel if I were this person at this time in this particular situation?" This might be done by relating a patient's experience to one's own. For example, a physician may hear a patient talk about fear of invasion by cancerous cells. The physician may be able to relate to similar feelings when faced with a life-threatening illness (or when a parent was), or the physician may relate to a story or movie in which an individual felt taken over or consumed by an alien force. The physician may imagine what such a loss will feel like in the future. Whatever the source, he or she will attempt to identify transiently with the patient in order to feel in part what the patient feels. Patients are correct when they say, "You don't know how I feel. You can't know how I feel." What you can do is experience an approximation of their feelings and, through words or expression, check out your perception with theirs in search of as close a match as possible. There are moments when the fit is very good, and at those moments an important bond is established in which the patient no longer feels as isolated or alone. An empathic exchange is, in itself, therapeutic and may go a long way to easing a patient's pain or to starting on the road to recovery.

To appreciate the power of such a connection, you have only to reflect on times in your life when someone has seemed to understand you. Attempting to understand another person takes time. However, it is a process that will save time in the long run. A patient who feels understood by the physician also feels she can trust the physician with her greatest worries. Instead of having to mask these worries, the patient may be able to talk with the physician about them and save precious time that would otherwise be spent on more irrelevant issues.

A sample dialogue may help clarify how one listens empathically.
JL said to her physician,

> I am frustrated with all of the disjointed care I am getting. No one is telling me what is going on with my body. First I have one reaction and then another, and no one seems to be aware of what anyone else is doing to me. I can't sleep, I'm exhausted, and I keep having one problem after another.

An unempathic response, and essentially the response the patient received, is the following:

> It's clear you are not handling your illness very well right now. I think you are depressed. I think you need to see a psychiatrist and try Prozac, which might help.

A response that tries to understand the patient's point of view is the following:

> You have had a number of side effects from the chemotherapy, and they haven't cleared up as readily as I would have liked. You seem understandably frustrated with how things are going including perhaps being frustrated with me for not being able to spend more time discussing reports from all the subspecialists you have seen lately. Let me tell you what I know about right now, and as soon as I get the rest of the reports, I will call you, and we'll meet again to go over them.
>
> You look and seem exhausted, and you're telling me you haven't been sleeping. Let's figure out what we can do to help you get the sleep you need in the short run. I also wonder how you are coping with all you've been through. You tell me you don't have much support at home, and I would think about seeing someone to talk to, like a psychiatrist. I frequently recommend talking with a psychiatrist to people with newly diagnosed cancer, and it often helps. Let me know if you're interested in that, and I'll get you a good referral.

What this second exchange did was directly address the concerns of the patient in a nondefensive way and in the physician's own words to see if they matched the patient's perceptions of the problem. It also attempted to resolve the patient's frustration by indicating that the physician was ready to take charge of the case in a personal way.

In attempting to teach empathic responses, there is a danger of encouraging students to make statements that seem canned or manipulative. "Oh, I can see that must be hard for you." Canned responses are the antithesis of genuine empathy and will leave the patient feeling patronized and the physician feeling inauthentic. It is the genuineness of the physician's response, however awkward, that is the hallmark of an empathic response. Patients don't care how you say what you feel; they are far more concerned with the honesty of your response and the depth of your efforts to understand them.

Empathic listening is essential in establishing a solid therapeutic alliance between physician and patient, and without this alliance, little effective treatment can be provided. Equally important in establishing this alliance is the way in which the physician relates to the patient.

STYLES OF RELATING

Physicians have varying approaches to patient care in terms of:

1. The quality of the interaction, e.g., warmth versus detachment
2. The nature of the communication, e.g., who does most of the talking
3. The decision-making process, e.g., who makes the decisions.

These factors can intermix in a number of ways, and different authors have used different designations for physicians' styles (Emanuel and Emanuel, 1992; Frankel, 1987; Kaplan and Sadock, 1991; Underwood and Owen, 1985). More important than the particular designations are the concepts that underlie them. See Table 1–1 for a summary of the categories described below.

The Paternalistic or Autocratic Style

The stereotypical image of the physician in the early 1900s was of a warm father figure who comforted the patient and gave advice (Book, 1991). With the explosion of scientific and medical knowledge in the mid-1900s, this style evolved into a more technical and often detached scientific approach to patient care in which the focus of the physician shifted from the patient to the disease.

Physicians who use the autocratic style may be warm or aloof, depending on their personalities. They provide information to the patient to the extent that they feel this is necessary or helpful. They typically dominate and control the interview process and will ask fewer open-ended questions and fewer questions in general than their more egalitarian colleagues. They make most or all decisions regarding patient care.

The critically ill patient requiring emergency procedures will do best with the physician who takes charge of the situation and makes the decisions necessary to save the patient's life. There are also some patients who relate best to this style in general. These may be patients who feel overwhelmed by their illness, are in crisis, or feel reassured by a strong authority figure who tells them what to do (LeBaron et al, 1985).

Table 1–1 **Physician Styles**

THE PATERNALISTIC OR AUTOCRATIC STYLE
May be warm or detached.
Decisions are made primarily by the physician.
Information is provided to the patient from the physician. The physician is dominant in the interview process.

THE SHARED DECISION-MAKING STYLE
Interaction is typically warm.
Decisions are shared based on expertise of each participant.
Information is shared. The physician asks more questions and is less dominant in the interview.

THE CONSUMER-BASED STYLE
Interaction may be warm or detached.
Decisions are made primarily by the patient.
Information is provided on the basis of the patient's questions. The patient may dominate the interview process.

The Shared Decision-Making Style

Many physicians find the autocratic role uncomfortable or unhelpful to their patients. They may use a more interactive approach in which both the physician and the patient bring their particular expertise to the interview process. The physician brings knowledge of the disease, treatment options, and possible outcomes. The patient brings personal experience with the illness, priorities, and specific concerns. Together, they work toward a consensus on treatment.

The interaction between physician and patient is typically warm and empathic (although, again, this depends upon the personalities of physician and patient). The communication is less dominated by the physician, who is more likely to ask questions, including those that focus on psychosocial concerns. This is the style of communication the patient is most likely to perceive positively (Bertakis et al, 1991; Buller and Buller, 1987).

The Consumer-Based Style

This third style coincides with the current "corporate" phase of medical care (Book, 1991). Using this approach, options are described by the physician, and decisions are left in the hands of the patient or others who will be paying the bills. This occurs most frequently, but not exclusively, in situations that do not involve serious illness. For example, the patient who wants plastic surgery to correct a perceived flaw may be left to make the ultimate choice.

The interaction will often be cordial and businesslike, and communication may be dominated by the patient. The physician is there essentially to answer questions.

Some physicians can readily shift their approach among these styles, depending upon the patient's needs or the situation. They recognize the patient who needs to be actively involved in decision making and the one who would be overwhelmed by such involvement. They also recognize situations that require an autocratic approach, versus those that do not.

Other physicians are less flexible. They have one approach to patient care and expect patients to adapt to them. A patient not satisfied with the physician's style may find another doctor who is more compatible. JL provides a fairly typical example of this solution. The oncologist's style was detached and autocratic. The patient wanted a physician who was warm and engaged and who would share the decision-making process with her. Because of this mismatch, the patient sought treatment elsewhere.

Sometimes, however, the mismatch may persist. This may be particularly true for indigent patients, patients who are easily intimidated, or patients in rural communities. Such patients may feel they have no options except to stay with their doctor or drop out of treatment altogether.

PROFESSIONAL BOUNDARIES

There is a fourth type of relationship between physician and patient that may overlap with any of the three styles previously mentioned. Whenever a physician uses a patient for his or her own end, an unethical relationship arises (Fromm-Reichman, 1950). This exploitation of the patient may be subtle or blatant. It is sometimes outside the physician's conscious awareness and may result from strong feelings on either side of the relationship. The physician may decide that he or she is in love with a particular patient or that a particular patient needs care beyond the normal parameters of the doctor–patient relationship. Often, these powerful emotions involve transference and countertransference feelings, which will be discussed in the next section of this chapter. The first infraction may be a small one, e.g., having the patient come at the end of the day so the physician can spend more time with the patient, or calling upon the patient for expertise in a particular field. These initial violations of boundaries have been called stepping onto "the slippery slope" (Gabbard and Nadelson, 1995) that leads physician and patient to serious compromise and results in harm to the patient. The boundary violations may be done ostensibly with the "consent" of the patient. For example, a physician may get a patient to agree to a sexual relationship. This remains an unethical arrangement because it has occurred in the context of the doctor–patient relationship (Nicholi, 1988).

The doctor–patient relationship is a fiduciary relationship that has at its center the element of trust. The dictionary defines a fiduciary relationship as one in which an individual stands in a "special relation of trust, confidence or responsibility in his obligations to others" (Morris, 1981). A patient trusts a physician to maintain professional boundaries, which includes keeping an appropriate distance from and concern for the patient despite what the patient does. There are many patients who will attempt to push the boundaries of the relationship. It is the physician's responsibility to set and maintain limits for the ultimate good of the patient.

The doctor–patient relationship is not an equal one no matter how egalitarian the physician may wish to be. Patients come to you for your expertise, and they come in a highly vulnerable and often regressed (childlike) state. Although some may come for wellness check-ups, most will see you in a state of fear and distress. They may invest you with superhuman powers. They will most certainly see you as an authority figure with skills and knowledge they lack. Because of this perception, there is an inherent power differential. This power can be easily and subtly misused by a physician. The doctor–patient relationship is clearly not the only relationship in which power can be misused. We could as well be talking about lawyer–client or teacher–student relationships. The difference, if there is one, may lie in the intensity of the emotional experience, which is inherent in the doctor–patient relationship. People come to you sick and afraid. They seek relief and reassurance and may well do whatever it takes to achieve that. It is your responsibility to maintain the boundaries that will allow the best treatment of the patient, and this is not always a simple task. Some emotional involvement with a patient is the mark of a good physician. Where does one draw the line about what is the "right" amount of concern?

The questions of ethical behavior with patients are ones that you will revisit and must revisit throughout your professional career. There are few simple answers to what constitutes unethical action. Most professional organizations have stated that a sexual relationship with a patient is unethical. This assertion is based on the breach of trust involved, the damage such a relationship does to a physician's objective judgment, and the power differential (Gabbard and Nadelson, 1995). Just as a child cannot give meaningful consent to a sexual relationship, neither can a patient who may be consumed with a variety of displaced and intense feelings based on the doctor–patient situation. Review boards are less clear about sexual relationships with former patients or about less blatant physical contact. Is it all right to hold a patient's hand when telling bad news or attempting to give comfort? Is it ever all right to hug a patient or to receive something in addition to money for your services, e.g., a gift, a stock tip, or some other service? The list of possible interactions is endless.

What you will need to develop as you grow in your sense of professional identity is a concept of your own professional boundaries. For some people, this is a relatively easy task. For others it is more difficult. As in any profession, there are people who routinely misuse others. Ideally, these people would be identified early and removed from the practice of medicine. Other people may get themselves in trouble more subtly. If there is a single question to ask yourself, it should be, "Is any action you take for the good of the patient alone?" Many situations are unclear and deserve to be discussed with a trusted colleague. Obviously, if you can keep your professional life clearly separate from your personal life, you will have an easier time maintaining boundaries that are in the best interest of your patients. To the extent that you can establish and maintain a rich and fulfilling life outside of your profession, you will be less needy within the confines of your office. Feeling that you need something from your patients to make your life happier should be seen as a signal of dangerous territory.

There are a variety of other ethical issues that do not directly involve the relationship between the doctor and the patient but are equally important. Many of these may become of increasing concern in the decades ahead as medical resources become more expensive. You may be asked to make decisions about which patients get which care. You may become involved in the controversy over assisted suicide or the right to die with dignity. You will need to make decisions about how much you will tell a patient and when, and how you will tell the patient. You will need to come to terms with your own convictions about what constitutes sound medical practice in the face of pressures from managed care for economic delivery of services.

It may be helpful to end this discussion with a case example.

A CASE STUDY

Dr. H. is a young physician with a growing practice in obstetrics and gynecology. He loves his work and is in great demand. Often, he sees his outpatients at the end of long days of surgery and deliveries. He will frequently fit a patient in either early in the morning or late at night, despite the fact he may need to do this at odd hours or when other staff are not present. His patients love him and frequently bring him gifts. He is very personable and will often discuss his life with interested patients. Sometimes patients will offer to fix him up with single women they know. Because he works so hard, he often feels lonely, with no opportunity to meet available women. On a few occasions, he has taken patients up on their offer to fix him up. He has refrained from dating any of his patients, although he finds several of them very attractive. He has thought about referring them to a colleague so that he might date them. His work is his life, and he occasionally feels he may be missing out on something. On the other hand, he feels lucky to have work that he so much enjoys and is so good at doing. While he knows many colleagues have been sued, he does not see this happening to him, because he is so popular with his patients and because he is such a good physician. He feels certain that his patients will not misconstrue his occasional pat on the arm or acceptance of tokens of appreciation.

Do you have any concerns about this physician's professional boundaries? What are they? You and your colleagues may have very different perceptions of this physician's behavior. Some of you may feel he is a good physician who cares about his patients' welfare, so there is no problem. Others may say he is asking for trouble, i.e., he is walking down the slippery slope toward ethics violations. Let's take a look at his behaviors individually. He appears to be a competent and hard-working physician who has respect for what he does and the patients he sees. There is no evidence that he demeans or devalues the patients. The pat on the arm may be viewed as reassuring or patronizing by the patients involved, and this is an example of one ambiguous area. The question of inappropriate sexual behavior often lies in the eyes of the beholder. In other words, to one patient, a pat on the arm or a hug may mean nothing more than a gesture of comfort. To another patient, it may mean the promise of a different sort of relationship, or it may feel demeaning or even like an invasion or an attack. The physician has no way of knowing how an individual will respond to such contact. He is naïve to assume that it will mean nothing more to the patient than he intends it to mean.

There are other examples of the naïveté of the physician in this vignette. One is that he will not be sued because he is so popular with his patients and is a "good" physician. Misunderstandings and miscommunication are as much a cornerstone of lawsuits as are misconduct and incompetence. Every physician wants to be liked and respected by his patients, but when this moves into the area of a popularity contest, the physician is on dangerous ground. Because of a desire to be liked by his patients, will the physician compromise his decisions regarding optimal care for a patient? Will he underestimate the powerful and often irrational components that go into a patient's "love" for her physician? There is a dangerous naïveté in the physician's decision to see patients whenever he wants, whether or not staff are present. The patient who adores or idealizes him today may feel betrayed or abused by him tomorrow. It is easy to underestimate the intensity of some patients' feelings. Other staff are needed both to verify what actually happens in the examining room and to help maintain a professional atmosphere that can become ambiguous when off-hour visits are arranged. Studies have suggested that inappropriate sexual behavior is more likely to occur with patients who are seen at the end of the day, which could suggest a conscious or unconscious collusion between physician and patient (Gabbard and Nadelson, 1995).

As a physician, you will find yourself responding to patients with a myriad of different feelings. To some, you will feel sexually attracted. There is nothing immoral in having these feelings. It is your response to this attraction that matters. This is often a difficult distinction to make. Some physicians feel so guilty about having sexual feelings toward their patients that they can never find a safe place to discuss them. What is not discussed or sorted through can often become acted upon instead, and that is where the trouble lies. The physician portrayed above has considered referring patients so that he might date them. Some people would find this an ethical resolution to a difficult problem. Others would say that because the relationship was born in the doctor–patient setting, it remains unethical, and that the physician is using his position of power unfairly for his own gain. It is also troublesome that this physician has little or no life outside of his work. This sets him up for a misuse of power, in that he seeks to find fulfillment in his life through relationships at work. While it has not gotten him into obvious trouble, it is likely to cause him problems in the future. He is tempted to use patients to fulfill his own needs and, in fact, has started along this path by accepting help from patients in the form of blind dates.

And what about the gifts? You will hear as many different opinions about gifts as there are physicians teaching this course. Most would agree that expensive gifts are inappropriate, but what about the smaller gift of gratitude? Don't you do as much damage to the doctor–patient relationship when you refuse a gift as you might conceivably do by accepting it? The meaning of the gift and the circumstances are what need to be considered. The first and foremost question in the physician's mind should be the meaning of the gift to the giver. Some psychiatrists refuse all gifts; other physicians, including psychiatrists, make their decisions on a case-by-case basis, focusing on the intent of the giver.

All this may seem like much ado about nothing, and certainly we are talking about different levels of concern when we are discussing sexual contact in contrast to the acceptance of a present. The common thread is the question of how best to maintain the trust and integrity of the relationship between physician and patient. It is a sacred trust that can be easily violated and less easily repaired. Patients will forgive their physicians a great deal, including honest mistakes. They will have a harder time forgiving a doctor for a breach of faith or a misuse of power, however much they seem to be pushing for such a violation. Professional boundaries are in place to protect both the patient and the physician, despite the powerful feelings that may sometimes push to disrupt these boundaries. These feelings are discussed below.

TRANSFERENCE, COUNTERTRANSFERENCE, AND THE REAL RELATIONSHIP

Individuals view one another through distorted lenses that have to do with past experience and early encounters. The more intense the relationship, the more likely it is to evoke feelings related to past relationships. This is called transference. In effect, the patients are "transferring" feelings toward others in their life onto the physician. If an individual has grown up perceiving people around him or her as unhelpful or even harmful, it should not be surprising the physician is viewed in much the same way.

Physicians also may have intense and sometimes distorted emotional responses to patients. These responses may be the result of the patient's attitude toward the physician, e.g., an adoring patient may elicit a sense of exaggerated concern on the part of the physician, or a hostile and demeaning patient may elicit an angry and defensive response from the physician. The physician also may respond to a patient according to the physician's history; for example, an older man may elicit a deferential approach in a physician who had a much-loved father and a young woman may evoke a protective stance in a physician who helped raise younger siblings. These feelings can be broadly defined as countertransference feelings. In simple terms, these are emotional reactions to the patient that often involve the physician's past experience.

Transference and countertransference are technical psychoanalytic terms that will be defined in more detail in Chapter 5 by Drs. Inderbitzin, Furman, and James. As noted above, they are the emotional responses between patient and physician that are influenced by unconscious factors related to past relationships. They usually surprise the physician with their intensity. Most physicians are disconcerted when the patient they are trying to help appears angry, seductive, or distrustful. They may be equally appalled when they discover there is a patient whom they particularly dislike or who makes them feel especially inadequate. A typical response to these unpleasant feelings is to try to deny or ignore them. While this may seem like a reasonable approach, it is one that can lead to more trouble in the long run. Doctors who are unwilling to recognize and understand their dislike for certain patients may instead try to avoid them. This will certainly compromise the relationship and ultimately the care provided.

In addition to transference and countertransference feelings, the nature of the *real* relationship also will affect behavior. Friction can occur between doctor and patient when either or both have difficult personality traits. Problems arise when physicians are rigid or overly controlling or have an inordinate desire to be "worshipped" or idealized by others. Physicians wishing for or expecting worship from patients find it particularly difficult to tolerate patients' anger. The oncologist working with JL is a case in point. The patient's descriptions depict a physician who was rigid and aloof. It is likely that the patient displaced some of her anger about the illness and the lack of certainty about her prognosis onto the physician. The displaced feelings may have been poorly tolerated by the physician, who then literally turned his back on her and sent her to a psychiatrist to get medicated.

It is also likely that there were more classic transference and countertransference elements in this relationship. The patient viewed important figures from the past as unhelpful and unsupportive. This past experience may have contributed to the intensity of her reaction to this physician. We know nothing about the physician's history and can only speculate about possible countertransference reactions. Because of his personal history, did this physician feel the patient's questions and requests were challenges to his authority and competence? Did he have a need to remain distant from a patient who might subsequently die despite his best efforts?

Transference and countertransference feelings always exist between patients and physicians, although they may vary in intensity. They are inherently neither good nor bad. The feelings themselves do not cause harm even when they are "negative" ones such as anger, hatred, or fear. When recognized and examined, these feelings can be a source of much useful and positive information. Harm can occur when they are ignored or denied. Physicians who cannot consciously acknowledge their dislike for certain patients may inadvertently and unconsciously harm them by dismissing them or by aggressively treating them with unnecessary tests or procedures.

When physicians can recognize these negative (and positive) feelings, they can explore their source through self-reflection and sometimes consultation with colleagues. Once they understand the meaning of the feelings, they can respond appropriately and consciously in a way that will ultimately be more therapeutic for the patient.

ISSUES OF COMPLIANCE

The ultimate goal of any interaction between physician and patient is to ensure that effective treatment is provided. This leads directly to the issue of compliance with treatment recommendations.

Poor compliance is a major problem in medical practice. It can be minimized or exacerbated by physician interventions and by the quality of the doctor–patient relationship (Fuller and Gross, 1990). As many as 50% of patients do not comply with treatment. One study showed that one third of patients complied with all treatment recommendations, one third complied with some recommendations, and one third were completely noncompliant (Sackett and Haynes, 1976). These figures do not change significantly with increasing severity of illness.

The statistics are demoralizing; they suggest that a correct diagnosis and treatment strategy is only half the battle. Far more complicated is the effort to get patients to comply with recommended treatment. It is easy to become frustrated with patients who do not comply with recommendations; for example, the obese patient who will not lose weight, or the smoker who will not quit. More dramatic are patients who do not make important life changes after significant events, such as the patient who cannot slow down after a myocardial infarction.

Change is a difficult proposition for everyone. The doctor who has had a serious illness or even a minor one will be in the best position to understand how difficult compliance can sometimes be. The simplest example of noncompliance might be the need for a full course of antibiotic medication to treat streptococcal pharyngitis. Every medical student knows the importance of completing the course of medication; yet, most can acknowledge how difficult it was for them to stick to the regimen without forgetting one or more doses.

The most effective approach to the problem of noncompliance is to look at factors that may impede compliance and those that seem to enhance it (Stoudemire and Thompson, 1983). The factors are numerous and patient-specific, but they can be categorized (see Table 1–2).

Table 1–2 **Factors Affecting Compliance**

FACTORS THAT IMPEDE COMPLIANCE
1. Low level of subjective distress.
2. Denial of illness.
3. Poor communication between physician and patient.
4. Complex regimens.
5. Treatment that is embarrassing or humiliating.
6. Outside factors that make compliance difficult.
7. Patient's perception that it is beneficial to remain ill.
8. Side effects that are significant for the patient.

FACTORS THAT ENHANCE COMPLIANCE
1. Good rapport between physician and patient.
2. Simple regimens.
3. Clear instructions that patient can repeat back to physician.
4. Positive feedback for adherence.
5. Increased level of distress.
6. Decreased waiting room time.
7. Increased time with physician.
8. Family support and involvement.

Factors Related to Noncompliance

1. *The patient may not feel ill.* Patients have a hard time taking their antihypertensive medications because they don't feel ill. Likewise, the patient being treated for an acute infection may stop taking medication as soon as symptoms are relieved.
2. *The patient may wish to deny the illness.* Taking medication or following some other treatment regimen is a reminder of the illness. A simple solution is to become noncompliant.
3. *The patient may not understand the rationale for the treatment or how the medication is to be taken.* This is particularly possible if the patient and physician do not communicate well.
4. *The patient may find the treatment regimen too difficult or disruptive to follow* (Stone, 1979). One patient reported that several different physicians were treating her, and she was asked to take 12 different medications throughout the day.
5. *The patient may feel embarrassed or humiliated by the treatment recommended.* This may be particularly true for young people who do not want to be seen as sick by their peers. They may find it difficult to take medications at school and therefore become noncompliant or "forget" to take their medications during the day.
6. *The patient's family, work pressures, or other outside factors may limit compliance.* For example, the woman in a high-pressure executive position may find it impossible to comply with her physician's advice that she cut back on her work hours. Family members may refuse to acknowledge illness in a relative, or they may give advice that contradicts that of the physician.
7. *The patient may perceive that he or she benefits from being ill.* He or she may get additional attention from family members, more time off work, or similar benefits. The patient may, on a conscious or unconscious level, wish to remain ill and therefore not comply.
8. *The patient may be noncompliant because of side effects from the medication.* If the medication makes patients feel worse, it is likely they will stop taking it.

There are undoubtedly other factors that contribute to poor compliance. A patient may let the physician know what these factors are if asked about them in a nonpunitive and nonjudgmental way. However, often physicians will need to ask repeatedly about compliance problems, especially those related to personal embarrassment or denial of illness.

Factors That Enhance Compliance

1. *Good rapport with the physician.* Patients who believe that their physician understands them and is interested in their welfare are far more likely to comply with the recommendations. It is also undoubtedly true that such a relationship will foster improved communication and greater mutual understanding. Shared priorities and styles of communicating enhance compliance.

2. *Simplifying treatment regimens.* Patients will have a far easier time with once-a-day dosing whenever possible, fewer pills, and a regimen that is easy to remember, e.g., taking medications at bedtime (Porter, 1969).

3. *Clear and simple instructions.* Physicians give directions regarding medication, but they do not always check to see what has been understood. Patients retain information better when it is presented at the beginning of a session rather than at the end (Ley, 1972). It is often useful to write down instructions if the patient can read, and to ask the patient to repeat the instructions. Misconceptions and misunderstandings can be readily cleared up if patients are asked to tell their physician what they understand about their illness and treatment regimen (Fuller and Gross, 1990).

4. *Positive feedback.* Compliance improves when patients are encouraged and praised for the progress they are making.

5. *Increased level of subjective distress.* Patients who feel bad tend to be compliant (Olson et al, 1985). Physicians can help patients understand the consequences of noncompliance by increasing their awareness of the disease and its impact on them.

6. *Decreased waiting room time.* While many physicians say there is little they can do about how long patients wait, it is well worth the effort to look at ways to make an office more efficient from a patient's perspective (Kaplan and Sadock, 1991).

7. *Increased time spent with the patient.* Good time-management practices can increase the amount of time spent with patients.

8. Family support and involvement.

Probably the single most important way to increase compliance is to identify the specific reasons why a particular patient finds it difficult to adhere to treatment. A useful approach to fostering compliance is to examine factors systematically as they relate to the patient, the medical regimen, the spouse and family, and the doctor–patient relationship. See Table 1–3 for specific questions to ask in examining each category.

DIFFICULT DOCTOR–PATIENT RELATIONSHIPS

This final section of the chapter focuses on particularly troubling aspects of patient care. These are the situations or types of patients that many physicians find especially frustrating or difficult to manage.

Difficult situations arise both in hospital and outpatient settings. Some of these difficulties relate to the situation itself, such as the patient who dies suddenly, leaving a bewildered and angry family behind. Others relate to the personality of the patient and how that personality style is affected by illness, such as the patient with obsessive-compulsive traits who is hospitalized with a myocardial infarction. Still others may relate to vulnerable areas for the physician, such as the physician who finds it personally threatening to work with a dying patient. Although the list of possibilities is endless, certain situations arise more frequently than others.

Table 1–3 **Fostering Compliance**

PATIENT FACTORS
1. Have the basic nature of the illness, rationale for treatment, benefits of compliance, and hazards of noncompliance been explained to and understood by the patient?
2. Does the patient appear appropriately concerned about the illness and motivated for treatment? (If not, why?)
3. Have major psychiatric syndromes been ruled out?
4. Can the patient recite the name of the medication and when and how to take it?
THE MEDICAL REGIMEN
1. Is the regimen as simple as possible in terms of the number of pills and the number of daily doses?
2. Are doses arranged around daily self-care rituals (at meals, at bedtime)?
3. Have frequent side effects been anticipated and explained in terms that will not frighten the patient?
THE SPOUSE AND FAMILY
1. Does the spouse or other support figure understand the illness and the need for medication? Will they support compliance?
THE DOCTOR–PATIENT RELATIONSHIP
1. Has continuity of care been established?
2. Has good rapport been established with the patient? (If not, why?)

(Reprinted with permision from Stoudemire and Thompson [1983])

The Seductive Patient

Patients often idealize their physicians. Sometimes this may take the form of an erotic or sexualized transference; patients may decide they are in love with their physician. These can be very powerful emotions that may both flatter and disturb the physician. They may elicit a variety of countertransference feelings ranging from uneasiness to sexual arousal to the feeling that this particular patient is, in fact, very special and in need of extra attention. Again, it is not the feelings themselves that cause trouble; it is what the physician *does* about the feelings that matter. By understanding that the source of the feelings is the patient's need to idealize the physician and to test the boundaries of their relationship, physicians may be better able to mitigate their own reactions. Many patients can act quite provocatively toward their caregivers. Erotic or provocative behavior will have a number of patient-specific meanings.

Physicians who are honest with themselves acknowledge that they may also have erotic feelings about some patients. Ethical obligations prohibit acting on these feelings, but they do not and cannot prohibit having the feelings themselves.

A CASE STUDY

SL was a young, attractive woman who went to see her internist with vague complaints of malaise and lightheadedness. While there, she acknowledged she was having difficulties with her marriage and did not want to move with her husband to another state where he had been transferred. The internist listened patiently to her account and suggested she talk with a therapist to sort out her feelings. The patient stated that it was difficult for her to talk to most people and that she was surprised at how much she had confided in the internist. She felt he had been enormously helpful and was all she needed at present. The physician found nothing physically wrong with the patient and asked her to call for a follow-up appointment if her symptoms did not abate. She hugged the physician "in gratitude" as she left his office.

The patient returned to the physician 2 weeks later attractively dressed in a tight-fitting blouse and skirt. She thanked him profusely for his attention on the previous occasions and said it had helped her feel more certain of her decision to leave her husband. She stated she felt much better but continued to have a light cough. She began unbuttoning her blouse, and the physician noted how attractive this woman was and how eager she seemed to be for his attention. There was a sexual tension in the air that was somewhat relieved by the internist's request for a nurse to step into the room. After the physician finished his examination, he left the room to allow the patient to dress. When he returned a few minutes later, he found she had only partially buttoned her blouse, leaving her bra exposed.

She motioned him to come in as she slowly finished buttoning her blouse. While he explained that there were no indications of a significant physical problem, she moved to a chair beside him and rested her hand on his arm. "I think you are very special," she said. "One of a kind, and it seems there is something between us." The physician moved away from the patient at this point and attempted to explain his professional responsibilities did not allow him to become romantically involved with patients. She protested, stating that they were both adults, and that this professional relationship surely did not extend to off-hour contact. He attempted to address the situation in terms of the boundaries he needed to maintain. It was not clear to the physician whether or not he could continue to treat this patient, and he asked how she felt about remaining with him or being transferred to another physician. The patient burst into tears and stated she could play by the rules. She also said she might be ready to take the referral to the therapist he had recommended earlier.

It is unfortunate that medical school typically does so little to help physicians deal with these often intense emotional responses. Talking to responsible colleagues is one way to sort out the feelings. A formal or informal psychiatric consultation can often help physicians deal more effectively with seductive patients. In rare circumstances, it may be necessary to transfer a patient to the care of another physician if it appears that the patient can no longer be treated objectively. It is also easier for physicians to deal with these feelings when they have fulfilling lives outside the office (Fromm-Reichman, 1950).

The "Hateful" Patient

There are certain patients that most physicians find hard to treat (Groves, 1978). Often, these are patients who are demanding and dissatisfied with treatment. They tend to blame their physician and others around them for their illness. They may alternate between idealizing their physicians and demeaning them. Physicians should feel wary when patients tell them they're the first doctor who ever understood them. It is likely that these patients will have unrealistic expectations and that they will subsequently devalue and demean their physicians. Doctors tend to pass these patients along to their colleagues as "interesting cases." This passing on is sometimes unfair to all concerned. Such patients can often benefit from a professional approach that maintains clear boundaries. These patients can also benefit from psychotherapy, although they frequently resist this form of treatment. A single example may serve as a template for the type of patient who tends to push physicians to their limit.

A CASE STUDY

A young woman was in the hospital with an asthma attack. She managed to stir up the ward by being demanding, childlike, and uncooperative. She considered some nurses to be "good staff" and others to be "bad staff." The same was true with her physicians. The "good staff" tended to reciprocate by viewing her as an unfortunate young woman who was being unfairly judged by other staff members. The "bad staff" saw the patient as manipulative, time-consuming, and ungrateful. Physicians tended to share these diverse opinions, depending on whether they were the "good" or "bad" doctor. A psychiatrist was called in to help settle the staff, who began to bicker among themselves. The primary physician asked the psychiatrist to "help with the management" of the patient.

In the psychiatric literature, this type of patient would probably be said to have a "borderline" personality disorder. These patients can generate a remarkable amount of turmoil. They have very contradictory views of themselves and others and tend to dump their inner turmoil into the world around them. What the psychiatrist did in this particular case was to get the staff to begin talking to one another. Their composite view of this patient was far more accurate than the view of any particular staff member. The psychiatrist recommended that the patient have one primary nurse and one primary physician with whom she was to discuss all of her concerns about care. This limited her ability to separate people into camps. Other staff were told to channel the young woman's concerns to the primary nurse and doctor. These individuals coordinated their information to avoid a split between the good doctor and the bad nurse, or vice versa. The patient remained difficult and demanding, but the staff were better able to function in her best interest because they were no longer caught up in her projections and turmoil.

The Patient with a Thousand Symptoms

These patients tax a physician as much as or more than the difficult patient just described. They appear to be invested in remaining ill. These are the patients who have multiple complaints that do not add up to a single disease picture. They often receive various diagnostic procedures, to no avail. They may doctor-shop or continue to come to the same physician despite their ostensible dissatisfaction that the doctor is unable to cure them. Doctors often respond to these patients with frustration and anger. Sometimes they respond aggressively by ordering unnecessary tests or performing unneeded procedures. It is not unusual for such patients to list ten or more procedures they have undergone for which there was only sketchy justification.

A CASE STUDY

ML was a nervous woman in her 40s who came to see her internist of many years complaining of an aching feeling behind her eyes. She was convinced this pain represented a brain tumor but was fearful of confirming this dire diagnosis through a computerized tomography (CT) scan. Her internist patiently examined her and discussed with her the lack of physical or laboratory findings suggesting that her diagnosis might be valid. The doctor referred her to an ophthalmologist to evaluate her symptoms further. The opthalmologist knew the patient and agreed to see her. He stated he did not see any indication of a brain tumor but acknowledged the only way to be absolutely certain of this could be to perform a CT scan. The patient felt sufficiently reassured to decline the offer of a CT scan. She returned home and, within a couple of days, she became fearful regarding pain in her right shoulder. She had previously suffered from a "frozen shoulder," which was the result of competitive tennis. Mobility had been restored, but now the pain recurred. The patient felt this pain might represent another tumor and requested an appointment with her orthopedist. This physician evaluated her and explained that the pain most likely represented a recurrent injury secondary to her return to active tennis practice. He advised a few days off the court and gave her a follow-up appointment.

The patient discussed the situation with her psychiatrist and acknowledged that she undoubtedly was overreacting, but that she could not silence the thoughts that she had some terrible disease. She was even able to make some connections between these obsessive worries and the fact that she grew up in a family obsessed with physical symptoms. The family communicated love, concern, and frustration through discussions of physical symptoms. The patient also recognized intellectually that when her frustrations with her husband worsened, her symptoms did likewise. She also acknowledged that she might use her symptoms to get some of the attention she felt she needed. Despite these insights, the patient continued to have new and recurrent fears related to her health. Trials of medication suggested by her psychiatrist were short-lived, as each medication gave her what she felt were intolerable side effects. Her internist of 15 years continued to see and evaluate her symptoms,

*without apparent frustration or annoyance. She was careful to take
the patient's concerns seriously, without resorting to invasive and
unnecessary procedures.*

This case illustrates the very chronic nature of these patients' complaints
and their need for consistent, competent, and nonjudgmental care. This patient had great faith in her internist, who managed her problems with respect
and conservative care. In short, the physician remained connected with the patient and tolerant of her style of relating. She treated her without mistreating
or abandoning her.

There are several important points to make about this type of patient.
These patients turn up frequently in general outpatient practice, accounting
for 5% to 10% of patients seen (Folks et al., 1994). Their need to be ill is often
unconscious, and their symptoms are real to them, not fabrications. In addition, even somatizing patients—i.e., patients who translate emotional problems
into physical symptoms—can develop genuine physical problems. Doctors
need to be alert to this possibility, at the same time refraining from unnecessary procedures. Such patients do best when they are seen frequently by one
personal physician on a long-term basis. They should be seen monthly whether
or not they have a problem. Often, this contact can eliminate the need to create a major health crisis to obtain the longed-for attention. These patients are
difficult to treat in psychotherapy despite the fact that their problems have an
emotional base. The best approach is one that combines frequent visits to a primary physician with adjunctive psychotherapy if the patient can tolerate it.
The focus of the medical approach is on management rather than cure (Folks
et al., 1994).

The Patient in the Hospital Setting

Unlike the type of patient just described, there are many other patients
who function well in the outpatient setting; they become problematic only
when hospitalized or when faced with a severe or debilitating illness.

Hospitals tend to rob patients of their sense of dignity and personal control. Even the most benevolent hospital has a schedule that is not the patient's
schedule. Patients also feel out of control because there is something wrong
with their body. It is difficult, if not impossible, to maintain a sense of autonomy in a hospital setting. In general, patients become more childlike when
hospitalized. How specific patients deal with hospitalization depends upon
their personality. Patients with rigid personalities and an obsessional style may
be overwhelmed by the perceived loss of control. They may become argumentative or noncompliant, or deny that they have a problem. If this type of patient
has a myocardial infarction, he or she may want to resume a full schedule of
work while still in the hospital. Alternatively, patients who tend to be depen-

dent may become completely submissive and helpless. The paranoid individual may become increasingly distrustful, demanding second opinions and threatening lawsuits.

A CASE STUDY

BT was a self-absorbed man in his early 70s who had been quite proud of his youthful appearance and vigor. After experiencing several months of increasing fatigue, he was evaluated by an internist and cardiologist, who informed him that he needed a heart valve replacement. BT had been prone to hypochrondriacal concerns throughout most of his life, and with this news he became very fearful that he would die from the surgery. He demanded constant reassurance from family members and his physicians and could talk about little else besides his upcoming surgery. The surgery was complicated by excessive bleeding, and the patient received a blood transfusion. In the ICU, he talked constantly and developed a brief paranoid psychosis, which resolved after 2 days. In the hospital, he remained very passive and refused even minimal efforts at self-care, relying on the nurses and his wife to take care of all his bodily needs.

When he was discharged home, he continued to remain in bed, stating he was too weak to walk and too weak to shave. He became extremely dependent on his wife and apparently unconcerned about his physical appearance or general well-being. His recovery was slow, with a number of partial relapses in which he would remain in bed and demand the total attention of his wife.

Clearly this patient had a number of factors that could have led to a slower recovery. These included his age and the complications that occurred during surgery, including significant blood loss requiring transfusion. Of greater significance, however, is the way in which this patient's coping style and regression hindered his recovery.

This case study illustrated the reactions of an emotionally fragile man who liked to be the center of attention when in good health. He often attempted to bolster his self-esteem through self-aggrandizing statements. One of his features about which he was justifiably proud was his youthful appearance and stamina. This view of himself was severely shaken by his need for surgery. The surgery undermined his sense of body integrity and left him feeling vulnerable and defenseless. His response to this narcissistic blow was to become completely passive and dependent. He could demand and receive attention for his illness, if not for his youthful good health. All of these emotional issues remained quite unconscious to the patient, who complained only of his weakness and discomfort.

The case also illustrates the severe behavioral regression that can be expected to take place when a person becomes seriously ill. There are few emotional injuries as great as the betrayal of one's body through severe or life-threatening illness. Regular coping mechanisms fail, and one is likely to regress to a more childlike state. Physicians need to be alert to regression and sensitive to the patient's wish that the physician and others provide what the patient feels he or she can no longer provide for him or herself. They will need to step into this gap without further infantilizing the patient. It is a delicate balance that can be most successfully negotiated by an empathic physician who is able to understand the patient's fears and anger while helping the patient maintain some sense of control over his environment (Nardo, 1987).

The Mentally Disturbed Patient

There are many patients requiring medical care who suffer from severe emotional illnesses. Some emotional illnesses may be related to the medical condition itself, such as depression due to hypothyroidism or depression related to a chronic and debilitating illness. Other conditions will be unrelated to the medical problem but may significantly interfere with medical care received. The patient who suffers from untreated paranoid schizophrenia may have a difficult time trusting the physician enough to allow treatment.

A CASE STUDY

CK was a 50-year-old man with chronic schizophrenia who was admitted to the hospital with newly diagnosed colon cancer. The patient was chronically delusional about a machine in his head planted there by extraterrestrial beings. His ability to function included holding down a job as a ticket taker in a local cinema and living fairly independently in a boarding house. He kept his mental health appointments and took his antipsychotic medication. He had required only one brief hospitalization for his schizophrenia in the past 5 years. This decompensation occurred shortly after the death of his mother.

The staff were initially quite upset that this patient had been admitted to their floor rather than the psychiatric service. They worried about the safety of other patients and were concerned that the patient might run off or become violent. In general, they avoided conversations with the patient regarding his physical condition as they felt he either could not understand what he was told or would decompensate under the stress of the diagnosis. A psychiatrist was called in to evaluate the patient and to determine whether or not he was mentally competent to make a decision regarding surgery.

In response to the psychiatrist's questions, the patient stated he knew why he was in the hospital. He said his doctor had explained

*the diagnosis to him as well as the need for surgery. He wondered
why none of the doctors or nurses in the hospital had talked to him
about the surgery. He acknowledged to the psychiatrist that the machine remained in his head and that occasionally it would try to
take over his thoughts. However, he stated that the machine did not
affect his understanding about his illness. He worried about why the
physicians were taking so long to operate.*

This patient's case represents a very common story and a common misunderstanding among health professionals about patients with chronic mental
illness. There is a false assumption on the part of many physicians that psychotic individuals cannot deal rationally with their physical illnesses. While this
occasionally may be true, it is likely that such an individual will be able to understand and make decisions about his illness that are as sound as anyone
else's. It is perhaps helpful to think of a patient's illness as a circumscribed part
of his mental functioning. Many other aspects of the patient's mental functioning are sound, rational, and grounded in reality. Even a person with severe psychosis is usually oriented to time, place, and person. His judgment is impaired
in relation to his delusional world, but not in relation to his physical symptoms.
There are, of course, exceptions to this generality, such as the patient with
delusions about his physical health. Even in this situation, however, it is often
possible for a patient to respond rationally to a diagnosed illness separately
from his delusional somatic concerns.

Often, physicians are frightened of patients who are mentally disturbed.
Most patients with serious mental illness can be treated successfully; they may
not be cured, and they may relapse, but they are not different from any patient
with a chronic illness. Physicians should treat such patients in the same way in
which they treat all other patients—with concern and respect.

Sometimes physicians err in the opposite direction. They may fail to recognize serious emotional illness when it is present, or fail to refer a patient for
psychiatric follow-up when referral is clearly indicated. The more exposure
physicians have to mentally ill patients, the more readily they will recognize
those who need psychiatric care and the more comfortable they will be in
working with them.

It is always appropriate to ask a psychiatric colleague for a formal or informal consultation regarding a patient who appears to have emotional difficulties.

The Dying Patient

How little we know about living until we take on the task of work with the
dying. It is a task that many physicians attempt to avoid. Even in the midst of a
specialty such as oncology, which is filled with dying patients, one may flee
from the work. One may turn to research and heroic efforts, all designed at sur-

vival, to avoid the harrowing task of living with a dying person. The reasons are not obscure. As physicians, we see ourselves as healers. We have come to the profession for a variety of conscious and unconscious reasons. Among those reasons may be our own fear of death. We become the Don Quixotes of the world who would eliminate death, and our American culture goes along with this belief that all things are possible. Even death can be avoided, and it is death that is the enemy. It is easy to become the keeper of this myth. The irony is that such a myth can eliminate some of the deepest meanings inherent in being alive and some of the finest aspects of being a healer.

When patients don't get well, and it is clear they will die despite every attempt to save them, many physicians see this as a personal failure. Their response may be denial or, more commonly, abandonment. They may distance themselves from their dying patients under the guise that there is nothing more they can do for them. In reality, this withdrawal may represent a wish to preserve their image as omnipotent healers or to spare themselves the pain of losing someone they have come to know and care about. They may hope to avoid facing such constant reminders of their own mortality, or they may wish to avoid the inevitable anger of the patient and family that such a thing could happen. Rarely are these motives conscious. Instead, physicians may tell themselves they must focus on the living, those who need their skill to survive. Work with the dying is better left to those more skilled at it, the chaplains and social workers.

The fear of dying has a unique meaning for each patient who is terminally ill. For nearly all, however, one of the preeminent fears is that they will die alone and in pain. Physicians remain healers when they make it clear through actions and words that they will stay with the patient and do everything possible to help them and make them comfortable and pain-free. Physicians who can make this commitment will find themselves rewarded in unexpected ways. It may be through the gratitude of a dying patient or the patient's family that a physician comes to experience the meaning of his work. More simply, by sharing the experiences of the dying patient, it may be that the physician comes to discover a greater reverence for life and death. When death is allowed to become part of the natural life cycle, however untimely, physicians may become both more humble and more humane in their work. They may discover that working with the dying is far from futile and is, in fact, enriching to both doctor and patient.

This is not to say that one can avoid difficult moments along the way or that all lives end well. Sadly that is not the case. People often die the way they live (but not always). An angry, hostile individual is unlikely to become docile and loving at the end of life to either the physician or anyone else, although a skilled physician may be able to discover what it is that such a patient needs in order to find some comfort.

There is much of practical value that a physician can do for a dying patient. For example, there is an assumption that every patient who is dying is bound to be depressed. While much has been written about the stages of grief, i.e., denial, anger, despair, bargaining, and resolution, less has been written about aspects of suffering that are not inherent in the dying process. The patient who remains depressed is not suffering an inevitable consequence of dying, but may, instead, be suffering from a depression that can be alleviated with medication. That may make all the difference in how such a patient lives out his last days or months or years. The patient who complains of intolerable suffering may, in reality, be talking about symptoms, such as nausea or pain, that a listening physician can respond to appropriately. There is often a fear of overmedicating dying patients, which can leave some in unnecessary pain. Other patients will attach a different meaning to their pain and will wish to limit and avoid such medication. A sensitive physician will attempt to hear the patient's complaints and wishes in the context of that particular patient's life story. In a wonderful book on empathy (Spiro et al, 1993), a contributor, Joanne Lynn, recounts a number of stories related to work with dying patients. One patient suffered terribly during bandage changes of her ulcerated lesions. Caregivers suffered along with her and begged her to take medication. She refused, finally explaining that she identified this suffering with the suffering of Christ and saw it as a noble and necessary part of her dying, which would be rewarded after her death.

Work with dying patients can be a source of enormous personal growth for both patients and physicians. There is no formula for the process. However, patients will tell their physician what they need if the physician is willing to listen. In this situation, it is the patient who is the guide. What most patients want to know is that their physician will support them to the end and will listen and accommodate their needs. Each patient will have a unique set of concerns about dying. For some patients, it will be the possible pain involved; for others, the focus may be on unfinished business or loved ones who will be left behind; still others may see it as a release from suffering. An example may help to highlight several issues.

A CASE STUDY

DM was a young man in his early 20s with AIDS. He had become severely depressed when he first learned a few years earlier that he was HIV positive. He recovered from this depression and resumed his normal lifestyle, which included a relatively monogamous, but often stormy, relationship with a lover who was also HIV positive. The patient came to see a psychiatrist after his second prolonged hospitalization, presumably to work on his relationship with his lover. He was finding it difficult to remain monogamous at the same time that he valued and needed his lover's support. His concerns about dying, which he alluded to infrequently, were related to pain and disfigurement.

Most of his work in therapy dealt with living rather than dying. The patient focused on straightening out his relationships with others and on finding pleasure and support in these relationships.

When his final illness came, he struggled with it for some time, often feeling frustrated with his primary physician when treatment was painful or unsuccessful. These moments of frustration were short-lived, however. For the most part he saw his physician as present and concerned. He used his psychiatrist to check out his feelings and his decisions regarding his care. Eventually, he chose to go home to die, which he did after several days. He died with unexpected grace after spending a good day with his family and lover.

This case illustrates a number of important issues. Patients who are dying are still very much concerned with life. There may be a transitional point in the process of dying, but until that moment is reached, a patient's concerns are mostly about living. A frequent complaint of patients who are terminally ill is that their caregivers stop talking to them. It is as if they are no longer considered among the living. This patient, through his own energy and with the cooperation of his family, lover, and doctors, remained very much in life until the end. He also maintained a sense that he could make decisions about how he lived. Toward the end of his life, he was concerned about his mother's attempts to force him to eat. This was a disagreement that was negotiated so that the patient was allowed to eat when and what he wanted. He decided when he wished to come home and discontinue further treatment. All of this contributed to the patient's feeling of autonomy, despite his debilitating illness.

In some cases, denial may help patients go on living. This raises the difficult issue of how and when patients should be told they are dying. Caregivers have a variety of opinions about this issue. Most would say it is important to know what the patient suspects or fears about the illness before you begin. Most physicians also would say it is important to leave room for hope. This hope should not take the form of false reassurances, but it should acknowledge the lack of certainty about any prognosis. The uncertainty regarding prognosis is one reason why a physician often may be reluctant to reply to a patient's question about how long he or she has to live. Some physicians do not routinely tell their patients that they have a fatal illness. This can lead to a fearful isolation in which family members, patient, and doctor can no longer communicate honestly and openly. Most patients are aware of how ill they are and often know they are dying (Burrows, 1991). For many, it is a relief when someone is willing to talk to them about it.

While physicians should be honest with their patients, they also should be respectful of each patient's coping style. A patient may be told the status of his or her illness and choose to live as if she or he had not received this news. The physician can respect this choice until and unless it appears to be harmful to the patient to maintain such a stance. Even in this situation, a sensitive physician will recognize that the patient has ultimate responsibility to make choices about living and dying. The patient DM had been told his diagnosis and knew intellectually that he probably would die from this illness. At that time, AIDS was a more certain short-term death sentence than it is today. Despite this intellectual knowledge, the patient used denial throughout much of the earlier stages of his illness, and this denial may have allowed him to fight off illnesses more successfully.

His primary concerns about his HIV status had to do with his fear of disfigurement and pain. This kept him from telling friends about his disease. He feared they would see him as wasting away. His isolation from others gave way slowly as an increasing number of friends knew about his illness and continued to accept and support him. Some of the support surfaced when others were willing to confide in him that they were HIV positive.

Finally, this patient contradicted the adage that people die the way they live. This was a fragile, anxious person who had lived much of his life in tumultuous relationships with little self-reflection. He often felt overwhelmed by minor difficulties. This was not how he reacted at the end of his life. Instead, he found a strength and acceptance that allowed him to die peacefully in the midst of people who loved him.

Dealing with death and the dying patient is discussed in some length in Chapter 10 by Drs. Wolman and Thompson.

SUMMARY

Every medical student knows that the decision to become a physician means enormous commitment and dedication. The learning process is unending. Part of this process involves a willingness to learn about oneself and one's patients. It is the human interaction that ultimately will be a major source of much pleasure and some frustration to the physician. The relationship the physician has with each patient serves as a cornerstone for that patient's treatment. The rest of this book will lay the groundwork for understanding human behavior, which is essential for establishing an effective and successful doctor–patient relationship.

ANNOTATED BIBLIOGRAPHY

Cassell EJ: The Nature of Suffering and the Goals of Medicine. New York, Oxford University Press, 1991

> Scholarly, well-written treatise on the need to shift the focus of medicine from the disease model to the sick person who is suffering. "Bodies do not suffer, people do."

Emmanuel E, Emmanuel L: Four models of the physician–patient relationship. JAMA 267(16):2221–2226, 1992

> The authors identify four types of relationships (the paternalistic, informative, interpretive, and deliberative models) and discuss the values and limitations of each.

Of equal or more interest are the letters in response to this article. See Rennie D, Dan BB (eds): Letters. JAMA 268(11):1410–1413, 1992

Fuller MG, Gross RT: Adherence to medical regimes. In Wedding D (ed): Behavior and Medicine. St. Louis, Mosby-Year Book, 1990

Comprehensive chapter that focuses on all aspects of patient compliance.

Groves JE: Taking care of the hateful patient. N Engl J Med 298(16):883–887, 1978

This article is a classic that discusses countertransference feelings in practical terms and offers useful suggestions for working with difficult patients. Includes "dependent clingers," "entitled demanders," "manipulative help rejecters," and "self-destructive deniers."

Nardo MJ: The personality in the medical setting: A psychodynamic understanding. In Michaels R (ed): Psychiatry, Vol. 2. New York, Basic Books, 1987

Well-written and practical guide to working with different personality types in the hospital setting. Includes compulsive, histrionic, depressive-masochistic, border-line, narcissistic, and paranoid personalities.

Spiro H., et al. (eds.): Empathy and the Practice of Medicine: Beyond Pills and the Scalpel. New Haven, Yale University Press, 1993

Excellent series of thought-provoking essays by eminent writers with medical backgrounds. Easy-to-read stories that illustrate various aspects of empathy and its importance in the education of medical students.

REFERENCES

Bertakis KD, Roter D, Putnam SM: The relationship of physician medical interview style to patient satisfaction. J Fam Practice 32(2):175–181, 1991
Book HE: Is empathy cost efficient? Am J Psychotherapy 45(1):21–30, 1991
Buller MK, Buller DB: Physicians' communications style and patient satisfaction. Health Soc Behav 28:375–388, 1987
Burrows A: A piece of my mind: The man who didn't know he had cancer. JAMA 266(18):2550, 1991
Cassell EJ: The Nature of Suffering and the Goals of Medicine. New York, Oxford University Press, 1991
Emanuel E, Emanuel L: Four models of the physician–patient relationship. JAMA 267(16):2221–2226, 1992
Folks DG, Ford CV, Houck CA: Somatoform disorders, factitious disorders, and malingering. In Stoudemire A (ed): Clinical Psychiatry for Medical Students, 2nd ed. Philadelphia, Lippincott, 1994
Frankel BL: The physician–patient relationship. In Wiener JM (ed): Behavioral Science. New York, John Wiley & Sons, 1987
Fromm-Reichman F: The psychiatrist's part in the doctor–patient relationship. In Principles of Intensive Psychotherapy. Chicago, University of Chicago Press, 1950
Fuller MG, Gross RT: Adherence to medical regimens. In Wedding D (ed): Behavior and Medicine. St. Louis, Mosby-Year Book, 1990
Gabbard GO, Nadelson C: Professional boundaries in the physician–patient relationship. JAMA 273(18):1445–1449, 1995
Groves JE: Taking care of the hateful patient. N Engl J Med 298(16):883–887, 1978
Kaplan HI, Sadock BJ: The doctor–patient relationship. In Synopsis of Psychiatry, 6th ed. Baltimore, Williams & Wilkins, 1991
LeBaron S, Reyher J, Stack JM: Paternalistic vs egalitarian physician styles: The treatment of patients in crisis. Family Practice 21(1):56–62, 1985
Ley P: Primary, rated importance and recall of medical information. J Health Soc Behav 13:311–317, 1972

Morris W (ed): The American Heritage Dictionary of the English Language. Boston, Houghton Mifflin, 1981

Nardo MJ: The personality in the medical setting: A psychodynamic understanding. In Michaels R (ed): Psychiatry. New York, Basic Books, 1987

Nicholi AM: The therapist–patient relationship. In Nicholi AM (ed): The Harvard Guide to Modern Psychiatry. Cambridge, Harvard University Press, 1988

Olson RA, Zimmerman JL, de la Roche SR: Medical adherence in pediatric populations. In Zeiner AR, Bendell P, Walker CE (eds): Health Psychology: Treatment and Research Issues. New York, Plenum Press, 1985

Porter AM: Drug defaulting in general practice. Br Med J 1:218–222, 1969

Rennie D, Dan BB (eds): Letters: Models of the physician–patient relationship. JAMA 268(11): 1410–1413, 1992

Sackett DL, Haynes RB: Compliance with Therapeutic Regimens. Baltimore, Johns Hopkins, 1976

Stone GC: Patient compliance and the role of the expert. J Soc Issues 35:34–59, 1979

Stoudemire A, Thompson TL: Medication noncompliance: Systematic approaches to evaluation and intervention. Gen Hosp Psychiatry 5:233–239, 1983

Underwood P, Owen A: Styles of doctoring and models of health. Australian Fam Physician 14(7):658–662, 1985

Zinn W: The empathic physician. Arch Intern Med 153:306–312, 1993

2

The Biopsychosocial Model in Medical Practice

Steven A. Cole,
Stephen M. Saravay,
and Richard M. Levinson

In Chapter 1, Dr. Shelton introduced the concept of the biopsychosocial model in medicine and discussed it in the context of the doctor–patient relationship. In this chapter, this model is discussed in a more expanded manner.

The following four postulates set forth the broad outlines of the biopsychosocial model of illness, which forms the fundamental underlying philosophy of this textbook.

1. Most illness, whether physical or psychiatric, is influenced and determined by biological, psychological, and social phenomena.
2. Biological, psychological, and social variables influence the predisposition, onset, course, and outcome of most illnesses.
3. Physicians who are able to evaluate the relationships of biological, psychological, and social variables of their patients' illnesses will be able to develop more effective therapeutic interventions and to achieve better outcomes.
4. To evaluate and manage medical problems adequately, physicians must be able to establish and maintain therapeutic doctor–patient relationships with many different types of patients.

Each chapter in this book will present a different perspective based on these four postulates. This book will provide students with practical approaches for integrating these variables into patient care. This chapter presents empirical and clinical data that support the four postulates described above, along with suggestions to help future physicians use this approach in the care of their patients.

WHY SHOULD PHYSICIANS STUDY EMOTIONS, BEHAVIOR, OR SOCIAL PROCESSES?

Many medical students may wonder what a course in human behavior really has to do with their future practice of medicine. They may feel that they have come to medical school to learn about disease: how to diagnose and treat ailments of the body. They may think that, while humanistic medicine (i.e., "caring for" and being "nice" or "understanding" to patients) is an important part of medical practice, the principles of a humanistic approach to medical practice are intuitive, self-evident, more or less "common sense," and cannot or do not need to be "taught." In addition, many practicing clinicians and students acknowledge that patients with psychiatric problems often come to physicians for help, but they feel that these patients can be referred elsewhere for help with their psychiatric problems and that medical practice should focus on physical illnesses.

This view of disease and medical practice, which many physicians endorse, has been described as the "biomedical model of illness" (Engel, 1977). It argues that psychological and social variables are of secondary importance in illness and the treatment process, and that physicians' major efforts should be primarily, if not exclusively, focused on the biological aspects of physical illnesses.

Focusing exclusively on biological aspects overlooks great variations in how people feel—how they experience the disease. After reviewing surveys of health in the United States, Barsky (1988) reported a paradox of health status in America. He noted that although there have been substantial improvements in the objective health status of the population, with increased life expectancy and a decline in mortality rates, people report higher rates of disability, symptoms, and general dissatisfaction with their health. Some of the increases in self-reported illness or disability could be associated with the success of medicine in sustaining the lives of persons who live with chronic health problems; yet Barsky believes that some of the deterioration in reported health is associated with a lower tolerance of symptoms, accompanied by a greater inclination to attribute uncomfortable feelings, such as lower back pain, to an "illness." Discomforts that were previously tolerated and overlooked are more likely to be defined as health problems requiring medical treatment. This tendency to attribute greater seriousness to minor physical symptoms, or to express emotions through physical complaints, is found to occur more commonly in patients with mental disorders, such as depression (Wells et al, 1989). Thus, how patients perceive and understand their feelings as the presence of disease may have much to do with variations in the actual reported health status of the population. To be effective, physicians must take into consideration how patients subjectively experience and understand their own "illnesses."

Therefore, this chapter disputes the position of a purist interpretation of the "biomedical" model and advocates an integrated approach to patient care by use of a "biopsychosocial model of illness." This view endorses a multidimensional or systems approach to the practice of medicine and conceptualizes illness and its outcomes as determined by multiple interacting biological, psychological, and social variables.

The biopsychosocial model maintains that emotional, behavioral, and social processes are implicated in the development, course, and outcome of illness. Medical students need to learn basic principles of psychosocial assessment and intervention to be able to practice multidimensional medicine and to be able to provide adequate and comprehensive care for their patients. Physicians who can integrate the psychological and social variables of their patients' illnesses will generally be able to develop more effective clinical interventions that will lead to better treatment outcome.

A body of research indicates that patients' satisfaction with physician visits is based primarily on the psychosocial dimensions of care. If patients perceive that their doctors care about them, show concern, and seem understanding, they are more satisfied and evaluate the quality of medical care more positively. On average, this "emotional" dimension appears more influential than the physician's technical competence in patients' assessment of the quality of their care (Ben-Sira, 1976). Even the satisfaction of patients who visit physicians with a primary interest in receiving procedures or medications is more influenced by the psychosocial aspects of the care received (such as counseling or education) than by the technical services (Brody et al, 1989). Therefore, physicians who endorse a biopsychosocial approach to medical practice generally will have better relationships with their patients and will find the practice of medicine less stressful and more personally fulfilling.

After the following case study, this chapter will then cover a wide range of topics related to biopsychosocial medicine, including:

1. Psychological and social factors related to the predisposition, onset, course, and outcome of physical illness
2. The use of psychosocial treatments for physical illness
3. A review of psychobiological mechanisms that might mediate between psychosocial processes and biological effects
4. Recent findings in psychiatric epidemiology, particularly as they relate to the general practice of medicine
5. Sociocultural influences on illness and illness behavior
6. The applicability of the biopsychosocial model to traditional psychiatric illnesses.

The following case study will provide a basis to begin a discussion of biopsychosocial assessment and treatment. The case will be presented, and a model biopsychosocial formulation will be developed along with multidimensional treatment recommendations. The case will demonstrate how the biopsychosocial model of illness is helpful in understanding and effectively treating a patient who has a major psychiatric disorder complicating the patient's primary physical condition.

A CASE STUDY

RF is a 47-year-old married man with a 60 pack/year history of cigarette smoking (i.e., two packs a day for 30 years) and a 5-year history of laryngeal cancer. He underwent several procedures on his neck 5 years ago and now reports that his life has "never been the same" since that time. Physical problems include difficulty talking and swallowing, with unpredictable and uncontrollable episodes of coughing and vomiting. These episodes are extremely embarrassing to him and have led him to restrict his activities. He no longer wants to go out and does not want to socialize with friends or family.

He and his wife report that he has been depressed for 5 years, but the depression has gotten much worse in the last year or so. He does not want to do anything and derives almost no pleasure in living. He has frequent crying spells and has great difficulty sleeping at night. He usually can fall asleep without too much trouble, but often awakens in the middle of the night and cannot fall back to sleep. He feels sad most of the time and believes that life is a burden. He often feels that he would prefer to be dead than to live in his current situation, but he says that he would not consider suicide. His appetite is poor, although he has not lost weight. He reports "no energy" and very low self-esteem. He is guilty about what he has done to his family as a result of this illness and blames himself for the illness because of his history of heavy smoking. He has trouble making decisions and reports trouble concentrating, as exemplified in his difficulty keeping his mind on books, television programs, or conversations.

He reports a sudden cessation of sexual activity since his diagnosis of cancer. He has no libido and feels unattractive to his wife. He and his wife report the almost total absence of physical intimacy from their relationship during the past 5 years. They do not hug each other anymore. There is little overt conflict, and the patient feels grateful to his wife and thinks that they have become "closer" since his illness. His wife, however, is very tearful in discussing the impact of the illness on her life. She feels guilty and responsible for her husband but does not want to have to restrict her own life unreasonably. She feels that she has retained the ability to enjoy life, and that if her husband cannot be motivated to go out, she has the right to go out without him. She spends time with her children and other friends.

RF and his wife are both worried about finances. Since his operations and his trouble talking, he has been unable to continue his work as a real estate agent. He has been denied Social Security disability payments. His wife works in retail sales, but her income is not sufficient to cover their household expenses, including the costs of their two children, a girl aged 14 and a boy aged 10. They are having trouble meeting the mortgage payments on their house, and they may need to sell the house and move into an apartment.

In addition, the patient is extremely worried about the impact of his illness on his children, especially because his own father died of lung cancer when the patient was 12. His mother, in addition, suffered from depressive illnesses, with two psychiatric hospitalizations for this problem.

He was referred for psychiatric evaluation. His internist felt that he was suffering from a rather severe depression and that his overall quality of life was more impaired than would be expected from the effect of the cancer itself.

CASE FORMULATION

Biological Variables

The biological variables are obviously the chief precipitants of RF's deteriorating condition. The cancer had a devastating impact on his life. He suffered from several difficult surgical procedures and afterward could no longer function as well as he had previously.

Some new physical symptoms have been troublesome. His talking has become more dysarthric (slurred, with poor enunciation). He has lost sensation on part of his tongue, and his coughing has become much worse. He is in the process of a new neurological evaluation to determine whether his cancer is recurring. He has just learned that he is also suffering from hypothyroidism secondary to neck radiation for the cancer.

The hypothyroid condition itself can cause a secondary mood disorder, which mimics major depression (O'Shanick et al, 1987). Similarly, the patient has been on the antihypertensive beta-blocker propranolol, which has also been implicated in causing mood disturbances (Hall et al, 1980). In addition, the patient's mother suffered from depressive illness. This family history suggests a biologically transmitted genetic predisposition to depression (see Chapter 13 by Dr. Baron on genetic vulnerability to psychiatric illness).

Psychological Variables

RF's psychological character traits play a prominent role in his current problems. He has always been a rather controlled, orderly person who depended on his intellect and a thorough, rational approach to problems to help him cope with life's vicissitudes. He has always disdained emotionality and felt that most of life's difficulties could be overcome if sufficient effort was put into working out practical solutions. He spent a great deal of effort organizing his work and his private life in order to arrange his affairs to be as predictable as possible. This personality style has been referred to as the "obsessive style" (MacKinnon and Michels, 1971) (see Chapter 5 by Drs. Inderbitzen, Furman, and James for a discussion of ego defenses and personality style).

The cancer, by itself, presented a major threat not only to his life but, by its very nature, to the predictability and certainty of his future. For a patient with an obsessive style of coping, the vagaries of cancer treatment and outcome present particularly troubling stresses. In addition, the patient's difficulty with eating and talking, as well as his unpredictable vomiting, compromised his control of his social circumstances and led to extremely embarrassing situations.

One episode on a trip to visit family was particularly disturbing. While eating dinner in an elegant restaurant, he suddenly and unpredictably vomited. This episode was so distressing to him that he now phobically avoids all social situations. His symptoms of depression have much worsened since then. The hopelessness, anhedonia (i.e., inability to experience interest or pleasure), and fatigue also have gotten worse since then. He refuses almost all activities.

In addition to these difficulties, the patient feels extremely guilty about his cigarette smoking and blames himself for his illness and its deleterious effect on his family. He worries about the psychological impact of the cancer on his children, especially if he dies of the disease. He cannot stop thinking about the death of his own father when he was young, and he is sad for himself and for his children at the same time.

Social Variables

The social variables are also prominent in this case. First of all, the loss of the patient's income has had a very negative impact on the family. Worries about finances have introduced new stresses into the family, and they are facing the loss of their home. The loss of the job also has had a negative impact on the patient's self-esteem in that he is no longer able to fulfill the "manly" role of "breadwinner" of the family.

In addition, the patient has cut himself off from several important sources of social support that might contribute positively to his current quality of life. Because of extreme vulnerability to social embarrassment, the patient does not see friends or children as much as previously. He may go for weeks without any outside contacts.

His withdrawal has had very negative effects on his wife and, in turn, has affected their marital relationship. There is no more sexual intimacy. His wife is tearful in discussing this problem and the absence of physical contact, including hugging, of any kind in their marriage. As we discussed this concern, the patient said that it is very hard for him to express emotional issues and added that he feels very unlovable in his present condition.

Biopsychosocial Formulation

The biopsychosocial formulation must evaluate and integrate the impact of different variables on the clinical problem. The patient is clearly suffering from "major depression," which is itself a biopsychosocial illness. Neurochemical, endocrine, and neurophysiological alterations are all part of this illness syndrome. RF's obsessive personality style makes adaptation to illness difficult because good coping with cancer requires some ability to live with uncertainty, as well as adequate self-esteem to cope with potentially embarrassing situations. The loss of his father at an early age may, in fact, predispose him to future depressive illness (see Chapter 11 by Dr. van der Kolk for a discussion of developmental trauma as factors predisposing to future anxiety and depression).

His marriage and social contacts also are threatened by his illness and his response to it. The possibility of a recurrence of the malignancy presents a new challenge to a very unstable psychological and social equilibrium.

It would be misleading, however, as well as dangerous, to conclude that RF has "good reasons" to be depressed. He certainly has many good reasons to be "sad," but the syndrome of major depression does not uniformly result from significant physical illness or any severe stress. Although the prevalence of psychiatric disorders is considerably higher among patients with chronic physical illness than in the general population (lifetime prevalence of 42% as compared with 33%) (Wells et al, 1988), the majority of patients with terminal cancer do not, in fact, develop major depressive syndromes (Cohen-Cole and Stoudemire, 1987). Major depression is associated with physiological and neurovegetative changes that occur in only a subset of individuals with severe physical illness (Cassem, 1988). When physical illness is complicated by a major depression, it should be vigorously recognized and treated. As Cassem (1988) has pointed out, "depression is a dread complication of physical illness." Physicians who suggest that patients may have "good reasons" to be depressed may do their patients a disservice because the incorrect assumption that depression is "normal" may lead to an acceptance of the syndrome without obtaining proper and effective treatment.

Biopsychosocial Management

Biopsychosocial management requires the integration of different therapeutic strategies along all three relevant dimensions.

Biological Interventions

Biological intervention for cancer evaluation must proceed rapidly and without delay. The depression must be treated similarly. First, the patient must receive appropriate thyroid replacement therapy. It is possible that this intervention may make a major difference in the patient's symptoms of depression. Similarly, the physician should consider substituting another antihypertensive agent for the propranolol, which might be exacerbating his depression. (Chapter 12 by Dr. Pedersen and colleagues discusses the biological influences on behavior, including mood regulation.)

If the patient does not respond rapidly to thyroid replacement or substitution of antihypertensive drugs, biological intervention for the major depression must be initiated. An antidepressant medication, such as nortriptyline or fluoxetine, should be prescribed to address the disruption in the patient's neurobiological mood and stress response system, and the drug should be monitored closely for effectiveness and side effects (Cohen-Cole and Stoudemire, 1987).

Psychological Interventions

Psychological intervention is just as important. Several different forms of psychotherapy for major depression, including interpersonal and cognitive approaches, have been demonstrated to be as effective as pharmacotherapy. The short-term interpersonal approach would focus on the difficulties the patient has experienced in making the transition from his role as breadwinner to the "sick role." The interpersonal approach also would focus on the new stresses on the marriage because of the cancer (see Chapter 10 by Drs. Wolman and Thompson on adult life-cycles and the stressful effects of illness on the family).

In contrast, a cognitive approach would emphasize the unrealistic expectations RF places on himself in the face of the devastating illness and help him maintain his self-esteem in spite of his new need to be more dependent on others (see Chapters 5 and 6 for a general overview of psychodynamic and behavioral/learning principles in psychotherapy).

Formal psychotherapy definitely would be indicated for RF, but many such patients will not accept this form of treatment. They may believe that the need for psychotherapy points to a character "defect," and they defend themselves against this view by refusing psychotherapy. Other patients refuse psychotherapy because of the expense involved.

Primary physicians can help such patients accept formal psychotherapy by legitimizing the process of therapy. Physicians can point out that depression is a medical illness that can be helped by expert treatment, including psychotherapy, as well as medications. Physicians also can help patients accept psychiatric referral by offering to collaborate with the treating psychotherapist and to remain in contact with the patient during the treatment. It is also often helpful to discuss examples of other patients with similar problems who have benefited from psychiatric referral.

Is there anything that the primary care physician can do with depressed patients with cancer who do not accept psychiatric referral? There is, in fact, a great deal that can be done (see Chapter 14 by Dr. Green on basic approaches to the psychological care of patients). As discussed in Chapter 1, a solid interpersonal relationship must be established and maintained, and it involves the use of good communication skills. *Careful listening* is essential, along with allowing the patient the opportunity to ventilate his or her feelings. Patients must be given *adequate opportunities to ask questions* as well. *Empathic comments,* which reflect the patient's feelings, can be quite helpful (e.g., "It is clear that you are especially worried about the impact that your illness may have on your children"). *Legitimizing* these feelings also is reassuring to patients (e.g., "I can certainly understand why you would find it so hard to think about the effect of your illness on your children"). Offering direct statements of support (e.g., "I will do what I can to help"), as well as statements of partnership ("Let's try to work on this problem together"), also can have a significant impact on the patient's ability to cope. Lastly, *respectful comments that praise* the patient's successful coping efforts are usually very comforting (e.g., "I am really impressed with how well you managed to cope with your children's fears last week") (Cohen-Cole and Bird, 1986a; Cohen-Cole, 1991).

The most important communication skill is the *flexibility* required to observe the patient's response to different interventions, and the ability and willingness to try interventions that will work for each patient. Some patients require more active support, whereas others prefer quiet listening. Physicians can learn the most effective approaches if they observe their patients closely and demonstrate a willingness to listen to their needs.

With respect to RF, physicians can help such obsessive patients by giving them as much control over their treatment as possible. Providing adequate detailed information is essential, and questions must be answered directly and as specifically as possible. Commenting directly on the difficulty of loss of control is usually perceived as empathic by obsessive or worry-prone patients (e.g., "I can certainly understand why this unpredictable illness is so particularly stressful to you, since you have always been able to manage your affairs in an orderly, predictable way").

Similarly, obsessive patients usually are frightened and resistant to becoming dependent on anyone. If this fear is acknowledged, physicians often can help their patients by indicating that sometimes accepting dependency takes unusual strength (e.g., "I know that it is hard to have to depend on someone else to provide for your basic needs, but I want you to realize that it takes particular strength and courage to be able to ask for and accept help that you, in fact, really do need. You actually can benefit your friends and family by accepting the help that they really do want to offer").

RF may be reexperiencing the grief he suffered as a child, as well as anticipatory grief over his own death. (Chapter 14 discusses in some detail the "grief model" of coping with illness, which relates directly to the type of supportive psychotherapy that the primary care physician may be able to provide.)

Social Interventions

Social intervention in this case is crucial. Vocational rehabilitation might be helpful in finding some productive employment for the patient. Social workers might help the patient find ways to appeal the decisions of the Social Security Administration, and, if necessary, legal assistance could be considered to appeal disability decisions.

RF's marriage is quite stressed. He and his wife are lonely, and they have not been able to talk to each other about their needs. A decrease in sexual activity is common after cancer is diagnosed, but this decrease need not herald the end of all physical intimacy (e.g., hugging). RF and his wife need the opportunity to talk to each other about their needs. A primary care physician can be very helpful in this regard simply by bringing up issues of intimacy and sexual relationships for open discussion. More open communication and ventilation of feelings often are sufficient to help resolve such problems. In more complicated cases, referral for sexual therapy can be essential (see Chapter 7 by Drs. Becker, Johnson, and Hunter on human sexuality).

The children are probably quite anxious themselves and may be suffering from psychological distress or even a psychiatric disorder. Every effort should be made to have them seen by the primary physician or by someone with special skills on the healthcare team who would evaluate the need for individual or family therapy (see Chapter 8 by Drs. Dell and Dulcan on how children cope with illness).

Mrs. RF has her own feelings of guilt, responsibility, and resentment, which have an impact on the overall quality of life of the couple as well as of the family. She could benefit from a chance to explore and work through some of these feelings, either with the primary physician or with a psychotherapist.

Summary

Many of the interventions suggested above for the adequate management of RF involve sophisticated and extensive psychosocial interventions. For physicians to be able to provide this type of comprehensive patient care, they must develop the knowledge and skill necessary in the course of their medical training.

The psychosocial interventions described above do in fact require more time than a mechanical and narrowly biological or "purely medical" approach, but they do not require the intensity or time demands of formal psychotherapy. Increasingly, time is a very costly commodity for physicians because insurers reimburse less well for patient visits than for diagnostic or surgical procedures (Eisenberg, 1992). It should be remembered, however, that patients with chronic illness return to primary physicians many times and that a great deal can be accomplished through short, supportive appointments spaced over long periods.

Thus, in addition to the prescription of antidepressants, adequate treatment of this patient necessitates numerous other psychological and social interventions. The physician who is interested and sufficiently well trained to provide this comprehensive care can function efficiently and effectively in this role. Physicians should make it clear to such patients that consultation with a psychiatrist may be necessary but would not disrupt their general medical care. In making a psychiatric or other mental health referral, the primary physician should always indicate willingness and interest in staying involved in the care of the patient.

The prognosis of improvement in functioning and quality of life for RF is quite good, assuming the patient complies with these multimodal treatment interventions.

THE BIOPSYCHOSOCIAL MODEL IN MEDICAL PRACTICE

Just as the biopsychosocial model of illness helps us understand and effectively treat patients such as RF, who have concurrent major *psychiatric* disorders that are complicating their primary physical condition, the biopsychosocial approach is just as helpful for treating patients with *medical disorders.* In other words, evaluation and management of psychological and social variables are critical in the care of the physically ill, *even if there is no major clinically significant psychiatric disorder present.* The following section will discuss the ways in which psychosocial variables have been shown to be significant in the predisposition, onset, course, and outcome of physical illness. Psychosocial interventions that lead to improved physical outcome and the psychobiological mechanisms by which some of these influences may operate also will be cited. The section will conclude with suggestions for the practice of clinical medicine.

Psychological and Behavioral Predisposition to Physical Illness

There are many psychological, behavioral, and social variables that play a role in the development of physical illness. In fact, life style and personal habits, such as tobacco use, alcohol and drug abuse, overeating, poor nutrition, lack of exercise, and so forth, account together for about 70% of all cases of illness and death in the United States (Houpt et al, 1980). Obesity, for example, is related to heart disease, diabetes, and hypertension. Nicotine addiction due to tobacco smoking is directly associated with lung cancer, emphysema, and coronary artery disease. Alcohol is related to cirrhosis of the liver, gastric ulcers, dementia, and half of the yearly fatal traffic accidents in the United States. The financial costs of these behaviorally related illnesses are staggering: the direct costs alone were approximately $250 billion in 1983 (70% of a healthcare expenditure of $355 billion) (Kamerow et al, 1986). This figure does not even include an estimate of the indirect costs (e.g., lost productivity).

Personality factors have also been thought to be factors predisposing to certain physical illnesses. Probably the best known is the so-called Type A behavior pattern and its relationship to coronary artery disease. Coronary artery disease is now the leading cause of death in this country, and any knowledge about predisposing or other risk factors should help us design appropriate interventions. Type A individuals feel under relentless pressure of time and usually are under a competitive and hostile strain with other people. Such persons are generally quite serious and ambitious in their work. They often find it hard to relax and to enjoy interpersonal pleasures. In general, Type A individuals walk and eat rapidly, hurry others along in conversation, speak with a very strong emphasis, clench their hands and teeth, try to do two things at once, and experience great time pressure (Friedman, 1969).

Early studies found that people with strong Type A behavior patterns have twice the incidence of coronary artery disease compared with persons without this pattern (Type B individuals). Similarly, once someone experiences a heart attack, the presence of the Type A behavioral pattern is associated with five times the likelihood of experiencing a second heart attack. Furthermore, the presence of Type A behavior is associated with twice the likelihood that a heart attack will be fatal (Rosenman et al, 1975).

There has been extensive controversy about the validity of the Type A behavior pattern and its hypothesized association with coronary artery disease. Some recent studies have failed to demonstrate the expected results (Ragland and Brand, 1988). Current conceptualization of the Type A behavior pattern now focuses more specifically on the dimensions of suspiciousness and hostility as the cardiotoxic component of this personality syndrome (Dembroski et al, 1989; Williams et al, 1980).

A major intervention study based on the Type A construct has recently lent some support to its validity. A 5-year controlled study examined the effects on cardiac recurrence of an elaborate stress-management intervention focused on reducing the strength of the Type A behavior pattern. At the end of the follow-up period, the recurrence rate of nonfatal infarctions in the intervention group was approximately half that in the other groups. Moreover, within the treatment group itself, the rates of recurrence were lowest among those with the greatest reduction in Type A behaviors (Friedman et al, 1984). In general, despite recent skepticism, some elements of the Type A construct seem to describe a robust and persisting relationship to coronary artery disease and may still be considered as a possible risk factor for this disease (Dimsdale, 1988). The Type A personality and its possible relationship to cardiovascular disease is also discussed in Chapter 3 by Drs. Walker and Katon.

Onset of Illness

The most common psychosocial variable associated with illness onset has to do with the sometimes illusive concept of "stress." Everyone `knows" that stress is related to disease; the stress–illness connection is widespread in popular mythology and the media. The concept of stress provides the philosophical linkage between the mind and the body. It is a fascinating, controversial, and pervasive concept in medical care today.

Conceptions of stress are controversial because they are sometimes very loosely defined and oversimplified. Exaggerated claims that stress causes all illness in a rather straightforward, mechanistic manner have led to skepticism. However, careful definitions and well-designed research have led to some remarkable findings about the relationship of stress to illness.

Generally speaking, the term "stress" has been used to describe emotional distress, the situational conditions that appear to provoke such distress, or both. For the purposes of clarity in this chapter, "stress" will denote the subjective state of distress, and the conditions that provoke this arousal will be termed "stressors." For conditions to cause subjective stress, they generally must tax the adaptive capacity of the person.

Holmes and Rahe (1967) postulated that major events in a person's life requiring change of any kind, whether positive or negative, would require adaptive efforts and readjustment of the organism. They argued that these effects can be cumulative and that the more readjustment required by the person, the more likely the person would be to develop physical illnesses. Holmes and Rahe developed the Social Readjustment Rating Scale to measure the impact of cumulative life events on the person (Table 2–1). As can be seen, a number associated with hypothesized readjustment is assigned to each of 43 different but common life events. The higher the number, the more readjustment is usually required after the event. Although there have been many methodological criticisms of this instrument, hundreds of subsequent investigators using better instruments have also demonstrated an association between life event "scores" and future development of physical illnesses (i.e., the higher the current scores for life events, the more likely the development of physical illnesses in the future [Cohen, 1981]). The psychobiological mechanisms through which life events or stressors can lead to illness are just beginning to be clarified and will be reviewed in a subsequent section.

A study conducted in Britain found strong evidence for a link between stress and the common cold (Cohen et al, 1991). Healthy men and women volunteers were given nasal drops containing a low infectious dose of one of five respiratory viruses resembling those commonly transmitted person-to-person that produce illnesses. Two days before and 7 days after exposure, the subjects

Table 2–1 **Social Readjustment Rating Scale**

RANK	LIFE EVENT	VALUE
1	Death of spouse	100
2	Divorce	73
3	Marital separation	65
4	Jail term	63
5	Death of close family member	53
6	Personal injury or illness	50
7	Marriage	47
8	Fired at work	46
9	Marital reconciliation	45
10	Retirement	44
11	Change in health of family member	40
12	Pregnancy	39
13	Sex difficulties	39
14	Gain of new family member	39
15	Business readjustment	38
17	Death of close friend	36
18	Change to different line of work	36
19	Change in number of arguments	35
23	Child leaving home	29
24	Trouble with in-laws	29
25	Outstanding personal achievement	28
27	Begin or end school	26
29	Revision of personal habits	24
31	Change in work hours or conditions	20
32	Change in residence	20
33	Change in school	20
36	Change in social activities	18
39	Change in family get togethers	16
43	Minor violation of the law	11

(Adapted from Holmes TH, Rahe RH: The social readjustment rating scale. J Psychosom Res 11:213–218, 1967)

were quarantined in apartments and examined daily by physicians for evidence of respiratory infections, such as signs and symptoms (e.g., sneezing, watery eyes, nasal stuffiness, sinus pain, sore throat, cough and sputum), number of facial tissues used, and a serum sample. Before exposure, subjects completed a series of measures of stress or stressful events in their lives over the past months. The investigators found that higher levels of stress were associated with a greater likelihood of viral infections and severity of cold symptoms. The findings suggest that stress compromises the immune system so that people are more vulnerable to viral infections.

Animal research has also been very illuminating in helping us understand the relationship of stressors to illness. A very large literature provides convincing data that a variety of stressors to animals (crowding, maternal separation, isolation, cold, immersion in water, electric shocks, and rotation stress) lead to increased incidence of hypertension, heart disease, ulcers, and decreased resistance to microbes, radiation, and transplanted tumor cells (Ader, 1981; Cassel, 1974; Weiner, 1977; Weiner et al, 1981). Psychobiological mechanisms leading to disease vulnerability are discussed in detail in Chapter 11.

There are several lines of investigation linking stress and mortality. One of the most replicable findings about stressful life events has demonstrated the risk of grief. Widows and widowers suffer a significantly increased risk of dying in the year after the death of their spouses (Middleton and Raphael, 1987). A study published in the *New England Journal of Medicine* demonstrates that psychological stress among patients with cardiac disease is associated with silent myocardial ischemia and ventricular dysfunction. The results strongly suggest that stress is related to undesirable cardiac events and possibly cardiac death (Rozanski et al, 1988). Sudden cardiac death is often precipitated by emotional distress (Dimsdale, 1987 and 1988). Psychological factors that affect vulnerability to medical illness, including a detailed discussion of the concept of "stress," are discussed in more detail in the following chapter.

Lack of social support also seems to be related to the occurrence of illness. One elegant epidemiological study demonstrated in a prospective fashion that persons with low social support suffered from a significantly increased mortality 5 years later. This correlation proved to be true even after controlling for the effects of smoking, health status, healthcare behavior, and all other health-related variables known to the investigators (Berkman and Syme, 1979).

Epidemiological studies of community populations in the United States, Finland, and Germany found that subjects who were socially isolated had two or three times the risk of mortality compared to those who were well integrated into their communities (House et al, 1988). For example, in the 1950s, researchers noted that residents of Roseto, Pennsylvania, had unusually low rates of mortality associated with heart disease. On closer investigation, they found a close-knit homogeneous community of Italian-Americans whose families immigrated to the United States in the 1880s. Evidence suggested that the high levels of social integration served to protect the community from heart disease leading to myocardial infarctions (Bruhn and Wolf, 1979). Interestingly, more recent studies (Egolf et al, 1992) found the "Roseto effect" diminished as Roseto became "Americanized." Rates of myocardial infarctions for men and women in Roseto have reached those of subjects of comparable age and sex in neighboring towns as close family ties and the community cohesiveness of their town have eroded. With proportionately fewer adults in the United States likely to have close community ties, supportive family relationships, or links through participation in voluntary organizations, vulnerability to various kinds of stressors and stress-related illnesses may increase.

Influence of Psychosocial Variables on the Course and Outcome of Illness and Use of Medical Services

Numerous psychosocial variables have been shown to relate to the course and outcome of physical illnesses. In particular, an accumulation of significant life events can herald a poor outcome. Social support in some circumstances has been shown to buffer the deleterious impact of stressful life events. A particularly ominous circumstance, then, is the combination of stressful life events without adequate social support to buffer these experiences. These two variables, particularly in combination, have been shown in numerous studies to predict poor outcome of physical illnesses.

High stresses, as measured by the presence of many significant life events, and low social support were associated with four times the subsequent risk of death in patients with myocardial infarctions. This order of magnitude was identical to the relative risk associated with other cardiac complications such as arrhythmias or congestive heart failure (Ruberman et al, 1984).

Social isolation is associated with an increased 10-year mortality among patients with stroke (Morris et al, 1993). Similarly, obstetric patients with high life-event scores and low social support have three times the rate of complications of pregnancy (Nuckolls et al, 1972). Patients with asthma experiencing high degrees of stressful life events and low social support are more likely to be using high-dose steroid treatments (de Araujo et al, 1972).

Just as high stress and social isolation can adversely affect the course and outcome of medical illness, so can specific mental disorders. Mental disorders may adversely affect the medical course and mortality rates of medical disorders and may increase the inpatient and outpatient utilization of general medical resources. Depression, the most common major group of psychiatric disorders associated with medical illness, has unique negative effects upon the medical conditions with which it is associated (Wells et al, 1989). Among patients with myocardial infarction, major depression is associated with a threefold increase in 6-month mortality (Frasure-Smith et al, 1993). Major depression is also an independent risk factor for first myocardial infarction, as shown in a prospective study (Pratt et al, 1996). Hypertensive patients with depression had an incidence of stroke 2.7 times higher than patients without depression. Depression with social isolation significantly increases the 10-year mortality rate in patients who have had strokes (Morris et al, 1993). Anxiety symptoms have been found to increase the mortality rate among patients who suffer a myocardial infarction (Kawachi et al, 1994).

Mental disorders also significantly increase the utilization of general medical resources in outpatient primary care settings and in general hospitals. For example, depressed patients will make seven times more emergency room visits and utilize two to three times the healthcare services and costs than do nondepressed patients (Johnson et al, 1992; Katon and Schulberg, 1992; Simon et al,

1995a, 1995b). Patients with panic disorder make 10 times the emergency room visits made by patients without panic disorder. The hospitalization rate of asthmatic patients with anxiety attacks can be triple the rate of asthmatic patients without anxiety attacks (Katon and Roy-Byrne, 1989). Patients with somatization disorder use up to nine times the healthcare services used by the general population (Smith, 1994). As these studies suggest, patients making high use of general medical care have a very high prevalence of mental disorders, especially depressive, anxiety, and somatoform disorders (Katon et al, 1990).

Studies of patients in general hospitals support these findings. Depression and delirium among general medical inpatients are associated with increased lengths of stay, increased use of hospital resources, an increased use of emergency room visits, and a higher rate of medical rehospitalization for at least 4 years after discharge (Saravay and Lavin, 1994; Saravay et al, 1996).

Psychosocial Interventions Make a Difference in the Outcome of Physical Illness

The research indicating that psychosocial variables have an impact on illness predisposition, onset, course, and outcome becomes particularly important when it comes to the point of designing interventions. Prediction, by itself, has an importance in medical care, but psychosocial interventions that can be shown to improve the prognosis of physical illness may well lower morbidity and mortality.

Numerous studies indicate that psychosocial interventions do indeed turn health outcomes in a positive direction. A meta-analysis of 34 controlled studies examining the effects of a supportive, educational, or psychotherapeutic intervention on patients after myocardial infarctions or surgery demonstrated that such interventions were associated with improved physical outcome (less pain, temperature, infection, and so forth), as well as improved emotional outcome (less anxiety and depression). Furthermore, subjects receiving the supportive interventions were discharged an average of 2 days earlier than control subjects (Mumford et al, 1982).

The study of cardiac patients with Type A behavior, discussed above, showed that behavioral intervention could halve the likelihood of future infarctions (Friedman et al, 1984). Providing a supportive companion to women in labor resulted in half the complications found among randomized control patients who did not receive this companionship. In addition, the women with the supportive companions achieved better bonding with their infants (Sosa et al, 1980).

Giving psychiatric treatment to patients with chronic physical illnesses, such as hypertension, diabetes, and chronic respiratory illnesses, has been shown to be associated with lower overall medical costs (Mumford et al, 1984). Psychiatric care also has been shown to have an "offset effect," lessening the use of medical services by patients. In a 5-year study of patients in a large health maintenance organization, Hankin et al (1983) found that providing psychiatric care to patients with mental health problems *significantly reduced* their use of nonpsychiatric care, especially their use of primary care medical services.

In addition, formal psychotherapy has been found effective in improving the outcome of patients with a wide range of physical illnesses (Cohen-Cole et al, 1986). For example, in a classic study, Spiegel and colleagues (1989) randomly assigned 50 women with metastatic breast cancer to therapeutic support groups that met over the period of 1 year; 36 women of comparable medical status were assigned to routine care as a control group. The support groups were intended to reduce feelings of social isolation and help women cope with their disease and its impact on their lives. There was considerable evidence that the participants appreciated the support groups because they improved the quality of life. The investigators also found that women randomly assigned to the therapy *lived longer.* Ten years after the study began, women in the therapy group lived a mean of 36.6 months, whereas the mean survival of the control group was only 18.9 months. In a similar study of psychoeducational group therapy given to patients with malignant melanoma, the treated group had longer-term, positive changes in affective state, coping, and the natural killer cell system, and at 5 to 6 years had a significantly lower mortality rate (Fawzi et al, 1993).

Psychobiological Mechanisms

How does stress lead to illness? How does low support lead to poor physical outcome? How does psychosocial intervention improve physical outcome?

Most of the mechanisms through which psychosocial variables exert their specific effects on illness processes cannot yet be elaborated in molecular detail. However, many psychoendocrine, psychoneurological, and psychoimmunological pathways are beginning to be discovered and described.

The hypothalamus recognizes threatening circumstances and responds with the secretion of releasing factors, such as corticotropin-releasing factor (CRF), which activate the anterior pituitary gland to release hormones, such as adrenocorticotropic hormone (ACTH), which, in turn, act on the adrenal gland to stimulate the production of cortisol. Cortisol has widespread bodily effects, including effects on glucose utilization, metabolism, and blood flow to large muscles. Cortisol, in addition, suppresses many immune functions.

Selye (1976) was one of the early investigators hypothesizing the mechanism of hyperadrenal function as a mediator of the relationship between stress and disease. Other endocrine activation, too, seems stress related. Studies have demonstrated that prolactin, growth hormone, thyroid hormone, and androgens also increase with subjective stress (Sachar, 1980) (see also Chapter 3).

The autonomic nervous system is also implicated in the axis between stress and physical problems. Hypothalamic recognition of danger is the originator of the mechanism. Hypothalamic stimulation activates the autonomic nervous system with the elaboration of epinephrine and norepinephrine, which have widespread bodily effects, including increased heart rate, blood pressure, and respiration. Such mechanisms may be related to the development of hypertension and related illnesses. Stress can cause myofibrillary degeneration and fatal ventricular arrhythmias in ischemic hearts. The neurophysiological connections between the environmental stressor, the internally perceived stress, and the impact on the end organ have been carefully worked out in animal and human studies. Stress activates the frontal lobes, which convey impulses through the frontal cortical brain stem pathways and hypothalamus through the autonomic nervous system to the heart. Blockade of this neurophysiological pathway at any point will prevent stress-induced ventricular fibrillation in ischemic hearts (Skinner, 1988).

In addition to endocrine and nervous system responses, psychoimmunological relationships may be implicated in the connection between psychosocial variables and illness outcomes. Grieving widows and widowers have been shown to have impaired lymphocyte responses to nonspecific mitogens. Persons under stress also show impaired natural killer cell activity (Dorian and Garfinkel, 1987). Numerous animal studies show the same associations linking stress with impaired immunity and increased illness outcomes (Dorian and Garfinkel, 1987). These mechanisms will be discussed in more detail in the following chapter.

Implications for the Practice of Medicine: Interviewing Skills

The importance of psychological and social variables in medical practice requires that physicians develop the knowledge and skills necessary to integrate these factors into general patient care. The skills necessary for this integration are complex and cannot be fully covered in this short introductory textbook.

The most important skill is the ability of the physician to communicate well with the patient. As discussed in Chapter 1, the doctor–patient relationship is the foundation of excellence in clinical medicine, and the interview is the building block of good relationships. Unfortunately, there is reason to believe that the general interviewing skills of physicians in practice are inadequate. One recent study demonstrated that physicians tended to interrupt their patients within the first *18* seconds of the interview. Patients did not get to tell their own stories, and physicians did not obtain an understanding of all the most important problems of their patients (Beckman and Frankel, 1984). Other studies have shown that the empathic skills that students demonstrate in their early years of training tend to diminish as they advance in their education (Maguire and Rutter, 1976). Physicians do not educate their patients well, and 50% of patients do not follow physicians' recommendations (Meichenbaum and Turk, 1987). It is likely that better educational and motivational skills among physicians would lead to better-informed patients who would adhere better to treatment recommendations. Such training has, in fact, been shown to lead to better patient outcome (Cohen-Cole and Bird, 1986b).

There are three basic functions of the medical interview:

1. To collect relevant data to develop and test hypotheses about illnesses
2. To develop and maintain therapeutic relationships with patients
3. To educate and motivate patients to adhere to treatment recommendations (Bird and Cohen-Cole, 1990).

Each of these interviewing functions is best served by specific skills in communicating with patients. While these cannot be reviewed here, they are discussed in detail elsewhere, and medical students have the opportunity to learn these skills in other settings (Cohen-Cole, 1991; Lipkin et al, 1995).

The development of adequate interviewing skills is only the beginning of what is required to be able to integrate psychological and social variables in medical practice. Physicians also must develop the disposition to collect relevant data concerning specific variables. For example, physicians should learn to ask patients about recent life stresses and levels of social support. Negative health habits, such as smoking, drinking, poor dietary habits, and not wearing seat belts, should be evaluated, and efforts should be made to educate patients and motivate them to change. Relevant knowledge of psychological processes should be mastered. Possible psychosocial treatment interventions should be learned and implemented where relevant. The task for physicians is large and complex. This book provides a starting point in this important process, and students are referred to standard textbooks on medical interviewing for more detail (Cohen-Cole, 1991).

EPIDEMIOLOGY OF PSYCHIATRIC DISORDERS IN GENERAL MEDICAL PRACTICE

Psychiatric Disorders in the Community

As discussed above, physicians need general psychosocial knowledge and assessment skills to be able to evaluate and appropriately manage relevant psychological and social variables in patients with *physical* disorders. However, it is important for medical students to realize that similar skills also are needed for the recognition and management of overt *psychiatric* disorders that present in the general medical sector.

Almost 30 million Americans suffer from mental disorders, alcohol abuse, or other substance abuse in any 6-month period. These illnesses cause untold suffering as well as enormous morbidity and mortality. The financial costs are staggering. The direct and indirect costs of these illnesses were estimated to be $218 *billion* in 1983. Mortality from alcohol and drug abuse, substance abuse–related accidents, and suicides related to other mental disorders all account for 108,000 deaths per year (Kamerow et al, 1986). Depression alone costs $44 billion annually (Greenberg et al, 1993a, 1993b).

The Epidemiologic Catchment Area study (ECA) provided data from a household survey of 20,000 persons in five states across the United States. About 28% of Americans suffered from a clinically significant and diagnosable mental disorder in the preceding year (Regier et al, 1993). Over one third (32%) of Americans have suffered from a mental disorder at some time in their lives. Phobias have the highest lifetime prevalence, followed by mood disorders (major depression and dysthymia) and alcohol abuse or dependence. Tables 2–2, 2–3, and 2–4 show the different prevalence rates of major mental disorders by social background characteristics (Robins et al, 1991).

It is interesting to note that anxiety and depressive disorders are much more common among women and that substance abuse is more common among men. Overall, the total prevalence of mental disorders is about the same in men as in women, although women are much more likely to seek help for their problems than are men. Another important finding is that, contrary to expectations, mental disorders *do not* increase with age. In fact, they seem to decrease after the age of 65. The "baby boom" generation now seems to be suffering from a dramatically increased prevalence of mood disorders in particular (Robins et al, 1991).

Table 2–2 **Selected Findings from the Epidemiologic Catchment Area Study**

	PREVALENCE (%)	
DISORDER	**Lifetime**	**1 Year**
Any disorder*	32.2	20.0
Schizophrenia	1.5	1.0
Mania	0.8	0.6
Major depression	6.4	3.7
Dysthymia	3.3	5.4
Alcohol abuse/dependence	13.8	6.3
Phobia	14.3	8.8
Somatization disorder	0.1	0.1
Antisocial personality	2.6	1.2

*Note: The ECA study systematically underestimates the true prevalence of mental disorders because the survey instrument (the "Diagnostic Interview Scale") did not include a number of important psychiatric disorders including posttraumatic stress disorder, somatoform pain disorder, hypochondriasis, conversion disorder, psychological factors affecting physical condition, and all personality disorders other than antisocial personality.
(Data from Robins L, Regier D (eds): Psychiatric Disorders in America: The Epidemiologic Catchment Area Study. Free Press, New York, 1991)

Table 2–3 **Selected Lifetime Prevalence by Sex**

	PREVALENCE (%)	
DISORDER	**Male**	**Female**
Any disorder	36.0	30.0
Major depression	2.6	7.0
Agoraphobia	3.2	7.9
Alcohol abuse	23.8	4.8
Antisocial personality	4.5	0.8

Besides the ECA study, there have been many other epidemiological studies of psychiatric disorders, in which prevalence in rural settings were compared with that in urban settings, and primitive with more advanced societies. These studies were undertaken to test the hypothesis that civilization and industrialization may be associated with increased rates of mental illness. Although there are some small differences, the most impressive finding of cross-cultural epidemiology has been that the prevalence of major mental disorders appears to be fairly stable across international boundaries (industrialized/nonindustrialized), as well as urban/rural boundaries (Murphy JM, 1988). There are some important exceptions, however, to these cross-cultural universals in the prevalence of the major mental disorders: schizophrenia is slightly *more* common in lower socioeconomic classes (in the United States) and *less* common in less developed societies; schizophrenia tends to have a better outcome in less developed societies; economic and social instability are both associated with higher rates and poorer outcome of mental illness; bipolar disorder is slightly more prevalent in more socially advantaged classes; depression is somewhat more common in urban areas; depression is more likely to occur in relatively powerless women, without emotional support and no outside employment (Boyd and Weissman, 1988; Kleinman, 1988; Murphy and Helzer, 1988).

As Brown, Gregg, and Ballard note in Chapter 4, the presentation of both physical and mental illness symptoms may vary in different cultures. For example, Kleinman and Kleinman (1985) describe how symptoms of mental disturbances are described as somatic complaints in Asian cultures far more

Table 2–4 **Selected Lifetime Prevalence by Age**

	PREVALENCE (%)			
DIAGNOSIS	**18–29 yr**	**30–44 yr**	**45–64 yr**	**65 + yr**
Major depression	5.0	7.5	4.0	1.4
Alcohol abuse/ dependence	33.5	33.4	24.3	15.0

than among Western cultures. Depressed patients often report a variety of diffuse and changeable physical symptoms, such as vague aches and pains, feeling tired all over, dizziness, and palpitations, and deny feeling depressed when asked. When Lau et al (1983) studied 213 cases of depression in Hong Kong, they found that 96 percent of the patients presented their symptoms as physical complaints, including headache, insomnia, feverishness, cough, and lower back pain. Kleinman (1980) notes that the languages spoken in China and Taiwan have few words referring to psychological states. Perhaps because Americans with little education also lack a psychological "vocabulary of discomfort," Kleinman finds that they, too, tend to present symptoms of mental disorders in somatic terms more than better educated persons (Kleinman and Kleinman, 1985). This characteristic of describing feelings and mood states in physical terms has been called "somatothymia" by Stoudemire (1991).

Although extreme mental disturbances such as psychotic depression, schizophrenia, and bipolar disorder are recognized throughout the world, they have different names and the expression of symptomatic behaviors varies. For example, a schizophrenic in a tribal society may say that his behavior is controlled by powerful sorcerers and witches, whereas his counterpart in the West might claim to be controlled by Martians or electrical impulses (Helman, 1990).

Locals generally differentiate "normal" controlled behaviors motivated by belief systems or rituals from similar behaviors not motivated by the sociocultural context and, therefore, labeled as "abnormal" and "pathological" (Helman, 1990). Edgerton (1977) reported a consensus among laypersons in four East African cultures that actions such as violent conduct, wandering around naked, talking nonsense, and sleeping and hiding in the bush—as long as they occurred "without reason"—are indicators of "madness."

Some disorders unique to other cultures share the symptoms of mental disorders with different labels in our own society. *Susto* (or "magical fright") is common throughout Latin America and among Hispanics in the southwestern United States. As Rubel (1977) described it, *susto* is based on the belief that an individual is composed of a physical body and of souls or spirits that can become detached from the body and wander freely. The loss of soul or spirit is believed to occur when someone is sleeping and dreaming or when one is shocked, frightened, or very surprised. The clinical presentations of *susto* are restlessness during sleep, loss of appetite, and lack of interest in dress or personal hygiene. Epidemiological studies of *susto* find that it is commonly preceded by a series of life stresses, including those that lead individuals to feel that they cannot meet the social expectations of their family or social group. Healing is carried out by a *curandero*, who devises various strategies for coaxing or entreating the soul or spirit to rejoin the body (Rubel, 1977).

Psychiatric diseases therefore exist and are recognized as abnormal or pathological in most societies. The experience of the disorder—or illness—may vary, as will the understanding of its causes or etiology. Cultural influences and provincial belief systems as they affect definitions of disease, illness, and illness "behaviors" will be discussed in more detail in Chapter 4.

Epidemiology of Psychiatric Disorders in Primary Care

Mental disorders are more common in patients who are medically ill. Patients with mental disorders tend to frequently visit general medical clinics. These patients use about twice as many general healthcare resources as those without mental disorders (Simon et al, 1995a and 1995b). Interestingly, these general healthcare costs can be reduced by proper treatment for substance abuse and mental disorder (Mumford et al, 1984). While the one-month prevalence of mental disorders is 16% in the general community, 21% to 26% of general medical outpatients will have a diagnosable mental disorder, and an even higher number (30% to 60%) will be found in the general medical hospital (Cole et al, 1996).

A significant proportion—an estimated 41% to 63%—of all mental health visits are made to *primary care* physicians rather than to mental health specialists (Mechanic, 1989). It has been found that 6% to 10% of medical patients meet criteria for major depression, and that 3% to 6% meet criteria for panic disorder. At least 10% of all medical patients are likely to have an alcohol problem (Kessler et al, 1985; Von Korff et al, 1987). Among hospitalized medical or surgical patients, patients with psychiatric problems had significantly longer hospital stays (Saravay and Lavin, 1994). Although 30% to 60% of medical inpatients will have psychiatric disorders, only 1% to 3% are likely to be referred (Saravay and Lavin, 1994). More than half of all these patients will *never* get help for their mental illnesses from mental health specialists. Their only chance for appropriate care will be their primary care physician (Shulman et al, 1985).

Are these patients being appropriately recognized and treated by their primary physicians? The data suggest not.

Only half of the population with mental disorders will seek help for them. Most will turn to their primary care physicians, who fail to make a diagnosis 50% of the time (Sartorius et al, 1993; Spitzer et al, 1994). Even after a diagnosis is made, patients with depression were prescribed antidepressants only 20% of the time, and of these, 40% received subtherapeutic doses (Wells, 1994). One study of major depression in the community determined that only 17% of patients with major depression were treated with an antidepressant medication, but over half were taking sedative hypnotic agents such as benzodiazepines for insomnia and other nonspecific complaints (prescribed in most cases by their primary care physician) (Weissman et al, 1981). Seventy percent of patients with panic disorder see 10 or more physicians before the correct diagnosis is made (Ballenger, 1987). Only 8% of patients with panic disorder were adequately treated. One study in Boston found that *none* of the patients whose disorders were diagnosed independently as meeting psychiatric criteria for alcohol abuse was recognized by the primary care physician (Borus et al, 1988). Of those patients seen by primary care physicians, relatively few are referred for specialty care. Patients also consistently underreport personal distress to their physicians (Eisenberg, 1992). The majority of people who commit suicide visit their primary physician in the month before they kill themselves. Their psychological distress is rarely recognized (Murphy GE, 1988).

Well-designed, prospective random controlled studies have demonstrated that psychiatric intervention programs can result not only in clinical psychiatric improvement but can also reduce utilization of general medical resources and reduce overall costs. The studies suggest that programs most likely to be effective will require an integration of mental health and general medical staff so that they can collaborate closely in diagnosis, triage, and treatment (Saravay, 1996). Persons hospitalized with hip fractures who were treated according to such models had improved psychiatric outcome, reduced length of stay, and reduced utilization of general medical resources after discharge (Strain et al, 1994). Similar findings have been demonstrated in medical outpatients with respect to depression and somatoform disorders (Katon and Gonzalez, 1994; Saravay, 1996). Models that combine collaboration of mental health and general medical care can improve clinical outcome while reducing overall cost (Saravay, 1996). Treatment of substance abuse such as alcoholism has been shown to reduce healthcare costs for family members as well as for the patient (Holder and Blose, 1992; SAMHSA 1995).

Why is so much mental illness missed in the primary care sector? The problem results from a combination of factors that relate to both the patient and the doctor. First of all, patients do not usually go to their doctor complaining of a mental illness. They generally present with somatic complaints that require a high level of suspicion, as well as diagnostic expertise on the part of the physician, to be diagnosed accurately. Many patients also do not want to believe that they may be suffering from a mental disorder. Finally, physicians must be able to educate patients skillfully concerning the current psychobiological understanding of mental illness in order to get them to accept proper treatment.

From the physician's point of view, psychiatric diagnoses often are missed because of time constraints as well as limited knowledge and skills to recognize such disorders (Cohen-Cole et al, 1982). Mental health training of primary care physicians is woefully inadequate. Residents in internal medicine receive an average of only 8 hours in the management of mental disorders over 3 years of residency training despite the fact that these problems occur in 25% of their patients (Strain et al, 1985). Family practice residents receive more mental health training, but almost none from psychiatrists (Goldberg et al, 1985).

Primary care physicians can increase their awareness of psychiatric illnesses and use this information to improve their quality of care. Physicians can communicate their interest and a willingness to listen—a cue many depressed people feel is lacking, thereby inhibiting the expression of their distress. Active listening may alert the physician to potential suicide risks, encourage more supportive behavior, and, if needed, lead to referral for specialty care. In this way, the doctor–patient relationship may enhance the quality of patient care (Mechanic, 1989).

Psychiatric illnesses are among the most common and troubling disorders in the country and represent the major problem of 25% of all medical patients. Surveys of practicing physicians indicate that they feel undertrained in recognizing and treating these disorders. Current research indicates that physicians underrecognize psychiatric problems. The need for further education is clear.

SOCIAL EPIDEMIOLOGY AND ILLNESS BEHAVIOR: SOCIOCULTURAL INFLUENCES ON DISEASE, MEDICAL UTILIZATION, AND OTHER ILLNESS-RELATED BEHAVIORS

Social Epidemiology

Further arguments for the biopsychosocial model can be made from the standpoint of social epidemiology, which represents the field of study of relationships between social groupings and patterns of illness. Four variables—age, sex, race, and socioeconomic variables—have been studied most intensively.

Age Factors

Physical Disorders. The incidence of illness is affected by age. In childhood, the majority of illnesses are acute infections and exanthemas, the latter being reduced through vaccinations against measles and rubella. The incidence of acute illness declines rapidly in adolescence and more gradually in old age, whereas chronic diseases increase in prevalence (Susser et al, 1985). Eighty-six percent of persons over age 65 have one or more chronic medical conditions, most commonly arthritis, hypertension, and heart disease. Hearing impairments, diabetes, cataracts, and varicose veins are also common ailments of the elderly (Cockerham, 1992a).

Life expectancy has increased dramatically. In 1900, an American could expect to live to age 47; present life expectancy is more than 70 years. Life expectancy after age 65 increased by only 2 years between 1900 and 1950 (from 11.9 to 13.9 years). Between 1950 and the mid-1980s, life expectancy at age 65 increased 3.8 years for women and 1.6 years for men, with overall mortality rates falling 29% in that period. Most of the decline was due to reduction of heart and cerebrovascular disease (Estes and Lee, 1986).

The overall decline in mortality, associated with declines in infant mortality and mortality associated with infectious diseases, accompanied by declining fertility rates, accounts for an increasing proportion of the population over age 65. In 1900, persons over age 65 were only 4% of the population; by 1987 they represented 12.3% of the population (or 29.8 million people). By 2050, 20% of the population is expected to be over the age of 65 (Cockerham, 1992a).

Mental Disorders. Age is also associated with the prevalence of mental impairments. Psychiatric disorders typically begin when people are young, the median age at first symptoms being only 16 years (the average age of the United States population is 40). Ninety percent of persons with mental disorders exhibit symptoms by age 38, with the exception of cognitive impairment disorders (such as Alzheimer's disease), which increase in frequency much later in life, especially after age 70. Particular disorders differ in their median age at onset. For symptoms of antisocial personality, the median age is 8 years; for phobias, age 10; somatization disorders, age 15; drug abuse, age 18; and schizophrenia and manic episodes, age 19. The median age for the onset of obsessive–compulsive disorders is 20 years; alcohol abuse/dependence, age 21; panic disorder, age 23; and major depression, age 25 (Robins et al, 1991).

Adolescence is an important period for the development of many disorders and most symptoms begin between the ages of 15 and 29 (Burke et al, 1990). The ECA studies suggest that the prevalence of depression, drug abuse, and alcohol dependence have been increasing among younger age groups over the past 40 years (Burke et al, 1991). Klerman (1976) hypothesized that Western societies were entering an "age of melancholy" characterized by changing family structures and increased urbanization, which has resulted in greater mental health problems among adolescents and young adults.

Gender Factors

Physical Disorders. As long as vital statistics have been available in the United States, men have had higher rates of mortality than women, but women have exhibited higher rates of morbidity and health services use (Verbrugge, 1985). Although women tend to report more morbidity, men tend to have a greater prevalence of life-threatening chronic diseases or behavioral and environmental risks. At all ages, death rates among male subjects exceed those of female subjects in heart disease, cancer, cerebrovascular accidents, and pneumonia, along with homicides, suicides, and accidental injuries (Cockerham, 1992a). Although the more frequent symptoms of women are generally minor, in later life women also die of the same diseases as men. For example, coronary heart disease is the leading cause of death among women after the age of 66, whereas it is the greatest killer of men after age 39. As Verbrugge notes (1985:163), "Men and women essentially suffer the same types of problems; what distinguishes the sexes is the frequency of those problems and the pace of death."

Differences in age-specific mortality are reflected in life expectancy (Table 2–5). In 1988, the average life expectancy at birth for white females in

Table 2–5 **Average Number of Years of Life Expectancy in the United States by Race and Sex, Since 1900**

YEAR	WHITE MALES	WHITE FEMALES	BLACK MALES	BLACK FEMALES
1900	46.6	48.7	32.5*	33.5*
1950	66.5	72.2	58.9	62.7
1960	67.4	74.1	60.7	65.9
1970	68.0	75.6	60.0	68.3
1980	70.7	78.1	63.8	72.5
1987	72.2	78.9	65.2	73.6
1988	72.3	78.9	64.9	73.4

(National Center for Health Statistics, 1991)
*Includes all nonwhites.

the United States was 78.9 years as compared with 72.3 for white males. For black females, life expectancy was 73.4 years as compared with 64.9 years for black males. A greater proportion of females than males survive at every age. For example, among males subjects the chances of fetal death during the prenatal stage are approximately 12% greater, and during the neonatal stage 130% greater (Cockerham, 1992a).

Table 2–6 details age-adjusted rates for causes of death, adjusted for sex and race, in the United States. Some of the gender differences in mortality are associated with lifestyles associated with sex roles in Western cultures. Expectations of aggression among males appear to be associated with greater rates of death and injury among adolescent men from accidents and violence. Men are also more likely to be employed in high-risk occupations and are more likely to use alcohol and other drugs and to experience health consequences as a result (Cockerham, 1992a).

Figure 2–1 presents the leading causes of death for adults 25 to 64 years old, but does not denote gender differences. Verbrugge (1985), however, has suggested that men and women may be moving toward greater equality in mortality rates as lifestyles change for women. For example, rates of cigarette smoking and alcohol consumption among women have been approaching that of men, and women are entering the labor force in occupations that have been dominated by men. Lung cancer, the eighth leading cause of death for women in 1960, became the leading cause of death for women in 1986, exceeding breast cancer.

As noted, women have higher rates of morbidity and utilize health services more than men, even when symptoms and services relating to reproductive health are excluded (Cleary et al, 1982; Cockerham, 1992a; Verbrugge, 1985). Women have higher morbidity from acute and nonfatal chronic conditions. Excesses are especially large (twofold or more) for varicose veins, frequent constipation, gallbladder conditions, chronic enteritis and colitis, corns and

Table 2–6 **Age-Adjusted Death Rates for Selected Causes of Death, According to Sex and Race, United States, 1988***

	WHITE MALES	WHITE FEMALES	BLACK MALES	BLACK FEMALES
All causes	664.2	384.4	1,037.8	593.1
Heart disease	220.5	114.2	286.2	181.1
Cerebrovascular diseases	30.0	25.5	57.8	46.6
Cancer	157.6	110.1	227.0	131.2
Pulmonary disease	27.8	14.5	26.0	10.0
Pneumonia and influenza	18.0	10.7	28.0	13.4
Liver disease and cirrhosis	12.1	5.0	20.7	9.3
Diabetes	9.6	8.4	19.8	22.1
Accidents	49.9	18.8	69.0	22.2
Suicide	19.8	5.1	11.8	2.4
Homicide	7.7	2.8	58.2	12.7
AIDS	9.9	0.7	31.6	6.2

(National Center for Health Statistics, 1991)
* Deaths per 100,000 resident population.

bunions, thyroid conditions, anemias, migraines, and chronic urinary diseases. Also more common among women are hypertensive disease, hemorrhoids, chronic bronchitis, chronic sinusitis, diverticula of the intestine, arthritis, and synovitis–bursitis–tenosynovitis (Verbrugge, 1985).

Women also restrict their activities because of health problems more then men—about 25% more days per year and 40% more days in bed per year, on average. Between the ages of 17 and 44, women have twice the number of physician visits and hospital stays as men do (if reproductive-related problems are excluded, the gap is 30%). Women are given substantially more prescription medications than men, especially psychotropic drugs (Verbrugge, 1985).

Considerable research has explored the reasons for the higher rates of morbidity among women as compared with men. A portion of the difference may be an artifact of reporting behavior. Some speculate that women are more sensitive to bodily discomforts as a result of childhood socialization, whereas men repress their reporting as they adhere to a cultural norm of stoicism. Furthermore, women are more often interviewed in home surveys on health status and may underreport the symptoms of their spouses relative to their own (Verbrugge, 1985).

The bulk of the research, however, suggests the differences in morbidity are not merely artifactual, but are real and associated with the demands of social role. In American society, the combined demands on women as caregivers, spouses, and employees apparently exceed those on men and, in some cases, such as employment, the rewards are fewer (Bird and Fremont, 1991). Women also perceive themselves as having less control in making decisions that affect their lives than men (Rosenfeld, 1989). The excessive role demands,

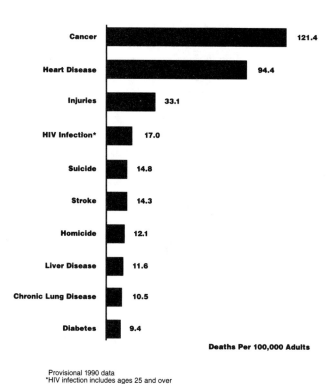

Cancer — 121.4
Heart Disease — 94.4
Injuries — 33.1
HIV Infection* — 17.0
Suicide — 14.8
Stroke — 14.3
Homicide — 12.1
Liver Disease — 11.6
Chronic Lung Disease — 10.5
Diabetes — 9.4

Deaths Per 100,000 Adults

Provisional 1990 data
*HIV infection includes ages 25 and over

Figure 2–1. *Leading causes of death for adults aged 25 through 64. (Centers for Disease Control, National Center for Health Statistics)*

lower rewards, and lack of control contribute to chronic stress, which is associated with a greater incidence and prevalence of symptoms. Studies in which role demands of men and women are comparable have found little or no differences in morbidity between them. In one study, when role demands were statistically controlled or held constant, morbidity among men exceeded that among women (Bird and Fremont, 1991).

Marital status interacts with gender in its association with both morbidity and mortality rates. Mortality rates among the married are less than those among subjects of comparable age who are single because they have been divorced, separated, widowed, or never married. Only a small portion of the difference is accounted for by selection—e.g., healthier persons are more likely to marry. The bulk of the difference is due to mortality associated with the use of legal but harmful substances (e.g., lung cancer with smoking, or cirrhosis of the liver with excessive alcohol use), with intentional or unintentional injuries (homicide, automobile accident, or suicide), and with conditions requiring prolonged care (tuberculosis or diabetes). Marriage has a significant impact on mortality rates for men, but hardly any effect on the health of women (Gove and Tudor, 1973).

The greater effect of marriage on the mortality of men probably occurs because the lifestyles of single men pose greater health risks than those of women. The lives of men change more dramatically with marriage. Evidence in support of this hypothesis was reported by Umberson (1987), who found changes in a variety of health-risk behaviors for men with marriage and even more with parenthood. Changes in the behavior of women with marriage and parenthood were minimal. In this culture, marriage provides men with care-givers—the traditional role of wives—and also acts as a form of social control. Women appear not to derive such health benefits from marriage in America (Umberson, 1987).

Mental Disorders. With respect to mental disorders, the picture is dif-ferent. The ECA studies mentioned earlier indicate that, contrary to previous research reporting greater levels of mental illness among women than men, more men than women report mental disorders during their lifetimes (36% as opposed to 30%). Men have excess amounts of alcohol abuse and antisocial personality, whereas women have higher rates of somatization, obsessive-compulsive, and major depressive disorders (Link and Dohrenwend, 1989; Robins and Regier, 1991). Community studies focusing more generally on mood disorders or depression scales find women with considerably more symptoms of mental disorders than men (Kessler, 1989). Although some of the gender differences have been attributed to reporting styles of men and women, the bulk of the research and the ECA studies suggest the differences for specific disorders are real.

As with general morbidity, research attributes some of the differences in psychiatric disorders to social roles and experiences. Women reportedly expe-rience greater chronic stress from their social roles, making them more vulner-able to stressful life events and contributing directly to symptoms of depression (Kessler, 1989). In general, married women employed outside the home enjoy better mental health than those remaining at home as housewives (Cockerham, 1992b). Additional research shows that the mental health bene-fits of employment are less for women when the family is very dependent on their income or when women are also expected to perform the full range of family roles. Thus, working-class or single parents receive fewer mental health benefits from working than middle-class women (Kessler and McLeod, 1984; Ross et al, 1983). Some (Thoits, 1987) attribute the greater vulnerability of women to depression to having less control over many situations or fewer resources with which to make decisions about their lives.

Rates of mental disorder are especially high among men and women who were separated, divorced, and never married as compared with those who are married. The never-married have much higher rates of drug abuse and higher rates of schizophrenia, bipolar disorder, alcohol dependency, and antisocial personality. Mental health can be both a cause and effect of marital status, since social competence is required for stable relationships. Widowhood is not necessarily associated with greater levels of psychiatric disorder, except that associated with bereavement. (Robins and Regier, 1991).

Social support associated with marriage may function to protect some from stressful life events and therefore help them resist the onset of mental disorders. A study of depression in London (Brown and Harris, 1978) found that, of women suffering comparable stressful life events, those who did not have a supportive, intimate relationship with their husbands were more likely to experience symptoms of depression. Although both women and men appear to derive mental health benefits from marriage, the advantages to men exceed those to women (Cockerham, 1992b). This finding may explain why women do not suffer as much as men from marital dissolutions. Women also adjust to the death of a spouse better than men, and adjust as well, if not better, to divorce (Kessler, 1989).

Race

Physical Disorders. Racial or ethnic groups manifest great differences in mortality and morbidity. Asian-Americans have the best health-quality levels, followed closely by whites, but blacks are especially disadvantaged relative to these groups. Black infants have had nearly twice the mortality rates as whites, and although the rates have diminished, the gaps between races persist (Cockerham, 1992a).

In the United States, blacks have a higher prevalence than whites of most life-threatening illnesses, such as AIDS, cancer, heart disease, and hypertension (Polednak, 1989). Although blacks make up 12% of the population, they account for 20% of persons with diagnosed hypertension. Between the ages of 25 and 44, hypertension kills black males 15 times more frequently than it does white males. Homicide is the leading cause of death of black men between the ages of 15 and 24 (Cockerham, 1992a).

Differences are reflected in life expectancies. In 1988, the average life expectancy of black males at birth was 64.9 years, 7.4 years less than white males (72.3 years) and 14 years less than white females (78.9 years) (Cockerham, 1992a). In Harlem, an area of New York City with a predominantly black population, a black male is less likely to survive to the age of 40 than a male in Bangladesh, one of the poorest nations in the world (McCord and Freeman, 1990).

Part of the difference due to race and ethnic group is accounted for by quality of life, availability resources, and behavior. Black people are more likely to smoke and drink alcohol excessively and have high cholesterol levels, excess weight, and diabetes (Otten et al, 1990). The problems are compounded by poor access to health services.

Relative to non-Hispanic whites, Hispanic subjects also have a disadvantaged health status with more diabetes, tuberculosis, hypertension, lung cancer, alcoholism, and deaths from cirrhosis of the liver and homicide. This ethnic group also contains disproportionate numbers of patients with AIDS, but lower mortality rates associated with heart disease and most forms of cancer. Hispanics are not a homogeneous population, and among those in the United States, Cubans have the best health status, followed by Mexican-Americans and Puerto Ricans (Cockerham, 1992a).

Native Americans, including American Indians and native Alaskans, have improved their overall health status over the past 40 years. American Indians still have a high mortality rate associated with diabetes. For example, the Pima Indians have rates that are 10 to 15 times higher than the general American population.

Many of the differences between ethnic or racial groups are confounded by social class. Several minorities, such as blacks, Hispanics, and Native Americans, are disproportionately from lower socioeconomic class backgrounds, which are also associated with higher morbidity and mortality rates.

Mental Disorders. The ECA studies find that blacks have higher rates of overall mental disorders than whites or Hispanics. Among older persons, blacks have higher rates of cognitive impairment and somatization. Blacks do not have higher rates of antisocial personality disorders or drug and alcohol abuse. Their overrepresentation in institutionalized populations for these conditions relates to a greater likelihood of vulnerability to criminal activity and prosecution associated with symptoms of these disorders (Robins and Regier, 1991).

Native Americans have rates of alcoholism two to three times higher than the general population and, relatedly, injuries and deaths associated with automobile accidents. Suicide rates are 20% higher than the general population, particularly among Native American youth (Cockerham, 1992b).

Hispanic-Americans are underrepresented in treatment populations of the mentally ill, perhaps partially because of language barriers to institutional care (Aneshensel et al, 1991). Some studies of Hispanics report that the Mexican-American culture contains supportive elements, particularly family and kinship ties, that reduce vulnerability to mental disorders (Mirowsky and Ross, 1984). Similarly, kinship and community ties may partially account for the low rates of mental disorder among Asian-Americans (Cockerham, 1992b).

Again, some of the differences in prevalence of mental disorders between ethnic groups may be accounted for by social class. Studies investigating overall rates of mental illness in communities, with the researchers controlling for (or holding constant) social class, found that differences between the ethnic groups were significantly reduced or disappeared (Thomas and Hughes, 1986; Warheit et al, 1975). Therefore, we next consider the relationship of social class to health.

Social Class

Physical Disorders. Social class, whether indicated by income, occupational prestige, or educational attainment, is associated with health status.

Persons from lower social classes have higher rates of morbidity, mortality, and disability than those of higher classes (Dutton, 1986; Dutton and Levine, 1989).

Part of the association may be caused by the inadequate access to health services by persons with low incomes, yet even in societies with universal access to services, social class is associated with mortality and morbidity (Reid, 1989). A remarkable 10-year study of 17,530 British men between the ages of 40 and 64, all employed by the civil service, found associations between civil service rank and health status. The highest-ranking administrators had the lowest death rates, and the lowest-status unskilled workers had the highest likelihood of death, most of it associated with coronary heart disease (Marmot et al, 1984).

Some of the class-related differences may be associated with conditions of life and risk behaviors, such as smoking, obesity, lack of intentional exercise, drug and alcohol use, and diet. Some unhealthy behaviors may represent adaptations or methods for coping with difficult life conditions associated with having few material or social resources. The physical or environmental conditions of low-income populations contain a high risk of harm from violence, unemployment, crowding, poor housing, social isolation, stress, and similar factors (Bunker et al, 1989; Dutton, 1986).

Ironically, coronary heart disease, traditionally associated with affluence and a higher incidence in wealthier countries, is more common among low-income populations (Cockerham, 1992a). In the United States, the incidence of coronary heart disease has been declining over the past 25 years. The advantages are disproportionately shared by persons of higher social class backgrounds, seemingly associated with healthier lifestyles and social and physical environments (Polednak, 1989; Stamler, 1985).

Mental Disorders. Like physical health, mental health is also directly associated with social class. The ECA study found that the least educated had the highest rates of mental disorders. The prevalence of mental disorders also were associated with other indicators of lower social class, such as receiving welfare payments, having unskilled jobs, or not being employed. The unemployed had at least double the rate of every major mental disorder except drug abuse. Bipolar disorder, schizophrenia, and panic disorder were particularly overrepresented among both unemployed and unskilled workers (Robins and Regier, 1991).

Of the various indicators of social class, education appears most associated with mental disorders in women and income levels most associated with men (Kessler, 1980). Of mental illnesses, schizophrenia clearly appears associated with lower social class along with most other disorders, whereas anxiety and bipolar mood disorders are apparently more prevalent in higher social classes (Link and Dohrenwend, 1989).

One of the classic studies interviewed adults in the midtown Manhattan area of New York City in nearly 2,000 randomly selected households. Using standard instruments designed to tap a range of mental disorders, the researchers found greater proportions of impaired persons with lower incomes. The authors argued that lower social status was responsible for disorder as a result of life conditions, but social status also increased the vulnerability of those exposed to stressors. Given similar levels of stress, persons from the lower social classes would be more likely to develop symptoms of mental disorders (Langner and Michael, 1963).

Attempts to determine why social class is associated with mental disorders, particularly schizophrenia, have offered several explanations. The "social causation" interpretation argues that deprivation produces more psychopathology (Kohn, 1972). Somewhat related is the argument that lower social class conditions undermine coping capacity or resources, making populations more vulnerable to mental illness (Kessler and Cleary, 1980).

A second explanation, "social selection," reverses the causal direction. It argues that persons who are mentally impaired may be selected into the lower social classes because of failures in life. An inability to achieve in occupation, education, or both causes individuals to "drift" down into the lowest social classes. A related version of this explanation is that persons predisposed genetically to schizophrenia disproportionately have lower social class origins, and they also fail to rise in social class through achievements in life (Kohn, 1972).

Evidence supports both explanations for schizophrenia (Dohrenwend et al, 1992), yet neither alone fully explains the association between class and mental disorder.

Utilization and Related Illness Behaviors

Definitions

To understand more fully the importance of human behavior in medical practice, it is important to distinguish among the concepts of "disease," "illness," and "illness behavior." *Disease* refers to a disturbance in physiological functioning of the organism. Such a disturbance can occur without the person's awareness. *Illness* refers to a state of poor health recognized by the person and usually treated by an expert. *Illness behavior* refers to the ways people respond to bodily indications and to the perceptions, values, attitudes, and interpretations that lead people to behave in particular ways in reference to their bodies (Kleinman et al, 1978).

From these definitions, it should be clear that disease and illness are not the same. Many patients may have "silent" disease—some physiological disruption of which they are not aware. Similarly, there are many people who have *illnesses* but no evidence of physiological *disease.* Finally, the behaviors of persons may vary greatly according to whether or not they perceive themselves as ill and according to their attitudes and values about how they should behave because of the presence of illness. As noted earlier, cultural influences are what constitutes "illness" and the determinants of variations in "illness behavior" are discussed in more detail in Chapter 4.

Physicians must deal as much with illness and illness behaviors as they do with disease itself. Physicians who understand something about cultural, social class, and personality differences in illness behavior will be able to provide more effective medical care. Patterns of illness behavior often make a great impact on the physical outcome of disease.

Decision Time: An Example of the Impact of Health Attitudes on Utilization and Outcome of Disease Processes

Deaths due to myocardial infarction represent the foremost killer of adult males from the ages of 30 to 60. Fifty percent of patients with myocardial infarction die before they ever reach a hospital (DiMatteo and Friedman, 1982). There is a great deal of variation, however, in the amount of time it takes such patients to reach the hospital. Fifty-six percent arrive within 4 hours after the onset of symptoms, 28% arrive within 4 to 14 hours, and 16% arrive more than 14 hours. Transportation issues relate to only about 10% of these cases. There are other factors that must be invoked to explain these great differences in the response to the initial awareness of chest discomfort. These variables account for the differences in decision time (DiMatteo and Friedman, 1982).

There are three general sets of factors that help explain differences in decision time.

Background Factors. Social class, age, sex, and ethnic group all have an impact on decision time. Persons of lower social class are less likely to seek medical help quickly. This response may have to do with rather objective access and financial issues: They are less able to afford care, they may have more difficulty finding transportation, they may not feel as well treated, and so forth.

Older patients are less likely to go for help quickly, and older women in particular are less likely to seek help quickly for symptoms of chest discomfort. This difference may relate more to the fact that women are less likely to think of cardiac events as explaining their chest symptoms than are men. Ethnic differences account for a great deal of variation in decision time. People of British descent have been trained to be more stoic about pain. They are much less likely to seek help rapidly for symptoms of chest discomfort. Such differences can account for a great deal of the variations in decision times and can account for many of the variations in the lethal effect of the heart attack itself (DiMatteo and Friedman, 1982).

Psychological Processes. Psychological issues are extremely important in determining the response time of the person to physical symptoms. Patients must make a "cognitive appraisal" of the meaning of their perceived symptoms and then make judgments regarding what to do about it. Many persons misinterpret their initial cardiac symptoms. In fact, 70% of persons who first experience the pain of cardiac ischemia originally consider the pain to result from abdominal indigestion or some source other than cardiac.

The psychological defense of *denial* can play an important part in decision time. Mechanisms of defense are psychological processes that enable persons to avoid the anxiety of facing certain issues. The defense mechanisms operate at unconscious levels so that persons may be unaware of their manifestations. Denial is one very powerful mechanism through which the awareness of certain anxiety-provoking issues can be minimized or unrecognized. Because heart attacks are so terribly overwhelming, many persons do not want to face the anxiety of coping with this reality. Persons who are able to maintain steadfast denial for long periods after the onset of cardiac symptoms are the ones most likely to have long decision times and are at more risk of cardiac death before reaching the hospital (DiMatteo and Friedman, 1982). (The concept of denial is discussed from the psychodynamic perspective in both Chapters 5 and 14.)

Social Variables. The social context or situation of the patient also plays an important role in the amount of decision time it takes from the first awareness of chest discomfort to the arrival in the hospital for care. The day of the week seems to play a role as well. Persons are more likely to arrive at the hospital sooner if the pain episode occurs during the week rather than on the weekend. Similarly, if the pain occurs at work, persons are more likely to seek care rapidly. It seems as if persons value their weekends and time at home and do not want to use this time in seeking medical help.

The presence of a spouse is another important determinant. When chest discomfort occurs in the presence of a spouse, the person is much more likely to get to medical help sooner. It seems much easier for persons to delay getting help if they are alone at the time the symptoms first occur.

In general, these variables—background, individual psychology or personality, and social variables—help determine the amount of time that a person takes from the time of first perception of chest discomfort to the time he or she decides to seek medical care. The seven most important variables all fall within these three categories:

1. Presence of the symptoms themselves
2. Recognition of the symptoms
3. Amount of social or physical disability
4. Perceived seriousness
5. Extent of cultural "stoicism"
6. Amount of relevant information or medical knowledge
7. Availability of sources of help.

These variables all contribute to the patient's decision time before going to the hospital. The most important of these variables are psychosocial in nature and account for a great deal of the ultimate variation in survival. For example, the mortality of "early" arrivals is about 10% as compared with the mortality of late arrivals, about 27% (DiMatteo and Friedman, 1982).

Demographic, Cultural, and Sociopsychological Variables Related to Utilization

The same type of variables that are related to the decision time to seek medical attention for chest pain symptoms are related to healthcare utilization, in general. Some term the behavior associated with defining symptoms and taking action "illness behavior."

Age and Gender. The findings for age and gender are fairly consistent. Utilization of health services is greatest among the elderly and the very young. Some of the more socially isolated elderly may seek medical care as a means of social contact and look forward to visiting their doctors for that purpose.

As noted, women utilize health services more than men. On average, they report more symptoms, make more physician visits, have more prescription drug use, and have higher rates of hospitalization, even with correction for maternity or reproductive health problems (Cockerham, 1992a).

In part, the greater utilization of services by women is associated with higher rates of morbidity. Evidence supports several additional explanations for greater use of health services by women. Women may be more sensitive to bodily discomforts as a result of childhood socialization when they were encouraged to express their discomfort and seek help. Boys, on the other hand, are discouraged from expressing pain or discomfort and are more likely to be rewarded for stoic behavior. Women are more apt to label their symptoms as physical illnesses and assess injuries as more serious and requiring care. As principal caregivers for their children and elderly parents, women become more knowledgeable about health and illness and are more accustomed to consulting physicians because they care for others. More flexible schedules, at least for women who are not employed outside the household, may allow greater use of health services. Women also are more likely than men to have regular doctors, another factor associated with greater use of physicians (Verbrugge, 1985).

Ethnicity and Social Class. Utilization of health services is influenced by ethnicity and social class background. Most of the differences in ethnicity are accounted for by social class, minority groups being disproportionately from lower social class backgrounds.

The availability of Medicare to persons 65 years of age and older and of Medicaid to some persons with low incomes has increased the capacity of people to contact physicians. By the mid-1980s, persons with low incomes had as many contacts with physicians per year as those with high incomes. This pattern does not indicate equity in access to care, because with higher morbidity, low-income persons actually needed to see physicians even more. Among those in need of care, low-income persons still received medical attention less often than higher-income persons (Dutton, 1986).

Access to care has actually deteriorated further throughout the 1980s, particularly among those with low incomes (Freeman et al, 1987). Currently, an estimated 32 to 37 million Americans lack any form of health insurance and rely primarily on overburdened public facilities, when available, for their care. Even in countries with national systems providing universal access to health services, persons from lower social class backgrounds have lower utilization rates (Cockerham, 1992a). Those from deprived backgrounds use fewer health services because they are less likely to recognize symptoms as requiring medical attention, lack transportation or the capacity to leave jobs to seek medical attention, find the facilities they attend to be rather unpleasant, and because they are more alienated from service delivery systems and bureaucracies (Dutton, 1978).

Ethnicity accounts for differences in utilization because varying cultural beliefs account for how diseases are understood, how symptoms are defined, and how sources of care are perceived. Chapter 4 describes some of these variations in more detail.

Some groups, such as rural Mexican-Americans in the Southwest, are suspicious of modern medical care and avoid seeking care until symptoms become very severe. Because their theories of disease etiology do not fit the conventional biomedical model, Mexican-Americans are likely to seek care from more familiar traditional healers such as a *curandero* (Cockerham, 1992a). Scott (1978) has described the diversity of services used in the Miami, Florida, area by Bahamian, Cuban, Haitian, Puerto Rican, and southern U.S. black populations. She finds, consistent with most studies, that the majority of these populations utilize a dual system of healing, patronizing a variety of lay and spiritual healers along with modern medical practitioners. Often, the modern Western practitioner is sought to treat the symptoms, whereas the traditional healer is expected to address the "real" causes of the illness—why the patient was somehow "selected" for disease, disability, or harm. Thus, some patients entering the office of a physician will already be under the care and treatment of a traditional healer.

Folk beliefs about the causes and treatments of illness are pervasive. Gillick (1985) points out that the way many educated, middle-class Americans think about the causes and cures of illness is alien to that of physicians. She describes a variety of "common sense" models about the educated populations' understanding of body functions and their beliefs about vitamin deficiency, disease resistance, stress, and causes of infectious diseases—most of them rather inaccurate. Each belief has led to popular treatments or preventive activities that are not helpful from a biomedical perspective.

A survey (Eisenberg et al, 1993) revealed that 34% of all Americans used "unconventional" therapies in the past year, and annual visits to practitioners providing unconventional therapies exceeded the number of annual visits to primary care physicians. Most persons (83%) using unconventional therapies also sought treatment from medical doctors, but three fourths of them did not disclose the use of unconventional therapies to their doctors. Persons using unconventional therapies represented the full range of social class and ethnicity, but the usage was more prevalent among better educated, wealthier Americans. Gillick (1985) echoes others carrying out cross-cultural research on health, in advising physicians to elicit their patients' theories and understanding of disease in order to be more effective in giving advice and fostering adherence to recommended therapies.

Social Networks. When people experience symptoms, they generally first describe their feelings to family, friends, and others before seeking care. Thus, patients act on symptoms with the reactions, advice, and guidance of laypersons in a social network. By the time patients enter a physician's care, they have proceeded through a "lay referral system" that has helped to define the appropriate response (Friedson, 1960).

If the social network is tightly integrated, as in a stable, multigenerational, culturally homogeneous community, the attitudes and beliefs of the social network will be very influential. If patients are suspicious of Western healers, as are some rural Mexican-Americans in the Southwest, they will not seek care from the Western healer, except as a last resort. If the tightly knit community is very accepting of modern medical care, such as Mormons in Salt Lake City, Utah (Geertsen et al, 1975), patients will readily seek care.

Social–Psychological Factors in Utilization. As discussed above in relation to decision time, individual psychological factors play an important role in healthcare utilization. Unconscious denial of the significance of physical symptoms can delay lifesaving medical intervention until it is too late.

In addition to the importance of mechanisms of psychological defense, individual health beliefs will influence the eventual utilization of medical resources. For individuals to seek care, they must first decide that the symptoms represent an "illness." This decision usually depends on the amount of pain or discomfort they are experiencing and the amount of impairment in role functioning caused by the symptoms. Other symptoms or changes in the biological state of the organism might also be seen as important, depending on the knowledge of the person and the implications of these changes for future activities.

In addition to defining the symptoms as indicative of illness, the person must also believe that there is something that can be done for the symptoms by a physician. Even then, the individual may not visit the physician if a visit is seen as too expensive, too painful or unpleasant, or too inconvenient.

Thus, decisions about medical utilization are made within the context of ethnic, social network, and social class matrices and modified by social–psychological factors that weigh benefits and costs of treatment against an individual's personal beliefs about health (Cockerham, 1992a; DiMatteo and Friedman, 1982).

These same sociocultural variables apply to a patient's ability to accept or reject or adapt to the "sick role" (described below), and they also have a great deal to do with the patient's ability or desire to adhere to the treatment rec-ommendations made by the physician. The issue of adherence to medical reg-imens is central to the overall outcome of medical care because most patients cannot be expected to recover from or avoid future disease complications unless they follow the physician's recommendations. Unfortunately, rates of nonadherence are extremely high: Hundreds of studies support the finding that about 50% of physicians' recommendations are *not* followed by their patients. This nonadherence cannot be explained by low education, low social class, or low intelligence. Ethnic, social network, social class, and health beliefs all seem more important (Meichenbaum and Turk, 1987).

In addition, other psychosocial factors are critical, in particular, the nature of the relationship between the doctor and the patient and the educa-tional skills of the physician (Meichenbaum and Turk, 1987). Here is yet another area where the communication skills of the physician are crucial to determining the illness outcome of the patient (Cohen-Cole and Bird, 1986b).

The Sick Role
Illness has a well-defined role in our society. Being sick is associated with a relatively clear set of obligations and responsibilities that were first described by the sociologist Talcott Parsons (1951). In Western societies, our social norms or expectations award the sick with two "rights" in exchange for two obligations.

The first right is that sick persons are exempted from normal social activ-ities. For example, people are not expected to work at their jobs, or work as effectively, and may be excused from meeting deadlines. The second right is that they are not blamed for their conditions; the sick are not held responsible for having an illness. In exchange, patients are expected to define their condi-tions as undesirable and not resign themselves to the illness. The second related expectation is that patients will cooperate with physicians in attempt-ing to get well.

Drawing on the "sick role" perspective generates some insights into the social nature of health and illness. For example, some conditions in our society are not fully accorded the status of sickness. Alcohol- and drug-dependent per-sons are sometimes not viewed as sick, perhaps because they are seen as resigning themselves to a condition rather than cooperating in order to get well, and hence are held responsible for their condition (Chalfant and Kurtz, 1971). Similarly, persons with AIDS may be viewed as responsible for their conditions and may be thought by some to deserve punishment rather than treatment.

A corresponding dynamic is the push by some groups to have their behaviors viewed or understood as medical conditions. Some (Barsky, 1988; Conrad and Schneider, 1980) describe the "medicalization" of various behav-iors or conditions in Western societies. For example, organized groups have been promoting the labeling of compulsive gamblers, alcoholics, and hyperactive children as "sick" rather than "bad," since the behaviors are attributed to an underlying illness rather than to willful behaviors.

Patients who do not cooperate with their treatment or who do not respond as expected to medical treatment may be viewed negatively by the medical profession. Labels such as "crock," "troll," and "gomer" are used to characterize these patients who do not fit into the sick role model (Leiderman and Grisso, 1985). Once patients are labeled in this manner, physicians often feel less obligated to follow through on the rest of their own responsibilities and obligations for taking care of the patients (Cohen-Cole and Freidman, 1983).

Although the sick role concept may offer some insights into understanding how society responds to those with illnesses, it does not offer a good description of many health problems. The norms absolving persons of responsibility for their illnesses may be less apparent as we learn more about the causes of chronic conditions. As people recognize that diet, exercise, smoking, alcohol consumption, and other factors are associated with the onset of chronic conditions, there may be a shift to seeing the ill as responsible and, perhaps, punitive actions will be taken— e.g., proposals to increase insurance premiums for smokers or to add taxes on alcohol and cigarettes, with the money to be used for medical services. Negative feelings of the general public or health workers toward persons with AIDS may in part reflect blaming sick individuals for the behavior that led to the health condition. The shift suggests a move away from the sick role toward "blaming the victim" on the part of some.

The expectation of the sick role that patients are not to be resigned to a condition and are to collaborate actively with a physician in treatment may be inappropriate for some disorders. It applies less well to chronic conditions such as hypertension or diabetes or to chronic degenerative or terminal conditions. In addition, it overlooks those actively engaged in self-care and those seeking care from a variety of nonphysician healers, or the culturally diverse ways people understand and react to their symptoms.

THE BIOPSYCHOSOCIAL MODEL FOR PSYCHIATRIC PATIENTS

This chapter has reviewed the many ways in which physicians must see patients with physical illnesses in a biopsychosocial context in order to understand their needs and to care for them adequately. Conversely, the same biopsychosocial perspective needs to be followed for patients with primary psychiatric disorders and *no other clear physical illnesses.* It is becoming clear that many, and perhaps most, major psychiatric disorders are characterized by genetic vulnerability and biological dysfunction (see Chapters 12 and 13). In others, the biological dysfunction can be linked to early environmental deprivations or stresses (see Chapter 11). Finally, biological treatments have been shown to be remarkably effective for treating many psychiatric disorders and for returning disabled patients to active functioning.

Although biological psychiatry has made great strides in the last few decades, it is crucial to note that psychological and social variables also are critical in the etiology and treatment of psychiatric disorders, even disorders with primarily biological underpinnings. Social variables can predict the course and outcome of many disorders, and psychosocial interventions can have profound effects on the outcome of psychiatric disorders.

Thus, *it should be clear that psychiatric disorders are not qualitatively different from any other medical illness.* They are, in fact, *medical illnesses* just like any other illness. The historic disjunction between the mind and the body is no longer true for modern medicine. Biological, psychological, and social variables are crucial for determining the etiology, onset, course, and outcome of all illness. This is just as true for illnesses with primarily physical symptoms, as well as for illnesses with primarily mental or behavioral symptoms.

SUMMARY

This chapter has presented and described the biopsychosocial model of illness, along with clinical and research findings that support its applicability to patients with physical as well as psychiatric symptoms. Physicians need to learn to integrate a wide variety of psychological and social data into their work with patients to provide adequate and comprehensive care. In fact, when medical care has been expanded to include this biopsychosocial perspective, patient outcome, as well as patient and physician satisfaction, has been shown to improve.

The remainder of this textbook provides a broad template for physicians to practice more integrated clinical medicine, according to these now well-documented biological, psychological, and social principles.

ANNOTATED BIBLIOGRAPHY

Balint M: The Doctor, His Patient and the Illness. New York, International University Press, 1957

> A classic text that discusses the role of the primary care physician in the management of psychological problems of general medical patients.

Cassel J: Psychosocial processes and "stress": Theoretical formulation. Int J Health Serv 4:471–481, 1974

> This paper represents an elegant integration of research findings related to stress and makes a very sophisticated theoretic argument about the illness process as it relates to stressful situations.

Cohen-Cole SA: The Medical Interview: The Three-Function Approach. St. Louis, CV Mosby, 1991

> This text provides a basic overview of the medical interview, appropriate for medical students and primary care physicians.

DiMatteo RM, Friedman HS: Social Psychology and Medicine. Cambridge, MA., Oelgeschlager, Gunn, and Hain, 1982

>   This excellent text covers a wide range of issues related to social and psychological issues in general medical practice.

Stoudemire A, Fogel B (eds): Psychiatric Care of the Medical Patient. New York, Oxford University Press, 1993

>   This text represents the "state of the art" of psychiatric issues in medical disorders. Sophisticated and up to date.

Usdin G, Lewis JM (eds): Psychiatry in General Medical Practice. New York, McGraw-Hill, 1979

>   This excellent source book for primary care physicians contains numerous articles on many illnesses. Good discussions of doctor–patient relationship issues throughout. It is a little dated on psychopharmacology, however.

Weiner, H: Psychobiology and Human Disease. New York, Elsevier, 1977

>   This book documents in exhaustive detail the research findings that demonstrate psychological and social contributions to the predisposition, onset, course, and outcome of seven physical illnesses. Weiner also synthesizes psychobiological understanding of these etiological relationships. Slightly dated but still relevant and consistent with more recent studies and reviews.

REFERENCES

Ader R (ed): Psychoneuroimmunology. New York, Academic Press, 1981

Aneshensel CS, Rutter CM, Lachenbruch PA: Social structure, stress, and mental health: Competing conceptual and analytical models. Am Sociological Rev 56:166–178, 1991

Ballenger JC: Unrecognized prevalence of panic disorder in primary care, internal medicine and cardiology. Am J Cardiology 60:39J–49J, 1987

Barsky AJ: The paradox of health. N Engl J Med 318:414– 418, 1988

Beckman HB, Frankel RM: The effect of physician behavior on the collection of data. Ann Intern Med 101:692–696, 1984

Ben-Sira Z: The function of the professional's affective behavior in client satisfaction: A revised approach to social interaction theory. J Health Soc Behav 17:3–11, 1976

Berkman LF, Syme SL: Social networks, host resistance, and mortality: A nine year follow-up of Alameda County residents. Am J Epidemiol 109:186–204, 1979

Bird CE, Fremont AM: Gender, time use, and health. J Health Soc Behav 32:114–129, 1991

Bird S, Cohen-Cole SA: The 'three function model' of the medical interview: An educational device. In Hale M (ed): Models of Teaching Consultation-Liaison Psychiatry. Basel, Switzerland, Karger, 1990

Borus JF, Howes MJ, Devins NP et al: Primary health care providers' recognition and diagnosis of mental disorders in their patients. Gen Hosp Psychiatry 10:317–321, 1988

Boyd JH, Weissman MM: Epidemiology of major affective disorders. In Michels R, Cavenar JO, Cooper AM, et al (eds): Psychiatry, revised edition, Vol. 3. Philadelphia, JB Lippincott, 1988

Brody DS, Miller SM, Lerman CR et al: The relationship between patients' satisfaction with their physicians and perceptions about interventions they desired and received. Med Care 27:1027–1035, 1989

Brown GW, Harris T: Social Origins of Depression: A Study of Psychiatric Disorders in Women. New York, The Free Press, 1978

Bruhn JG, Wolf S: The Roseto Story: An Anatomy of Health. Norman, OK, University of Oklahoma Press, 1979

Bunker JP, Gomby DS, Kehrer BH (eds): Pathways to Health: The Role of Social Factors. Menlo Park, CA, Henry J. Kaiser Foundation, 1989

Burke KC, Burke JD, Regier DA, Rae DS: Age at onset of selected mental disorders in five community populations. Arch Gen Psychiatry 47:511–518, 1990

Burke KC, Burke JD, Rae DS, Regier DA: Comparing age at onset of major depression and other psychiatric disorders by birth cohorts in five U.S. community populations. Arch Gen Psychiatry 48:789–795, 1991

Cassel J: Psychosocial processes, and "stress": Theoretical formulation. Int J Health Serv 4:471–481, 1974

Cassem N: Depression secondary to physical illness. In Frances AJ, Hales RE (eds): Review of Psychiatry., Vol. 7. Washington, APA Press, 1988

Chalfant HP, Kurtz R: Alcoholics and the sick role: Assessments by social workers. J Health Soc Behav 12:66–72, 1971

Cleary PD, Mechanic D, Greenley JR: Sex differences in medical care utilization: An empirical investigation. J Health Soc Behav 23:106–119, 1982

Cockerham WC: Medical Sociology, 5th ed. Englewood Cliffs, NJ, Prentice-Hall, 1992a

Cockerham WC: Sociology of Mental Disorder, 3rd ed. Englewood Cliffs, NJ, Prentice-Hall, 1992b

Cohen F: Stress and bodily illness. Psychiatr Clin North Am 4:269–286, 1981

Cohen S, Tyrrell DAJ, Smith AP: Psychological stress and susceptibility to the common cold. N Engl J Med 325:606–611, 1991

Cohen-Cole SA: The Medical Interview: The Three-Function Approach. St. Louis, CV Mosby, 1991

Cohen-Cole SA: On teaching the new (and old) psychobiology. In Friedman C, Purcell EF (eds): The New Biology and Medical Education. New York, Josiah Macy Foundation, 1983

Cohen-Cole SA, Bird J: Interviewing the cardiac patient. II. A practical guide for helping patients cope with their emotions. Quality of Life and Cardiovascular Care 3:53–65, 1986a

Cohen-Cole SA, Bird J: Interviewing the cardiac patient. III. A practical guide to educate patients and to promote cooperation with treatment. Quality of Life and Cardiovascular Care 3:101–112, 1986b

Cohen-Cole SA, Bird J, Freeman A et al: An oral examination of the psychiatric knowledge of medical housestaff: Assessment of needs and evaluation baseline. Gen Hosp Psychiatry 4:103–111, 1982

Cohen-Cole SA, Friedman CP: The language problem: Integration of psychosocial variables into routine medical care. Psychosomatics 24:54–57, 1983

Cohen-Cole SA, Pincus HA, Stoudemire A et al: Recent research developments in consultation-liaison psychiatry. Gen Hosp Psychiatry 8:316–329, 1986

Cohen-Cole SA, Stoudemire A: Major depression and physical illness: Special considerations in diagnosis and biological treatment. Psychiatr Clin North Am 10:1–17, 1987

Cole SA, Sararay SM, Hall R et al: Academy of Psychiatric Medicine Pamphlet Mental Disorders in General Medical Practice, Adding Value to Healthcare through Consultation Liaison Psychiatry. Dubuque, IO. Kendall/Hunt, 1996

Conrad P, Schneider JW: Deviance and Medicalization: From Badness to Sickness. St. Louis, Mosby, 1980

de Araujo G, Dudley DL, Van Asdel PP Jr: Psychosocial assets and severity of chronic asthma. J Allergy Clin Immunol 50:257–261, 1972

Dembroski TM, MacDougall JM, Cosa TT, Grandits GA: Components of hostility as predictors of sudden death and myocardial infarction in the multiple risk factor intervention trial. Psychosomatic Med 51:514–522, 1989

DiMatteo RM, Friedman HS: Social Psychology and Medicine. Cambridge, MA, Oelgeschlager, Gunn, and Hain, 1982

Dimsdale J, Ruberman W, Carleton R et al: Sudden cardiac death: Stress and cardiac arrhythmias. Circulation 76 (Suppl 1): 1198–1201, 1987

Dimsdale, JE: Research links between psychiatry and cardiology: Hypertension, Type A behavior, sudden death, and the physiology of emotional arousal. Gen Hosp Psychiatry 10:328–338, 1988

Dohrenwend BP, Levav I, Shrout PE et al: Socioeconomic status and psychiatric disorders: The causation-selection issue. Science 255:946–952, 1992

Dorian B, Garfinkel PE: Stress, immunity, and illness: A review. Psychol Med 17:393–407, 1987

Dutton DB: Explaining the low use of health services by the poor: Costs, attitudes, or delivery systems? Am Sociological Rev 43:348–368, 1978

Dutton DB: Social class, health, and illness. In Aiken LH, Mechanic D (eds): Applications of Social Science to Clinical Medicine and Health Policy. New Brunswick, NJ, Rutgers University Press, 1986, pp. 31–62

Dutton DB, Levine S: Overview, critique, and reformulation. In Bunker JP, Gomby DS, Kehrer BH (eds): Pathways to Health: The Role of Social Factors. Menlo Park, CA, Henry J Kaiser Foundation, 1989, pp 29–69

Edgerton RB: Conceptions of psychosis in four East African societies. In Landy D (ed): Culture, Disease and Healing: Studies in Medical Anthropology. New York, Macmillan, 1977, pp 358–367

Egolf B, Lasker J, Wolf S et al: The Roseto effect: A 50-year comparison of mortality rates. Am J Public Health 82:1089–1092, 1992

Eisenberg DM, Kessler RC, Foster C et al: Unconventional medicine in the United States. N Engl J Med 328:246–252, 1993

Eisenberg L: Treating depression and anxiety in primary care. N Engl J Med 326:1080–1084, 1992

Engel G: The need for a new medical model: A challenge for biomedicine. Science 196:129–136, 1977

Estes CL, Lee PR: Health problems and policy issues of old age. In Aiken LH, Mechanic D (eds): Applications of Social Science to Clinical Medicine and Health Policy. New Brunswick, NJ, Rutgers University Press, 1986, pp 335–355

Fawzi FI, Fawzi NW, Hyun CS et al: Malignant melanoma: Effects of an early structured psychiatric intervention, coping and affective state on reoccurrence and survival six years later. Arch Gen Psychiatry 50:681–689, 1993

Frasure-Smith N, Lesperance F, Talajic M: Depression following myocardial infarction: Impact on 6-months survival. JAMA 270 (15):1819–1825, 1993

Freeman HE, Blendon RJ, Aiken LH et al: Americans report on their access to care. Health Affairs 6:6–18, 1987

Friedman M: Pathogenesis of Coronary Artery Disease. New York, McGraw-Hill, 1969

Friedman M, Thoresen CE, Gill JJ et al: Alteration of Type A behavior and reduction in cardiac recurrences in post-myocardial infarction patients. Am Heart J 108:237–248, 1984

Freidson E: Client control and medical practice. Am J Sociology 65:374–382, 1960

Geertsen R, Klauber MR, Rindflesh M et al: A re-examination of Suchman's views on social factors in health care utilization. J Health Soc Behav 16:226–237, 1975

Gillick MR: Common-sense models of health and disease. N Engl J Med 313:700–703, 1985

Goldberg RJ, Novack DH, Fulton JP et al: A survey of psychiatry and behavioral science curriculum in primary care residency training. J Psychiatric Education 9:3–11, 1985

Gove WR, Tudor JF: Adult sex roles and mental illness. Am J Sociology 78:812–835, 1973

Greenberg TE, Stiglin LE, Finkelstein SN et al: Depression: A neglected major illness. J Clin Psychiatry 54(11):491–424, 1993a

Greenberg TE, Stiglin LE, Finkelstein SN, et al: The economic burden of depression in 1990. J Clin Psychiatry 54(11):405–418, 1993b

Greenley JR, Mechanic D, Cleary PD: Seeking help for psychological problems: A replication and extension. Med Care 25:1113–1128, 1987

Hall RCW, Stickney SK, Gardner ER: Behavioral toxicity of nonpsychiatric drugs. In Hall R (ed): Psychiatric Presentation of Medical Illness: Somatopsychic Disorders. New York, SP Medical and Scientific Books, 1980, pp 337–353

Hankin JR, Kessler LG, Goldberg ID et al: A longitudinal study of offset in the use of nonpsychiatric services following specialized mental health care. Med Care 21:1099–1110, 1983

Helman CG: Culture, Health, and Illness. London, Wright, 1990

Holder HD, Blose JO: The reduction of health care costs associated with alcoholism treatment: A 14-year longitudinal study. J Studies Alco 53:292–302, 1992

Holmes H, Rahe RH: The social readjustment rating scale. J Psychosom Res 11:213–218, 1967

Houpt JL, Orleans CS, George LK et al: The role of psychiatric and behavioral factors in the practice of medicine. Am J Psychiatry 137:37–47, 1980

House JS, Landis KR, Umberson D: Social relationships and health. Science 241:540–545, 1988

Johnson J, Weissman M, Klerman GL: Service utilization and social morbidity associated with depressive symptoms in the community. JAMA 267:1478–1483, 1992

Kamerow DB, Pincus HA, Macdonald DI: Alcohol abuse, other drug abuse, and mental disorders in medical practice. JAMA 255:2054–2057, 1986

Katon W, Gonzales J: A review of randomized trials of psychiatric consultation-liaison studies in primary care. Psychosomatics 35:268–278, 1994

Katon W, Roy-Byrne PP: Panic disorder in the medically ill. J Clin Psychiatry 50(8):299–302, 1989

Katon W, Schulberg H: Epidemiology of depression in primary care. Gen Hosp Psychiatry 14:237–247, 1992

Katon W, VonKorff M, Lin E et al: Distressed high utilizers of medical care: DSM-III-R diagnoses and treatment needs. Gen Hosp Psychiatry 12:355–362, 1990

Kawachi I, Sparrow D, Vokonas PS et al: Symptoms of anxiety and risk of coronary disease: The normative aging study. Circulation 90:2225–2229, 1994

Kessler LG, Cleary PD, Burke JD Jr: Psychiatric disorders in primary care: Results of a follow-up study. Arch Gen Psychiatry 42:583–587, 1985

Kessler RC: Sociology and psychiatry. In Kaplan HI, Sadock BJ (eds): Comprehensive Textbook of Psychiatry, Vol. 1, 5th ed. Baltimore, Williams & Wilkins, 1989, pp 299–301

Kessler RC, Cleary PD: Social class and psychological distress. Am Sociological Rev 45:463–478, 1980

Kessler RC, McLeod JD: Sex differences in vulnerability to undesirable life events. Am Sociological Rev 49:620–631, 1984

Kleinman A: Patients and Healers in the Context of Culture. Berkeley, CA, University of California Press, 1980

Kleinman A: Rethinking Psychiatry: From Cultural Category to Personal Experience. New York, The Free Press, 1988

Kleinman A, Eisenberg L, Good B: Culture, illness, and care. Ann Intern Med 88:251–258, 1978

Kleinman A, Kleinman J: Culture and care. In Kleinman A, Good B (eds): Culture and Depression. Berkeley, CA, University of California Press, 1985, pp 429–490

Klerman G: Age and clinical depression: Today's youth in the twenty-first century. J Gerontol 31:318–323, 1976

Kohn ML: Class, family, and schizophrenia: A formulation. Soc Forces 50:295–304, 1972

Langner T, Michael S: Life Stress and Mental Health: The Midtown Manhattan Study. London, The Free Press of Glencoe, 1963

Lau BWK, Kung NYT, Chung JTC: How depressive illness presents in Hong Kong. Practitioner 227:112–114, 1983

Leiderman DB, Grisso J: The gomer phenomenon. J Health Soc Behav 26:222–232, 1985

Link BG, Dohrenwend BP: The epidemiology of mental disorders. In Freeman HE, Levine S (eds): Handbook of Medical Sociology, 3rd ed. Englewood Cliffs, NJ, Prentice-Hall, 1989, pp 102–127

Lipkin M, Putnam S, Lazare A (eds): The Medical Interview. New York, Springer-Verlag, 1995

MacKinnon RA, Michels R: The Psychiatric Interview in Clinical Practice. Philadelphia, WB Saunders, 1971

Maguire GP, Rutter DR: Training medical students to communicate. In Bennett AE (ed): Communication Between Doctors and Patients. London, Oxford University Press, 1976

Marmot MG, Shipley MJ, Rose G: Inequalities in death: Specific explanations of a general pattern. Lancet 83:1003–1006, 1984

McCord C, Freeman HP: Excess mortality in Harlem. N Engl J Med 322:173–177, 1990

Mechanic D: Mental Health and Social Policy, 3rd ed. Englewood Cliffs, NJ, Prentice Hall, 1989

Meichenbaum D, Turk DC: Facilitating Treatment Adherence: A Practitioner's Guidebook. New York, Plenum Press, 1987

Middleton W, Raphael B: Bereavement: State of the art and state of the science. Psychiatr Clin North Am 10:329–345, 1987

Mirowsky J, Ross CE: Mexican culture and its emotional contradictions. J Health Soc Behav 25:2–13, 1984

Morris PLP, Robinson RG, Andrzejewski P et al: Association of depression with ten-year post-stroke mortality. Am J Psychiatry 150:124–129, 1993

Mumford E, Schlesinger H, Glass G: The effects of psychological intervention on recovery from surgery and heart attacks: An analysis of the literature. Am J Public Health 72:141–151, 1982

Mumford E, Schlesinger HJ, Glass GV et al: New look at evidence about reduced cost of medical utilization following mental health treatment. Am J Psychiatry 141:1145–1158, 1984

Murphy GE: Suicide and attempted suicide. In Michels R, Cavenar JO, Cooper AM et al (eds): Psychiatry, revised edition–1988, Vol. 1. Philadelphia, JB Lippincott, 1988

Murphy JM: Cross-cultural psychiatry. In Michels R, Cavenar JO, Cooper AM et al (eds): Psychiatry, revised edition–1988, Vol. 3. Philadelphia, JB Lippincott, 1988

Murphy JM, Helzer JE: Epidemiology of schizophrenia in adulthood. In Michels R, Cavenar JO, Cooper AM et al (eds): Psychiatry, revised edition–1988, Vol. 3. Philadelphia, JB Lippincott, 1988

Nuckolls CB, Cassel J, Kaplan BH: Psychosocial assets, life crises and the prognosis of pregnancy. Am J Epidemiol 95:431–441, 1972

O'Shanick GJ, Gardner DF, Kornstein SG: Endocrine disorders. In Stoudemire A, Fogel BS (eds): Principles of Medical Psychiatry. Orlando, Grune & Stratton, 1987

Otten MW, Teutsch SM, Williamson DF, Marks JS: The effect of known risk factors on the excess mortality of black adults in the United States. JAMA 268:845–850, 1990

Parsons T: The Social System. New York, The Free Press, 1951

Polednak AP: Racial and Ethnic Differences in Disease. New York, Oxford University Press, 1989

Pratt AL, Ford BE, Crum RM et al: Depression, psychotropic medication and risk of myocrdial infarction. Prospective data from the Baltimore ECA follow-up. Circulation 94:3123–3129, 1996

Ragland D, Brand R: Type A behavior and coronary heart disease case-fatality. N Engl J Med 318:65–69, 1988

Regier DA, Boyd SH, Burke JD Jr et al: One month prevalence of mental disorders in the United States. Arch Gen Psychiatry 45:977–986, 1988

Regier DA, Narrow WE, Rae DS et al: The de facto US mental and addictive disorders service system: Epidemiologic Catchment Area prospective one-year prevalence rates of disorders and services. Arch Gen Psychiatry 50:85–94, 1993

Reid I: Social Class Differences in Britain, 3rd ed. Glasgow, UK, Fontana Press, 1989

Robins LN, Locke BZ, Regier DA: An overview of psychiatric disorders in America. In Robins LN, Regier DA (eds): Psychiatric Disorders in America: The Epidemiologic Catchment. Area Study. New York, The Free Press, 1991, pp 328–366

Robins LN, Regier DA (eds): Psychiatric Disorders in America: The Epidemiologic Catchment Area Study. New York, The Free Press, 1991

Rosenman R, Brand R, Jenkins C et al: Coronary heart disease in the Western Collaborative Group Study: Final followup experience of 8 and a half years. JAMA 233:872–877, 1975

Ross CE, Mirowsky J, Ulbrich P: Distress and the traditional female role: A comparison of Mexicans and Anglos. Am J Sociology 89:670–682, 1983

Rozanski A, Bairey N, Krantz D et al: Mental stress and the induction of silent myocardial ischemia in patients with coronary artery disease. N Engl J Med 318:1005–1012, 1988

Rubel A: The epidemiology of folk illness: Susto in Hispanic America. In Landy D (ed): Culture, Disease and Healing: Studies in Medical Anthropology. New York, Macmillan, 1977, pp 119–128

Ruberman W, Weinblatt E, Goldberg J et al: Psychosocial influences on mortality after myocardial infarction. N Engl J Med 311:552–559, 1984

Sachar EJ: Advances in Psychoneuroendocrinology. Psychiatr Clin North Am. Philadelphia, WB Saunders, 1980

Saravay SM: Psychiatric interventions in the medically ill: Outcome and effectiveness research. Psychiatr Clin North Am 19:1–14, 1996

Saravay SM, Lavin M: Psychiatric comorbidity and length of stay in the general hospital: A critical review of outcome studies. Psychosom 35:233–252, 1994.

Saravay SM, Pollack S, Steinberg MD et al: Four-year follow up of the influence of psychological comorbidity on medical rehospitalization. Am J Psychiatry 153:397–403, 1996

Sartorius N, Ustun TB, Costa e Silva JA et al: An international study of psychological problems in primary care: Preliminary report from the WHO collaborative project on psychological problems in general health care. Arch Gen Psychiatry 50:819–824, 1993

Scott CS: Health and healing practices among five ethnic groups in Miami, Florida. In Bauwens EE (ed): The Anthropology of Health. St. Louis, Mosby, 1978, pp 61–70

Selye H: The Stress of Life, rev ed. New York, McGraw-Hill, 1976

Shulman RA, Kramer PD, Mitchel JB: The hidden mental health network: Treatment of mental illness by nonpsychiatric physicians. Arch Gen Psychiatry 42:89–94, 1985

Simon GE, Ormel J, VonKorff M et al: Health care costs associated with depressive and anxiety disorders in primary care. Am J Psychiatry 152:353–357, 1995a

Simon GE, Von Korff M, Barlow W: Health care costs of primary care patients with recognized depression. Arch Gen Psychiatry 52:850–856, 1995b

Skinner JE: Brain involvement in cardiovascular disorders. In Elbert T, Langosch W, Steptoe A, Vaitl D (eds): Behavioural Medicine in Cardiovascular Disorders. New York, John Wiley & Sons, Ltd., 1988

Smith GR Jr: The course of somatization and its effects on utilization of health care resources. Psychosomatics 35:263–267, 1994

Sosa R, Kennell J, Klaus M et al: The effect of a supportive companion on perinatal problems, length of labor, and mother-infant interaction. N Engl J Med 303:597–600, 1980

Spiegel D, Kraemer HC, Bloom JR et al: Effect of psychosocial treatment on survival of patients with metastatic breast cancer. Lancet 2:888–891, 1989

Spitzer RL, Williams JBW, Kroenke K et al: Utility of a new procedure for diagnosing mental disorders in primary care: The PRIME-MD 1000 study. JAMA 272:1749–1756, 1994

Stamler J: Coronary heart disease: Doing the "right things." N Engl J Med 312:1053–1055, 1985

Stoudemire A: Somatothymia: Parts I and II. Psychosomatics 32:365–381, 1991

Strain JJ, Hammer JS, Fulop G: APM Task Force on psychological intervention in the general hospital inpatient setting: A reveiw of cost-offset studies. Psychosomatics 35:253–262, 1994.

Strain J, Pincus HA, Houpt JL et al: Models of mental health training for primary care physicians. Psychosom Med 47:95–110, 1985

Substance Abuse and Mental Health Services Administration (SAMHSA): Cost of Addictive and Mental Disorders and Effectiveness of Treatment. Rockville, MD, U.S. Dept of Health and Human Services, 1995

Susser MW, Watson W, Hopper K: Sociology in Medicine, 3rd ed. New York, Oxford University Press, 1985

Thoits PA: Gender and marital status differences in control and distress: Common stress versus unique stress explanations. J Health Soc Behav 28:7–22, 1987

Thomas ME, Hughes M: The continuing significance of race: A study of race, class, and quality of life in America, 1972–1985. Am Sociological Rev 51:830–841, 1986

Umberson D: Family status and health behaviors: Social control as a dimension of social integration. J Health Soc Behav 28:306–319, 1987

Verbrugge LM: Gender and health: An update on hypotheses and evidence. J Health Soc Behav 26:156–182, 1985

Von Korff M, Shapiro S, Burke JD et al: Anxiety and depression in a primary care clinic. Arch Gen Psychiatry 44:152–156, 1987

Warheit GJ, Holzer CE, Avery SA: Race and mental illness: An epidemiologic update. J Health Soc Behav 16:243–256, 1975

Weiner H: Psychobiology and Human Disease. New York, Elsevier North-Holland, 1977

Weiner H, Hofer MA, Stunkard AJ (eds): Brain, Behavior, and Bodily Disease. New York, Raven Press, 1981

Weissman MM, Myers JK, Thompson WD: Depression and its treatment in a US urban community 1975–1976. Arch Gen Psychiatry 38:417–421, 1981

Wells KB: Depression in general medical settings: Implications of three health policy studies for consultation-liaison psychiatry. Psychosomatics 35:279–296, 1994

Wells KB, Golding JM, Burnam M: Psychiatric disorder in a sample of the general population with and without chronic medical conditions. Am J Psychiatry 145:976–981, 1988

Wells KB, Stewart A, Hays R et al: The functioning and well-being of depessed patients: Results from the medical outcomes study. J Am Med Assoc 262(7):914–919, 1989

Williams R, Haney T, Lee K et al: Type A behavior, hostility, and coronary atherosclerosis. Psychosom Med 42:539–549, 1980

3 Psychological Factors Affecting Medical Conditions and Stress Responses

Edward A. Walker
and Wayne J. Katon

In keeping with this book's emphasis on the biopsychosocial model, we now consider in somewhat more detail how psychological variables may interact with social factors and biological systems in the pathogenesis of disease and illness. In that regard, the concept of "stress"—whether it is considered in relation to biological, psychological, or social systems—is critical. Although the concept of stress is difficult to define, it is an ubiquitous, if not unavoidable, component of life. Although most people have an intuitive belief that "too much of it" makes them ill, only in the last two decades have methodologically sophisticated studies firmly established a link between stress and medical illness. This research has elucidated several important concepts:

1. Stressful life events are correlated with increased risk of becoming medically ill.
2. Some stressors can be perceived *positively* and others *negatively,* and this perception is mediated by cognitive "coping" mechanisms.
3. Maladaptive ways of coping with stress, such as smoking, heavy drinking, and substance abuse, may alter susceptibility to illness.
4. A strong network of social support seems to buffer patients against the effects of stress.
5. The central nervous, endocrine, and immune systems appear to have numerous interconnections.

6. An individual's response to physical and psychological illness depends on both genetic and acquired (developmental and learning) factors.

The *Diagnostic and Statistical Manual of Mental Disorders* (DSM-IV) (American Psychiatric Association, 1994) provides the category of "Psychological Factors Affecting Medical Condition" under which to include psychological processes influencing the initiation or exacerbation of physical disease (Table 3–1). The category can be used to describe conditions that in the past have been deemed to have a "psychosomatic" or "psychophysiological" component, and may include tension headache, diabetes, angina pectoris,

---

Table 3–1 **Diagnostic Criteria for 316: Psychological Factors Affecting Medical Condition (PFAMC)***

A. The presence of a general medical condition (coded on Axis III)
B. Psychological factors adversely affect the general medical condition in one of the following ways:
    (1) The factors have influenced the course of the medical condition as shown by a close temporal association between the psychological factors and the development or exacerbation of, or delayed recovery from, the general medical condition.
    (2) The factors interfere with the treatment of the general medical condition.
    (3) The factors constitute additional health risks for the individual.
    (4) Stress-related physiological responses precipitate or exacerbate symptoms of the general medical condition.

Choose name based on the nature of the psychological factors (if more than one factor is present, indicate the most prominent):
    Mental Disorder Affecting Medical Condition (e.g., an Axis I disorder such as Major Depressive Disorder delaying recovery from a myocardial infarction)
    Psychological Symptoms Affecting Medical Condition (e.g., depressive symptoms delaying recovery from surgery; anxiety exacerbating asthma)
    Personality Traits or Coping Style Affecting Medical Condition (e.g., pathological denial of the need for surgery in a patient with cancer; hostile, pressured behavior contributing to cardiovascular disease)
    Maladaptive Health Behaviors Affecting Medical Condition (e.g., non-compliance with medication or diet; overeating; lack of exercise; unsafe sex)
    Stress-related Physiological Response Affecting Medical Condition (e.g., stress-related exacerbations of chest pain, hypertension, arrhythmia, or tension headache)
    Other or Unspecified Psychological Factors Affecting Medical Condition (e.g., interpersonal, cultural, religious)

* Adapted from DSM-IV (American Psychiatric Association, 1994) obesity, gastric ulcer, rheumatoid arthritis, asthma, ulcerative colitis, and many others. In each case, environmental factors must be temporally related to the onset or worsening of the disease.

This chapter will examine the evidence concerning the role of psychological and psychosocial variables in altering individual susceptibility to disease processes. Although biological and genetic factors play a primary role in disease onset, the development of disease is a multifactorial process involving a complex interplay between the environment and humans as psychobiological organisms. We will review the historical development of the mind–body relationship, the evidence linking stress to disease modulation, and the physiological connections between mind and body, namely the autonomic nervous system, the neuroendocrine system, and the immune system.

A CASE STUDY

Mr. R. is a 30-year-old man who presented to his physician with a 2-month history of abdominal bloating and epigastric pain. Over the preceding 14 days, he had noticed increasing fatigue, passed several black, tarry stools, and had been having trouble running his business as a fence builder because of a lack of energy. He had a family history of peptic ulcer disease. On physical examination, he was found to be quite pale and had epigastric pain to palpation and tachycardia. Laboratory examination revealed guaiac-positive stool and a low hematocrit. The patient was admitted to the hospital, where a duodenal ulcer was diagnosed. He made a rapid recovery with medical therapy despite his refusal of blood transfusion because of religious beliefs.

Many stressful events were noted in the months before admission. The patient had undergone a traumatic divorce, and he and his wife shared joint custody of their two children. Despite the divorce, however, the patient employed his wife in his business. In addition, he discovered 1 year before admission that his wife had embezzled $12,000 from his business and that he was already several thousand dollars in debt to the Internal Revenue Service.

The patient was raised in a family with little emotional support and a distant, critical father. He worked very hard to win his father's affection, but was constantly frustrated. His style of coping with stress, based on this family experience, was to trust few people, to work hard, and to rely only on himself and perhaps his wife. He perceived his wife's embezzlement as a disaster both financially and emotionally and felt he no longer could trust anyone. He fired his staff and increased his own workload to 12 to 14 hours a day, 7 days a week, to handle the threat and anxiety of potential bankruptcy. Thus, he coped by withdrawing from people, relying even less on others, working harder, and trying to deny his pain and anger toward his wife. He began to feel progressively worn out approximately 6 months before admission and admitted to having depressed mood, anxiety, insomnia, decreased energy, and, at times, feelings of hopelessness. Clinical depression developed as his coping mechanisms were overwhelmed. Nevertheless, the patient continued to work hard and, approximately 2 months before admission, began to experience abdominal pain. He admitted, however, to distrusting doctors ("they're only out to rob you") and therefore waited until he could "barely drag" himself to work to come into the clinic, again using coping mechanisms of denial and minimization toward his physical condition.

Because illness onset is multifactorial in origin (see Fig. 3–1), treatment must be targeted specifically at biological, psychological, and social problems. For instance, the family physician treated this patient's peptic ulcer medically. When attempts at counseling him regarding his depression, anxiety, and rigid personality traits were not successful, the patient eventually accepted his doctor's recommendation to get psychiatric help. In psychotherapy, the patient gained insight into his behavior and used his illness experience as a chance for growth. He began to take more recreational time off from work, ultimately hired help for his business, and was able to get a bank loan to stabilize his business. At

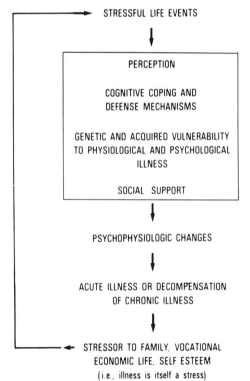

Figure 3–1. Model of illness onset.

follow-up 6 months later he had no symptoms and felt he was coping with interpersonal and family problems better than he had before his illness.

THE HISTORICAL DEVELOPMENT
OF THE MIND–BODY RELATIONSHIP

Our current concepts of mind and body are the products of a long evolutionary process that naturally followed the sociocultural, scientific, and philosophical trends of each historical period. Our early ancestors confronted many of the same diseases we know of today, without the aid of the scientific method or the knowledge of anatomy, physiology, and behavior that we take for granted in modern medicine. Theological explanations were frequently invoked, such as possession by evil spirits, and rituals were used to rid the body of evil influences. The powerful attraction of these early beliefs as explanatory models is apparent in their continued appeal to many people in an otherwise scientific twentieth-century society.

The ancient Greek physicians developed the beginnings of a rational approach to our understanding of disease and how it affects mind and body. Although they discriminated between *soma* (body) and *psyche* (soul), this distinction was often blurred. Hippocrates believed that many diseases and mental states were caused by emotions, or passions as they were known, and theorized a mind–body physiology based on combinations of four basic humors (yellow bile, black bile, phlegm, and blood) with the four basic elements (air, earth, fire, and water). Various combinations of these building blocks produced different diseases and mental states. The physical manifestations of such mental states as fear and anger were hard to ignore, and when strong emotions precipitated symptoms such as chest pain or death, it provided "evidence" for the physical potency of the passions.

A major conceptual change occurred in the seventeenth century. Causality, observation, and measurement were given new emphasis as the desire to understand the structure of the universe and its component parts increased. Against the background of this new scientific method, René Descartes advanced his philosophy of distinguishing the thinking mind (*res cogitans*) from the physical body (*res extensa*), a division that fundamentally influenced the way physicians thought about the mind and body. Descartes' theory, misinterpreted for centuries as a rigid dualism, formed the basis for contemporary misunderstandings about the nature of mind and body. The heritage of this conceptual confusion is seen in the thinking of many modern physicians who seek to divide "organic" from "psychological" disease and who speak of "psychiatric overlays" on physical conditions, as if, by removing the "overlay," the patient would return to a state of pure organic disease.

Current theories of mind–body interaction were most markedly influenced in the late nineteenth century by Sigmund Freud and his contemporaries.

Freud, originally a neurologist seeking to find a scientifically unified theory of biology and behavior, became interested in patients with somatic symptoms in whom no physical pathology could be found. These patients, known as "hysterics," were problematic to his physician colleagues, who tried various remedies without results. His followers began to postulate the existence of specific personality types and, later, unconscious psychodynamic conflicts and attitudes as the causes of specific physiological conditions.

The belief that stress and psychological conflict could not only *influence* but actually *produce* specific physical diseases became a focus of many of these physicians. Several, most notably Franz Alexander, formulated theories involving particular diseases that would result from specific psychological conflicts and defenses, the so-called "specificity theory" of psychosomatic disorders. Thus, the chronic suppression of emotional tension would lead to discharge in autonomic nervous system pathways and cause structural change in specific tissues and organs. The so-called organic neuroses (essential hypertension, bronchial asthma, neurodermatitis, ulcerative colitis, peptic ulcer, rheumatoid arthritis, and thyrotoxicosis) became the classic paradigms of psychosomatic illness of this new school, with the idea that each was caused by a specific type of neurosis.

Experimental evidence has never supported this degree of specificity, and the theory is no longer widely held. On the other hand, while psychiatric disorders and stress do not appear to cause diseases directly, these conditions can seriously alter the patient's perception of, and adaptation to, chronic disease. In addition, treatment of a comorbid psychiatric disorder may be an important step in assisting the patient to adjust to the aversive symptoms of chronic medical illness. For example, patients with ulcerative colitis (a disease caused by stress, according to the specificity theory) who also have a major depression have significantly more functional impairment than patients without depression who have a comparable degree of gastrointestinal disorder (Walker et al, 1996).

One of the important enduring contributions of this specificity theory, however, is the finding that the Type A behavior pattern—characterized by a sense of urgency, striving for achievement, and hostility—is a risk factor for coronary artery disease. Recent critiques of this behavior pattern have found that not all its personality characteristics are equally associated with this increased risk, but that *hostility, cynicism,* and *antagonistic relationships* appear to be most strongly correlated with vulnerability to coronary artery disease (Goldstein and Niaura, 1992; Koskenvuo et al, 1988; Niaura and Goldstein, 1992).

The early promise of psychiatric research in providing specific connections between mind and body gradually fell into disrepute as the fragile underpinnings from research by and large did not stand the test of time. There were many exceptions, such as Pavlov's studies on conditioned reflexes, Cannon's work on the fight-or-flight response, Wolff's studies of gastric acid secretion, and Selye's work on stress and cortisol. With the tremendous technological thrust of modern medicine, however, much of this psychosomatic framework fell into disregard. Medicine was taught as the study of physiological "organic" illness and psychiatry as the study of psychological illness. A patient's illness was worked up biomedically, and when a physical cause was not found, the patient could then be referred to a psychiatrist.

This dualistic view of mind and body was built on a model of the physical universe that used the linear cause-and-effect rules of classical mechanics. During the mid-twentieth century, a new model of causality was developed in the ideas of von Bertilanffy and Bateson, who saw the universe from a systems perspective: Systems have self-regulating, homeostatic properties that create a circular cause–effect. All living things depend on this type of *homeostatic equilibrium,* nesting systems within systems to maintain life.

Noting this complexity of living things, George Engel (1977), an internist with training in psychoanalysis, proposed the *biopsychosocial model* as a paradigm for explaining the multiple ways in which an organism's physical health could be modified not only by physical pathogens but also by learning, cultural norms, and mental processes. Similar to earlier psychobiological theories of psychiatrist Adolf Meyer, Engel's model viewed disease not simply as a reductionistic chain of physical events, but more as a complex summation of organic, psychological, and social variables, each capable of exerting profound effects on the outcome of disease. Although patients might intuitively grasp the connections between mind, body, and stress, many contemporary physicians continue to maintain an archaic, reductionistic philosophy that sacrifices common sense for the sake of "scientific" biomedical method.

The lesson from history is that the challenge to contemporary medical students will be mastering the technical biomedical aspects of medical treatment without sacrificing the psychological, social, and environmental factors that are an important part of holistic patient care. Acquiring all of this information may seem to be an enormous burden early in medical school, as a tremendous weight is put on memorization of large amounts of factual information; however, practicing physicians draw heavily on their knowledge of behavior, stress, and mind–body interactions to devise practical, effective treatment plans that help their patients cope with medical illness. (The biopsychosocial model is also discussed in Chapter 1 by Dr. Shelton, in Chapter 2 by Drs. Cole, Saravay, and Levinson, and in Chapter 14 by Dr. Green.)

WHAT IS STRESS AND HOW DOES IT INFLUENCE DISEASE?

The concept of "stress" was originally imported to medicine from physics by Hans Selye to describe the actions of forces against an object in equilibrium. With reference to behavior, it has been used to refer to (1) an aversive stimulus event, (2) a specific physiological or psychological response, or (3) a special type of transaction between the person and the environment (Cohen, 1981). Confusion is avoided if each of these is considered separately. We will distinguish *stressors* (or stressful life events) from the *psychological state of stress* (feelings of threat, harm, or loss) and from *stress responses* (on physiological, psychological, or social levels).

Stressors are defined as those life events that induce *change in routine*, the *persistence of positive or negative environmental conditions*, or specific types of *situations of monotony* where no change has occurred when change might have been expected (i.e., not getting an anticipated promotion at work).

Although there has been a growing awareness of the ability of stress to influence morbidity and mortality since the mid-nineteenth century, it was not until the 1950s that well-designed studies investigated this relationship. In a pioneering prospective study of patients with pulmonary tuberculosis, Holmes (1961) found that the predictors of recovery were psychosocial assets such as strong family ties, steady employment, adequate income and job satisfaction, regular recreation, frequent social participation, flexibility and reliability, and realistic goals. He soon moved from the study of predictors of recovery to predictors of the onset of illness.

As previously mentioned in Chapter 2, on the basis of this experience, Holmes and Rahe (1967) developed the Schedule of Recent Life Events (SRE) to allow quantitative definition of life crises. The SRE (Table 3–2) is a checklist of 43 events requiring various degrees of adaptation (e.g., losses, childbirth, catastrophe, and success). Each life change is assigned a particular number of life-change units (LCUs) (the death of a spouse, for example, is rated at 100 LCUs), and within a particular period the individual accumulates an LCU score. Holmes and Rahe found a nearly linear relationship between LCU scores and the number of illnesses experienced, with the highest correlation in the 6 months following these life events. Thus, the more LCUs were accumulated, the more likely were illnesses of all kinds in a subsequent 2-year period.

In later retrospective studies, Holmes and Rahe found that illness developed within 2 years in 30% to 35% of subjects with low life-change scores (in the range of 100), 50% of those with intermediate scores (200 LCUs), and 80% of those with high scores (300 LCUs). In prospective studies, a very similar picture emerged; sickness developed in about 80% of the people in the high-risk group, about 50% of the medium-risk group, and about 30% of the low-risk group. Since then, several studies have validated this relationship between life changes and the onset of a number of psychiatric, medical, and surgical diseases.

Across all cultures, the death of a spouse is consistently rated as the most significant life change correlated with increased morbidity and mortality. Numerous studies have shown that during the first 6 months after bereavement, there is a significant increase in death and illness among the surviving spouses,

Table 3–2 **The Social Readjustment Rating Scale**

LIFE EVENT	MEAN VALUE
Death of a spouse	100
Divorce	73
Marital separation	65
Jail term	63
Death of a close family member	63
Personal injury or illness	53
Marriage	50
Fired at work	47
Marital reconciliation	45
Retirement	45
Change in health of family member	44
Pregnancy	40
Sex difficulties	39
Gain of new family member	39
Business readjustment	39
Change in financial state	38
Death of a close friend	37
Change to different line of work	36
Change in number of arguments with spouse	35
Foreclosure of mortgage or loan	30
Change in responsibilities at work	29
Son or daughter leaving home	29
Trouble with in-laws	29
Outstanding personal achievement	28
Spouse began or stopped work	26
Begin or end school	26
Change in living conditions	25
Revision of personal habits	24
Trouble with boss	23
Change in work hours or conditions	20
Change in residence	20
Change in schools	20
Change in recreation	19
Change in church activities	19
Change in social activities	18
Change in sleeping habits	16
Change in number of family get-togethers	15
Change in eating habits	15
Vacation	13
Christmas	12
Minor violations of the law	11

especially widowers, as compared with the expected rates for age (Raphael and Middleton, 1987). Emerging evidence that this phenomenon involves a process of alteration of immune system function is addressed later in the chapter.

Although most investigators now agree that there is a statistical correlation between life-change scores and the development of illness, the correlations are relatively low, i.e., life-change units are probably only one of the variables involved. Although most researchers agree that stress-induced illness may be caused by chronic physiological arousal, the final response to stress may be mediated by several factors that can either buffer or intensify the stressor. These are the person's (1) perception or *cognitive appraisal* of the events, (2) *coping* or defense mechanisms, (3) *social support* systems, and (4) degree of *genetic vulnerability.* We shall look at each of these factors in more detail.

Cognitive Appraisal of Life-Change Events

Events that are stressful for one person may not be for another. Thus, if a person has adequate resources to meet a challenge or does not believe that danger exists, a stress reaction may not occur. Lazarus (1977) has pointed out that a stimulus can evoke a stress reaction by psychophysiological means only if it is interpreted by the individual as *harmful or threatening* so that coping processes are brought into play to minimize potential harm. The LCU theory of Holmes and Rahe made no attempt to separate negative from positive life events, yet there is evidence they may have different physiological consequences. For example, although levels of cortisol, catecholamines, and growth hormone rise after negative life events, only catecholamines show a rise after events of a pleasurable nature (Rose, 1980). Furthermore, undesirable life events are stronger predictors of disease outcomes (Vinokur and Selzer, 1975). Rahe, recognizing the impact of perception of life change, has modified the SRE so that in recent prospective studies subjects now not only list their life changes but score their own LCUs subjectively according to the degree of life adjustment needed to handle the event.

Hinkle and Wolff (1958) also found that episodes of illness are not randomly distributed among the population. They found in several large populations that 25% of the people had 50% of the episodes of illness over a 20-year period. These illnesses often appeared in a cluster during life, and the clusters of illness episodes were most apt to occur when the individuals perceived that they were having difficulty adapting to the environment.

Coping and Defense Mechanisms

Coping is defined by the dictionary as "struggling" or "contending." It describes behavior involving special physical and emotional energy and attention that is required to deal with some difficult circumstances. Lazarus (1977) defined two types of coping or self-regulation of a perceived stress. One that he calls "direct action" occurs when the person tries to alter or master the troubled interaction with the environment, as when one attempts to demolish, avoid, or flee the harmful agent or to prepare somehow to meet the danger. Thus, if a student faced with an important and potentially threatening examination spends the anticipatory interval immersed in preparation, he or she is engaged in a direct-action form of coping. This sense of mastery and readiness, regardless of whether or not it is realistic, mitigates the stress reaction before the time when the threat must be faced.

A second coping mechanism, called palliation, occurs when direct action is too costly to undertake or when the person is unable to manage the environmental challenge successfully. Such modes of control include ego defenses (i.e., denial, rationalization); taking tranquilizers, alcohol, or sleeping pills; or engaging in a variety of techniques such as muscle relaxation, jogging, or yoga. These palliative forms of coping are focused on possible ways of reducing the affective, visceral, or motor disturbances that are distressing the person, as opposed to attempts to master the environmental challenge on which the stress reaction depends. This decrease in distressing symptoms may enable individuals to think more clearly and problem-solve or even confront situations they would normally avoid.

Numerous studies have shown that the way an individual copes may reduce physiological arousal in the face of stressful events. For example, patients with myocardial infarction who adopt the use of an appropriate amount of denial and minimization as major ways of coping with their anxiety about death and disability have fewer potentially fatal arrhythmias (Freeman and Folks, 1987). It is also known that patients whose coping ability has become overwhelmed are prone to the development of mental illnesses such as depression, anxiety attacks, or psychosis and subsequently have two to four times the prevalence of medical illness (Hankin and Oktary, 1979). Patients who inherit or acquire (through traumatic early childhood experience) susceptibility to mental illness under stress also are more likely to develop medical illness.

Social Support

Recent research evidence suggests that those who have social supports are protected in crisis from a variety of pathological states (Bebbington, 1987). It is thought that supports buffer the individual from the potentially negative effects of crisis and can facilitate coping and adaptation. Patients with social supports and assets may live longer and have a lower incidence of somatic illness, as well as more positive mental health. Studies of marital and health status consistently reveal that those who are married have lower mortality rates than those who are single, widowed, or divorced (Ortmeyer, 1974). These risks are consistently higher for men than women and seem to decline with age (see also Chapter 2).

In a prospective study of 10,000 adult men, Medalie and Goldbourt (1976) found seven risk factors (anxiety, severe family problems, age, total serum cholesterol, systolic or diastolic blood pressure, certain electrocardiographic abnormalities, and diabetes mellitus) associated with the development of new angina pectoris. They found that the husband's subjective perception of a high degree of love and support from his wife reduced the risk of angina pectoris even in the presence of high-risk factors. Similarly, in a large prospective study of men after myocardial infarction, Ruberman et al (1984) found that socially isolated men with high life stress had four times the risk of death from cardiac causes as their low-stress, nonisolated counterparts. Thus, life stress, loss of control, and job strain can combine with decreased social support to increase the risk for morbidity and mortality due to coronary artery disease (Goldstein and Niaura, 1992; Niaura and Goldstein, 1992).

Lack of family support also has been shown to influence the incidence of streptococcal pharyngeal infections. Meyer and Haggerty (1962) prospectively studied 76 families for a 1-year period by means of systematic throat cultures for hemolytic streptococci. Acute or chronic family stressors appeared to influence not only whether an individual became ill after colonization, but also the degree of postinfection immune titers.

Brown and Harris (1978) studied the incidence of major depressive disorder in 458 women who had been exposed to stressful life events. Women with high degrees of stress and little support had four times the rate of depression than women with equal degrees of stress but much support. The researchers concluded that a confiding, intimate relationship with a spouse buffered the person from the effects of high levels of stress.

Finally, the long-term influence of childhood developmental stressors has been shown to be important in modifying the pathogenesis of disease. In Chapter 11, on the psychology and psychobiology of developmental trauma, Dr. van der Kolk outlines a model of how early abuse (presence of a negative factor) and neglect (absence of a positive factor) can cause lasting changes in homeostasis and physiological reactivity to disease. Thus, particular traumatic events during critical periods of central nervous system development can lead to an irreversible failure to achieve developmental milestones because central nervous system plasticity is reduced. Although we are just beginning to understand the specific neurological deficits, they appear to be present both on anatomical and neurochemical levels, suggesting that social support has a direct effect on the expression of biological structure.

Biological Predisposition to Stress-Induced Illness

Another component in the multifactorial causation of onset of illness is the patient's health and organ susceptibility to illness. We have already referred to biological and learned predispositions to mental illness. Many patients also have diseases such as angina pectoris, duodenal ulcers, and juvenile-onset diabetes mellitus. Stress may play a contributing role in causation, especially in the first two illnesses, but there is no doubt that once the disease is present, symptoms of these disorders can be exacerbated by stress. That is, once end-organ damage has occurred, the patient is more likely to respond to stressful events with an exacerbation of symptoms of chronic illness, despite a prior history of adequate coping with an identical stressor. On the other hand, some patients exhibit a biological hardiness, sometimes called *resilience,* that appears to protect them from stress-induced physical pathology.

Acute stressors appear to be greater risk factors for sudden cardiac death for individuals who already have some form of cardiac disorder, usually ischemic heart disease (Lown et al, 1980). Similarly, acutely stressful life events may not necessarily predispose individuals to schizophrenia; however, they are associated with exacerbation or precipitation of an episode of the illness in some vulnerable individuals (Bebbington, 1987).

PSYCHOPHYSIOLOGICAL PATHWAYS

Evidence has been presented that stressful life events are important factors in the onset of illness, but what are the pathways and mechanisms that mediate the body's reaction to stress? Recently, many of the pathways of this stress response have been illuminated. The hypothalamus appears to act as a central mediator for the coordinated regulation of the autonomic nervous, immune, and neuroendocrine systems (see Fig. 3–2). This phylogenetically ancient part of the brain integrates cortical (cognitive), limbic (emotional), and autonomic (visceral) inputs and controls many of the neural and endocrine systems required for both homeostasis and rapid adaptation. The affected tissues and organs complete the cycle by feeding back to the higher initiating and regulating centers. The hypothalamus, therefore, appears to be the locus where psychological stress may be converted into physiological function. Neuroendocrine mechanisms regulating mood and behavior are discussed in detail in Chapter 12 by Dr. Pedersen and colleagues; this chapter focuses on stress-related factors involved in neuroendocrine and immune systems.

The hypothalamus contains the nuclei of the autonomic nervous system, which are grouped into two divisions—the sympathetic and parasympathetic—that innervate the viscera and many hormone-secreting cells. For example, the pancreatic insulin cells are contacted directly both by sympathetic and parasympathetic nerves that respectively suppress and stimulate insulin secretion (Sterling and Eyer, 1981).

The brain also influences the body's hormones by means of its own chemical messengers. Some act directly on peripheral tissues; others act on peripheral hormone-secreting cells. Still others act on the pituitary, which controls both peripheral tissues and endocrine organs. The balance of corticotropin-releasing hormone (CRF) in the hypothalamus and norepinephrine in the brain stem locus ceruleus modulates both the tone of the autonomic nervous system as well as the production of adrenocorticotropic hormone (ACTH), which consequently regulates serum levels of cortisol, a principal hormone in the stress

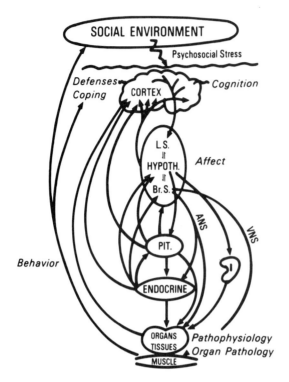

L.S.=Limbic System
Br.S.=Brain Stem
HYPOTH.=Hypothalamus
PIT.=Pituitary
ANS=Autonomic Nervous System
VNS=Voluntary Nervous System
I=Immune System

Figure 3–2. Psychophysiological pathways of the stress
response. (Reproduced with
permission from Reiser MF:
The psychophysiology of
stress and coping. In
Psychophysiology–Report
Number 1. Philadelphia,
SmithKline, 1980)

response. Both the cellular and humoral arms of the immune system also appear to be under the control of the brain through these hormones.

What is the reason for having these central controls since there are local self- regulating controls of physiological homeostasis (such as blood pressure and the serum glucose level)? Neural controls permit hormonal and organ changes to occur in anticipation of changes in local feedback systems; such anticipatory changes then can reduce the size and length of metabolic fluctuations. In addition, most processes in the body cannot be kept constant and must vary according to the demands of the environment on the organism. Blood pressure must be able to vary with changes in demand (e.g., sudden fright, sexual intercourse, or taking a test). If the only controls over blood pressure were local, then it would be impossible to have such adaptive changes in blood pressure because every deviation from the "normal" would be corrected automatically (Sterling and Eyer, 1981).

BROAD PATTERNS
OF NEUROENDOCRINE
AND NEUROIMMUNE RESPONSE

Probably as a result of the experience of our primitive ancestors, we have evolved a complex but efficient energy management system that reacts flexibly to changes in our environment. Our nervous, endocrine, and immune systems have two basic states of readiness—one vegetative and reparative, the other highly responsive to impending or actual danger. The evolutionary value of both of these states is obvious in a hostile, unpredictable environment, but our primordial physiology, designed for coping with episodic, intense stress, may be ill-equipped to deal with modern life with its chronic, variable-level stressors.

These hormonal, autonomic, and immune system changes are under central nervous system control through an elaborate network of cell groups found in and around the hypothalamus that have the role of maintaining a flexible homeostasis. Kiely (1974) has labeled these reciprocally balanced components the *ergotropic* and *trophotropic* systems.

The Ergotropic System

The *ergotropic system* integrates functions that prepare the individual for positive action. It is characterized by alerting, arousal, excitement, increased skeletal muscle tone, and sympathetic nervous system activity and the release of catabolic hormone products. It is similar to Cannon's description of the fight-or-flight responses but includes many changes in sympathetic nervous system discharge as well as neuroendocrine and behavioral parameters (see Table 3–3).

This system must mobilize energy quickly to deal with unexpected environmental demands. Complex molecules are broken down into component parts such as free fatty acids and glucose that can be rapidly converted into energy. Reproductive and reparative processes are slowed. The thymus shrinks, and the levels of antibodies and white cells in the blood fall. Increased cardiac output and blood pressure speed extra blood to the tissues. Flow to the heart, muscle, and brain must be maintained or increased, but flow to the gut, kidney, and skin is decreased because the blood is needed elsewhere (Sterling and Eyer, 1981).

In the early part of the century, Cannon noted that during arousal, as in preparation for fight or flight, there was not only an increase in blood pressure

Table 3–3 **Characteristics of the Ergotropic and Trophotropic Systems**

	ERGOTROPIC	TROPHOTROPIC
Predominant autonomic nervous system branch	sympathetic	parasympathetic
Blood flow	brain and muscle	gut, kidney, and skin
Skeletal muscle	increased tone	decreased tone
Immune function	decreased	increased
Reproductive function	decreased	increased
Metabolism	catabolic	anabolic

but also a change in blood flow. More blood was delivered to the heart and skeletal muscle, and less to the skin, gut, and kidneys. Later, Selye showed that cortisol also is secreted during arousal and makes an important contribution to this mobilization. The levels of several other behaviorally activating hormones also increase during arousal, with corresponding decreases in hormones whose functions include energy storage, growth, renewal, repair, and maintenance of surveillance against infectious agents and the body's own malignant cells.

The Trophotropic System

The *trophotropic system* reverses this ergotropic process and integrates systems that promote withdrawal and conservation of energy: raising the stimulus barrier to perceptual input, decreasing skeletal muscle tone, and increasing parasympathetic nervous function and the circulation of anabolic hormones. This system is turned on by relaxation or lack of perceived threat.

The anabolic hormones promote energy storage, growth, renewal, repair, and maintenance of surveillance against infectious agents and the body's own malignant cells. In the anabolic state, the body stores energy or glycogen, fat, and protein by polymerization of glucose, fatty acids, and amino acids. Bone is replaced by reabsorption and redeposition of calcium salts. Wounds are healed by production of new cells and by extracellular deposition of proteins. The immune system is maintained by continuous cell and antibody production in the bone marrow, lymphoid tissue, and thymus.

These two systems have reciprocal activity and are maintained in a flexible balance. With mild to moderate degrees of excitation of the ergotropic system, there is a corresponding degree of inhibition of the trophotropic system, and vice versa. Therefore, mild to moderate arousal turns on the catabolic hormones of the sympathetic system and inhibits parasympathetic discharge with its anabolic hormones. At moderate to high degrees of trophotropic or ergotropic activation, the facilitory effects are more sharply increased, and reciprocal inhibition of the opposite system is maximal. Thus, during moderate to high levels of arousal, the level of ergotropic tuning is very high and trophotropic responsiveness becomes nil. At this level of arousal, an ergotropic response may be elicited by a stimulus that normally would produce a trophotropic response: for example, having a difficult day at work, coming home irritable and uptight, and kicking the affectionate cat or "snapping" at the spouse or children.

Finally, at maximal degrees of arousal, both the ergotropic and trophotropic systems discharge simultaneously (Kiely, 1974). A clinical example is the state of anxiety wherein a variety of skeletal, visceral, and psychic disturbances effect simultaneous discharge of both systems. Flooding of the cerebral cortex by afferents from both systems may be experienced as dread; weak knees may coexist with tremulous hands, representing effects on skeletal muscle tone of the mixed ergotropic and trophotropic system discharge. Simultaneous activation of sympathetic and parasympathetic divisions may be expressed as sweating, tachycardia, nausea, vomiting, and bowel and bladder hyperactivity.

In summary, accompanying the shift from relaxation to arousal, there is a shift in a whole pattern of hormonal secretions, accompanied by an increase in sympathetic nervous system discharge. The endocrine pattern in arousal promotes the mobilization of energy at the expense of maintenance and repair processes. The catabolic processes are accompanied by auxiliary mobilization of the renovascular system for conservation of salts and water. All of these shifts are initiated by the brain through its control over the autonomic and endocrine systems.

For a person to remain healthy, however, these periods of arousal must be balanced by periods of relaxation in order to replenish the resources exhausted by catabolism. Without this replenishment, there would be no repair of accumulated damage, no vigilance against pathogens. In some patients, stress may become chronic as coping mechanisms are overwhelmed, and a psychiatric illness such as depression or anxiety attacks, physical illness, or both, develops.

In summary, balance between the sympathetic and parasympathetic nervous systems is essential for maintenance of homeostasis. We now focus on two areas of clinical research in which the articulation of the linkage between stress and disease is most clearly delineated, cardiovascular health and immune system function.

CARDIOVASCULAR DISEASE AND STRESS

We have previously discussed the effects of acute sympathetic nervous system activation on cardiac function, specifically increases in cardiac rate and output as well as in blood pressure. These effects are usually transitory and limited to the period during which the acute stressor is present. We are now learning that longer periods of less intense stress can have important consequences as well.

Major depression, a psychiatric disorder that is associated with prolonged periods of stress, has been linked to both increased medical disease as well as higher risk for death. Barefoot and Schroll (1996) followed a cohort of 730 Danish community residents for 25 years and noted that patients with high scores on measurements of depression had nearly twice the risk for death from heart attacks. Barefoot et al (1996) also followed a cohort of 1,250 patients with coronary artery disease for almost 20 years and found that patients with major depression had an 84% greater risk of cardiac death 5 to 10 years after their initial heart attack. Finally, Frasure-Smith et al (1993) found that patients who became depressed after a heart attack were five times more likely to die in the next year than were depression-free controls.

Pathways for these effects are slowly being uncovered. For example, depressed patients have been shown to have "sticky" platelets that are more easily activated in clotting mechanisms (Musselman et al, 1996). Also, depression is associated with increased activation of the sympathetic nervous system, which leads to elevated levels of plasma norepinephrine (Veith et al, 1994).

PSYCHONEUROIMMUNOLOGY

There is an increasing body of evidence that the central nervous system, the endocrine system, and the immune system may have multiple bidirectional interconnections that allow mutual modulation and feedback (Stein et al, 1987). Since the coining of the term "psychoneuroimmunology" by Ader in 1964, there have been numerous studies of the relationship between the immune system and stress, psychiatric illness, and environmental factors. Although these data are as yet inconclusive, strong patterns have emerged that suggest a coherent theory of interaction between the central nervous system and the immune system.

One of the most impressive examples of this linkage has been the investigations of the ability of the immune system to be *classically conditioned* (Ader and Cohen, 1975) (see Chapter 6 by Dr. Dorsett on behavioral concepts). For example, in experiments repeatedly "pairing" oral saccharin with cyclophosphamide (an immunosuppressant), significant immunosuppression could be demonstrated upon presentation of the saccharin stimulus *alone*. This is an important finding because it involves a purely behavioral stimulus engaging the immune response, with a noxious effect.

In a double-blind study (Smith and McDaniel, 1983), subjects underwent repeated skin testing with tuberculin antigen on one arm and saline on the other. After five trials the sequence of syringes were reversed, and marked diminishment or absence of reaction was noticed where the saline was expected by the subject. Upon explanation of the identity of the test substances, the previously vigorous response was obtained. Whether this was due to conditioning or cognitive set, the influence of higher cortical centers in modulation of the response is evident.

In three separate controlled studies, Kiecolt-Glaser (Kennedy et al, 1988) examined the immunological function of 75 first-year medical students during final examinations, 38 recently separated or divorced women, and 34 persons giving long-term care to relatives with Alzheimer's disease. She observed similar quantitative and qualitative changes in immune cells in these three groups undergoing acute and chronic stress, including decreases in the percentages of T helper cells, decreased numbers and function of natural killer (NK) cells, and changes in the latency of herpes virus. Psychological variables, including loneliness, attachment, and depression, were related to the decrements in immunological surveillance.

Both humoral and cell-mediated immunity seem to be modulated by stress. Stress has been reported to influence the courses of certain illnesses, such as asthma, streptococcal infection, and arthritis that involve B-cell systems, but the more robust findings involve T-cell mechanisms (Stein et al, 1987). The importance of T-cell regulation of the entire immunological response has been underscored recently by the epidemic of AIDS. Studies have shown that stressors such as death of a spouse, sleep deprivation, and inability to escape from chronic physical threat can alter T-cell regulatory patterns and response to mitogens. The protective effects of coping seem to prevent this alteration. Rats exposed to a tail-shock paradigm over which they had no control had markedly diminished T-cell mitogen response as compared with a second group of rats that were able to control the termination of the shock. This difference existed, despite the fact that all animals received the same total amount of shock (Stein et al, 1987).

Three recent studies show the important clinical implications of stress reduction on the immune system. Innoculation of 394 volunteers with cold viruses showed a direct relationship between stress level and serological evidence of infection and symptoms. This dose–response effect was present for four other experimental viruses (Cohen et al, 1991). Meijer et al (1988) showed that adolescents who had clinical influenza were more likely to have had preceding psychiatric symptoms than adolescents who did not have clinical illness but did have positive serological evidence of infection. Finally, several replicated studies of *in vivo* immunological function have shown that, as compared with patients without depression, those with major depression have both reduced numbers of natural killer cells and diminished natural killer cell capacity (Irwin et al, 1992).

The current state-of-the-art research in psychoneuroimmunology shows it to be in its scientific infancy. Many substances, such as cortisol, growth hormone, substance P, endorphins, opioids, and somatostatin, have been shown to be immunomodulators. Innervation of the thymus, spleen, and lymph nodes has suggested possible direct central nervous system effects, and the continued study of the immune-cell surface has demonstrated receptors for adrenergic and cholinergic neurotransmitters (Stein et al, 1987). Solomon (1987) has proposed more than 30 "postulates" of immune–endocrine–central nervous system interaction analogous to Koch's postulates of infectious disease; yet, despite the relatively small amount of data in this area, preliminary controlled studies are increasingly implicating stress in the modulation of the immune system. Correspondingly, behavioral strategies that decrease the influence of stressors continue to show promise in the repair and strengthening of the immune system (Kiecolt-Glaser and Glaser, 1992). Recent work in patients with cancer has even demonstrated the potential of behavioral interventions to shape the clinical course of malignancies (Anderson et al, 1994). As our understanding of this complex system increases, it can only add to the continued unraveling of the mystery of stress and disease. Chapter 11 discusses the scientific evidence that traumatic stress early in life can neurobiologically alter the individual's neuroimmune system.

TREATMENT STRATEGIES

Although a thorough discussion of treatment approaches is beyond the scope of this chapter, the application of certain general principles can be useful. The overall strategy is a careful understanding of the potency of the biopsychosocial model as both a diagnostic aid and a treatment guide. The biopsychosocial model is, in reality, an integrated alliance of three major models: biomedical, psychological, and social–behavioral. Although the treatment plan needs to reflect the physician's understanding of the mutual interdependence of these approaches for the sake of evaluation and planning, they can be usefully separated with a biomedical diagnosis, a psychological diagnosis, and a social–behavioral diagnosis, followed by a treatment plan for each.

Let us take, for example, the case of a 29-year-old woman with chronic strep throat infection and major depression. From a *biomedical* standpoint, the following observations arise:

Biomedical data:

1. Neurovegetative symptoms secondary to hypothalamic dysregulation
2. Decreased immunological surveillance
3. Poor nutritional status

Biomedical diagnoses:

1. Major depression
2. Streptococcal pharyngitis
3. Impaired nutrition

Biomedical treatment:

1. Antidepressant therapy
2. Antibiotic therapy
3. Dietary counseling

Next, the *social–behavioral* viewpoint:
Social–behavioral data:

1. Husband abuses patient physically
2. Cigarette smoking
3. Drinks too much alcohol

Social–behavioral diagnoses:

1. Physical abuse by spouse
2. Nicotine abuse
3. Alcohol abuse
4. Maladaptive coping

Social–behavioral treatment:

1. Referral to women's shelter
2. Behavior modification plan to reduce and stop smoking
3. Referral to Alcoholics Anonymous
4. Supportive counseling by physician to suggest new ways of coping

Finally, the *psychological* aspect:
Psychological data:

1. Patient repeatedly chooses to return to abusive partner
2. Adult child of alcoholic parents

Psychological diagnoses:

1. History of childhood abuse by father
2. ACOA (adult child of alcoholic) syndrome

Psychological treatment:

1. Referral for insight-oriented psychotherapy
2. Education about ACOA syndrome
3. Referral to ACOA group

By combining the distinctive viewpoints afforded by the model, an integrated treatment plan emerges that accounts for many aspects of the patient's functioning. The prescription of an antidepressant may be less effective in the face of continued physical assault, just as progress in insight-oriented psychotherapy would be hampered by the cognitive slowing typical of pharmacologically untreated major depression. Not all aspects of this plan would be immediately implemented in the first visit; however, the longitudinal perspective of primary care allows a gradual unfolding of this strategy over time, thus allowing patients to proceed at their own pace.

SUMMARY

The onset of disease appears to be multifactorial. Over the past century we have learned a great deal about the biological components of susceptibility to illness, yet it has been only in the last 20 to 30 years that we have rigorously examined the psychosocial factors. We no longer view the psychosocial problems as causative of disease, but rather as important factors in altering susceptibility to illness. The challenge to future physicians is to integrate this biopsychosocial view of patients into diagnosis and treatment in a pragmatic and compassionate manner.

ANNOTATED BIBLIOGRAPHY

Vitaliano PP, Maiuro RD, Russo J et al: A biopsychosocial model of medical student distress. J Behav Medicine 11:311–331, 1988

> An excellent overview of the stress and coping of medical students, illuminating many of the concepts in this chapter.

Engel GL: The clinical application of the biopsychosocial model. Am J Psychiatry 137:535–544, 1980

> One of the best illustrations of the biopsychosocial model comparing the management of a myocardial infarction patient using the biomedical and biopsychosocial models.

Kiecolt-Glaser JK, Glaser R: Psychoneuroimmunology: Can psychological interventions modulate immunity? J Consult Clin Psychol 60:569–575, 1992

> An excellent summary of recent research concerning behavioral modification of immune system activity.

Lipowski ZJ: Psychosomatic medicine: past and present. Can J Psychiatry 31:2–21, 1986

> A historical overview of the development of the concept of "psychosomatic," including a summary of current and future research trends.

Chrousos GP, Gold PW: The concepts of stress and stress system disorders. JAMA 267:1244–1252, 1992

> A timely scholarly review of "what's new" in the physiology of the stress response, aimed at clinicians.

Kennedy S, Kiecolt-Glaser JK, Glaser R: Immunological consequences of acute and chronic stressors: Mediating role of interpersonal relationships. Br J Med Psychol 61:77–85, 1988

> A thorough review of social support and its modulating effect on the production of medical illness.

Sternberg EM et al: The stress response and the regulation of inflammatory disease. Ann Intern Med 117:854–866, 1992

> A well-written, concise summary of recent developments with respect to behavioral influences on immune system function.

Stoudemire A, Hales RE: Psychological and behavioral factors affecting medical conditions and DSM-IV: An overview. Psychosomatics 32:5–13, 1992

> The introduction to a 12-part series of scholarly reviews used in revising the DSM-IV criteria for psychological factors affecting medical condition.

Anderson BL, Kiecolt-Glaser JK, Glaser R: A biobehavioral model of cancer stress and disease course. Am Psychologist 49:389–404, 1994

> A summary of recent thought about the relationship between stress and the development of cancer, and the implications for behavioral management of cancer patients.

McEwen BS: Protective and damaging effects of stress mediators. New Eng J Med 338:171–179, 1998

> A superb state-of-the-art review of the physiological effects of stress on humans and the basic neurobiological mechanisms involved. Documents that adverse stress can alter brain functioning and immunological competence as well as impair cardiovascular functioning.

REFERENCES

Ader R, Cohen N: Behaviorally conditioned immunosuppression. Psychosom Med 37:333, 1975

American Psychiatric Association: Diagnostic and Statistical Manual, 4th ed. Washington, DC, American Psychiatric Association, 1994

Barefoot JC, Helms MJ, Mark DB et al: Depression and long-term mortality risk in patients with coronary artery disease. Am J Cardiol 78:613–617, 1996

Barefoot JC, Schroll M: Symptoms of depression, acute myocardial infarction, and total mortality a community sample. Circulation 11:1976–1980, 1996

Bebbington PE: Psychosocial etiology of schizophrenia and affective disorders. In Michels R, Cavenar JO (eds): Psychiatry. Philadelphia, JB Lippincott, 1987

Brown GW, Harris T: Social Origins of Depression. London, Tavistock, 1978

Cohen F: Stress and bodily illness. Psychiatr Clin North Am 4:269–286, 1981

Cohen S, Tyrrell DA, Smith AP: Psychological stress and susceptibility to the common cold. N Engl J Med 325:606–612, 1991

Engel GL: The need for a new medical model: A challenge for biomedicine. Science 196:129–136, 1977

Frasure-Smith N, Lesperance F, Talajic M: Depression following myocardial infarction: Impact on 6 month survival. JAMA 15:1819–1825, 1993

Freeman AM, Folks DG: Psychiatric aspects of cardiovascular disease. In Michels R, Cavenar JO (eds): Psychiatry. Philadelphia, JB Lippincott, 1987

Goldstein MG, Niaura R: Psychological factors affecting physical condition: Cardiovascular disease literature review. Part I. Psychosomatics 33:134–145, 1992

Hankin J, Oktary JS: Mental Disorder and Primary Care: An Analytic Review of the Literature. U.S. Department of Health, Education and Welfare (HEW Publication No. (ADM) 78–661). Washington, DC, U.S. Government Printing Office, 1979

Hinkle LE, Wolff HG: Etiologic investigations of the relationships between illness, life experiences and the social environment. Ann Intern Med 49:1373–1388, 1958

Holmes T, Joff JR, Ketchan JW, Sheehy TF: Experimental study of prognosis. J Psychosomat Res 5:235–252, 1961

Holmes TH, Rahe RH: The social readjustment rating scale. J Psychosomat Res 11:213–218, 1967

Irwin M, Lacher U, Caldwell C: Depression and reduced natural killer cytotoxicity: A longitudinal study of depressed patients and control subjects. Psychol Med 22:1045–1050, 1992

Kennedy S, Kiecolt-Glaser JK, Glaser R: Immunological consequences of acute and chronic stressors: Mediating roles of interpersonal relationships. Br J Med Psychol 61:77–85, 1988

Kiecolt-Glaser JK, Glaser R: Psychoneuroimmunology: Can psychological interventions modulate immunity? J Consult Clin Psychol 60:569–575, 1992

Kiely WF: From the symbolic stimulus to the pathophysiological response: Neurophysiological mechanisms. Int J Psychiatr Med 5:517–529, 1974

Koskenvuo M, Kaprio J, Rose RJ et al: Hostility as a risk factor for mortality and ischemic heart disease in men. Psychosomat Med 50:330–334, 1988

Lazarus RS: Psychological stress and coping in adaptation and illness. In Lipowski ZJ, Lipsitt DR, Whybrow PC (eds): Psychosomatic Medicine. New York, Oxford University Press, 1977

Lown B, Desilva RA, Reich P et al: Psychophysiologic factors in sudden cardiac death. Am J Psychiatry 137:1325–1335, 1980

Medalie JH, Goldbourt U: Angina pectoris among 10,000 men. Am J Med 60:910, 1976

Meijer A, Zakay-Rones Z, Morag A: Post-influenzal psychiatric disorder in adolescents. Acta Psychiatr Scand 78:176–181, 1988

Meyer RJ, Haggerty RJ: Streptococcal infections in families: Factors affecting individual susceptibility. Pediatrics 29:539–549, 1962

Musselman DL, Tomer A, Manatunga AK: Exaggerated platelet reactivity in major depression. Am J Psychiatry 153:1313–1317, 1996

Niaura R, Goldstein MG: Psychological factors affecting physical condition: Cardiovascular disease literature review. Part II. Psychosomatics 33:146–155, 1992

Ortmeyer CF: Variations in mortality, morbidity and health care by marital status. In Erhardt CF, Berlin JE (eds): Mortality and Morbidity in the United States. Cambridge, Harvard University Press, 1974

Raphael B, Middleton W: Current state of research in the field of bereavement. Isr J Psychiatry Relat Sci 24:5–32, 1987

Rose RM: Endocrine responses to stressful psychological events. Psychiatr Clin North Am 3(2):251–276, 1980

Ruberman W, Weinblatt E, Goldberg JD et al: Psychosocial influences on mortality after myocardial infarction. N Engl J Med 311:552–559, 1984

Smith RG, McDaniel SM: Psychologically mediated effect on the delayed hypersensitivity reaction to tuberculin in humans. Psychosomat Med 45:65–70, 1983

Solomon GF: Psychoneuroimmunology: Interactions between central nervous system and immune system. J Neurosci Res 18:1–9, 1987

Stein M, Schleifer SJ, Keller SE: Brain, behavior and immune process. In Michels R, Cavenar JO (eds): Psychiatry. Philadelphia, JB Lippincott, 1987

Sterling P, Eyer J: Biological basis of stress-related mortality. Soc Sci Med 15E:3–42, 1981

Veith RC, Lewis N, Linares OA et al: Sympathetic nervous system activity in major depression. Basal and despiramine-induced alterations in plasma norepinephrine kinetics. Arch Gen Psychiatry 51:411–422, 1994

Vinokur A, Selzer ML: Desirable versus undesirable life events: Their relationship to stress and mental distress. J Perspect Soc Psychol 32:329–337, 1975

Walker EA, Gelfand MD, Gelfand AN, Creed F, Katon WJ: The relationship of current psychiatric disorder to functional disability and distress in patients with inflammatory bowel disease. General Hosp Psychiatry 18:220–229, 1996

4 Culture, Ethnicity, and the Practice of Medicine

Peter J. Brown, Jessica Gregg,
and Bruce L. Ballard

> Disease and its treatment are only in the abstract purely biologic processes. Actually such facts as whether a person gets sick at all, what kind of disease he acquires and what kind of treatment he receives largely depend upon social factors.
>
> Erwin Ackerknecht

Culture is the fundamental source of the diversity in thought and behavior among different human groups. If you were to travel around the world, you would undoubtedly be struck by the cultural diversity you found—in food, architecture, dress, religious beliefs, ideas about sex and marriage, and so on—and those differences would make the trip exciting and fun. There are similar advantages of living in a multicultural society like the United States. At the same time, however, the fact that we live in a society with marked cultural variations represents a challenge to the physician and the practice of medicine. People's ideas about the causation of their illness, the proper roles of doctors and patients, as well as rules about what to do when a person is ill also vary with culture and among subcultural groups. In the United States and Canada, much of this cultural variation is subsumed under questions of ethnicity. The purpose of this chapter is to demonstrate how culture affects illness behavior and medical care; this discussion builds on the biopsychosocial model of health introduced in the first two chapters of this book, particularly as it deals with illness behavior. We also argue here that sensitivity to cultural variation is a learnable skill that has practical benefits for effective medical care as well as for the practice of preventive medicine.

Special consideration of the impact of culture and ethnicity on behavior is warranted because of the simple, but often unrecognized, fact that the United States is one of the most culturally heterogeneous nations. The ethnic diversity of patients who may come into a major metropolitan hospital is remarkable. We are a nation of immigrants, irrespective of a national ideology (the "melting pot" myth) that minimizes the importance of ethnic and class differences. Clinical training is the first time many medical students must interact regularly with people whose backgrounds are very different from their own. In the context of healthcare, a strict application of a biomedical model of disease also minimizes the importance of social diversity because all cases (like all Americans) are expected to be alike. There is a single correct answer for the scientific questions on examinations. In the complex world of actual medical care, however, it is necessary to have effective communication and mutual trust between healers and patients, and this trust is possible only with flexibility and adaptability by practitioners.

Perceptual and behavioral differences based on ethnicity, subculture, or class are not simply "noise" that can be ignored by a physician. From an epidemiological standpoint, ethnicity and class are clearly related to lifestyle patterns such as diet, smoking, or stress, which are major causes of morbidity and mortality. As described in Chapter 2, basic elements of a patient's interaction with the medical system—for example, the interpretation of symptoms, the decision to seek care, or even the manner in which pain is experienced and reported—are things that people learn through the processes of socialization and enculturation in a society. Social science research suggests that patient *noncompliance* often arises from a conflict between the patient's view of what is going on and the physician's view. There is a danger of *ethnocentrism* when one simply "explains away" noncompliance in terms of the personality of the patient. Understanding the patient's point of view and effectively communicating with patients from different cultural backgrounds represent a central challenge to the practice of medicine today.

In this chapter, we stress the importance of two fundamental and related concepts that must be applied to the understanding of patients and their illness behaviors: culture and ethnicity. The first part of the chapter outlines some conceptual underpinnings of medical anthropology regarding the relationship of culture to health. We show that culturally prescribed behaviors shape epidemiological risk. We also argue that cultural beliefs are central to socially constructed definitions of health and disease. In other words, culture provides definitions of what is normal or healthy, as well as explanations of how and why people get sick. The second half of the chapter focuses on ethnicity, briefly describing the range of cultural beliefs about health and illness found in major ethnic groups in the United States. Sensitivity to variation in cultural beliefs can improve the serious problem of patient noncompliance. The chapter concludes with practical suggestions for improving cross-cultural communication between physicians and their patients.

THE FUNDAMENTAL CONCEPT OF CULTURE

Human societies, unlike those of other animals, are distinguished by *culture*—learned patterns of thought and behavior. The ability to adapt through the nonbiological mechanism of culture is the primary reason for the remarkable success of our species. Culture is transmitted from one generation to the next through the symbolic communication of language. It includes not only directly observable behaviors such as patterns of diet and social organization, but also more subjective ideological components of beliefs and values. As such, culture provides a context of *meaning* to individuals. Both cultural behaviors and beliefs can have important adaptive functions.

One useful model of culture, the materialist model seen in Fig. 4–1, divides culture into three mutually dependent layers. The material foundation of a cultural system is the economic mode of production, which includes the technology and the population size that the productive economy allows and requires. Contingent on the first layer is the system of social organization, which includes kinship and marriage practices, politics, and status differentiation. Contingent upon the social structure is the ideology or belief system, including ideas, beliefs, and values, both secular and sacred. Most anthropologists believe that ideology is an extremely important part of culture, in part because it rationalizes and reinforces the economy and social structure. Ideology enables people to make sense of their world and to share their common world view. A culture is an integrated system: a change in one part causes changes in the other layers. The materialist model indicates that the direction of causal change is from the bottom layer upward (the thicker arrows in Fig. 4–1). An economic change has drastic implications for population size, social organization, and associated beliefs. On the other hand, most people within a society tend to explain things from the top down (the thin arrows in Fig. 4–1), i.e., from the view of their cultural beliefs.

One important universal in human cultures is that all societies have ethnomedical systems that attempt to combat the inevitability of disease and death. All medical systems include, at a minimum, three logically coherent elements: (1) a theory of the etiology of illness, (2) techniques for the diagnosis of illness, and (3) methods for appropriate therapy. In many societies, it is difficult

Figure 4–1. *A materialist model of culture.*

to distinguish between the ethnomedical and religious systems. For a physician practicing in a multiethnic context, it is important to be aware of these preexisting medical beliefs and to avoid the fallacy of seeing patients as "empty vessels" waiting to be filled with biomedical knowledge (Polgar, 1963). Recognition that, from the patient's point of view, multiple medical systems may be operating within a single clinical encounter may be the first step in effective cross-cultural communication.

CULTURE AND HEALTH

Culture Shapes Epidemiological Risk

Disease is never randomly distributed–either within or among societies. The kinds of diseases we are exposed to (and will die from) depend on the kind of culture we live in and our particular role within society. Economic production systems can change particular ecological settings to increase or decrease the risk of contracting a particular disease. People living in small hunting and gathering bands have different health risks than do peasant farmers engaged in irrigation-agriculture or urbanites working in an industrial setting.

Brown and Inhorn (1996) have described the epidemiological distribution of a wide variety of infectious diseases from the viewpoint that disease distribution is determined largely by particular cultural behaviors. For example, the slow virus *kuru* has been found only among the Fore tribe of the highlands of Papua New Guinea. It is hypothesized that the transmission of this virus was a result of ritualized mortuary behaviors, including cannibalism of the brains of infected individuals. Less dramatic cultural behaviors have been linked to diseases such as malaria, schistosomiasis, echinococcosis, and sexually transmitted diseases. Larson (1989) demonstrated how labor migration and patrilineal kinship systems in central Africa put women at high risk for contracting AIDS. The culture of sexuality in Brazil, examined by Parker (1987), adds to the problem of sexually transmitted diseases because of the high cultural value placed on different sexual behaviors, including anal intercourse.

The most common causes of death in affluent societies such as the United States, the cardiovascular diseases, are also shaped by cultural traditions of high-fat diets, small amounts of exercise, and high-stress working conditions. Such epidemiological risks are linked not only to cultural traditions, but more important, to social class.

Culture Defines Normality, Disease, and Health

Cultural behaviors and beliefs are usually learned during childhood, and they are often deeply held and seldom questioned by adults, who pass their "obvious" knowledge and habits to their offspring. In this regard, cultural beliefs and values are largely unconscious factors in the motivation of individual behaviors. Cultural beliefs define "what is normal" and, therefore, constrain the choices of behaviors available to an individual.

Members of all societies are *ethnocentric* in that they use their own arbitrary beliefs and values to judge people from other cultures. What is considered "normal" and "abnormal," acceptable and unacceptable, disease and health varies from culture to culture and even within subcultures of society. Thus, for example, in the social context where their prevalence is endemic and high, malaria, *pinta,* and diarrhea have all been described and treated in certain cultures as "normal" (Brown and Inhorn, 1990).

Understanding a patient's cultural norms is particularly important in the context of mental illness because what is considered a mental disorder should represent a significant deviation from local standards of expected behavior (Cockerham, 1986). Hence, societies vary as to what falls out of the realm of "normal" behavior and becomes "abnormal"—the latter often being labeled as some form of psychiatric or mental illness. There is little doubt that social labels of abnormality can function as mechanisms of social control (Szaz, 1974), even as political tools to control dissidents. This idea, however, has been subject to controversy. There appear to be boundaries on the relative range within which societies define normality. Cross-cultural studies of the objective characteristics of "crazy" behavior in societies as diverse as the Eskimo and the Yoruba of Nigeria have been shown to be remarkably similar (Konner, 1989; Murphy, 1976), suggesting that some psychiatric illnesses (including schizophrenia) may be universal.

Certain cultures have special manifestations of mental illness or aberrant behavior that have been described as "culture-bound syndromes" (Favazza, 1985; Simons and Hughes, 1985), in that some mental illnesses are linked inextricably to a particular cultural context.[1]

Classic examples of these "culture-bound syndromes" (or culture-specific) include the conditions *koro, latah,* and *amok.* Initially described in Southeast Asia (but also reported in Nigeria and the United States), koro is described as the perception that the penis is shrinking and retracting into the abdomen. A man with koro fears that death will occur once the penis has sunk all the way into his abdomen. Panic accompanies the experience of koro, and epidemics of this syndrome have been reported in India, Thailand, and Singapore. Latah, found in Malaysia, involves an elaborated startle reflex during which startled individuals say obscene things or their attention can be captured so that their behavior temporarily matches that of the person who startled them. Women who are latah sometimes are startled many times a day, primarily for the entertainment of on-lookers. Amok ("running amok") is a

---

[1] There has been considerable debate concerning some of these culturally limited disorders, and it now appears that the general pattern may fit within DSM categories, although the content of symptoms must be culturally interpreted (Hahn, 1995).

syndrome first reported in Malaysia and characterized by a period of brooding followed by extreme violence and homicidal attacks, ending with exhaustion and amnesia. This pattern also has been labeled the "sudden mass assault" taxon. Episodes of behavior resembling all of these syndromes have been reported in other areas of the world, and it now appears likely that they are "culturally constructed," rather than culturally limited. Although these syndromes sound bizarre, one should note that most standards for health and illness are dependent on the observer's own frame of reference and expectations. Indeed, it was not long ago that homosexuality was officially diagnosed as a mental illness in the United States. Similarly, before the Civil War, slaves who had an "inordinate" desire to escape were diagnosed with the mental illness called "drapetomania."

Some anthropologists have argued that certain culture-specific illnesses may serve as a way for oppressed individuals to protest against cultural norms and/or values. For example, during illness attributed to spirit possession in the Zar cults in Northern Sudan, Ethiopia, Somalia, Arabia, and Southern Iran, possessing spirits housed in the bodies of female victims cause their victims to fall ill and to behave erratically, often cursing men, smoking, drinking, and demanding gifts of food and clothing from the victim's husband or father before agreeing to leave. It has been argued that illnesses contracted through Zar cults enable Islamic women to express opposition to patriarchal aspects of Islamic culture (Boddy, 1989; Lewis, 1971). In Northern Sudan, local Islamic cultural practices often include regulation of women's behavior, female seclusion, and female circumcision, and it has been noted that Zar spirit possession expanded in this area at the same time that local Islamization increased (Boddy, 1989:35). According to Boddy, Zar victims use their illnesses to vent frustrations about their lives. They also exact a penance from male family members on whom they often blame their suffering.

Interestingly, some anthropologists have argued that hysteria and anorexia nervosa have served somewhat similar purposes in the United States and Europe. In contrast to spirit possession, which allows women to protest their condition in ways otherwise forbidden to them, hysteria and anorexia nervosa channel women's protest into exaggerations of prevailing ideals of female behaviors and attitudes. Hysteria, which became epidemic among middle and upper class women in the second half of the nineteenth century, was an elaboration of the dominant culture's feminine ideals of delicacy, dependency, and languid domesticity. The middle and upper class woman, hysterical or not, was expected to remain in the home, to be somewhat sickly, to confine her interests to domestic life, and to remain generally inactive (Bordo, 1986; Ehrenreich and English, 1973). Hysterics elaborated this role, suffering nervous fits and complaining of weakness, headaches, and the inability to exert themselves. They focused the attention of the household on themselves, often reigning as a "petty tyrant" over husbands, servants, and children (Ehrenreich and English, 1973:40). Barbara Ehrenreich and Deidre English explain:

With hysteria, the cult of female invalidism was carried to its logical conclusion. Society has assigned affluent women to a life of confinement and inactivity, and medicine had justified this assignment by describing women as innately sick. In the epidemic of hysteria, women were both accepting their inherent 'sickness' and finding a way to rebel against an intolerable social role. Sickness, having become a way of life, became a way of rebellion (1973:42–43).

Similarly, many scholars argue that anorexia nervosa appears to be both an elaboration of, and a protest against, current social ideals of femininity (cf. Bordo, 1986, 1989; Brumberg, 1988; Chernin, 1981; Scheper-Hughes and Lock, 1987). Susan Bordo (1989) argues that anorexia nervosa develops in response to the conflicting messages received by contemporary women concerning their role as women. On the one hand, women are told that they can do anything and be anything, while on the other hand, they continue to learn the "feminine" virtues of nurturance of others and domesticity. Through anorexia, women see the opportunity to meet both demands through the simultaneous exercise of self-denial, self-control, and discipline. As such, women also are able to lodge silent but visible protests against demands that often seem mutually exclusive and, therefore, impossible to meet.

Culture Affects Personality Development

Anthropologists have examined the relationship between cultural practices, particularly early childhood experiences, and later adult personality. This area of inquiry, begun in the 1930s and heavily influenced by psychoanalytic theory, led to descriptions of "national character," some of which had weaknesses of stereotyping. Cross-cultural comparative studies show a covariance between a society's environmental circumstances and subsistence ecology, which, in turn, constrain the social learning contexts of childhood, adolescence, and ultimately adult personality. Such a "modal personality" ultimately is reflected in the art, rituals, and religion of the society. For example, John and Beatrice Whiting (1975) have demonstrated how "husband-wife intimacy" (including sleeping arrangements and paternal involvement with children) is correlated with the degree to which a society is involved in war or its preparations.

The essential contribution of cultural factors to child development relates to the socialization and learning environment of the child (Favazza, 1985; Konner, 1989). That environment includes techniques of discipline, stressors the child may be exposed to, initiation rituals, behavioral expectations of the child, and skills of the parents and other caretakers. Children develop into adults, having had most of their values and standards of behavior transmitted to them by the family. The behavior and personality of the individuals along with the values inculcated by the family are absorbed from the cultural milieu and, thus, at least partially, determine how the individual interacts with society.

Until recently, it was generally accepted that culturally determined child-rearing practices affect adult personality development in three ways. First, excessive childhood deprivations predispose people to adult psychopathology; second, the sharing of childcare responsibilities by the mother may be beneficial; and third, conflicts within a family concerning love and hate and dependence and independence are more important than conflicts about toilet training or sexual behavior (Favazza, 1985:250). A problem with this area of research is the absence of any cross-culturally valid definitions of the independent variables (i.e., deprivations) or the dependent variables (i.e., psychopathology). Despite the tremendous variety of child-rearing practices used throughout the world, including cultures characterized by physical abuse (Scheper-Hughes, 1987) and institutionalized homosexuality in initiation rituals (Konner, 1989), a central conclusion from cross-cultural research must be that the majority of children grow up to be relatively well-adjusted adults.

Cross-cultural research on child development has forced the reconsideration of important concepts in psychiatry and psychology, such as the universality of the childhood Oedipus complex (which, according to Malinowski [1927], does not fit the social dynamics of a matrilineal society like the Trobriands) or the universality of social stress related to sexuality in adolescence, which, according to Mead (1928), did not fit a permissive society like Samoa. In recent years, both of these classic examples have been questioned: the Oedipus case by Spiro (1982) and the Samoa case by Freeman (1983). Indeed, the entire model of early childhood influences on adult psychological features has been questioned seriously in the work of Kagan (see Konner, 1989).

There is little doubt that certain cultural and socioeconomic contexts may engender increased psychopathology as well as medical disease. Enormous stress is placed on people when social processes change rapidly or situations are created in which people have little control. For example, in a classic study, Kardiner and Ovesey (1951:308) emphasized the impact of oppression and discrimination on the personality development of African Americans. They stated:

> The result of the continuous frustrations in childhood is to create a personality devoid of confidence in human relations, of an eternal vigilance and distrust of others. This is a purely defensive maneuver which purports to protect the individual against the repeatedly traumatic effects of disappointment and frustration. He must operate on the assumption that the world is hostile.

The study was notable for its identification of the impact of social discrimination on personality development in certain individuals, yet the observations may have overemphasized psychopathological findings while not adequately recognizing the adaptive strength of African Americans to social oppression.

In a different context, in rural Western Ireland, Scheper-Hughes (1979) has described the cultural setting for the unusually high prevalence of serious mental illness, particularly schizophrenia. Economic stresses in the region are severe and have resulted in female emigration and depopulation. The traditional pattern of land inheritance is linked to markedly delayed ages of marriage for men and high rates of celibacy. The culture displays an ethos of severe sexual repression, as well as ridicule and scapegoating of children. In the historic past, the Irish tolerated eccentrics, including people who had visions, but today there is little such tolerance; the result is high rates of hospitalization. Scheper-Hughes argues that these conditions contribute to the region's high prevalence of schizophrenia, as well as the specific symbolic themes in which disturbed thought patterns are presented by Irish patients.

Culture Provides Explanatory Models of Illness

Medical anthropologists sometimes distinguish between *disease* and *illness*. Disease refers to the objective clinical signs and pathophysiological process that can result in a recognized diagnostic label from the *International Classification of Disease* (ICD) or from the *Diagnostic and Statistical Manual* (DSM). Illness refers to individuals' perceptions of being "not well" to the degree that they act upon those perceptions. Although illness refers to a subjective experience, physicians should recognize that it is no less "real" than disease. Of course there can be disease without "illness," as in hypertension, and illness without "disease," as in the common case of a patient who complains of not feeling well, but for whom no physical abnormality can be identified. Hence, the terms *disease* and *illness* are *not* synonomous.

Ethnomedical systems provide both a categorization scheme for illnesses and, more important, explanations for their cause (Fabrega, 1974). From a cross-cultural perspective, Foster (1976) distinguished between *personalistic* and *naturalistic* medical systems based on the predominant orientation of their etiological theory. This distinction is summarized in Table 4–1, although, in complex societies such as our own, elements of both types co-exist. In personalistic systems, illness is thought to be the result of supernatural forces aimed at the patient for a particular reason, either through sorcery or spirit possession or because of a breach of taboo. In these systems, diagnosis and therapy largely involve shamanistic trance and ritual, aimed at correcting and counteracting the supernatural causes of illness; therapy is thought to be effective largely because of the belief of the patient in the power of the curer. Naturalistic ethnomedical systems, which include the traditional medicine of complex civilizations (India, China, and Greece), are based on a principle of balance between elements of the body. Diagnosis based on the examination of symptoms and therapy involve the adjustment of humors to re-create the body's natural balance and health. A widely dispersed concept in naturalistic

Table 4–1 **Typology of Ethnomedical Systems**

	PERSONALISTIC	NATURALISTIC
Causation	Active agent	Equilibrium loss
Illness	Special case of misfortune	Unrelated to other misfortune
Religion/magic	Intimately tied to illness	Unrelated to illness
Prevention	Positive action	Avoidance
Responsibility	Beyond patient control	Resides in patient
Societies	'Primitive' bands/tribes	Ancient "great traditions"

(Adapted from Foster GM: Disease etiologies in non-Western medical systems. Am Anth 78:773–782, 1976)

systems is the hot/cold theory of disease (discussed below for Hispanic patients).

In the context of modern medical care, it is more important for a clinician to be able to elicit the patient's "explanatory model" of illness (Kleinman, 1988), rather than to memorize details of an ethnomedical belief system. *An explanatory model for disease is an individual's personal interpretation of disease.* As such, an explanatory model allows a person to understand the causes, consequences, and prognosis of an illness experience; an explanatory model can give meaning to life-threatening conditions. As lay explanations, explanatory models often differ from biomedical explanations for disease, and this disparity between belief systems may underlie problems with communication and noncompliance between patients and healers. When physicians recognize and acknowledge alternative explanatory models, then they have the ability to identify both areas of potential treatment noncompliance and areas where the belief systems converge and can reinforce appropriate therapy (Chrisman and Maretzki, 1982; Snow, 1993).

While lay explanatory models show significant individual variation, research indicates that ethnicity is an extremely important factor (Harwood, 1981). A patient's explanatory model can be learned through a few additional questions asked during the taking of a patient's history. Kleinman and colleagues (1978) have suggested eight questions (listed in Table 4–2) for eliciting such information. Some patients may view the physician as the ultimate expert on diagnosis and treatment and find these questions inappropriate. However, these questions are very useful for understanding why a particular patient with a particular constellation of symptoms is seeking medical care. Asking such questions during a clinical interaction can get important social and cultural concerns "on the table" for discussion. When there is not a context of mutual understanding and respect, it is more likely that a patient's psychosocial and cultural concerns will not receive attention and, as the following case history illustrates, the patient is more likely to be "noncompliant."

Table 4–2 **Questions for Eliciting a Patient's Explanatory Model of illness**

1. What do you think has caused your problem?
2. Why do you think it started when it did?
3. What do you think your sickness does to you? How does it work?
4. How bad [severe] do you think your illness is? Do you think it will last a long time, or will it be better soon, in your opinion?
5. What kind of treatment would you like to have?
6. What are the most important results you hope to get from treatment?
7. What are the chief problems your illness has caused you?
8. What do you fear most about your sickness?

(Adapted from Kleinman A, Eisenberg L, Good B: Culture, illness and care. Ann Intern Med 88:251–258, 1978)

Dona Enilda[2] lives with her grandson at the top of a steep hill in a one room shack without plumbing or electricity in a large city in northeastern Brazil. She looks much older than her 54 years. She walks with a shuffling gate and a limp, making it seem almost miraculous that she manages to climb up and down the slick muddy sides of the hill every day to catch the bus that takes her to her radiation therapy. Dona Enilda used to clean houses for a living, but now she is in treatment for stage IIIB cervical cancer, and she must depend on her 14-year-old grandson to pick up odd jobs to buy the beans and rice they eat every day.

She says her disease began with itching and bleeding from her vagina, although she felt no pain until "the doctors kept sticking things in there." She only went to the doctor at all, she says, because her *patroa,* her employer, made the appointment and brought her to the clinic herself. From the clinic, she was sent to another doctor, who in turn sent her to radiation therapy. He didn't tell her what the therapy would be like, but he said it was the only way to save her life.

Half-way through the treatment, however, Dona Enilda has decided that she will no longer continue. The treatment ". . . makes me want to vomit. Even the coffee which I love, and which I drink all day, I can't stand to see it. It makes me sick. . . ." Rather than helping, the treatment seemed to be making her worse, and she is now convinced that her illness must have "been sent" on her by a spiteful neighbor. The only cure, she has determined, will be to visit a spiritualist center and have the spell removed. It will be expensive and time consuming, and she can't afford the time or the bus money to do both the radiation therapy and the spiritual cleansing, so she will stop radiation therapy. She will not discuss this decision with her doctor, she says. He barely speaks to her anyway, and he will be angry with her for believing in *macumba,* the black magic that allowed this disease to be sent.

[2] This case is based on the ethnographic field research of Jessica Gregg. Pseudonyms are used (Gregg, 1997)

The LEARN Model for Improving Cross-Cultural Communication

If a physician is dealing regularly with patients from an ethnic group different from his or her own, it is valuable to be aware of the *range* of health beliefs and practices of that group. Readings suggested at the end of this chapter can provide the student with coherent summaries of the ethnomedical systems for some ethnic groups. Effective communication skills are important and learnable.

Berlin and Fowkes (1983) suggest the mnemonic LEARN (Table 4–3) to improve cross-cultural communication in the clinical setting; the mnemonic stands for listen, explain, acknowledge, recommend, and negotiate. The first suggestion is the most important—*listen* to the patient's perception of the problem. This goal can be accomplished by eliciting the patient's "explanatory model" through the questions indicated in Table 4–2. Research on patient satisfaction with physician consultation indicates that active verbal interaction, particularly the time spent listening to the patient, was the strongest predictor of satisfaction (Korsch and Negrete, 1972). When the physician *explains* his or her view of a patient's problem, it is important to use terms that can be understood. The *acknowledgment* of possible differences between the views of the patient and the physician needs to be accomplished in such a manner that the patient's ideas are not demeaned but, rather, treated with respect. In this regard, the physician must *recommend* (rather than order) a particular treatment plan. The idea of recommending actions to a patient is important because it reframes the concept of compliance. Mutual respect, coming from both sides of a cultural boundary, is the only way that a therapeutic alliance between patient and healer can be created. If there is a difference of opinion between the two parties, and if there is a context of mutual respect, then it is possible to *negotiate* a treatment plan that is acceptable to both patient and physician.

The following case from a New Mexico hospital illustrates the often complicated process of listening, acknowledgment of cultural differences, and negotiation that must occur to achieve care that is satisfactory to participants on both sides of a cultural divide. Medical practitioners in the Southwest have had

Table 4–3 **LEARN: A Guideline for Improved Communication**

L	*Listen* with sympathy and understanding to the patient's perception of the problem.
E	*Explain* your perceptions of the problem.
A	*Acknowledge* and discuss differences and similarities.
R	*Recommend* treatment.
N	*Negotiate* an agreement.

(Adapted from Berlin ED, Fowkes WC: A teaching framework for cross-cultural health care. West J Med 139:130–134, 1983)

a long history of working effectively in a multicultural setting and cooperating with Native American people (Adair et al, 1988).

Mrs. W., a 78-year-old Navajo sheepherder, was transported from her home on the Arizona–New Mexico border to a large hospital in Albuquerque after presenting at a local clinic near her home with signs of severe respiratory distress. Although she spoke no English, her daughter who accompanied her explained that Mrs. W. had not been feeling well for the last several days and had become significantly worse over the last 24 hours. The report of the clinic on the border suggested that the doctors were afraid that Mrs. W. may have been exposed to the Hantavirus, a dangerous respiratory pathogen.

Given her clear distress and rapidly deteriorating condition and the potential severity of the infection, Mrs. W. was taken immediately to the intensive care unit, where she was placed in a room with sliding glass doors that faced a common hall, and where physicians hoped to begin aggressive management, including immediately starting several intravenous lines and placing her on a respirator. They explained to the daughter that while her mother was not currently in acute need of centrally administered drugs or artificial help in breathing, the measures were precautionary in case her condition deteriorated even further. Saying that she would have to discuss it with family members first, the daughter denied permission for the procedures, and no amount of explanation regarding the medical necessity of the procedures could sway her. As the night wore on, Mrs. W.'s breathing became increasingly labored, and caregivers pressured the daughter for a decision. Finally, the daughter agreed that initial procedures could begin, but that any other major medical decisions would have to involve the entire family.

By the next day, all of Mrs. W.'s children and siblings had arrived at the hospital and, for the next month, made their home in the waiting room. The eldest son, a member of the military, pulled one of the nurses aside and explained to her that if other procedures needed to be performed in the future, the staff should not present them to the family as precautionary. He said that talking about bad things that might happen in the future suggested that those things were wished for, or somehow being "called on" his mother. Rather, to communicate more effectively with the family, the staff should always refer to his mother's present condition and the need to address current problems.

Over the course of the next several days, Mrs. W. became increasingly ill, developing blisters over most of her body and becoming febrile and incoherent. Laboratory results showed that she was negative for the Hantavirus, and medical personnel were baffled as how best to handle a case that was becoming less and less hopeful. When hospital workers attempted to communicate their fears to the family, however, they were told that there was nothing to worry about, and that Mrs. W. would live. Her son had consulted a healer in his community, who had discovered the source of the illness and was working on a cure.

According to the traditional healer, Mrs. W. had been very successful with her sheep for the last few years and, in addition, had woven a large rug that she sold for several thousand dollars a few months earlier. This good fortune had ignited the envy of her clan sisters, who has visited this illness on her. They had sent the illness through Mrs. W.'s back. As evidence, Mrs. W.'s son pointed to a large, red burn-like mark that had appeared on her back during the course of the hospital stay.

Importantly, Mrs. W.'s son explained, in order for her to be healed, the hospital staff would need to follow certain rules. First, the curtains on the glass doors in the front of Mrs. W.'s room would have to remain shut, shielding her from the gazes of outsiders. In addition, no one, except her immediate family and regular nurses and doctors, would be allowed to look at her. Third, the family requested that they be able to rub Mrs. W. with herbs provided by the healer, and they asked that Mrs. W. not be washed afterwards. Finally, they stated that no menstruating women could be allowed to care for her.

The hospital staff agreed that they would do their best to protect Mrs. W.'s privacy and would attempt to assign the same nurses to her every shift. They explained, however, that they would have to compromise on some of the other conditions. Negotiating with the family, the staff agreed not to wash Mrs. W.'s hair ever and to wash her body only when they needed to change the dressings over her blisters. The family agreed to the necessity of the dressing changes and to the occasional washings. The staff also noted that they could not both provide continuity of care and, given that most of the nurses and half of the medical staff were females, ensure that no menstruating women would enter the room. The family agreed to waive that condition.

Mrs. W. remained in the hospital for 2 months. She was found to be positive for Rocky Mountain Spotted Fever, but physicians were never able to fully understand why her condition became so severe so quickly, She did recover, however, and at the time of this writing,[3] she is in transitional care, getting ready to move back home to her family and sheep herd.

CULTURE, ETHNICITY, AND MEDICAL CARE

In complex societies such as our own, ethnicity is a fundamental source of cultural diversity and, for the medical practitioner, of potential misunderstanding. The concept of ethnicity has three fundamental aspects: (1) it establishes ties by reference to common origins, (2) it implies that members of the collectivity share particular patterns of behavior and interpersonal interaction, and (3) it implies that ethnic groups participate with one another in a larger social system (Harwood, 1981). Ethnic groups, then, participate and reflect to different degrees the cultural attitudes of both the dominant culture and the specific subculture.

[3] March 1997. Case reported by Jessica Gregg.

It is important to emphasize that this is a discussion of ethnicity rather than "race." The idea of race has been abandoned by nearly all biological anthropologists and human biologists (Goodman and Armelagos, 1996). Race is a commonplace and politically powerful social concept that has no practical utility in biological studies. Indeed, there is genetic and phenotypic variation among human populations, but these differences simply cannot be forced into discrete or relevant categories as required by the concept of race; the idea of race is simply folk biology. In a powerful recent analysis, Hahn (1992) has shown that the use of race in health statistics is full of politically relevant contradictions devoid of biological validity and falsely implies that health differentials stemming from class or ethnic inequalities actually have a genetic basis. Importantly, in comprehensive analyses of sociomedical problems such as infant mortality, it is social class that has the strongest explanatory power.

It is useful to remember that there is much variation in the degree to which members of ethnic groups share cultural standards or publicly express their ethnicity. Indeed, the concept of ethnicity brings with it a serious danger of stereotyping, the mistaken notion that all members of another group are alike. Even among recent immigrants, there is much cultural variation based on regional, educational, and class differences in the country of origin. The length of time a person has been in the United States, his or her socioeconomic milieu, and the language spoken at home all make cultural stereotyping a dangerous enterprise.

It is important, nevertheless, that practitioners become culturally sensitized to the range of cultural beliefs and behaviors present in the ethnic groups they serve. This information can be clinically valuable in a medical setting, for example, in terms of interpreting a patient's complaints. In a classic study, Zborowski (1952) described ethnic variation in attitudes toward pain and cultural standards for communicating about the pain. Whereas both Jewish and Italian-American patients were described as having an "emotional" response to pain, the Italian Americans in the sample were more concerned with the immediate relief from pain, while Jewish patients were anxious about the implications of the pain in terms of the future health and welfare of the family. On the other hand, "WASP" patients reflected a cultural belief that it was "no use" to complain about pain and preferred to describe or report the experience. Patients from this cultural background attempt to avoid being a "nuisance" in the hospital setting, thinking of themselves as part of a team. A serious report of pain from this group, because it is based on different cultural standards about interpersonal communication of unpleasant things, must also be evaluated differently. Recently, Bates (1992, 1993) has completed methodologically rigorous studies of pain and ethnicity focusing on Puerto Rican Americans, WASPs, and African Americans. The studies demonstrate the influence of ethnicity on the actual perception of pain, as well as rules about communicating distress. Similarly, medical anthropologists have offered detailed ethnographic descriptions of patients who experience pain, and this research has re-emphasized the importance of sociocultural factors in the experience and communication of pain (Good, 1992).

The experience of pain can only be communicated to the physician through the patient and his or her cultural beliefs and standards. The physician must be aware of both the danger of stereotyping and individual variation and the characteristic health beliefs and behaviors of ethnic groups. The multicultural diversity created by the large number of African-American and Hispanic patients already present in the United States, as well as recent immigrants from Caribbean countries, Central America, the former Soviet Union, and Southeast Asia, has increased the importance of the physician's evaluation of the role of sociocultural factors that may influence disease vulnerability, attitudes toward illness and medical treatment, and, for our purposes, manifestations of presumed mental illness.

With this in mind, a brief summary of some ethnic minorities in the United States is appropriate. (For more detailed discussions see Clark, 1983; for general clinical issues, see Barker, 1992; Galanti, 1991; Harwood, 1981; or Spector, 1985; for psychiatric disorders, see Gaw, 1982, 1992.)

African-American Culture

African Americans consist of a very heterogeneous social category; yet, as a group, they have been historically distinct, suffering from slavery in the past and recurring racism to the present time. Thus, while it is important to avoid the danger of stereotyping, it is also important to recognize that historical pressures and racism affect the culture of all African Americans. As Bell Hooks (1990) notes, "there is a radical difference between a repudiation of the idea that there is a black 'essence' and recognition of the way black identity has been specifically constituted in the experience of exile and struggle."

African-American religion and healing developed simultaneously as slaves attempted to create both meaning for their suffering and the methods to alleviate it. The lifeview in which African-American medicine operated considered the universe a hostile place where the forces of good and evil, God and Satan, struggled for control in both the natural realm of human and God and in the unnatural realm of sorcery and the devil (Mathews, 1987). Within this universe, illnesses may have natural or unnatural causes. Natural events occur according to the laws of God and nature and may, therefore, be explained as resulting from extreme behaviors that upset the balance of nature, such as too much drinking or eating, or as the result of God's will, perhaps as punishment for sinful behavior. Unnatural events are supernatural, caused by the devil or some other force of evil, and are therefore unpredictable, and are both caused and cured by magic (Snow, 1983: 821). This categorization and interpretation of disease provided illnesses with context and meaning and thus made them more tolerable.

Given that African Americans continue to struggle with racism and social inequity, it is perhaps not surprising that many elements of this meaning–

providing system continue to exist in African-American culture. Recent ethnographic studies of the health beliefs and practices of urban, lower-class African Americans include several observations useful for clinicians (Flaskerund and Rush, 1989; Heurtin-Roberts and Reisin, 1990; Mathews, 1987; Snow, 1983, 1993). Illnesses continue to be categorized as "natural" and "unnatural." Unnatural causes of illness include "hexes" (voodoo, hoodoo, and rootwork) and satanic influence. The hex can cause a variety of symptoms, particularly gastrointestinal problems, and is often thought to be the malevolent work of a close relative or friend. The idea of hex can be a predominant theme in the presentation of psychiatric cases. Jordan reports that a belief in the power of the hex has led some African Americans to use voodoo for therapy (Jordan, 1975). Snow reports that many African Americans believe medical doctors cannot help in the case of a hex, and patients seek the care of traditional religious healers with the power to cure them (Snow, 1993). Unless belief in rootwork (evil magic) is identified as part of the patient's presentation by the evaluating physician, extensive medical and psychiatric evaluation may prove to be frustrating. In general, however, African Americans rely almost entirely on orthodox biomedicine for their care (Jackson, 1981).

Importantly, biomedical definitions are frequently integrated into traditional belief systems, creating conditions with similar names but different perceived etiologies and cures, which may contribute to serious (and potentially dangerous) miscommunication between physicians and African-American patients. This problem is especially true for those illnesses considered "natural."

For example, an extremely important concern for those who believe in the traditional African-American model is the condition of the blood. Healthy blood is "at rest" or "quiet" (Heurtin-Roberts and Reisin, 1990), and illness results when blood begins rising in the body toward the head. Research among low income African-American women in New Orleans, Louisiana, for example, reveals two conditions, "high-blood" and "high-pertension," which may result from movements of the blood. High-blood is the result of too much or too-thick blood. Excessive blood slowly rises toward the head and "works on the heart too hard" (Heurtin-Roberts and Reisin, 1990). The condition is thought to be hereditary, but is believed to be exacerbated by rich diets and red meat. It is treated with medically prescribed antihypertensive drugs and vinegar bitters or epsom salts, which should "thin out" the blood (Heurtin-Roberts and Reisin, 1990; Snow, 1993).

"High-pertension" is perceived as a more acute condition than high-blood. In an individual suffering from high-blood, the blood stays elevated, slowly damaging the heart. High-pertension, on the other hand, causes the blood to shoot up suddenly to the head, often causing immediate death. Like high-blood, high-pertension is also considered the result of excessively thick blood, but the rapid ascendance of the blood to the head (as opposed to the moderately elevated condition of blood in high-blood) is produced by acute anxiety or nervousness. Treatment for high-pertension stresses the importance of relaxation and rarely includes medication, although tranquilizing pills are perceived as somewhat effective. Changes in diet and weight loss are considered ineffective treatments (Heurtin-Roberts and Reisin, 1990; Snow, 1983). Physicians treating African-American patients with hypertension need to remain cognizant of these folk models in order to avoid confusion and severe miscommunication in treatment.

At the same time, in working with African-American patients from higher social classes who have accepted current biomedical approaches to disease, it is important for the physician to recognize that there can be circumstances of racism and discrimination occurring in the work environment that increase job stress. This can be an aspect of the current culture of African Americans. These stress factors would be important if one is treating hypertension in a patient from that background, since such stress might influence the response to treatment. For example, Dressler (1991) has demonstrated how "status incongruity" between self-identification of status and the way in which a person is treated can be an important factor in upwardly mobile people, both in Brazilians and among African Americans in the South.

Where folk models overlap with physician models of illness, clinicians may find an important ally in folk models for the prevention and treatment of disease. For instance, Flaskerund and Rush (1989) note that low-income African-American women in Los Angeles have integrated AIDS into their traditional beliefs about illness and healing practices. Defining AIDS as a "natural" illness, the women advised that to prevent the disease, a person must live moderately, refrain from excessive sexual activity, eat right, and keep clean. The authors note that AIDS prevention programs among these women, then, should focus less exclusively on using condoms and not sharing needles and should broaden to include more frequent advice on the importance of monogamy to a moderate lifestyle (Flaskerund and Rush, 1989).

In addition, the long history of racism in the United States has left some African Americans suspicious of advanced biomedical explanations of disease. In the case of AIDS, there are some African Americans who, when made aware of the increasingly endemic incidence of AIDS in inner city African-American communities, reject current information on transmission because of a belief that the appearance of this disease is part of a conspiracy or plot to destroy African Americans. These patients will not readily accept the concept of a virally transmitted disease that requires epidemiological control through changes in behavior. Unless the physician maintains some cognizance of this belief, education efforts connecting AIDS transmission to intravenous drug use and unprotected sexual contact may, in certain instances, fall on deaf ears.

Hispanic-American Cultures

The Spanish-speaking population of the United States is made up of a variety of ethnic groups, including people with cultural roots in Puerto Rico,

Mexico, and Cuba, as well as in both Indian and Mestizo groups of Latin America. The cultural heterogeneity within this category is significant and important, yet there are several key commonalities. First are the obvious problems of language and problems of communication, which can be particularly critical in a healthcare setting. Other commonalities include general conditions of poverty and migration-associated stress; a cultural emphasis on the extended family; interactional norms linked with notions of respect and modesty for women; and some basic philosophic premises about the relationship of body and mind. The health beliefs and behaviors of these groups have been the subject of much social scientific research (Bauwens and Spicer, 1977; Schreiber and Homiak, 1981).

With respect to Mexican Americans, Murillo (1972) notes that there is no specific Mexican-American family type, but thousands of different families, depending on regional, historic, political, socioeconomic, and acculturation factors. The Spanish language may or may not be spoken in the home. For example, some Mexican Americans have very little familiarity with Spanish, whereas others are bilingual and deal with differing nuances of communication, depending on the language being used. With the mixture of European, Spanish, and Indian influences, Mexican Americans may have a range of religious beliefs; therefore, it may be erroneous to assume, for example, that a patient is unduly influenced by Catholicism.

Research on the folk medical beliefs of all Hispanic groups indicates that both natural and supernatural cases of illness are thought to operate. Natural causes include drafts (*mal aire*), fallen fontanelle in children (*mollera caida*), intestinal obstruction (*empacho*), but, most important, an imbalance of hot and cold elements (see Pachter, 1993, for the most comprehensive treatment of this subject). The hot/cold theory of disease is based on traditional Hippocratic beliefs of four humors (the moist/dry distinction is essentially ignored in these folk beliefs). Illnesses, foods, and remedies are classified in the hot/cold system in terms of their essential character; illnesses represent either an excess or surfeit of hot or cold humors. Therefore, in this cultural conception, a cure involves readjusting the body's humors to recreate a healthy balance.

Harwood (1971, 1981) has shown that, for Puerto Rican patients, the hot/cold theory can present problems of compliance when, for example, a "hot" illness such as rheumatic fever is treated with a "hot" remedy such as antibiotics. From the patient's perspective, such an incongruence may defy their own cultural logic. Harwood shows, however, that the "principle of neutralization," in which the "hot" nature of an antibiotic can be balanced by taking the pill with a "cool" substance such as fruit juice or tea, can resolve the cultural incongruence and improve results (see Harwood, 1981, for detailed clinical suggestions). It is important to remember, however, that Puerto Rican and other Hispanic patients vary in the degree to which they give credence to the folk model, and, therefore, the clinician must try to determine, for individual patients, whether this folk conceptualization may affect treatment outcome.

Because of language problems, there may be mislabeling of some symptoms as "psychotic" in Hispanic patients, especially in patients who present with pseudohallucinations or the syndrome of *ataque* (also called Puerto Rican syndrome; see Harwood, 1977). The ataque syndrome includes anxiety, hyperventilation, and occasional behavior resembling a seizure disorder; it is usually transient (Pachter, 1993).

According to Harwood, the belief system of *espiritismo* (spiritism) is a common feature of Puerto Rican health culture in the Northeast. Espiritismo is a belief based on the reality and power of spirit possession, communication through mediums, and removal of harmful influences by spiritist specialists. It is practiced in neighborhood *centros,* which resemble a "clinic" with mediums and assistants. Patients are reported to present with a variety of somatic and anxiety-related symptoms, including nightmares and mood disturbances. The "therapy" of the patients is conducted by the medium, who communicates with a spirit who essentially conducts an exploratory psychotherapeutic interview with the patient to determine areas of emotional pain and conflict. Various types of malevolent spirits, which may possess the body, can control the patient. The work by Harwood (1977) shows that spiritists provide valuable mental health services to this underserved community and that their work can be successfully integrated with the biomedical approach.

Mention should also be made of the mental health conditions of *susto* (soul loss, or magical fright) and *nervios* (nerves). The symptoms of susto are similar to those of depression, although the condition is thought to be the result of the inadvertent separation of the soul from the body. The ritual cures of *curanderos* have been shown to relieve symptoms (Rubel et al, 1984). Hispanic ideas of curing appear to be linked to several philosophical premises (Table 4–4).

Although the concept of good and evil spirits occupying and controlling one's body and behavior may sound primitive, it is quite similar to commonly held beliefs about spiritual life prevalent in Christianity and that persist in many Christians. Even psychoanalysis uses concepts of "good and bad objects" that are "introjected" or "internalized" intrapsychically from one's environment. More-

Table 4–4 **Latino Philosophical Premises about Health and Curing**

1. Illness can result from strong emotional states.
2. Illness can be caused by being out of balance with the environment.
3. Patients can be the innocent victims of malevolent forces.
4. The body and soul are separable.
5. Cure requires participation of the entire family.
6. The natural world cannot be distinguished from the supernatural.
7. Sickness of a member can bring a family closer.
8. A healer should be open and treat you with respect.

(Adapted from Maduro P: Curanderismo and Latino views of disease and curing. West J Med 139:64–71, 1983) over, classic psychoanalysis has its own ritualistic traditions of initiation and training; techniques of therapy are thus heavily influenced by cultural factors.

Asian-American Groups

Asian Americans represent a very wide array of cultural traditions with such remarkable variation that generalizations are difficult to make. Some Southeast Asian groups, such as the Hmong who are concentrated in parts of Minnesota and California, still retain active folk medical systems based on shamanism. In these places, cooperation between this ethnic minority and the biomedical community is a process in which anthropological interventions have been helpful.[4]

Traditional Asian ethnomedical systems, including traditional Chinese medicine, Japanese medicine, as well as South Asian Ayruvedic medicine and its Muslim analogue, Unani medicine, represent written professional traditions that are thousands of years old (Leslie and Young, 1992). In general, these are naturalistic ethnomedical systems based on the principle that health is based on the balance of elements attributed to organ systems in the body. In traditional Chinese medicine, organ systems are paired in complementary oppositions of *yin* and *yang* in complex patterns of mutual reinforcement (creation) or conflict (destruction). A balance in this complementarity is necessary for the healthy flow of life energy, *chi*, through the body. Illness occurs when balance is disrupted, and equilibrium must be restored either by building up particular parts of organ systems or by stimulating and adjusting the flow of energy between organ systems through particular pathways or meridians. Such interventions are the purpose of acupuncture.

It should be noted that body fluids, especially blood and semen, are important elements of healthful physiology. Berlin and Fowkes (1983:133) provide this example of the utility of the LEARN model in this context:

> A 25 year-old Vietnamese woman was seen for a routine prenatal examination. As part of her evaluation, she had blood drawn for laboratory testing. Within the next few days, she returned with a variety of symptoms, including weakness, fatigue, and coryza. She attributed this to having blood removed, feeling the removal of blood weakens the system and causes illness.

Her physician knew Vietnamese medical beliefs and acknowledged them, but he also explained how much blood volume was actually taken, and gave examples of blood donors who had much larger volumes taken with no symp-

---

[4] This work is associated with the efforts of Peter Kunstadter (1997). Problems with Hmong reaction to surgical interventions have been studied by Hu (1997).

toms. After this discussion, the woman seemed pleased with the explanation and became less fearful; her symptoms went away.

The context of this episode seems to be related to ethnomedical theories of physiology in which bodily substances are linked in an ascending order. For example, Edwards (1983) reports that, in Chinese medicine, it takes seven units of a precursor product to produce one unit of the subsequent product:

$$\text{Food} \to \text{blood} \to jing \to chi \to shen$$

in which *jing* is semen or sexual fluid, *chi* is life energy, and *shen* is ethereal energy. Because several physiological systems are involved in this interaction, symptomology can vary. What is most important, however, is the idea that an interruption of the cycle—for example, through the taking of blood—can have a geometric effect on each subsequent element. As such, in the context of these ethnomedical beliefs, it "makes sense" that this patient would be concerned about the blood that had been drawn. Similarly, it is important to note that many cultures make no distinction between food and medicine.

The work by Kleinman (1980) on traditional Chinese culture is aimed at understanding how cultural beliefs influence the experience of illness and the patient role. He has shown a general reticence on the part of Chinese to verbalize distressful effects and a tendency of anxiety and depression to be manifested in predominantly physical or somatic symptoms. However, the extent to which these characteristics appear in Chinese Americans, including the effect of acculturation, is not clear.

Other Ethnic Groups

Cultural summaries of health beliefs and behaviors relevant to clinical care are available for a wide variety of ethnic groups, including Haitians, Italians, and Navajos (Harwood, 1981); Filipinos, Japanese, Jamaicans, Pacific Islanders, Middle Easterners, Soviet Jews, and Alaskan Eskimos (Clark, 1983); and Chinese Americans, Afghan refugees, East Indians, Iranians, Korean Americans, Laotian refugees, Ethiopians, Russian emigres, and seasonal farm workers (Barker, 1992). Spector (1985) and Bauwens and Spicer (1977) provide similar discussions for lower-income whites.

Biomedical Culture

Clearly, it is important for physicians to understand the cultural models of disease held by their patient populations. It is also important that physicians and their patients recognize that biomedicine (medicine as it is practiced in hospitals, universities, and clinics in most industrialized nations) itself forms a subculture containing culture-specific values, beliefs, and practices. Patient–physician interactions may, in fact, be viewed as cross-cultural communication, with each participant struggling to understand the worldview of the other.

Although practitioners and patients of biomedicine often tend to regard this system as based purely in scientific fact and therefore as beyond or above culture, anthropologists studying biomedicine have made it clear that the system is as much a product of a particular cultural milieu as are other types of healing. They do not argue that biomedical notions of anatomy, physiology, and disease etiology are only applicable to individuals and populations in particular cultural systems. Rather, they emphasize that the environment in which biomedical ideas and practices are generated influences both the type of idea that is generated and the ways in which that idea is eventually implemented.

The influence of culture on biomedicine may be explored in two ways: (1) by examining the social and historical context in which biomedicine has developed, and (2) by examining the influence of specific cultural contexts on the biomedicine subculture. Most historians trace the origins of biomedicine to the philosophy of Rene Descartes, which was previously discussed in Chapter 3. Descartes postulated a possible separation of the mental and the social worlds from the physical body, although Descartes' theories have been interpreted in a simplistic manner. The "dualism" attributed to Descartes was an intrinsic concept in Greek philosophy dating to Socrates and Plato and involved metaphysical, not scientific, concepts. Nevertheless, mind-body dualism permeated much of Western thought. It formed an essential component of traditional biomedical theory (Scheper-Hughes and Lock, 1987) in which diseases afflict the bounded, physical body, and, therefore, the body alone is the focus of the therapeutic encounter (see also Chapter 2). Social and mental disorders are considered outside the realm of biomedicine (Rhodes, 1990; Scheper-Hughes and Lock, 1987). Critics argue that Cartesian thinking in biomedicine leads to an unfortunate reluctance on the part of physicians to adopt a more integrated approach to illness, one that understands disease as the product of a mind–body–society interaction. They contend that an understanding of illness as a product of social environment and mental state, as well as the product of biological malfunction, would allow physicians the ability to comprehend more fully the causes and consequences of illness (Cassell, 1991; Cousins, 1979; Finkler 1991; Scheper-Hughes and Lock, 1987.)

Even as biomedicine can be understood as a distinct system that developed out of a specific cultural historical context, it also can be analyzed as several varied systems, each uniquely affected by a different cultural context. For instance, it is possible to make distinctions between biomedical cultures in France, England, and the United States (Hunt, 1992). Physicians in England and the United States, diagnosing and treating heart conditions, differ markedly in their assessment of the need for patients to undergo heart surgery. Unlike physicians in any other biomedical system, French physicians prescribe lactobacillus from yogurt cultures in conjunction with prescriptions for antibiotics in order to counteract stomach distress from those medicines (Hunt, 1992).

In the study by Finkler (1991) on biomedicine in Mexico City, the author notes that while biomedicine in Mexico "is practiced along the lines of a world-wide biomedical model that focuses on the body and its anatomical lesions and depends chiefly on pharmacological treatments," individual physicians combine biomedical understandings with traditional folk understanding to explain sickness. Thus, common folk conditions such as *nervios* and *susto* (traditionally believed to be caused by anger, anxiety, and/or fright, and to result in numerous symptoms, such as jabbing pains in the heart, trembling, tiredness, insomnia, and headaches) were often translated by the physicians in Finkler's study into organic dysfunctions. Finkler (1991:80) explains that "physicians frequently diagnose patients with problems of the spine. Their emphasis on the spinal column may reflect a reinterpretation of nerves as a dysfunction of the nervous system that is lodged in the spine and that causes a nerve sickness." Here, then, culture clearly influences how physicians interpret symptoms and how illnesses are addressed in the biomedical system.

Several analysts have noted that, in the United States, the North American emphases on the individual and on technology give rise to a biomedical culture that is focused more on treatment than on alleviation of suffering. Suffering is experienced by persons, not simply by bodies (Cassell, 1991). However, increasing reliance on advanced technology focuses physician efforts more narrowly on the body and away from the sufferer and his or her subjective needs.

Farmer and Kleinman (1989) illustrate this point through a study of the AIDS-related deaths of two individuals, Anita in Haiti and Robert in Boston. Having suffered from AIDS for 2 years, Robert entered the hospital after being barred from air travel home to Chicago because of his medical condition. Weary of treatment, Robert made clear to the hospital staff that he wanted no additional invasive care. At most, he wanted enough care to enable him to board an airplane, and if that was not possible, he requested that he just be "kept clean." Instead, he was given a feeding tube, an endoscopy, and a CT scan of the neck. He died a few hours after the last procedure.

Anita died in Haiti. She was given almost no medical care and died in the house of her godmother, who refused to take her to the clinic:

> Why should we take her there . . . She will not recover from this disease. She will have to endure the heat and humiliation of the clinic. She will not find a cool place to lie down. What she might find is a pill or an injection to make her feel more comfortable for a short time. I can do better than that . . . for some people a decent death is as important as a decent life. (Farmer and Kleinman, 1989)

In a culture in which advanced technology is scarce and, therefore, rarely perceived as the solution to most problems, and social ties are perceived as more important than individual autonomy, Anita's life was not extended through technological advances, but neither was her suffering deepened by social isolation and invasive and ultimately useless therapy. The point the authors make here is not that technology is bad or that biomedicine as practiced in the United States is wrong. Rather, they argue that North Americans have allowed cultural biases toward technology and treatment of the individual to permeate notions of healing to the extent that physicians often ignore other equally vital and much more elemental aspects of healing.

DISCUSSION

Social and cultural factors are essential for understanding human behavior because they provide both context and meaning for action. Human thought and behavior encompasses such diversity among social groups because of culture. In childhood, all people learn their social group's beliefs about health, illness, and what to do when sick. Because such beliefs can influence the interpretation of symptoms and effective communication between the patient and physician, they are very important.

Learned cultural behaviors, for example, in diet or notions of "ideal body type," can influence the social epidemiological distribution of disease. Higher prevalence of disease in minority ethnic groups, however, is better understood in terms of social class than culture itself. The social stresses of poverty have a large impact on physical and mental health.

In most social situations, stereotyping is used to distance ethnic groups by creating barriers of misunderstanding between them. Physicians and other healthcare personnel must recognize the impact of their own sociocultural backgrounds on attitudes, perceptions, and prejudices that they may have toward persons of social, educational, ethnic, cultural, and lifestyle backgrounds different from their own. Physicians must be able to listen to the patient as well as respond in an emphatic and nonjudgmental manner. It is also valuable to remember that the medical community itself has a culture—a set of values and beliefs about health and illness—which can simply be foreign and poorly understood by patients.

It is important to know and understand the cultural background of patients in both medical and psychiatric practice. Failure to do so will complicate understanding the patient's symptoms, making a correct diagnosis, and planning and communicating an effective treatment plan. Errors that may occur include stereotypic labeling of minority patients, drawing premature conclusions regarding the patient based on the patient's ethnic group and cultural and socioeconomic background, and failure to use interpreters when major language and cultural barriers exist between physician and patient.

ANNOTATED BIBLIOGRAPHY

Barker JC: Cross-cultural medicine: A decade later. West J Med 157: 1992

This special issue summarizes cultural information and clinical problems on 16 ethnic groups in northern California, including recent political refugees.

Clark MM: Cross-cultural medicine. West J Med 139: 1983

>This special edited issue contains excellent summaries on the health beliefs and behaviors of 12 different ethnic groups, as well as more theoretical summaries of issues surrounding culture and medicine.

Gaw A: Cross-Cultural Psychiatry. Boston, John Wright-PSG, 1982

>This book includes papers by a number of writers and elucidates aspects of psychiatry as applied to minority groups in the United States. It is useful for acquiring some general background information that is important in the clinical assessment of patients.

Harwood A: Ethnicity and Health Care. Cambridge, Harvard University Press, 1981

>An excellent collection of articles on major ethnic groups and their demographic and social epidemiological characteristics and health beliefs. The article by Jackson on lower-class urban blacks is particularly recommended.

REFERENCES

Acosta FX, Yamamoto J, Evans LA: Effective Psychotherapy for Low Income and Minority Patients. New York, Plenum Press, 1982
Adair J, Deuschle KW, Barnett CW: The People's Health: Medicine and Anthropology in a Navajo Community. Albuquerque, University of New Mexico Press, 1988
Bates MS, Edwards WT, Anderson, KO: Pain. J Intl Association Study Pain 52(1):101–112, 1993
Bates MS, Edwards WT: Ethnicity and disease. Intl J Population Differences Disease Patterns 2(1):63–83, 1992
Bauwens E, Spicer EH: Ethnic Medicine in the Southwest. Tucson, University of Arizona Press, 1977
Berlin ED, Fowkes WC: A teaching framework for cross-cultural health care. West J Med 139:130–134, 1983
Boddy J: Wombs and Alien Spirits: Women, Men, and the Zar Cult in Northern Sudan. Madison, University of Wisconsin Press, 1989
Bordo, S: Unbearable Weight: Feminism, Western Culture, and the Body. Berkeley, University of California Press, 1993
Bradshaw WH: Training psychiatrists for working with blacks in basic residency programs. Am J Psychiatry 135:1520–1524, 1978
Brown P, Inhorn M: Disease, ecology and human behavior. In Sargent CF, Johnson TM (eds): Medical Anthropology: Contemporary Theory and Method. Westport, CT, Praeger, 199X.
Brumberg JJ: Fasting Girls: The Emergence of Anorexia Nervosa as a Modern Disease. Cambridge, Harvard University Press, 1988
Cassell EJ: The Nature of Suffering and the Goals of Medicine. New York, Oxford University Press, 1991
Chernin K: The Obsession: Reflections on the Tyranny of Slenderness. New York, Harper and Row, 1981
Chrisman NJ, Maretzki TW: Clinically Applied Anthropology: Anthropologists in Health Science Settings. Dordrecht, Reidel Publishing Company, 1982
Clark MM: Cross-cultural medicine. West J Med 139: 1983
Clark MM: Cross-cultural medicine: A decade later. West J Med 157(3): 1992
Cockerham WC: Medical Sociology, 3rd ed. Englewood Cliffs, NJ, Prentice Hall, 1986
Cousins N: Anatomy of an Illness as Perceived by the Patient. New York, Bantam Books, 1979
Dressler W: Stress and Adaptation in the Context of Culture: Depression in a Southern Black Community, Albany, State University of New York Press, 1991
Edwards JW: Semen anxiety in South Asian cultures: Cultural and transcultural significance. Med Anth 7(3):51–67, 1983
Ehrenreich B, English D: Complaints and Disorders: The Sexual Politics of Sickness. New York, Feminist Press, 1973

Eisenberg L, Kleinman A: The Relevance of Social Science for Medicine. Dordrecht, Reidel Publishing Company, 1981

Fabrega H: Disease and Social Behavior: An Interdisciplinary Perspective. Boston, MIT Press, 1974

Farmer P, Kleinman A: AIDS as Human Suffering Daedalus Spring: 1989

Favazza AE: Anthropology and psychiatry. In Kaplan HI, Sadock BJ (eds): Comprehensive Textbook of Psychiatry, 4th ed. Baltimore/London, Williams & Wilkins, 1985

Finkler K: Physicians at Work, Patients in Pain: Biomedical Practice and Patient Response in Mexico. Boulder, CO, Westview Press, 1991

Flaskerund JH, Rush CE: AIDS and traditional health beliefs and practices of black women. Nursing Res 38(4):210–215, 1989

Foster GM: Disease etiologies in non-Western medical systems. Am Anth 78:773–782, 1976

Freeman O: Margaret Mead and Samoa. Cambridge, Harvard University Press, 1983

Galanti G: Caring for Patients from Different Cultures: Case Studies from American Hospitals. Philadelphia, University of Pennsylvania Press, 1991

Gaw A: Chinese Americans. In Gaw A (ed): Cross-Cultural Psychiatry. Boston, John Wright-PSG, 1982

Gaw A, Ed. Culture, Ethnicity, and Mental Illness. Washington, DC, American Psychiatric Press, 1992

Good MJD (ed): Pain as a Human Experience: An Anthropological Perspective, Berkeley, University of California Press, 1992

Goodman A, Armelagos, G: The resurrection of race: The concept of race in physical anthropology in the 1990s. In Reynolds LT, Lieberman L (eds): Race and Other Misadventures. Dix Hills, NY, General Hall,1996

Hahn HA: The state of federal health statistics on racial and ethnic groups. JAMA 267(2):268–271, 1992

Harwood A: The hot-cold theory of disease: Implications for the treatment of Puerto Rican patients. JAMA 216:1153–1158, 1971

Harwood A: Rx-Spiritist as Needed: A Study of a Puerto Rican Mental Health Resource. New York, Wiley, 1977

Harwood A: Ethnicity and Medical Care. Cambridge, Harvard University Press, 1981

Heurtin-Roberts S, Reisin E: Folk models of hypertension among black women. In Coreil J, Mull JD (eds): Anthropology and Primary Health Care. Boulder, CO, Westview Press, 1990

Hooks B: Yearning: Race, Gender, and Cultural Politics. Boston, South End Press, 1990

Hu, J: Medical encounter as cultural conflict: Perceptual differences and consequences of the interaction between Hmong immigrants and surgeons. Seattle, WA, Meetings of the Society for Applied Anthropology, 1997

Hunt GJ: Social and cultural aspects of health, illness, and treatment. In Goldman HH (ed):Review of General Psychiatry, 3rd ed. Norwalk, CT, Appleton and Lange, 1992

Jackson JJ: Urban black Americans. In Harwood A (ed): Ethnicity and Medical Care. Cambridge, Harvard University Press, 1981

Johnson TM, Sargent CF (eds): Medical Anthropology: Contemporary Theory and Method. New York, Praeger, 1990

Jordan WC: Voodoo medicine. In Williams RA (ed): Textbook of Black-Related Diseases. New York, McGraw-Hill, 1975

Kardiner A, Ovesey L: The Mark of Oppression. Cleveland, World Publishing, 1951

Kleinman A: Patients and Healers in the Context of Culture. Berkeley, University of California Press, 1980

Kleinman A: Rethinking Psychiatry: From Cultural Category to Personal Experience. New York, The Free Press, 1988a

Kleinman A: The Illness Narratives. New York, Basic Books, 1988b Kleinman A, Eisenberg L, Good B: Culture, illness and care. Ann Intern Med 88:251–258, 1978

Konner M: Anthropology and psychiatry. In Kaplan HI, Sadock BJ (eds): Comprehensive Textbook of Psychiatry, 5th ed. Baltimore, Williams & Wilkins, 1989

Korsch BM, Negrete VF: Doctor–patient communication. Sci Am 227(2):66–74, 1972

Kunstadter P: Health and health services in Southeast Asia and among Southeast Asians in Thailand and California. Seattle, WA, Meetings of the Society for Applied Anthropology, 1997

Larson A: Social context of human immunodeficiency virus transimssion in Africa: Historical and cultural bases of East and Central African sexual relations. Rev Infect Dis 11:716–731, 1989

Leighton AH: Relevant generic issues. In Gaw A (ed): Cross-Cultural Psychiatry. Boston, John Wright-PSG, 1982

Leslie C, Young A (eds): Paths to Asian Medical Knowledge. Berkeley, University of California Press, 1992

Lewis IM:Ecstatic Religion. London, Penguin, 1971

Maduro R: Curanderismo and Latino views of disease and curing. West J Med 139:64–71, 1983

Malinowski B: Sex and Repression in Savage Society. London, Routledge and Kegan Paul, 1927

Mathews H: Rootwork: Description of an ethnomedical system in the American South. Southern Med J 80(7):885–891, 1987

Mead M: Coming of Age in Samoa. New York, Morrow, 1928

Murillo N: The Mexican-American family. In Wagner NN, Haug MJ (eds): Chicanos: Social and Psychological Perspectives. St. Louis, CV Mosby, 1972

Murphy JM: Psychiatric labeling in cross-cultural perspective. Science 191:1019–1028, 1976

Pachter LM: Latino folk illness. Med Anthropology 15(2): 1993

Parker R: Acquired inimunodeficiency syndrome in urban Brazil. Med Anthropology Q 1:155–175, 1987

Polednak AP: Host Factors in Disease: Age, Sex, Race, and Ethnic Group. Springfield, MA, CC Thomas, 1987

Polgar S: Health action in cross-cultural perspective. In Freeman HE, Levine S, Reader LG (eds): Handbook of Medical Scoiology. Englewood Cliffs, NJ, Prentice Hall, 1963

Rhodes LA: Studying biomedicine as a cultural system. In Johnson TM, Sargent CF (eds): Medical Anthropology: Contemporary Theory and Method. New York, Praeger, 1990

Rubel AJ, O'Nell CW, Collado-Ardon R: Susto: A Folk Illness. Berkeley, University of California Press, 1984

Scheper-Hughes N: Saints, Scholars and Schizophrenics. Berkeley, University of California Press, 1979

Scheper-Hughes N: Child Survival: Anthropological Perspectives on the Treatment and Maltreatment of Children. Dordrecht, Reidel Publishing Company, 1987

Scheper-Hughes N, Lock M: The mindful body: A prolegomenon to future work in medical anthropology. Med Anthropology Q 1(1):6–41, 1987

Schreiber JM, Homiak JP: Mexican Americans. In Harwood A (ed): Ethnicity and Medical Care. Cambridge, Harvard University Press, 1981

Simons RC, Hughes CC: Culture-Bound Syndromes: Folk Illnesses of Psychiatric and Anthropological Interest. Dordrecht, Reidel Publishing Company, 1985

Snow L: Traditional health beliefs and practices among lower class black Americans. West J Med 139:16–24, 1983

Snow LF: Walkin' Over Medicine. Boulder, CO, Westview Press, 1993

Spector RE: Cultural Diversity in Health and Illness. Norwalk, CT, Appleton-Century-Crofts, 1985

Spiro M: Oedipus in the Trobriands. Chicago, University of Chicago Press, 1982

Spurlock J: Black Americans. In Gaw A (ed): Cross-Cultural Psychiatry. Boston, John Wrigh-PSG, 1982

Spurlock J, Lawrence LE: The black child. In Noshpitz JD (ed): Basic Handbook of Child Psychiatry. New York, Basic Books, 1979

Szaz TS: The Myth of Mental Illness. New York, Harper & Row, 1974

Whiting JW, Whiting BB: Children of Six Cultures: A Psychocultural Analysis. Cambridge, Harvard University Press, 1975

Wilson ED: On Human Nature. Cambridge, Harvard University Press, 1978 Zborowski M; Cultural components in response to pain. J Soc Issues 8:16–30, 1952

Zola IK: Structural constraints in the doctor-patient relationship: The case of non-compliance. In Eisberg L, Kleinman A (eds): The Relevance of Social Science for Medicine. Dordrecht, Reidel Publishing Company, 1981

II

Major Psychological Theories of Human Behavior

5 *Psychoanalytic Psychology*

Lawrence B. Inderbitzin,
Andrew C. Furman,
and Mark E. James

Chapters 5 and 6 focus on several major psychological approaches that have been developed to understand human behavior. This chapter examines *psychoanalytic* theory, and Chapter 6 explores *behavioral/ learning* schools of psychology. The decision to present only these two major branches of psychology is based on (1) the practical limitations of space imposed by the length of this book; (2) the goal of focusing on the *essential* principles of understanding human behavior; (3) the fact that psychoanalytic and behavioral/ learning approaches to behavior are fundamental in understanding other schools of psychology; and (4) the fact that these theories have received the most widespread application in understanding and managing the problems of psychiatric and medical patients.

Important psychological concepts derived from other theories, however, are discussed and integrated into other chapters in the text. For example, the cognitive psychology of Jean Piaget is discussed in Chapter 8 by Drs. Dell and Dulcan, family systems theory is discussed in Chapter 9 by Drs. Kaslow, Aronson, and Wootten, the life cycle developmental theory of Erik Erikson is discussed in Chapter 11 by Dr. van der Kolk, and theories of attachment behavior are elaborated in Chapter 10 by Drs. Wolman and Thompson. Therefore, while Chapters 5 and 6 present the two most widely used *fundamental* theories for understanding human behavior, other important concepts are integrated throughout the text, emphasizing the importance of reading this text as a whole rather than in parts.

For a more thorough introduction to psychoanalytic concepts, the introductory texts by Brenner, Nemiah, Engel, and Malan are recommended (see Annotated Bibliography). Readers are referred to standard comprehensive textbooks of psychiatry for information regarding contributions to understanding human behavior by individuals such as Allport, Maslow, Lewin, Adler, Rank, Klein, Reich, Horney, Sullivan, Fairbairn, Balint, and Winnicott. We begin now with a comprehensive discussion of psychoanalytic theory.

PSYCHOANALYTIC THEORY

There are three fundamental aspects to psychoanalytic psychology. (1) a *method of investigation* of the mind; (2) a *general theory* of human behavior; and (3) a *method of treatment* for certain psychological disorders. This chapter discusses basic concepts primarily related to the latter two. Psychoanalysis grew from medical roots and was begun and initially developed by the neurologist Sigmund Freud. From its beginning, psychoanalysis was oriented toward seeking the *origins* of psychological disturbances and understanding how the biologically endowed infant developed in interaction with the environment. Contrary to popular belief, Freud emphasized the importance and interplay of *both* biological and environmental influences throughout his writings (1905, 1916–1917), a view that is consistent with the general biopsychosocial philosophy of this text.

While psychoanalytic concepts facilitate a comprehensive approach to understanding personality, they also have many practical applications in understanding the emotional reactions of patients during the stress of physical illness. For example, under the stress of physical illness, some patients will "regress" to more childlike behavior and have intense emotional reactions directed toward their physicians that often require specific interventions. The following case study demonstrates some of these principles.

A CASE STUDY

A 45-year-old woman was hospitalized for the evaluation of pelvic pain. She was eventually diagnosed with ovarian cancer in an early stage, and her physicians felt she was a good candidate for surgery. As the diagnosis and nature of her illness were explained, she listened quietly with a passive, bland facial expression. When asked if she had any questions, she said simply that there must have been a mistake "during all the testing," and that she was sure she did not have cancer because she could "just feel" that she did not. Over the next 24 hours, she began to insist that there would have been a clear message from "the Lord" directly to her if such a serious illness were present and that she could not allow surgical treatment for "something that isn't there anyway." She had been a religious woman in a traditional manner all her life and had not spoken of such direct communications from God in the past. She had no history of psychiatric illness and was described by her husband as "very strong and always in control of her emotions."

Her primary physician had several interviews with her over the next 2 days, listening patiently as she expressed her certainty that everything was "ok" and no treatment was needed. Without argument or confrontation, the physician calmly repeated his diagnostic impressions and recommendations at the close of each meeting. On one occasion, the patient became slightly tearful as she was assuring the physician that there had been an error in the tests. The physician remarked that it would be very frightening, in any case, to be told that one had cancer and needed an operation. The woman cried more deeply and apologized for "acting like a baby." As she felt permission to cry and to be afraid, she sobbed with the physician and then with her family as she began to agree that the evaluation had been carefully performed and the appropriate treatment should begin.

In the face of the extreme stress of learning she had cancer, this patient had regressed to a more childlike level of functioning. Her defensive denial was not characteristic of her previous personality style and represented her effort to maintain her sense of strength and emotional control. To acknowledge illness and fear was to "act like a baby" and might have felt like risking the loss of the love of her family members around whom she was always strong and in control. The physician was empathic and respectful of his patient's psychological needs and conflicts. He tried to understand the feelings behind the patient's defenses, and he allowed the patient to maintain her defensive posture and resulting equilibrium until she felt safe and supported enough to accept the painful current reality.

As will be seen in the subsequent sections of this chapter, certain psychoanalytic concepts such as regression, defenses, ego strength, and transference can assist and deepen an understanding of the patient's behavior and facilitate the most effective way of helping a patient such as this through the course of an illness (see Table 5–1).

FUNDAMENTAL CONCEPTS

In developing psychoanalysis, Freud's methodology was essentially empiric, or based on data from clinical observations of his patients. Because his theories were influenced by the science of his time (Helmholtz School), it is easily overlooked that the fundamental concepts are firmly rooted in clinical observa-

[*continued on p. 146*]

Table 5–1 **Glossary of Key Concepts**

Adaptive point of view

The human organism has evolved to adapt to external reality; the ego has developed as an internal regulator of behavior and as an "organ" of adaptation.

Anal

This psychosexual stage occurs from 18 months to 3 years, during which anal sphincter control evolves and the child is aware of bowel function; pleasure is attained from anal and rectal stimulation through defecation and retention of feces; at this time, the child is involved with issues of mastery and autonomy, and conflicts emerge between obedience and defiance.

Character (personality) disorder

A disturbance of the personality involving habitual inflexibility of patterns of behavior without significant subjective discomfort; behavior is *ego-syntonic* in that the patient views it as appropriate, reasonable, and justified; yet the outcome of such behavior often results in problems for the patient.

Compromise formation

Activity or product of the functioning of the ego that balances the gratification of drives with the opposition against such gratification; although the instinctual drives and their associated unconscious wishes continually push for expression, this is opposed by the adaptation of the person to reality and by inner standards and morals; the ego allows for the gratification of drives in a disguised, substitute, or partial form, which is consciously unrecognizable as such; most mental events are the product of compromise formation; those that come to attention clinically are referred to as neurotic symptoms.

Conscious

Mental processes consisting of the ordinary stream of thoughts and emotions, which are actively experienced as they occur; these obey rational, secondary process logic; used as a noun or adjective.

Countertransference

The feelings and attitudes of the therapist toward the patient, which may arise from activation of conflicts from the therapist's own past, or which may be a result of the patient's projections onto the therapist; countertransference may negatively impact the therapeutic approach toward the patient or may provide a source of data about unconscious processes occurring in the patient.

Defense mechanisms

Specific unconscious mental methods used by the ego to protect against the danger of conscious awareness of repressed drives or wishes associated with the real or imagined punishments of childhood.

Developmental point of view

Behavior is a product of both intrinsic factors and interaction of the person with the environment, but these change in an expectable sequence during the course of development; all behaviors form a continuum dating back to earliest infancy, and most symptoms relate to past experience during development.

Dynamic–motivational point of view

Psychoanalysis explains human behavior and mental phenomena as being motivated by goal-directed forces (wishes or needs inherent in the nature of humans), which may be in opposition to one another, resulting in conflicts and compromise formations.

(continued)

Table 5–1 *(continued)*

Dynamic unconscious

The processes and contents of the "system unconscious" held out of conscious awareness by the action of repression; they strive for discharge but are abhorrent or threatening morally, so this resulting conflict causes anxiety; if the repression fails, neurotic symptoms may result.

Ego

In Freud's structural model, it is the agency of the mind that mediates between id drives, external reality, and the prohibitions of the superego, working to facilitate maximal gratification while simultaneously adapting to external and internal moral standards; its complex set of functions includes reality testing, regulation of drives, relationships with other people and mental representations of others, thought processes (organizing perceptions, forming conclusions, remembering, concentrating, learning, judgment, and so forth), defense mechanisms, autonomous functions (perception, motor function, intention, intelligence, language), and synthetic, integrating, and organizing functions.

Ego–Ideal

Subgroup of superego functions that includes goals, ideals, and standards of exemplary achievement; it serves to regulate mood, behavior, and self-esteem through the generation of affects or shame.

Empathy

A special way of knowing or perceiving the emotional psychological state of another; one person momentarily shares the feelings possessed by another person.

Free association

The method of operation by the patient in psychoanalysis in which he or she thinks freely and reports everything that comes to mind without the usual selectiveness used in conventional discourse.

Id

In Freud's structural model, unconscious collection of drives, urges, and wishes that continually push for complete gratification despite the constraints of reality.

Insight

The subjective experiential knowledge of formerly unconscious pathogenic mental content and conflicts that occurs during the process of psychoanalysis and is accompanied by adaptive behavioral changes.

Instinctual drives

Innate inner stimuli that motivate the organism toward gratification, usually through another person; the two basic instinctual drives are the *sexual* and the *aggressive.*

Interpretation

Therapeutic intervention by the analyst to assist the patient to become aware of inner mental conflicts and ideas that had been excluded from consciousness, with the goal of accomplishing self-knowledge and symptomatic improvement.

Latency

This stage lasts from approximately age 5 to 12; the sexual drives and conflicts are less apparent in that the major activities of this time period are learning and other socially approved channels of gratification; this is a period of considerable development of the ego.

(continued)

Table 5–1 *(continued)*

Metapsychology

A highly abstract conceptual framework for organizing, systematizing, and orienting clinical data.

Neurosis

A mental disturbance involving abnormalities of thought, behavior, attitudes, and emotions; classic neuroses include hysteria, obsessions, phobias, and depression; the symptoms of neurosis are *ego-dystonic* (i.e., they are recognized by the patient as abnormal and alien to the self).

Object

A person or thing through which instinctual needs can be gratified or expressed; the inner mental schemas that conceptualize other persons are referred to as *object representations;* the area of study that explores the relationship of the self to inner objects is the theory of *object relations;* some include interpersonal relations in this definition.

Oral

The psychosexual phase during the first 18 months of life during which the mouth, lips, and tongue are the major source of sensual pleasure; because the infant is dependent on the mother during this stage, optimal development allows the infant to acquire a sense of trust and a sense that the world is safe and needs will be met.

Phallic–oedipal

The psychosexual stage occurring between the ages of 3 and 6; this phase begins as the penis or clitoris becomes the major source of sensual pleasure; the child develops an intense desire to possess exclusively the parent of the opposite sex and to eliminate the perceived rival other parent; the jealous conflict of a triangular relationship, with attendant fantasies related to castration, leads eventually to identification with the parents and the development of the superego.

Pleasure–unpleasure principle

The tendency of the mind to work toward achieving pleasure and avoiding unpleasure; according to Freud, this serves to reduce the amount of drive tension or mental stimulation, because pleasure represents a discharge of mental energy, and unpleasure represents an increase in undischarged mental energy.

Preconscious

In Freud's topographic model, psychic material not occurring as "deeply" in the mind as conscious or unconscious material; can be experienced consciously through attention.

Primary process

Type of thought occurring in the unconscious, characterized by irrationality, wishfulness, and domination by emotions and instinctual drives; the logic of primary process uses mechanisms seen in dreams such as displacement, condensation, and symbolism.

(continued)

Table 5–1 *(continued)*

Psychic determinism

All psychological events in the present are influenced and shaped by past experiences; nothing in mental life occurs solely by chance.

Repetition compulsion

The tendency to repeat periodically the same, usually painful, experience; this is also referred to as the "neurosis of destiny"; because repetition compulsion is closely linked historically and conceptually with Freud's idea of death instinct, the more recent term "compulsion to repeat" may be preferable.

Resistance

The automatic opposition to free association that is activated to protect against the emergence of awareness of inner unconscious conflicts.

Secondary process

Rational, logical, controlled thinking that characterizes the ordinary conscious stream of thought.

Stages of psychosexual development

(See *oral, anal,* and *phallic*—the three stages.) Regular sequence of development of the instinctual drives; the expression of drives centers on and is organized around specific sensual anatomical regions (oral, anal, and phallic), which change in pleasurable emphasis in a specific inborn order as the infant grows and develops; multiple other developmental phenomena occur during these stages and are interwoven with the psychosexual phenomena during each phase. (See Fig. 5–1).

Structural model

Freud's later model (following topographic model) of psychic functioning, which categorizes three mental structures (see *ego, id,* and *superego*) defined as collections of psychological processes and functions.

Superego

In Freud's structural model, the group of mental functions that represent morals, standards (see also *ego-ideal*), prohibitions, and conscience, and generate the affects of guilt and shame; it is acquired through internalization of parental figures through identification.

Therapeutic alliance

The rational, nonneurotic, conscious relationship between patient and doctor based on the mutual agreement to work together for the patient's benefit.

Topographic model

Freud's first model (the structural model followed) of psychic functioning, which classifies three "regions" (see *conscious, preconscious,* and *unconscious*) of mental operations in terms of their relationship to consciousness.

Transference

The unconscious displacement of feelings, attitudes, and expectations from important persons in the patient's childhood to current relationships.

Unconscious

Everything in the mind outside of normal conscious awareness; processes here are irrational, obey primary process logic, and may be revealed through dreams, a slip of the tongue (parapraxis), or free associations.

tions. In any scientific theory there is an interrelationship between the various hypotheses and concepts, with some being more basic and better established than others. In psychoanalytic theory, its various components are sometimes referred to as "points of view" (Rapaport, 1960).

The concept of *psychic determinism* provides the orienting attitude and groundwork on which everything else in psychoanalytic theory rests. It means that *all psychological events are determined by antecedent ones and that nothing occurs by chance in mental life.* The *unconscious* or *topographic point of view,* like psychic determinism, is so well established that these two hypotheses have been described as "established laws of the mind" (Brenner, 1974: 2). The term *unconscious* means *unnoticeable* and refers to mental processes and content that are significant and important in determining behavior but of which the person is *unaware. Unconscious* is used in psychoanalysis both as an adjective and a noun, and the latter refers to a portion of the mind sometimes called the *dynamic unconscious,* which contains drives, feelings, and ideas held out of conscious awareness by countering forces.

Freud's first theory of the mind and of intrapsychic conflict was the *topographic model* in which the mind was divided into *conscious, unconscious* (repressed), and *preconscious* (the preconscious being capable of becoming conscious under directed attention). The *conscious* province of the mind was governed primarily by what was referred to as *secondary process* (rational, logical thinking). The unconscious, on the other hand, was governed by different laws referred to as *primary process*—irrational thought processes that defy Aristotelian logic and are closely linked to emotional states; primary process includes the type of symbolic thought that characteristically occurs in dreams.

Freud (1900) wrote *The Interpretation of Dreams* within the framework of the topographic model, which subsequently (Freud, 1923) became subordinate to the *structural model* (discussed later). Freud's monumental discoveries about the meaning of dreams also served to confirm the significant findings from his earlier research with hysteria, such as the importance of the unconscious, the instinctual drives, and the influence of past developmental experiences on the present. His understanding of dreams led to the formulation of a new general psychology.

Dreams

With respect to dream theory, current evidence indicates that dreams serve a variety of purposes, including activation of brain circuitry to maintain the functional integrity of dendritic and synaptic connections, storage of memories, and the integration of data about new life experiences with preexisting cognitive and emotional response patterns (Winson, 1985). According to classic Freudian psychoanalytic theory, one of the most important functions of dreaming is the expression, fulfillment, or gratification of unconscious infantile wishes or impulses in a disguised or difficult-to-recognize form. Put simply, the dream may be a coded message and *represents a wish fulfillment.*

On awakening, the dream that is consciously remembered is referred to as the *manifest dream.* It is never what it seems to be, but rather, is a product of the action of dream activity on the *latent dream content,* which consists of unconscious infantile urges, wishes, and conflicts. The dream is also shaped by one's ongoing daily concerns, known as the *day residue,* and by any physical sensations occurring during sleep, such as discomfort or noise.

The mental activity that transforms the latent dream content into the manifest dream is referred to as the *dream work.* Unconscious impulses, memories, day residue, and physical sensations are reworked, disguised, and distorted during the dream work by specific mechanisms described by Freud. *Condensation* is the process by which a large amount of unconscious material is combined and expressed in a single event or image in the manifest dream. Often one thing in the manifest dream represents the simultaneous expression of multiple unconscious urges, conflicts, or thoughts and feelings. *Displacement* is the mechanism that disguises the meaning of the dream by changing the object toward which the impulse is directed or the person to whom the feeling is attached. This results in the strange or illogical quality of dream imagery. The emotional charge belonging to an important latent idea is transferred to a more neutral or innocuous manifest image. Foreground material in the *manifest* dream may then represent less significant *latent* content, whereas some of the lesser events in the manifest dream may be associated with more important latent content. *Symbolism* is the mechanism by which an unconscious idea is represented metaphorically in the manifest dream by something else. Finally, in the *dream work,* the various distorted themes and images are woven into a relatively coherent story line, a process known as *secondary elaboration.*

In psychoanalysis, dream analysis can lead to insights about defensive processes and resistances, the state of the transference, and important childhood events in addition to unconscious instinctual strivings (wishes). In early psychoanalytic history, dreams were considered *the* "royal road to the unconscious," in contrast to the current view that dreams are *one* important and unique source of data for analysis.

A CASE STUDY

A young man in psychotherapy had often described the anger he felt as a child toward his mother, and a dream helped to provide a better understanding of this anger. He depicted his mother as self-centered, inhibited, and depressed. He suspected she was sexually frigid with his father. In recent sessions he felt envious of his psychiatrist. He reported a dream: "I was in a hospital and realized I was an intern. I was wheeling a woman on a gurney. She was supposed to have a complicated operation but it's like she was going to die anyway. She looked like my friend's mother. Then I was in my parents' basement where my father had a workshop, and the woman was lying on the workbench. I was supposed to perform the operation but didn't know what to do. I put a big pill into her mouth. Then I woke up. I felt anxious."

He noted that certain aspects of the woman in the dream also reminded him of his mother. He began talking for the first time about a wish he had had throughout much of his life—that he could somehow make his mother feel better, make her happier, so she would love him and respond to him. The psychiatrist made a mental note of the oedipal wish also expressed in the dream, of the patient operating on his mother on his father's workbench, and its similarity to his replacing his father in the parental bed. Toward the end of the session the patient stated, "I'd like to bring her here so you could cure her, but there's something about the idea of her lying on your couch that makes me angry."

The Dynamic Point of View

The description of the unconscious and the topographic model continues with the *dynamic or motivational point of view.* Freud's belief that behavior is in part determined by *wishes* or *needs* ("instinctual drives" in psychoanalytic theory) that are biologically derived was based on two familiar observations: (1) that behavior is *not always triggered by external stimulation* but often occurs without it, as though spontaneously; and (2) behavior, in general, may be observed to have causally determined goal-directed components (Rapaport, 1960:48).

Experienced as an inner pressure, the instinctual drives in Freud's theory aim toward satisfaction, guided by the compass of "the pleasure-unpleasure principle leading toward activities that provide gratification and away from those that provide pain" (Cooper et al, 1989:2). Instinctual drives require something (usually termed *object* in psychoanalytic theory) through which or in regard to which they can achieve their aims, and the coordination between drive and object are now assumed to be guaranteed by evolution (i.e., the infant's need to nurse at the mother's breast).

It is important to note that the instinctual drives of humans differ significantly from the instincts of other animals. *"Instincts" refers to innate, biologically inherited propensities to respond in stereotypic ways that have individual or species survival value.* Certain complex behaviors of animals, such as mating rituals and migrations of birds, have survival value and are *unlearned.* The instinctual drives of humans, while they may have great compelling force, do not always *necessarily* have survival value. In addition, because of intelligence factors, humans have a great capacity for learning and problem solving (an *ego* capacity in psychoanalytic terms) that, coupled with a long and complex process of social and emotional development, leads to extensive plasticity and adaptability.

Two basic drives are most often emphasized by psychoanalysts, the *sexual* and the *aggressive.* Although Freud defined sexual in a broad way, equating it with sensual or pleasurable (1905), the term sexual drive has continued to be *erroneously* used as a synonym for sex and/or for sexual intercourse. In most of the manifestations of the drives that we can observe, the sexual and the aggressive components are intermingled. Although part of our constitutional endowment, the instinctual drives undergo a complex development (psychosexual development) and will be described later in conjunction with the *developmental point of view.*

The **adaptive point of view** in psychoanalytic theory refers to external reality as a source of stimuli, and this thesis has undergone greater change in psychoanalytic psychology than any other (Rapaport, 1960). Of central importance are the contributions of Hartmann (1948, 1958). The human organism from this point of view is considered to be a product of evolution and is born preadapted to reality. The ego develops as an internal regulator of behavior and becomes the human's "organ of adaptation." Reality and adaptation "are the matrix of all behavior" (Rapaport, 1960:60–61).

The **developmental hypothesis,** or the *genetic point of view* (the term *genetic* referring here to a process of development—not in the sense of cell biology) was implicit even in Freud's earliest work. From this point of view, every behavior is the product of two basic interacting factors: (1) intrinsic forces, which are *antecedent* to and *independent* of experience; and (2) *experiential* factors, which are based on learning or other forms of environmental influence. In this conception, all behaviors are part of a continuum extending back to earliest infancy. Furthermore, development is not a straight line process forward but rather occurs in a series of progressions and regressions. The clinically important concepts of regression and fixation are interrelated and are intrinsic aspects of the developmental hypothesis.

Regression, mentioned earlier as a frequent behavioral reaction observed in patients during the stress of both physical and psychiatric illness, refers to the *turning back* from a more mature pattern of behavior to a more immature or childlike state of feeling and thinking. The process of regression often serves a self-protective or defensive purpose. The following case history is illustrative of this process.

A CASE STUDY

A 55-year-old university professor was transferred to the oncology unit after being diagnosed with colon cancer. After surgery that resulted in a colostomy, he became increasingly withdrawn and uncommunicative. He told his physician that he was certain his wife of 30 years no longer loved him, and he wondered if she would continue to visit. He became apathetic and uninvolved in his treatment,

> *even though his physicians were optimistic about his prognosis. He begin to depend on the nurses for bathing and feeding, acting as if he were physically incapable of managing himself. A formerly proud, independent, and dignified man, his behavior became more dependent and helpless. He complained, whined, and became angry when his demands were not met immediately.*
>
> *This patient "regressed" to an earlier mode of functioning in reaction to the diagnosis of cancer. Such regression of ego functioning is often associated with the development of depression, increased dependency needs, and preoccupation with the fears characteristic of early childhood. In this case, the patient subsequently revealed that he experienced his surgery not only as a mutilation of his body but was ashamed and embarrassed by the loss of control of his bowels imposed by the colostomy. He also felt helpless, afraid, and had an intense need to be cared for, but hated these feelings of dependency at the same time.*

The concept of *fixation* refers to an arrest or failure in the developmental process. There is a tendency for areas of development that are not fully mastered to retain a component of continued or unresolved emphasis in the person's behavior that plays a role in later personality functioning. The concepts of fixation and regression are strongly linked to each other because under stress there is a tendency of patients to *regress* to stages of developmental immaturity in which they may be *fixated*. In Freud's thinking, the degree of *regression* was determined in part by the level of the patient's developmental immaturity or "point of fixation" in psychosexual development. These ideas were central in his thinking about the etiology of neurosis. The following elaboration of the developmental hypothesis will help to clarify these concepts further.

PSYCHOSEXUAL DEVELOPMENT

Based on evidence from adult and childhood analyses as well as child observations, Freud postulated an inborn developmental sequence of *psychosexual stages* according to which areas of the body progressively achieved primacy in regard to certain pleasurable sensations and activities. He termed these modes of functioning *oral, anal,* and *phallic*. Under normal circumstances, Freud postulated that there is a more or less orderly progression from one "zone" to the next, with each phase merging into the next as psychosexual development proceeds. However, conflicts at any stage of development could result in fixation and regression to an earlier unmastered developmental phase.

The *oral stage* of psychosexual development in this theory occurs approximately during the first year and a half of life. During this stage, the mouth, lips, and tongue are the primary areas of pleasurable sensations and gratification; and the majority of the child's activities and relationships to others occur principally through the oral cavity and mucosa. The prototype of oral pleasure is the baby nursing at the breast. This is a period of absolute dependence on the mother for nourishment, pleasurable sensation, and a secure atmosphere. A sense of trust should develop that the world is a safe place and that the child's basic needs will be met. Evidence of difficulties encountered during the oral period of development are sometimes revealed in the personalities of adults, especially during times of stress, as in the following case.

A CASE STUDY

A 30-year-old woman was followed as an outpatient in a general medical practice. She tended to be unusually clinging and dependent on the physician for reassurance, although she recognized that she was basically physically healthy. She was extremely sensitive to the slightest delay and sometimes remarked that her physician was not "warm enough," never gave her enough time, and probably "really didn't care." She often made demands for medication and had a tendency to become dependent on tranquilizers and sleeping pills. In expressing her need for a secure, consistent, and dependable caretaker, she was both clinging and needy but, at the same time, was unable to trust her physician, and was silently resentful toward him. Exploration of her early family life revealed evidence of a cold, inconsistent, and neglectful mother who gave little emotional nurturance to her children, leaving them with unmet yearnings to be cared for, nurtured, and protected.

Such personality traits and modes of interpersonal behavior may result from fixation at and/or regression to the oral phase of development. This period of infancy is marked by feelings of helplessness, dependency, and need for nurturance and protection. Children who are neglected, deprived, or abused, either physically or emotionally, during this period of development may experience a lifelong unmet intense "hunger" for love and may feel a sense of insecurity accompanied by a basic mistrust of others; they often both expect and fear that they will be hurt or rejected in interpersonal relationships. These difficulties with trust, attachment, and commitment may be complicated by a sense that they are unlovable or not worthwhile. When unmet needs for love, mixed with fear of rejection and feelings of anger, frustration, low self-esteem, and depression become intrinsic parts of the personality makeup, there are often also difficulties establishing stable adult relationships. This stage of development is also discussed in the context of attachment theory in Chapters 8 and 9 and

Eriksonian psychosocial theory in Chapter 10. The neurobiological effects of developmental trauma in this phase of development are discussed in Chapter 11.

The *anal stage,* which Freud termed *sadistic–anal* to emphasize the importance of the *aggressive* drive in this stage, occurs from about *18 months to 3 years.* The anal and rectal mucosa, as well as the feces themselves, are a main source of both pleasurable and unpleasurable sensations, which become a focus of the child's interest. During this period, anal sphincter control develops, and the child acquires a sense of mastery and autonomy. Struggles for control often ensue as the child has more freedom to produce or withhold bowel movements. The child simultaneously begins to experience some degree of independence and a new sense of control over other aspects of life.

Developmental issues at this stage are marked by struggles over control versus lack of control, obedience versus defiance, protest versus submission, and giving versus withholding, leading to the unfortunate labeling of this period as the "terrible twos." The frequent use of the word "no" is not necessarily a sign of defiance and stubbornness but a way of the child to assert his or her own needs and wishes, resist unwanted intrusion of the parents, and protect self-interests independent of the wishes of the parents. It is a time when the child is testing his or her assertion, aggression, and independence, and represents an effort to exert some degree of independent control. Problems during this stage of development are often associated with family environments that are strict, rigid, overly controlling, critical, and emotionally constricted. Children's early attempts at expressing anger and assertiveness are sometimes responded to with severe criticism and punishment in such settings, resulting in the perception that certain emotions are bad, dangerous, or unacceptable. The resentment and frustrations of being unable to express their own angry feelings are then repressed and may require rigid personality defenses to maintain a sense of control. Such persons as adults may appear to be emotionally rigid, aloof, and constrained, and have difficulties expressing affectionate as well as angry feelings. In psychiatric terminology these traits are characteristic of *obsessive–compulsive* personalities.

A critical, demanding, perfectionistic family atmosphere may contribute to smoldering resentment. This situation, combined with a fear of expressing their feelings, makes the core problem of obsessive–compulsive patients one of unresolved anger and fear of both punishment and loss of the parent's love and approval. Attempts to gain parental love by achieving and being "perfect" may become a driving force in the personality. Hence, the person's self-esteem becomes overly dependent on productivity and approval from external sources. The following is illustrative.

A CASE STUDY

A 40-year-old businessman was admitted to the hospital for evaluation of abdominal pain. He was polite, but his manner was formal, tense, controlled, and emotionally distant. While undergoing diag-

nostic procedures, he appeared constantly indecisive, demanding a thorough and logical explanation for each step in the diagnostic process. He was stubborn at times and submitted slowly and reluctantly to the most routine recommendations and requests. He experienced the medical workup as an issue of control and as being "forced" into something he did not want to do.

This patient's behavior indicated a central conflict reflecting ambivalence over the childhood issue, "Should I obey or say 'no'?" If the physician respects this sort of patient's need for control and independence and provides careful detailed explanations, "power struggles" and treatment failures can often be avoided.

According to Freud, the *phallic,* or the *phallic–oedipal* stage, is next to occur and extends from about age 3 to age 6. The leading organ of pleasure during this stage is the phallus (the penis for the boy and the clitoris for the girl), and masturbatory stimulation results in pleasure that more closely approaches the usual sense of the word "sexual" (see also Chapters 7 and 8).

Freud considered the *Oedipus complex,* which occurs during this stage of development, to be of central importance in both normal and pathological psychological development. The central defining features of the Oedipus complex relate to the attitude of the child toward the parent of the opposite sex. From the little boy's perspective, he wishes to possess mother exclusively and eliminate father; from the little girl's perspective, the wish is to eliminate mother and take her place with father. In order to fully understand and appreciate the Oedipus complex and its decisive influence on subsequent development and functioning, several factors need to be further emphasized.

By the age of 4 or 5, the child has reached a level of development of conceptual thinking characterized by a *qualitative* as well as a *quantitative* difference in perceptual and cognitive capacities. Children are able to fantasize and to recognize within themselves the existence of feelings of love, hate, jealousy, and fear, much as they occur in later life. Furthermore, they are able to perceive their parents not only in terms of their sexual differences but also in terms of the parents having some kind of relationship, including a sexual one, from which the child is excluded. This *triangular* relationship is characteristic of the oedipal phase and differentiates it from the "preoedipal" child's relationships, which are predominantly dyadic or "two-wayed." In addition, the intensity of the feelings associated with the Oedipus complex is comparable to the most passionate love affair in adult life. The child's situation may be further complicated by the fact that the jealously hated rival—the parent of the same sex—is also someone who is loved. Wishes to eliminate the feared and hated rival may result in intense fears of punishment for these hostile wishes but also the threat of the loss of the parent's love.

As the little boy enters the oedipal phase, his primary attachment is already to his mother, and his developing mental fantasy life begins to center on wanting to possess her exclusively in some sexual way, which is still poorly defined in his mind. The stirrings within him are expressed in wishes such as to look at her, touch her, and marry her. He may show increasing jealousy and hostility toward his father, who is viewed as a rival for mother's affections, that culminate in wishes to get rid of father in some way. Resultant fears that father will find out about his wishes and retaliate by punishing him, possibly by even castrating him, combined with his wishes to maintain his loving relationship with his father, lead him to renounce his wishes for mother and to strengthen his *identification* with father. It is as if the little boy says to himself, "I can't have Mommy, so I'll give up my wishes for her and grow up to be like Daddy and marry someone like Mommy."

The situation with the little girl is more complicated and also extremely controversial. Freud (1925) thought that the little girl's first "phallic" impulses were directed toward the mother just like the little boy's and that her attention was focused on her clitoris much like the little boy's is focused on his penis. Thus, the little girl's oedipal phase *begins* with masculine strivings. When the little girl discovers the little boy's penis, she feels that her clitoris is "inferior" and experiences this as a "narcissistic injury," a degrading humiliation that leads both to "penis envy" and a blaming of her mother for the plight. According to classic Freudian theory, this leads to a relinquishing of mother as the primary source of love and a turning to the father in hopes that he will provide her with a penis or a baby as a substitute. In the little girl's mind, her mother now becomes the jealous rival. Freud (1925:256) thought, *"Whereas in boys the Oedipus complex is destroyed by the castration complex, in girls it is made possible and led up to by the castration complex."* The oedipal dynamics of girls tend to be repressed relatively less than the oedipal conflict of boys, possibly due to the relatively lesser quantity of anxiety over the threat of genital damage in comparison to boys. Hence girls continue during development to be more noticeably attached to their fathers and more openly in conflict with their mothers. Freudian theory holds that threats of punishment, loss of love, or the fantasy of genital damage by the father's penis normally contribute to repression and resolution of this conflict.

Freud believed, then, that feminine identification is a developmental byproduct of a primary sense of *genital inferiority,* and that *penis envy,* the discontent with one's own genitals and the desire to possess a penis or other masculine qualities, persists unconsciously as a core determinant of personality in women. This theory emphasized only what the little girl does not have rather than what she does have. Although many psychoanalysts have reported findings from selected patients that tended to confirm Freud's view of female sexual development, others such as Stoller (1968, 1976), Blum (1976), and Kleeman (1976) have emphasized a girl's *primary femininity* as had been proposed much earlier by Horney (1926), Jones (1948), and Fenichel (1945). Current theory derived from clinical work and observation of children (Chehrazi, 1986) indicates that early in development girls recognize and form mental representations of their genitals and experience them in a positive and pleasurable way. Identifying with the mother and expressing wishes for a baby occur prior to the oedipal conflict. (Additionally, a boy may also experience a sense of genital inferiority as he recognizes in fantasy that "his penis is much too small for his mother's genital and [he] reacts with the dread of his own inadequacy, of being dejected and derided" [Horney, 1932].)

The recognition of anatomical differences is an important event for both sexes. Some girls may experience curiosity and envy for the penis as a transient phase specific reaction, which is normally worked through and resolved. Derivatives relating to conflicts at this stage of development have been observed to reemerge in some women in the context of regression, neurosis, or narcissistic character pathology, and is evidenced by hostile rivalry toward men with feelings of inadequacy and sexual dysfunction. Freud also suggested that the development of the superego, which occurs as a consequence of resolving the Oedipus complex, is inadequate in women. However, this component of his theory has been discarded, and, in contemporary theory, the female superego is not inferior to the male counterpart but differs in content. Obviously, these Freudian theories of female development have incited controversy and severe criticism.

Resolution of the Oedipal Stage

Eventually, for both boys and girls, reality dictates that an exclusive relationship with the parent of the opposite sex is not possible, resulting in the so-called oedipal defeat. Sexual identity becomes crystallized as identifications with the parent of the same sex are solidified. The wish to possess the parent of the opposite sex and the intensely competitive feelings toward the parent of the same sex become repressed. A variety of possible traumas during this period (such as disturbed family interactions; emotional, physical, or sexual abuse; loss of a parent; and illnesses and operations) may contribute to neurotic pathology.

Disturbances in development prior to the oedipal stage often distort the oedipal situations. For example, if a girl has a cold, unavailable, or rejecting mother, she may turn to the father prematurely and intensely for nurturance and support, resulting in an overly sexualized attachment to him in the oedipal period. Anger toward the unempathic or emotionally rejecting mother may persist with an inner core of unmet needs for love and acceptance. In an effort to get father's attention and compete with mother, the prototypical theatrical, dramatic, attention-seeking, seductive "little girl" routine may become a persistent and ingrained adult personality trait. While these persons may be "seductive" in a sense, the behavior relates unconsciously to the use of their femininity and sexual attractiveness to gain love and attention to compensate for the frustrating relationship with their mother. Hence, adult sexualized relationships have as a fundamental goal securing maternal nurturance and closeness and controlling men.

In boys, another variant of the oedipal conflict results when a cold, rejecting, or unavailable father provides an untenable model for identification. The boy, therefore, becomes intensely involved with mother and also identifies predominantly with her, leading to the so-called effeminate male or male hysteric. Special problems may result if the father is demeaning, humiliating, or abusive, thereby compounding the sense of anger and frustration in the child through further injuries to his sense of self-esteem. Hence, little boys who are subjected to intense teasing, criticism, and humiliation by their fathers (where the father is competitive with his son for the wife's attention) may develop painful self-doubts about their basic masculinity, adequacy, and competence. The hypermasculine "macho" personality sometimes represents an attempt to compensate for and deny traumatic shame and humiliation experienced during the phallic–oedipal stage of psychosexual development. These persons are recognized in adulthood as always needing to prove their masculinity in various types of hyperaggressive, hypersexual, and risk-taking behaviors.

One classic example of behavior that indicates unresolved oedipal issues in both adult men and women is the repetitive pattern of becoming intensely attracted to persons of the opposite sex whom they "cannot have" or who are in some way unavailable or inappropriate. This is a repetition of the effort to competitively secure the love of the unavailable parent of the opposite sex, which was never resolved. The typical dilemma for such persons is that, even if they are eventually able to secure the love of their longed-for romantic object, they may soon lose interest and move on to another "conquest" in an effort to again win love, approval, and affirmation of their self-worth.

There are many other variations on the oedipal theme. Personality characteristics that are often evidence of unresolved oedipal-related issues in adults include intense concerns over competitiveness, rivalry, jealousy with underlying feelings of insecurity, excessive guilt, and conflicts about success.

Massive trauma in psychosexual development can occur if children are subjected to overt sexual molestation, abuse, or incest, or if the parent is covertly and overtly sexually seductive with the child. While sexual abuse was once thought to be a rare event, it has been estimated that as many as 10% to 25% of female children may have been subjected to some form of sexual abuse, with alcoholism in the family being a primary risk factor. While a discussion of the pervasive impact that sexual abuse may have on children's psychosexual development and their later interpersonal and sexual relationships is beyond the scope of this text, one may say that the effects are often devastating and cause lasting problems if psychotherapeutic treatment is not received.

A CASE STUDY/OEDIPAL

Mr. H., a 24-year-old medical student, sought consultation with the student health psychiatrist for his inability to perform successfully on two successive medical licensing examinations, a requirement for graduation. Prior to the current difficulties, he was an accomplished student with an impressive academic record and no history of test failures. His current failure interfered not only with his becoming a physician, but also with his upcoming marriage, which, his fiancee said, was contingent upon his obtaining his medical degree.

Over the course of several evaluation sessions, the psychiatrist and Mr. H. discussed many issues, including Mr. H.'s relationship with his parents and peers. His father was described as competitive and angry, bitter about not having a college education; his mother as kind and compassionate, "too good for my father." Socially, Mr. H. had numerous friends and described several casual sexual encounters during college but no sustained relationships with women other than the current engagement of 2 years.

A course of psychoanalytically oriented psychotherapy was begun, and it became evident that Mr. H. feared his father's anger. Mr. H. was unconsciously fearful that if he were to become more successful than his father, his father would react in a hostile and competitive way. By not passing his examination and graduating, and thus not besting his father, Mr. H. avoided any imagined paternal reprisals. Not graduating also served to postpone indefinitely Mr. H.'s wedding, for the marriage was viewed as a further triumph over his father, an Oedipal victory by a union with a woman who unconsciously represented Mr. H.'s mother. This fantasized victory brought with it guilt, guilt that could be warded off by his failure in the examination. With therapy, Mr. H. eventually came to view his failure as a compromise formation, a vestige of Oedipal triangulation, and saw that his unconscious fears were inhibiting his happiness and success.

THE DEVELOPMENT OF THE EGO AND THE STRUCTURAL MODEL

We now turn from the subject of the stages of psychosexual development to the concept of the *ego.* In Freud's earliest work, the term *ego* stood for the person, self, or consciousness, which, in turn, was equated with "the dominant mass of ideas" (Freud, 1893–1895:116). *Defenses* or *ego defense mechanisms* were associated with consciousness, and the unconscious was used to refer to that part of the mind in which unacceptable wishes, feelings, and ideas were sequestered from conscious awareness.

As Freud developed his psychoanalytic techniques with an increasing emphasis on free association, and his clinical experience expanded, he observed that psychological defenses against forbidden or painful unconscious material were also unconscious. Furthermore, he recognized that self-punitive tendencies could also be outside of awareness (such as unconscious sense of guilt). These and other observations led to Freud's elaboration of the *structural model* in 1923. "Structure" is not being referred to here in a physical or anatomical sense; in psychoanalytic theory mental structures are defined as those determiners of behavior whose rate of change is slow; therefore, they have a relatively stable, enduring, or permanent quality. The structures of the structural model are *hypothetic constructs* that are defined by their psychological functions in mental life. The three major components of the structural model are the *id, ego,* and *superego,* which are discussed below.

The *id* is closely tied to biological endowment and is considered the source of motivation (instinctual drives). Wishes are considered to be derived from the drives. The id functions unconsciously and in accordance with the *pleasure principle;* that is, it strives for immediate and complete gratification without regard for reality.

The *superego,* which also functions in a largely unconscious manner, includes the moral values, standards, and prohibitions that are internalized in the course of development. The superego or conscience prohibits and is punitive (i.e., by guilt). The superego also includes the *ego ideal,* which embodies the goals and aspirations of the person and is important in the regulation of self-esteem and mood. It originates during early development and is modified during subsequent developmental phases as the idealized qualities of significant others are internalized. Although major internalization of the ego ideal occurs as the oedipal conflict is resolved, this structure reaches its definitive quality during late adolescence (Blos, 1974).

Some analysts consider the ego ideal to be a substructure of the ego rather than the superego, and others think it is an altogether separate mental structure. One major function of the ego ideal is protection against narcissistic injury (damage to self-esteem), because a person can compare his or her thoughts and behavior against internal standards rather than with idealized others. Pathology of the ego ideal contributes to disorders of self-esteem regulation as observed in patients with narcissistic personality disorder and depression (Bibring, 1953; Reich, 1960). Conflict of the ego with the superego can produce the emotions of guilt and/or shame.

Although most analysts agree that the superego as an autonomous, structured, functional entity is established in conjunction with the resolution of the Oedipus complex, its development does not begin or end at this point. The superego is developmentally closely linked to the ego, and both agencies evolve through processes known as *identification* and *internalization*. The external prohibitions and restraints of the parents are transformed into internal regulators by the child because of fear of punishment and need for the parent's love (to offend or displease the parent would bring about rejection). Thus, precursors to the superego begin during the anal stage of development, if not even earlier, and are evidenced by a change from pleasure in messiness and rebellion to pride in cleanliness and control. The postoedipal (approximately ages 6 to 8—early latency) superego is characteristically harsh and severe but not fully reliable in controlling behavior. This severity of superego tends to decrease in late latency (ages 8 to 12). Further transformation in the superego based on new identifications with peers and cultural standards during adolescence results in more autonomy and the ability to make one's own decisions and regulate self-esteem internally. Hence, one begins to make choices based more on one's own value judgment and moral standards rather than being controlled by the dictates of the internalized parental superego developed during childhood. The ego's functions include those that relate to reality (i.e., reality testing and adaptation to reality), regulation of drives and feelings, defensive reactions, relationships to other people, intellectual synthesis and integration, and autonomous activities (perception, cognition, and motility, and so forth). All of these functions undergo a gradual development beginning in infancy. Although some of the ego's functions are conscious, many are unconscious. No sharp line can be drawn between id and ego; they exist on a continuum and cannot be separated except in situations of conflict (Freud A, 1966).

A CASE STUDY

A young married man presented at his doctor's office with symptoms of a urinary tract infection (UTI). Physical examination and laboratory studies verified the diagnosis of a UTI, which responded well to antibiotic therapy. He returned later, however, complaining of unusual sensations in his penis and said that he was certain he had AIDS. Additional testing, including HIV serology, was negative. He insisted that despite the test results he must have AIDS. He complained that he had low energy, felt amotivated, had lost his appetite, and couldn't sleep. As the medical interview continued, he noted that he was feeling depressed and worried. About 8 weeks prior to the interview, he had attended a bachelor's party for his best friend at a local establishment where nude dancers performed. He left rather intoxicated and sexually aroused. On the way home he solicited a prostitute to perform oral sex on him. Afterward he immediately felt guilty and ashamed and lapsed into despair. He tortured himself with how he could do such a thing to his wife and young son. During the following weeks he kept secret what had happened but ruminated constantly how "dirty, depraved, and disgust-

*ing" he was. Later, when he developed dysuria, he somehow knew
he was doomed and had contracted AIDS.*

*He was referred to a psychiatrist who prescribed antidepressant
medication and a course of psychoanalytically oriented psychotherapy. During the psychotherapeutic work it became evident that he
set very high standards for himself as a husband and father. He
often longed for the freedom of his high school days, but he resolved
not to think about it and dedicated himself to his family responsibilities. He had a very strict conscience and often felt guilty in many
spheres of his life. He came to realize that believing he had AIDS was
in essence a form of self-punishment by which he sentenced himself
to death for the "sexual crime" he had committed. His subsequent
therapy revealed and highlighted the interaction of the psychic
agencies id, ego, superego, and ego ideal in his acute conflicts. He
was eventually able to view his sexual indiscretion in a more realistic light, and although he harbored regret and took responsibility
for his actions, he realized that his obsession with HIV reflected an
unconscious wish for punishment that was out of proportion to his
actual behavior.*

THE ROLE OF ANXIETY
IN PSYCHOANALYTIC THEORY

In conjunction with the structural theory, Freud described the *central
role of anxiety* in mental conflict in another of his major works, *Inhibitions,
Symptoms, and Anxiety* (1926). The concept of anxiety is inextricably linked
to his theories of neurosis. In two classic psychoanalytic case studies ("Little
Hans" and the "Wolf Man"), he recognized that anxiety causes repression
(forcing of ideas and feelings into the unconscious) and related the development of anxiety to *four typical danger situations,* each characteristic of a
particular stage of development. Freud postulated that when more stimuli
occur than can be adequately mastered by the immature ego, the situation
becomes traumatic for the child, and anxiety develops.

The first danger situation is loss of the nurturing or caretaking parent,
the primary "object" of the child's dependency and love (*loss of the object*). In
this situation, the fear is loss of or abandonment by the mother. The next
danger situation is fear of the *loss of the parent's love.* By the third or fourth
year, the fear is loss of the penis or *castration* in the boy and the analogous
fear of *genital damage* in the girl. The fourth danger, according to Freud,
occurs in conjunction with the resolution of the Oedipus complex and is the
fear of disapproval or punishment by the superego (*guilt*).

An additional aspect of Freud's theory of anxiety is the ego's ability to *anticipate* a danger situation and actively produce a small alerting amount of anx-

iety, which he called *signal anxiety*. Other feelings, such as depression, can also function in a warning capacity. This signal not only warns of danger but initiates psychological defensive activities to regulate, control, and ward off the threat from conscious awareness and protect against further disturbing feelings.

THE MECHANISMS OF DEFENSE

In the structural theory, intrapsychic conflict and anxiety are central. According to the *principle of multiple function*, all behavior serves several functions, is responsive to many pressures, or is a solution for many tasks. Thus, for the psychoanalyst, no behavior is *only* what it manifestly seems to be. Instinctual drives, defenses, unpleasurable affects (including guilt from the superego) are the components of psychic conflict that combine to form what Brenner has referred to as "*compromise formations*" (Brenner, 1982). All compromise formations are overdetermined (i.e., more than one wish or defense is represented simultaneously in all behaviors).

Ego *mechanisms of defense* are various automatic, involuntary, unconsciously instituted psychological activities that are activated in response to signals of anxiety or other unpleasurable feelings. The phenomenon of *repression* is considered the primary ego defense, and Anna Freud (1936) in her influential book, *The Ego and the Mechanisms of Defense*, describes other mechanisms of defense used by the ego, such as identification, isolation of affect, reaction formation, regression, undoing, projection, reversal, turning against the self, and sublimation (Table 5–2). She also notes defenses are often mistakenly equated with psychopathology, even though they are a necessary and adaptive aspect of personality development and functioning. The term *defense mechanisms* can be misleading because there are no special ego functions that serve *only* purposes of defense, and any aspect of ego function can be used for defensive purposes (Brenner, 1982).

As previously noted, signal anxiety alerts the ego to a conflictual situation that may lead to a danger situation or a combination of danger situations. The term *defense* indicates the ego's opposition to other components of the conflict, such as unacceptable wishes, painful affects, or self-punitive impulses. The ego's action may be conscious or unconscious and may result in observable behavior or in an inhibition and/or absence of expected behavior. It is important to remember that the ego may defend against a wide range of painful affects, such as depression, guilt, or shame, and that both the objects of defense and the defensive actions are numerous and diverse. For example, one feeling can be used to defend against another, such as an angry contempt of someone to ward off a sense of admiration and envy. Denial may be directed at an aspect of internal reality such as sexual longing or at an external reality such as the death of a loved one. The complex nature of conflict and the principle of multiple function described earlier make it impossible to categorize defenses completely.

Table 5–2 **Defense Mechanisms**

Delusional projection

Frank delusions about external reality, usually of a persecutory type.

Denial (psychotic)

Denial of external reality.

Distortion

Grossly reshaping external reality to suit inner needs.

Projection

Attributing one's own unacknowledged feelings to others.

Schizoid fantasy

Tendency to use fantasy, autistic retreat, and imaginary relationships for the purpose of conflict resolution and gratification.

Hypochondriasis

The transformation of reproach toward others arising from bereavement, loneliness, or unacceptable aggressive impulses into first self-reproach and then complaints of pain, somatic illness, and neurasthenia.

Passive-aggressive behavior

Aggression toward others expressed indirectly and ineffectively through passivity.

Acting out

Direct expression of an unconscious wish or impulse in order to avoid being conscious of the affect or the ideation that accompanies it.

Dissociation

Temporary but drastic modification of the integration of consciousness or memory, or of one's character or sense of personal identity, to avoid emotional distress.

Repression

Seemingly inexplicable naïveté, memory lapse, or failure to acknowledge input from a selected sense organ.

Displacement

The redirection of conflicted feelings toward a relatively less important object than the person or situation arousing the feelings.

Reaction formation

Conscious affect and/or behavior that is diametrically opposed to an unacceptable instinctual (id) impulse.

Intellectualization

Thinking about instinctual wishes in formal, bland terms that leave the associated affect unconscious.

(continued)

Table 5–2 **(continued)**

Altruism

Vicarious but constructive and instinctually gratifying service to others.

Humor

Overt expression of feelings without individual discomfort or immobilization and without unpleasant effect on others.

Suppression

The capacity to hold all components of a conflict in mind and then to postpone action, emotional response, or worrying.

Anticipation

Realistic anticipation of or planning for future inner discomfort.

Sublimation

Indirect or attenuated expression of instincts without adverse consequences or marked loss of pleasure.

(Adapted from Vaillant GE (ed): Empirical Studies of Ego Mechanisms of Defense. Washington, DC, American Psychiatric Press, 1986, pp 105–117)

Defenses develop in an approximate chronology, and empiric studies demonstrate that defensive styles correlate with independent measures of mental health and certain diagnostic categories (Vaillant, 1986). This has led to systems of classifying defenses (immature, neurotic, and mature) that tend to be oversimplified and perhaps misleading. The most mature person uses "immature" defense at times and vice versa (see Table 5–2). If defenses that are "normal" in early childhood, such as denial, projection, and splitting, persist into later years, severe psychopathology may result, such as that seen in patients with borderline personality disorder discussed later in this chapter.

THEORY OF NEUROSIS

The psychoanalytic theory of neurosis is grounded in the structural model. The basic tenet of the structural theory of neurosis is that intrapsychic conflict leads to *compromise* among the agencies of the mind. The extent to which the compromise is "neurotic" is determined by the degree of anxiety or other painful affect involved and the amount of maladaptive behavior entailed.

Any time the ego is confronted with impulses that, if gratified, would lead to psychic danger, the ego signals a conflict. It allows a small discharge of anxiety to initiate defenses against the threatening impulse and accommodates to the pressure of the drives, superego, and external reality with a compromise. It is the success of such compromises in terms of feelings and behavior that determines the health and stability of the person. Ideally, anxiety should be experienced primarily in its *signal function* (i.e., as an appropriate signal to possible danger), and the person's conduct should afford pleasure while being generally acceptable to others. A defense against an impulse can also help satisfy the impulse in a more acceptable way (e.g., displacement or sublimation). In cases of pathological guilt, the aggressive drive may be involved in superego acts of self-punishment. Every compromise has aspects of drive satisfaction, moral values, and accommodation to reality.

In what is known as a *symptom neurosis,* the compromise is felt as painful and maladaptive, and although the person may feel unable to alter the pattern, there is conscious acknowledgment of suffering and motivation to change. In *character neurosis,* the situation is somewhat different. The essence of character is in the repetitive and incessant use of certain defenses that gives the person a particular "stamp." Although character traits and defenses may be rigid and automatic, they often are relatively comfortable to the person and are termed *ego-syntonic,* indicating that they are not a source of distress. For these reasons, conflicts stemming from maladaptive character defenses may be more difficult to treat, and efforts to change such mechanisms are met with a great deal of resistance. From the patient's point of view, these characteristic compromises are familiar and sensible and may be described as "part of the way I am." The reasons for interpersonal conflicts are externalized and are believed to be due to the faults of others. An important insight from the study of character is the need to transform such defenses into *ego-dystonic* experiences with a subsequent motivation to change.

OBJECT RELATIONS THEORY OF DEVELOPMENT

The term *object* first appeared in psychoanalytic theory as an essential aspect of the definition of drive. Freud defined the term *object* as the thing toward which a drive is directed, and there could be no drives without objects. The term is often used to describe real people existing as a part of external reality, as well as images of those people within the mind. A multiplicity of object relations theories have evolved, and there are great differences, even among object relations theorists, as to how the term *object* or *object relations theory* should be defined.

In this presentation, we distinguish interpersonal relations, which refer to relationships with people in the real world, from internalized object relations, which is our main focus. The child's earliest experiences have dyadic (self-object) features even before there is clear differentiation between the self and object.

We have chosen to present the work of Spitz and Mahler to illustrate how the earliest structures of the psychic apparatus are built up during specific stages of development through the process of internalization of object relations. Their work is strongly empirically based and consistent with the important clinical and theoretical contributions of Jacobson and Kernberg. It must be remembered, however, that there are other, very different approaches to object relations theories, such as those of Klein, Fairbairn, Guntrip, Balint, and Winnicott.

Rene Spitz (1965) was probably the first major psychoanalytic investigator who used direct observations of the early mother–child relationships to study the development of object relations. (The term *object relations* in psychoanalytic terms usually refers to the relationship of the infant to anything other than him- or herself, which is at least initially the mother, then father, and later other "objects" of the person's attention and desire.)

Although Spitz was not the first investigator to note the smile of the infant that appears at around 6 weeks, he placed it in the context of social significance and considered it the *first organizer* of the psychic structure (Spitz, 1965). Spitz believed that during the first few weeks of life, neonates lived in a relatively undifferentiated, disconnected state, primarily perceiving only internal stimuli and little beyond their own bodies. This phase of development between birth and about 1 month of age was described similarly by Mahler, who called this period the *normal autistic phase* (Mahler et al, 1975). The mother's attuned responses to the child's needs are provided in such a way as to promote a sense of safety and to protect the infant from any excessive internal and external stimulation, stress, or discomfort.

Awareness of something other than oneself—initially the mother—who satisfies one's needs begins at about the second month of life, the beginning of the phase called *normal symbiosis.* As a result of the mother's helpful ministrations, infants begin to retain mental representations of her associated with reduction of tension and with pleasurable sensations such as satiety and cuddling. The infant's perception of mother, however, is still only fragmentary and not clearly differentiated from his or her own sense of self. It was postulated that infant and mother identities "share a common boundary" and sense of fusion or merger (symbiosis). The term *part-object* was used to designate that, at this time, the mother is only "partly" recognized in terms of her nurturing and/or frustrating functions, which could at times be perceived by the infant as inconsistent. "Good-mother" representations become associated with the all-fulfilling, nurturing, and pleasurable aspects of mother, and "bad-mother" representations become associated with aspects of mother that may be frustrating or do not meet the infant's demands for immediate gratification or are punitive or rejecting. Ideally, the child would integrate these separate aspects and responses of mother into a coherent unified mental representation so that the child realizes that one and the same mother can be both gratifying but occasionally frustrating as well. In addition, the child would also realize that seemingly conflicting emotions (anger and love) could be felt toward the same person at alternating times or that these two emotions could be experienced simultaneously (ambivalence).

The two earliest stages of relative nondifferentiation between infant and mother (normal autism and normal symbiosis) end at about 5 months in this model of development, and the formal phase of *separation-individuation* proper begins (Mahler et al, 1975; see Table 5–3 and Fig. 5–1).

The period of 6 to 36 months is a critical stage of development when a discrete self-concept and identity are developed based on a sense of awareness of separateness from mother. Patients with so-called *borderline* personality disorders have been associated with major developmental difficulties at this stage of development.

There are four *subphases* of separation–individuation. The first is called *differentiation* (5 to 7 months). It is heralded by the tendency of the increasingly alert child to push himself or herself back from the usual position

Table 5–3 **The Separation–Individuation Process**

PHASE/AGE	COMMENT
Normal autistic (Birth–1 month)	No differentiation of inside versus outside, "me" versus "not me."
	Experience of need-satisfying activities of mother blend with the experience of needs themselves.
	Establishment of physiological homeostatic equilibrium in new postpartum conditions.
Normal symbiotic (1 month–5 months)	Increased attention and interest in outside world.
	Dawning awareness of mother and establishment of specific bond with her (or primary caretaker).
	Specific smiling response.
Subphases	
A. Differentiation (5 months–7 months)	Increasing manual, tactile exploration of mother's face.
	Efforts to push back to take a look at mother.
	Comparison of mother with "other," familiar and unfamiliar (comparative scanning).
	Curiosity and wonder about external world with frequent "checking back to mother."
	Development of stranger anxiety.
B. Practicing (7 months–16 months)	"Early" practicing period with motility away from mother by crawling, climbing, and righting self.
	Practicing period "proper" heralded by free, upright locomotion.
	Rapid development of autonomous ego functions in close proximity to mother.
	Active exploration of environment with mother as "home base" and frequent trips back to her for "emotional refueling."
	Development of separation anxiety.
	Beginning of representational intelligence and first level of self-identity.

(continued)

Table 5–3 **(continued)**

C. Rapprochement (16 months–24 months)	Toddler more aware of loss of "ideal sense of self" when separated from mother.
	Experience of separateness as relative helplessness.
	Efforts made to regain union with mother by bringing and sharing objects with her, seeking attention and "wooing."
	Wish to be helped and soothed by mother immediately when needed while simultaneously wishing to retain autonomy and self-control (ambitendency).
	Frequent "no-win" situations for mother as she tries to foster autonomy and also provide safety and assistance for child.
D. Object constancy (24 months–36 months)	Establishment of self-representation as predominantly positive in spite of child's imperfections and limitations.
	Internal representation of mother as basically "good" and reliable, even though occasionally frustrating and disappointing.
	Recognition of mother as a separate person with wishes and preferences of her own.
	Increasing tolerance of separations and more trusting of adult substitutes.
	Continued development of a variety of ego functions allowing greater frustration tolerance, understanding of limits, and ability to obey simple rules for personal safety.

of molding to the mother's shoulder and "take a look." This early deployment of physical measures to "push back" from mother and scan and explore her visually is labeled the *hatching process.*

Practicing, the second subphase, encompasses a period of 7 to 16 months. It is evidenced by a dramatic maturation of motor function. The child can now crawl and explore and exhibits the joy of discovery. Toddlers at this stage feel omnipotent and oblivious to harm as they experience a "love affair with the world." Children during this phase often become so absorbed in and delighted with their activities that they are oblivious to mother, only occasionally needing to return to her for "refueling" and reassurance that she is consistently there to protect and nurture them as the need arises.

Rapprochement is the third phase of separation–individuation. It extends from about 16 months until 18 to 24 months. Mother is no longer taken for granted by the child. The child's increased awareness of being separate and having her own limitations in meeting all of her own needs threatens the child with a traumatic loss of self-esteem. For example, if the child is upset, hurt, or unable to carry out a task, he or she may be torn between wishes to be near

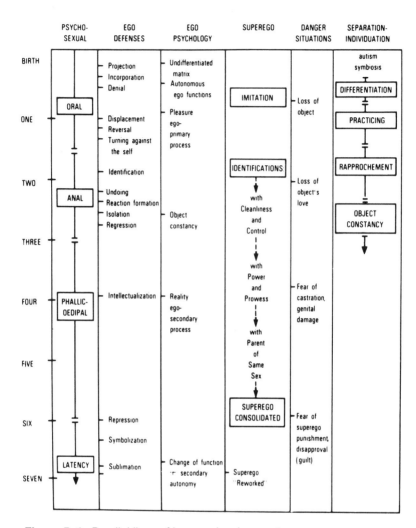

Figure 5–1. *Parallel lines of human development.*

mother and be comforted by her and a compulsion to move away from her and function independently. There may be periods of increased irritability and an increase in stranger and separation anxiety during this time. Mahler (1975) referred to the rapprochement period as a "crisis" because of the deep ambivalence and conflict within the toddler about dependence–independence issues. The mother, at this time, is confronted with frequent "no-win" situations. The resolution of this phase depends in large part on her ability to allow the child sufficient separation and autonomy while still being flexibly available for support "on demand." Difficulties in negotiating this period of great vulnerability have been associated with serious personality problems in adults. The following example illustrates the rapprochement phase.

A CASE STUDY

A 20-month-old boy was admitted to the pediatric unit for an asthma attack. This was his fourth admission in 5 months, and it was evident that there were problems with his taking medication at home. The mother felt that her son had become "impossible to handle." She stated, "He wants to take the medicine himself but he spills it, and when I try to help he resists and spits it out." The nurses observed that the mother quickly limited the child's appropriate explorations of the ward and was overly protective, and the child was frequently seen trying to free himself from her "hugs."

In this characteristic rapprochement phase conflict of separation–individuation, the mother needed to be supported in her efforts to do things for her son that he could not safely do alone, while also loosening the restraints on his explorations, curiosity, and attempts at independence.

In the third year of life, the fourth and final subphase unfolds, and the child ideally obtains what is known as *object constancy*. A secure sense of self is developed with differentiation between the self and a stable mental representation of the mother who can be seen as a distinct person with wishes and preferences of her own and experienced as "good" even when she is frustrating or disappointing.

The term *object constancy* has been used in two different ways, which has led to some confusion. In the cognitive sense, the term has been used to refer to the capacity to maintain a stable inner image of a person even when the person is not present. This use is derived from Jean Piaget's (see Chapter 8) concept of "object permanence" and is a prerequisite for the establishment of object constancy. Object constancy, which should solidify during the third year of life, refers to the ability to maintain an inner image or representation of the mother, the thought of which enables the child to experience a sense of safety, comfort, and love even in the mother's absence. Problems in the adult personality stemming from difficulties in attaining "object constancy" during separation–individuation are exemplified by the following case.

A CASE STUDY

A 25-year-old man was admitted to intensive care after taking an overdose. When he was alert, he described taking the pills "on impulse" after a fight with his girlfriend precipitated by her wish to leave him. His history revealed a pattern of self-destructive actions, particularly after frustrations and disappointments in close relationships. His relationships were usually stormy and chaotic, with frequent outbursts or rage when he felt rejected or disappointed by the other person. Although the young man saw people frequently and had a number of superficial friends, none of the relationships endured, and he usually felt painfully empty and depressed when alone. He was intolerant of the shortcomings of others and the inevitable disappointments in human relationships. He appeared to be unable to maintain an idea of another person as basically "good" when he felt that his needs were not being totally met. His emotional reactions to such frustrations alternated between rage and despair, and characteristically, his aggression became directed toward himself in a self-destructive manner.

In medical settings, persons of this sort often oscillate between idealizing and devaluing their physicians, depending on how thoroughly they feel their needs are being met at any given moment. It can be very difficult for the physician who is feeling unfairly attacked by an ungrateful patient to avoid responding by retaliating, by becoming angry, or by rejecting the patient. Some physicians will acquiesce to unreasonable demands to avoid feeling guilty in response to provocations, thereby avoiding the full blast of the patient's anger. The general pattern of alternating between idealization and devaluation of others is a general characteristic of borderline personalities. Separation–individuation theory will be discussed again in Chapters 8 and 10.

SELF THEORY AND THE DEVELOPMENT OF THE SELF

Another psychological theory that has developed out of the general framework of the psychoanalytic tradition is *self psychology*. It offers some important insights into certain aspects of personality development. The primary focus of self psychology as elucidated by Kohut (1971) is on the development and psychopathology of the core sense of self. Kohut defined and used the terms *self* and *narcissism* in a way that differed from other psychoanalysts. He considered the self to be a psychic structure, but not one of the "agencies" of the mind such as the ego or superego as described by Freud.

In attempting to understand patients with narcissistic personality disorders, Kohut observed and described specific kinds of psychological reactions, known as *transferences,* that emerged during his treatment of such patients. First, he described an "idealizing" transference that corresponds to the patient's image of the idealized parent; second, he described a "mirroring transference" that represents a component of the patient's own self-aggrandized image. Developmentally, Kohut postulated that the child's "grandiose" sense of self is the equivalent of "I am perfect; look at me"; the idealized image of the parent is "You are perfect, and I am a part of you." From these two structures, Kohut postulated a *separate developmental line* for the development of one's sense of "self." For example, the grandiosity, sense of invincibility, and exhibition-ism often seen in children (hence, the popularity of and identification with "super hero" cartoon characters) are the forerunners of initiative, ambition, and healthy self-esteem in the adult when developmental disturbances do not seriously interfere.

Kohut placed great emphasis on the need for the mother to be *empathic* with the child for the development of a healthy sense of self. The mother must provide "mirroring" or approving responses of pleasure and excitement to the child's exhibitionism and prevent sudden severe traumatic disappointments when the inevitable frustrations of reality are met and children painfully real-ize their own limitations. Thus he emphasized the mother's functions as a necessary regulator, modulator, and protector of the child's self-esteem through empathic responsiveness. The failure of the mother to help the child attenuate the infantile grandiosity and transform it into a realistic and healthy sense of self-esteem leads to pathology of the self as evidenced by a retention of grandiosity in the adult.

Persons with narcissistic personalities may display an air of arrogant grandiosity and entitlement. Their lives are a desperate search for power, at-tention, or money to shore up their sense of self and their basic sense of value. Patients with narcissistic personality disorders are often characterized by ego-centricity, self-importance, grandiosity, selfishness, and arrogance in varying degrees. They tend to relate to other people in an exploitive manner and use others primarily to embellish or meet their own needs. Persons with narcissis-tic personalities tend to be exquisitely sensitive to real or perceived injuries, slights, or losses. Physical injuries or illnesses are particularly troublesome, for the narcissist's fragile sense of self is often intimately tied to the body and physical appearance, and the physical loss is felt as an assault on the integrity of the self. Such losses are often met with profound rage. The following case illustrates the point.

A CASE STUDY

A middle-aged business executive came to the hospital with minor facial lacerations and a broken ankle after falling from his motor-cycle. After being triaged by the nurse and determined to have only relatively minor, non-life-threatening injuries, he was placed in a cubicle and asked to wait for the emergency room (ER) resident. He quickly became angry and abusive, demanding to know the qualifications of the ER physicians who have "obviously underesti-mated the severity of the injuries" and not attended to him quickly enough. He demanded to speak with the hospital administrator and the Chief of Staff. Reassurance by the ER resident that the injuries were minor and would heal quickly and without sequelae only fur-

ther enraged the patient. The Chief Resident, somewhat more psychologically sophisticated than the resident, knew that for this narcissistically vulnerable individual, no injury was minor and that all injuries were perceived as a threat to a fragile sense of self. The rage was fueled by the unconscious fear of irreparable damage. She communicated to the patient that she appreciated the severity of the injuries and that she takes them very seriously. The patient then became calm enough to be attended to by the ER staff.

Kohut considered the development of the self as *the* central issue in psychic development and thought the sexual and aggressive drives, so crucial in classic Freudian theory, were by-products of disturbed development of the self. His theory of psychopathology emphasizes defects in the development of self rather than intrapsychic conflicts. Classic Freudian analytic approaches based on resolving intrapsychic conflict are not necessarily incompatible with Kohut's emphasis on empathy and healing of the self in the therapeutic process. Empathy on the part of the therapist has always been an intrinsic part of traditional psychoanalytic treatment. Kohut's contributions not only emphasize the importance of empathy but also focus attention on narcissistic psychopathology and personality types who are considered unlikely to benefit from traditional psychoanalytic approaches.

A CASE STUDY

A middle-aged woman came for an appointment with her doctor, whom she described as "the best specialist in town." Her doctor actually found her annoying, as she often spoke disparagingly of others and tended to prolong appointments with seemingly endless descriptions of her bodily functions. Because of a busy schedule, the doctor cut her appointment short and laughed uncomfortably when she protested. She looked hurt but composed herself and walked stiffly out of the office. Two days later she called for an urgent appointment for a severe headache, backache, and several other symptoms. She complained that her body was "falling apart," and she appeared enraged. Physical examination was essentially unremarkable. On further conversation, she described feeling humiliated at her last appointment. She drove home, yelled at her husband, cursed her doctor for being "a jerk," and sat for hours in front of the TV "feeling dead." These feelings persisted and her aches and pains escalated so she again called to see her doctor. Since her physician knew something about psychological theories of narcissism, she realized on further reflection that her hurried manner and laughter with the patient had been received as a failure of empathy and a severe injury to the patient's self-esteem, causing a state of self-

fragmentation experienced as emotional and physical "falling-apart." When she conveyed this awareness to the patient in a caring and empathic manner, the patient immediately felt remarkably better.

PSYCHOANALYTIC THEORY AND THE PHYSICIAN–PATIENT RELATIONSHIP

Now that the basic concepts in psychoanalytic theory have been reviewed, how may they be practically helpful in clinical medicine? One may begin to address this question by examining the nature of the physician–patient relationship, which was discussed in Chapter 1.

The therapeutic importance of the relationship between the physician and patient has been known and emphasized throughout recorded medical history. Hippocrates insisted that the physician know the patient "as an individual and [know] all the relevant circumstances of his life" (Hutchins, 1952: 117). However, the remarkable technological advances in medicine, which have greatly increased our knowledge about diseases, make it easy to forget that for each patient the experience of illness is different, depending on the person's specific circumstances.

Psychoanalysts, beginning with Freud, considered the physician–patient relationship to be a subject for explicit study. As introduced in Chapter 1 by Dr. Shelton, the phenomenon of *transference* is an essential and extremely valuable concept that explains various aspects of the physician–patient relationship that may appear to be inexplicable and unreasonable. The term *transference* is defined as unconsciously applying feelings, attitudes, and expectations from important persons in one's *past* to people in one's *current* life. Freud first learned about the role of transference in the psychoanalytic situation in a manner that would be ultimately helpful for all practicing physicians in caring for their patients. His singular focus on the interesting psychopathology of his patient Dora (1905) led to his overlooking an important aspect of the physician–patient relationship, the *transference,* aspects of which were subsequently responsible for failure of her treatment. Freud described it this way: "Owing to the readiness with which Dora put one part of the pathogenic material at my disposal during the treatment, I neglected the precaution of looking out for the first signs of *transference,* which was being prepared in connection with another part of the same material—a part of which I was in ignorance. . . . In this way the transference took me unawares, and because of the unknown quantity in me, which reminded Dora of Herr K., she took her revenge *on me* as she wanted to take her revenge *on him,* and *deserted me* as she believed herself to have been *deceived and deserted by him*" (Freud, 1905: 118–119). Freud failed to recognize a particularly painful and problematic aspect of a past relationship that Dora transferred onto and repeated with Freud during the treatment. This led Dora to reject Freud as a therapist as once she had been rejected by Herr K., and thus the treatment failed.

Transference reactions stem from early childhood experiences with the parents and include a broad range of dependent, sexual, and aggressive feelings and wishes. Transference occurs, to some extent, in all human relationships and forms the substrate for one's emotional reactions to other people throughout life. Transference often develops with special intensity between patient and physician due to the dependency on the physician that often develops in the context of painful and anxiety-provoking medical illness. Transference feelings may lead to childlike expectations for the physician to protect and nurture the patient back to health as would a parent.

Freud divided transference into positive and negative (hostile) types and further subdivided positive transference into an "unobjectionable" positive transference and the "erotic" transference. Negative transference and erotic transference function as resistances to the psychoanalytic treatment process. However, the "unobjectionable" positive transference was considered by Freud to be necessary and especially useful in the physician–patient relationship (Freud, 1911–1913:139).

Countertransference refers to the displacement *onto the patient by the therapist or physician* of feelings, wishes, and attitudes derived from the therapist's or the physician's own early childhood experiences. Hence, countertransference may be thought of as the physician's own transference to the patient.

It is not uncommon for patients to have or develop transferences to their physicians, and the vast majority of such reactions are positive if patients are capable of basic trust in other people and are capable of forming a cooperative relationship with the physician. Evidence of problematic (negative) transference reactions are evidenced by patients who appear unreasonably suspicious, hostile, litigious, antagonistic, provocative, excessively dependent or clinging, or sexually seductive. Hence, a mistrustful patient may have been traumatized or hurt in early stages of life when especially vulnerable to a person from whom he or she sought help or was dependent—usually a parent figure. This mistrust and anger can be transferred onto the physician because the patient may react to the physician (unconsciously) in a similar manner. Problematic erotic transferences can also seriously disrupt the doctor–patient relationship.

Likewise, physicians may suddenly experience intense, seemingly inappropriate reactions to patients—either hostile, affectionate, or sexual—if the patient comes to represent a conflicted significant figure from their own life. Awareness that such reactions on either the patient's or physician's part may be complicating the physician–patient relationship should give rise to self-inspection on the part of the physician and possibly a psychiatric consultation (formal or informal) to gain an objective view of the situation. Problematic transference reactions in the medical setting are usually most pronounced when patients are severely regressed under the stress of a medical illness or the patient (or physician) has evidence of a preexisting personality disorder. Transference and countertransference reactions have been discussed in Chapter 1, especially in regard to distinguishing unconscious versus "realistic" emotional interactions between doctor and patient.

A CASE STUDY/COUNTERTRANSFERENCE

A middle-aged internist was seeing an elderly woman patient with vague abdominal complaints. The patient had a long history of fleeting somatic complaints and would present to her physician with these symptoms during particularly stressful periods in her life. She usually responded favorably to gentle reassurance and support after a careful physical examination. During her last visit, the physician uncharacteristically ordered an extensive battery of exams involving a number of complicated and uncomfortable diagnostic procedures, procedures that were medically defensible but extremely unlikely to produce any meaningful results. Several weeks later, after the tests were found to be all within normal limits, the physician asked herself why she had ordered these painful procedures when she knew their likely result. Upon careful reflection, the physician determined that the patient reminded her of her own mother, a cold and distant woman who likewise was prone to multiple somatic complaints. Fear of her unconscious anger at her own mother led to a countertransference enactment on the part of the physician characterized by an unconscious displacement of her anger onto her patient.

The Treament Alliance

Another aspect of the physician–patient relationship derived from psychoanalytic therapy applicable to the medical setting is the *treatment alliance,* which is also referred to as the therapeutic alliance or working alliance. In general, these terms all refer to the rational, conflict-free, conscious relationship between the patient and physician, which is based on their agreement to work together for the patient's benefit. It is probably based in part on the existence of a positive transference.

In general, an attitude of concern, respect, honesty, and courtesy combined with empathy and protection of privacy and confidentiality will foster a positive relationship in any physician–patient relationship. Studies indicating why therapist/ physician–patient relationships fail have tended to confirm this observation. If the physician is able to convey a genuine interest in being helpful to the patient, and there is a congruence between the patient's own current, crucial interests and the interests of the physician, the treatment, medical or psychiatric, is most likely to continue on a positive track and not be prematurely interrupted by the patient (Inderbitzin, 1990; Nicholi, 1978). (See also Chapter 1.)

Illness, and especially hospitalization, tend to create a situation of *forced dependency* and certain types of regressive, childlike behavior in patients, which may pose a threat to the physician–patient relationship and the ongoing treatment. The specific nature of the patient's reaction in such instances is determined by a variety of factors, including the circumstances of the current situation (such as the nature and severity of the illness), the current state of the physician–patient relationship, and previous experiences with caretakers in similar situations. A major determinant, however, is the nature of the underlying personality structure of both the patient and physician.

The applications of psychoanalytic concepts and psychodynamic-based therapy in the care of the medically ill patient are discussed further in Chapter 14 by Dr. Green.

PSYCHOANALYSIS AND PSYCHOANALYTIC PSYCHOTHERAPY

Psychoanalytically oriented psychotherapy is a method of treatment based on psychoanalytic theory and technique and is the most widely practiced form of psychotherapy in the United States (Henry et al, 1973; Parloff, 1979). It is most often described in terms of comparisons and contrasts with its parent discipline, classic Freudian psychoanalysis. As described first by Freud (1911–1913), psychoanalysis is the treatment of choice for patients who suffer from chronic symptoms or characterological problems reflecting intrapsychic conflict, developmental arrests or deviations, and/or personality deficits not inconsistent with growth potential. Psychoanalysis is particularly preferable over other treatment methods if chronic symptoms have not improved or are not likely to improve with briefer, less intense forms of psychotherapy. Furthermore, if some other treatment would provide temporary relief but with high risk of recurrence of the chronic symptoms, psychoanalysis should be considered. In addition to these criteria for psychoanalysis, patients must also fulfill certain criteria for analyzability, which include the capacity to form a treatment relationship, maintain it in the face of a therapeutic regression, and then ultimately relinquish it.

The overall goal of psychoanalysis is to foster the greatest change in personality structure that is possible. Psychotherapeutic goals vary widely, but an overall goal is the resolution of symptoms and some degree of behavioral change. Patients suffering from acute symptoms, even if they reflect evidence of intrapsychic conflict, are treated more appropriately with psychotherapy than psychoanalysis, unless the symptoms are embedded in a rigid character structure, or there is evidence of developmental distortions or arrested development. The psychoanalytic treatment situation is designed in such a way as to intensify the transference relationship and center the patient's infantile neurotic conflicts around the person of the analyst. Although this may occur also in other forms of treatment, *it is not an aim* of routine psychotherapy; some psychotherapies, such as brief psychotherapy, are designed to minimize transference manifestations. Patients who show evidence of not being able to distinguish between transference reactions to the analyst and reality should, in general, be treated by psychotherapeutic rather than psychoanalytic methods. In psychoanalytic technique, the analyst tries to avoid becoming a model for the patient and uses interventions primarily intended to promote insight. The psychotherapist, however, sometimes deliberately tries to provide a model for the patient and offers suggestions and other supportive measures.

Psychoanalysis requires four to five sessions per week, use of the couch, and is open-ended with a usual duration of at least 3 years. The technique of free association is central to the methodology of classic psychoanalysis (Kris, 1989). The psychoanalytic situation is structured in such a way (including the analyst's neutrality and relative personal anonymity) to foster a temporary therapeutic regression, allowing intrapsychic conflicts to be observed by analyst and patient. The analytic situation is, in a sense, artificially contrived to enable patients to reexperience and remember in the here and now as much of their painful and problematic past as is possible and to bring past experiences to the conscious surface where insight can be used for change. In his or her interventions, the psychoanalyst is guided primarily by the manifestations of transference and resistance (Freud, 1914), and *interpretation* is the primary technique applied to gain insight and foster change in the intrapsychic balance.

Modifications of classic psychoanalytic technique and the development of other psychoanalytically oriented psychotherapies resulted from efforts to shorten psychoanalytic treatment and adapt it to a wider range of patients, including those too disturbed to tolerate classic psychoanalysis. Insight-oriented (expressive) psychotherapy and so-called supportive psychotherapy are not dichotomous methods of treatment. Supportive elements exist even in the most insight-oriented classic psychoanalysis, and, at times, interpretations, which are usually thought of as an expressive therapeutic technique, can be the most effective supportive intervention. Books by Luborsky (1984) and Werman (1987) emphasize that supportive and expressive therapies exist on a continuum, and these authors illustrate the flexible application of psychoanalytic concepts to different kinds of patients with various types of goals and at different stages of treatment.

Psychoanalytic psychotherapy (dynamic psychotherapy), including psychoanalysis, has been shown to be effective for a wide variety of problems and disorders (Bachrach, 1991; Bergin and Lambert, 1978; Luborsky et al, 1975; Smith et al, 1980, Wallerstein, 1986). Results of efficacy studies of psychoanalytic psychotherapy demonstrate target symptom improvement rates of 86% to 92%, and that this is maintained at 7-year follow-up (Crits-Christoph, 1992; Luborsky et al, 1988). Nevertheless, there are many unanswered questions and remaining problems. We need to learn much more about what therapy, administered by what therapist, is effective for which patients with what conditions, as well as the differences in outcomes between brief dynamic psychotherapy and longer-term treatments such as psychoanalysis (Luborsky, 1984). Like any other effective treatment in medicine, psychotherapy has the potential to cause great harm as well as much benefit to patients. It is essential that an experienced clinician who is knowledgeable about both psychopathology and various treatment modalities perform a careful diagnostic evaluation and assess the need for medical and neurological evaluation, and the possible need for psychopharmacological agents, before any form of psychotherapy is recommended. Many authors, such as Levine (1952) and Malan (1979), have emphasized the crucial role of diagnosis and have described diagnostic evaluation processes that begin with a clinical psychiatric diagnosis but necessarily go far beyond that. Such a diagnostic process always includes a psychodynamic understanding of the conflicts within the patient and between the patient and his or her environment, as well as how these conflicts developed out of the patient's past. Study of the precipitating factors of the present illness are particularly useful in this endeavor. Furthermore, it is necessary to know about the patient's strengths and highest level of functioning, weaknesses and most severe disturbances, and the balance between the two.

Only the clinician who is able to grasp empathically the patient's inner world and way of being in the world is able to prescribe effectively. Many of the principles and practices of psychotherapy that are especially helpful in understanding and helping patients with emotional difficulties in coping with medical illness are discussed in Chapter 14.

ANNOTATED BIBLIOGRAPHY

Brenner C: The Mind in Conflict. Madison, CT, International Universities Press, 1982

> In this work, Brenner elaborates on the theory of psychic conflict—how infantile wishes come into conflict and lead to various compromise formations. Along the way he reviews his own revisions of important psychoanalytic concepts.

Brenner C: An Elementary Textbook of Psychoanalysis, rev ed. New York, International Universities Press, 1973

> This book is a widely recommended and thoroughly comprehensive introduction to the fundamental concepts of classic psychoanalytic theory. Brenner discusses the fundamental hypotheses, the drives, psychosexual stages of development, the topographic and structural models, ego functioning, object relations, parapraxes, wit, dreams, psychopathology, and psychic conflict.

Engel G: Psychological Development in Health and Disease. Philadelphia, WB Saunders, 1962

> This is a distillation of George Engel's thinking about human psychological functioning derived from many years of teaching medical students and residents. The development of the psychic apparatus is described as resulting from the interaction of biological, psychological, and social processes. Engel also discusses how psychological adaptations affect body functions in health and disease. The first half of the book delineates the stages of development in considerable detail; the second half

presents a unified concept of health and disease, explaining the role of psychological processes in medical and psychiatric illnesses.

Freud A: (1936). The Ego and the Mechanisms of Defense, rev ed. New York, International Universities Press, 1966

> This classic work by Anna Freud, originally published in 1936, advanced the theory of the role and functioning of the ego. It examines various ego defense mechanisms, including how and why they operate, and is illustrated with many clinical examples from the author's psychotherapeutic work with children.

Greenberg JR, Mitchell SA: Object Relations in Psychoanalytic Theory. Cambridge, Harvard University Press, 1983

> This scholarly work provides a detailed, comprehensive description of various theories of object relations, including those of Freud, Sullivan, Klein, Fairbairn, Winnicott, Guntrip, Hartmann, Mahler, Jacobson, Kernberg, Kohut, Sandler, and others. The authors contrast and compare theories based on a drive/structure model and those based on a relational/structure model.

Levy S: Principles of Interpretation. New York, Jason Aronson, 1984

> This book is concerned with the technical theory of interpretation used in psychoanalytically oriented psychotherapy. Levy describes how the interviewer or therapist listens to the productions of the patient, and then formulates and verbalizes interventions that best facilitate the therapeutic process. Many clinical vignettes illustrate the technical points described.

MacKinnon R, Michels R: The Psychiatric Interview in Clinical Practice. Philadelphia, WB Saunders, 1971

> The authors provide a discussion of basic principles of the psychodynamic interview, then focus on how these are applied in the interviewing and psychotherapy of patients with specific types of psychopathology. Their discussions describe the core psychodynamic issues present in these patients, how these will manifest in the interview, and how the interviewer can therapeutically intervene.

Malan D: Individual Psychotherapy and the Science of Psychodynamics. London, Butterworths, 1979

> Malan describes the principles and techniques of intensive psychotherapy, beginning with basic psychoanalytic principles. He stresses the observational data and the psychodynamic formulations that can be generated to explain the data and test the hypotheses. This book is structured around many illustrative case examples and explains a method of brief psychotherapy as well as long-term therapy. The theoretical orientation of the author includes attention to object relations and the role of the vicissitudes of infantile experience in shaping adult psychopathology.

Nemiah J: Foundations of Psychopathology. New York, Oxford University Press, 1961

> This book reviews the basic concepts of psychoanalysis, then provides an explanation of the psychodynamic bases of various types of psychopathology. It is strongly empiric in its approach, and the concepts are richly illustrated with many clinical cases, which clearly demonstrate the applicability of psychoanalytic principles in the management of medical and psychiatric patients. One especially useful element is the emphasis on the role of fantasy in mental life.

Ursano RJ, Silberman EK, Diaz A: The Psychotherapies: Basic Theoretical Principles and Techniques. In Stoudemire A (ed): Clinical Psychiatry for Medical Students, 2nd ed. Philadelphia, Lippincott, 1994

> An excellent overview of the various types of psychotherapies, giving a theoretical basis for each as well as clinical indications.

Waelder R: Basic Theory of Psychoanalysis. New York, International Universities Press, 1960

> The author reviews many fundamental concepts of psychoanalysis, with elaboration on the topics of the sexual and aggressive instincts, anxiety, ego psychology,

and basic principles of psychotherapy. Waelder effectively addresses many of the criticisms that have been leveled at psychoanalysis over the years.

Zetzel E, Meissner W: Basic Concepts of Psychoanalytic Psychiatry. New York, Basic Books, 1973
This book reviews psychoanalytic theory, including discussions of anxiety, repression, developmental theory, primary and secondary process, narcissism, ego functions and development, object relations, identity formation, neurosis, and therapy. Like most of the books on this list, it evolved out of years of teaching these principles to residents and medical students.

REFERENCES

Bachrach H, Galatzer-Levy R, Skolnikoff A, Waldron S: On the efficacy of psychoanalysis. J Am Psychoanal Assoc 39:871–916, 1991

Bergin A, Lambert M: The evaluation of therapeutic outcomes. In Garfield S, Bergin A (eds): Handbook of Psychotherapy and Behavioral Change: An Empirical Analysis. New York, John Wiley & Sons, 1978

Bibring E: The mechanism of depression. In Greenacre P (ed): Affective Disorders. New York, International Universities Press, 1953

Blos P: The genealogy of the ego ideal. Psychoanal Study Child 29:43–88, 1974

Blum G: Masochism, the ego ideal, and the psychology of women. J Am Psychoanal Assoc 24(Suppl):157–191, 1976

Brenner C: The Mind in Conflict. New York, International Universities Press, 1982

Brenner C: An Elementary Textbook of Psychoanalysis, rev ed. New York, Doubleday, 1974

Chehrazi S: Female psychology: A review. J Am Psychoanal Assoc 34:141–162, 1986

Cooper A, Francis A, Sacks M: The Psychoanalytic Model. In Michels R, Cavenar J, Cooper A et al (eds): Psychiatry, Vol. 1. Revised New York, Basic Books; Philadelphia, JB Lippincott, 1989

Crits-Christoph P: The efficacy of brief dynamic psychotherapy: A meta-analysis. Am J Psychiatry 149:151–158, 1992

Erikson E: Configurations in play—clinical notes. Psychoanal Q 6:139–214, 1937

Fenichel O: The Psychoanalytic Theory of Neurosis. New York, W.W. Norton, 1945

Freud A: (1936). The Ego and the Mechanisms of Defense, rev ed. New York, International Universities Press, 1966

Freud S: Inhibitions, Symptoms and Anxiety. SE 20, 1926

Freud S: Some Psychical Consequences of the Anatomical Distinction Between the Sexes. SE19, 1925

Freud S: The Ego and the Id. SE19, 1923

Freud S: General Theory of the Neuroses. SE16, 1916–1917

Freud S: On the history of the psycho-analytic movement. SE14, 1914.

Freud, S. Papers on Technique. SE12, 1911–1913

Freud S: Fragment of an Analysis of a Case of Hysteria. SE7, 1905

Freud S: The Interpretation of Dreams. SE4 & 5, 1900

Freud S: Studies on Hysteria. SE2, 1893–1895

Hartmann H: (1939). Ego Psychology and the Problem of Adaptation. New York, International Universities Press, 1958

Hartmann H: The mutual influences in the development of the ego and id. Psychoanal Study Child 7:9–30, 1952

Hartmann H: Comments on the psychoanalytic theory of instinctual drives. Psychoanal Q 17:368–388, 1948

Hartmann H, Kris E, Loewenstein R: Comments on the formation of psychic structure. Psychoanal Study Child 2:11–38, 1946

Henry W, Sims J, Spray S: Public and Private Lives of Psychotherapists. San Francisco, Jossey-Bass, 1973

Horney K: The dread of women: Observations on a specific difference in the dread felt by men and women respectively for the opposite sex. Intl J Psycho-analysis 13:348–360, 1932

Horney K: The flight from womanhood: The masculinity complex in women as viewed by men and women. Intl J Psycho-Analysis 7:324–339, 1926.

Hutchins R (ed): Great Books of the Western World. Chicago, University of Chicago Press, 1952

Inderbitzin L: Treatment alliance in acute schizophrenia. In Levy S, Ninan P (eds): Schizophrenia: Treatment of the Acute Psychotic Episode. Washington, DC, American Psychiatric Press, 1990

Jones E: The early development of female sexuality. In Papers on Psycho-Analysis. London, Balliere, Tindall and Cox, 1948

Kleeman J: Freud's views on early female sexuality in the light of direct child observation. J Am Psychoanal Assoc 24 (Suppl):3–28, 1976

Kohut H: Analysis of the Self. New York, International Universities Press, 1971

Kris A: Psychoanalysis and psychoanalytic psychotherapy. In Michels R, Cavenar J, Cooper A et al (eds): Psychiatry, Vol. 1. Revised New York, Basic Books; Philadelphia, JB Lippincott, 1989

Levine M: Principles of psychiatric treatment. In Alexander F (ed): Dynamic Psychiatry. Chicago, University of Chicago Press, 1952

Luborsky L: Principles of Psychoanalytic Psychotherapy. New York, Basic Books, 1984

Luborsky L, Crits-Christoph P, Mintz J, Auerbach A: Who Will Benefit from Psychotherapy? Predicting Therapeutic Outcomes. New York, Basic Books, 1988

Luborsky L, Singer B, Luborsky L: Comparative studies of psychotherapies: Is it true that "Everybody has won and all must have prizes"? Arch Gen Psychiatry 32:995–1008, 1975

Mahler M, Pine F, Bergman A: The Psychological Birth of the Human Infant. New York, Basic Books, 1975

Malan D: Individual Psychotherapy and the Science of Psychodynamics. Boston, Butterworths, 1979

Nicholi A: The therapist-patient relationship. In Nicholi A (ed): The Harvard Guide to Modern Psychiatry. Cambridge, The Belknap Press of Harvard University Press, 1978

Parloff MB: Can psychotherapy research guide the policymaker? A little knowledge may be a dangerous thing. Am Psychol 34:296–306, 1979

Rapaport D: A historical survey of psychoanalytic ego psychology. Introduction in Erikson E: Identity and the Life Cycle. Psychological Issues 1(1). New York, International Universities Press, 1959

Rapaport D: The Structure of Psychoanalytic Theory. Psychological Issues 2(2). New York, International Universities Press, 1960

Reich A: Pathologic forms of self-esteem regulation. Psychoanal Study Child 15:215–232, 1960

Smith M, Glas G, Miller T: The Benefits of Psychotherapy. Baltimore, Johns Hopkins Press, 1980

Spitz R: The First Year of Life. New York, International Universities Press, 1965

Stoller R: Primary femininity. J Am Psychoanal Assoc 24 (Suppl):59–78, 1976

Stoller R: Sex and Gender. New York, Science House, 1968

Ursano RJ, Silberman EK, Diaz A: The Psychotherapies: Basic Theoretical Principles and Techniques. In Stoudemire A (ed): Clinical Psychiatry for Medical Students, 2nd ed. Philadelphia, Lippincott, 1994.

Vaillant G: Empirical Studies of Ego Mechanisms of Defense. Washington, DC, American Psychiatric Press, 1986

Wallerstein R: Forty-two Lives in Treatment: A Study of Psychoanalysis and Psychotherapy. New York, The Guilford Press, 1986

Werman D: The Practice of Supportive Psychotherapy. New York, Brunner/Mazel, 1987

Winson J: Brain and Psyche: The Biology of the Unconscious. New York, Vintage Books, 1985

6 Behavioral and Social Learning Psychology

Pamela G. Dorsett

The preceding chapter was an overview of the basic principles of psychoanalytic psychology and its application to the care of patients. In this chapter, the contributions of behavioral theory will be discussed. While the concluding section of this chapter compares psychoanalytic with behavioral theory and therapy, no attempt will be made necessarily to reconcile or integrate psychoanalytic and behavioral theory, although serious efforts have been made to do so (Marmor and Woods, 1980). It is the position of this text that both perspectives have value and clinical importance in understanding human behavior. The two approaches are presented recognizing that appreciation of diverse models may facilitate selection and the integrated use of the most appropriate techniques for each patient's given needs.

CHARACTERISTICS OF BEHAVIORAL THEORY

The philosophy of the science of human behavior called behaviorism has evolved from a rich, albeit relatively brief, history. There are several basic characteristics and assumptions common to most positions within what is known as *behavioral psychology*.

First, the subject matter for study is *objectively measurable behavior*, particularly relationships between behavior and other verifiable events. Behaviors may be external and directly observable, such as social interactions, or internal, such as emotions and cognitions. Physiological responses are internal events that can be monitored through instrumentation.

A second characteristic of behavioral psychology is a commitment to *experimentation* and the *empirical method.* Behavior is defined objectively and in such a way that it can be measured reliably. The nature of the relationships between behavior and variables such as environmental events are explored, described, and analyzed by means of experiments using methodology similar to that employed in the study of the natural sciences. Through experimentation, general laws or principles of behavior can be discovered such that behavior can be predicted and controlled.

Third, *learning* is emphasized. Further, it is assumed that adaptive and maladaptive behaviors are acquired in basically the same ways. The behavioral perspective rejects the notion of traits and underlying processes (e.g., conflicts) in explaining behavior. Personality development, whether "normal" or "abnormal," is seen as the result of the unique contributions of learning experiences and genetic endowment. Maladaptive behavior that is not learned can be affected by learning principles, and significant environmental factors can be changed to alter this behavior. As such, the behavioral view is optimistic regarding change.

Many figures have made significant contributions to the behavioral movement. An overview is presented in Table 6–1 and several key figures and their respective contributions are discussed in more detail in the sections that follow. (See Kazdin [1978] for a complete history of the behavioral psychology movement.)

CLASSICAL OR RESPONDENT CONDITIONING

Ivan Pavlov (1849–1936) and two other neurophysiologists in Russia, Ivan Sechenov (1829–1905) and Vladimir Bechterev (1857–1927), played significant roles in promoting application of the experimental method to the study of psychological phenomena and formulating the principles of classical or respondent conditioning (Table 6–2). Pavlov studied digestion and developed a surgical technique that made it possible to obtain secretions directly from the glands and, therefore, to observe and measure the secretions outside the animal's body. He had already begun to direct his research toward elucidation of the variables affecting the acquisition and elimination of "psychic secretions" (i.e., gastric secretions elicited by stimuli such as the sight of food rather than by direct physical stimulation) when he received the Nobel Prize in 1904 for his work in digestion. His initial attempts to explain the secretions on the basis of "expectancies" were not productive, so he set about the task of analyzing the nature of the responses and their relationship to other events.

Table 6–1 **Major Contributors to the Behavioral Movement**

Ivan Sechenov (1829–1905)	Proposed that behavior was reflexive to external stimuli and advocated the use of experimental methodology for the study of behavior.
Vladimir Bechterev (1857–1927)	Focused on aversive stimuli and reflexes with humans and other species.
	Attempted to apply principles of reflexology to psychiatric disorders.
	Advocated objectivism, empiricism, and experimentation in psychology.
Ivan Pavlov (1849–1936)	Formulated principles of classical (respondent) conditioning.
	Advocated objectivism, empiricism, and experimentation in psychology.
John B. Watson (1878–1958)	Advocated objectivism, empiricism, and experimentation in psychology with observable behavior as the subject matter.
	Publicized the behavioral position. "Father of Behaviorism."
	Extended application of the classical conditioning model to the development of emotions in humans.
Edward L. Thorndike (1874–1949)	Studied patterns of behavior in trial-and-error learning.
	Formulated the Law of Effect and emphasized the consequences of behavior.
Edward C. Tolman (1896–1961)	Maintained that behavior is purposive and referred to subjective states in accounting for behavior.
	Proposed that reinforcement serves as information and not to strengthen behavior directly.
B. F. Skinner (1904–1991)	Shifted focus of explanations for behavior from stimuli to consequences.
	Formulated principles of operant conditioning.
	Advocated a methodology for studying behavior called the experimental analysis of behavior.
	Presented the radical behaviorism position.
	Helped distinguish operant and respondent (classical) conditioning.
	Had great impact on the development of behavior modification.
Joseph Wolpe (1915–)	Used an animal model to study the development of emotional reactions and ways of treating such problems.
	Developed treatment techniques based on the principle of reciprocal inhibition.
	Generated research and contributed to the development of behavior therapy through his techniques.
Albert Bandura (1925–)	Emphasized reciprocal determinism and cognitive and self-regulatory processes.
	Elucidated variables affecting observational learning.

Table 6–2 **Classical or Respondent Conditioning**

TERM	DEFINITION	EXAMPLE
Unconditioned stimulus (UCS)	Elicits an unconditioned response or reflex.	Blast of air into eye causes eye blink.
Unconditioned response (UCR)	Reflex elicited by an unconditioned stimulus.	Eye blink in response to blast of air.
Conditioned stimulus (CS)	Previously neutral stimulus that comes to elicit an unconditioned response through pairings with an unconditioned stimulus.	Tone presented immediately before blast of air into eye. Tone alone comes to elicit eye blink.
Conditioned response (CR)	Response elicited by the conditioned stimulus.	Eye blink in response to tone.
Discrimination	The conditioned response is elicited by some stimuli similar to the conditioned stimulus but not by others.	Tones of a particular frequency range elicit the eye blink but others do not.
Generalization	Stimuli similar to the conditioned stimulus elicit the conditioned response.	Tones most similar to the original one elicit the eye blink.
Extinction	Conditioned stimulus loses the power to elicit the conditioned response by no longer being paired with the unconditioned stimulus.	After repeated presentations of the tone without the blast of air, the tone alone no longer elicits the eye blink.

Pavlov found that by repeatedly pairing a stimulus that elicited the salivation reflex, the previously neutral stimulus would also elicit a reflexive-type response. For example, a tone would not elicit salivation. However, if the tone was presented with food for several conditioning trials, then, when presented alone, the tone did elicit salivation. In this paradigm, the food is called an *unconditioned stimulus* (UCS), and the response it elicits is called an *unconditioned response* (UCR) or reflex. The tone, a previously neutral stimulus that comes to elicit salivation through conditioning or pairing with the UCS, is called a *conditioned stimulus* (CS). The response it elicits is a *conditioned response* (CR).

Pavlov determined that the CS loses its power to elicit a CR if it is no longer paired with the UCS, a process called *extinction*. After some period of time has elapsed following extinction, the presentation of the CS may again temporarily elicit the CR. This phenomenon is called *spontaneous recovery*.

In his work, Pavlov demonstrated that, once a CS had been established, similar stimuli also elicited the CR, a phenomenon called *generalization*. Tones of similar though different frequencies, for example, elicited a salivation response. However, if *different* tones were presented *without* being followed by the food and only *one* tone was paired with the UCS, then only *one* *stimulus* elicited the CR. This is the process of *discrimination.*

A very practical clinical example of this phenomenon may be observed in patients receiving chemotherapy for cancer. Anticipatory nausea and vomiting in cancer patients receiving chemotherapy can be explained by *respondent conditioning.* The UCS is the chemotherapy agent that produces nausea and vomiting, the UCRs, as side effects. Various neutral stimuli such as the smell of the hospital or sight of the treatment room become associated with the UCS. After several pairings, the neutral stimuli become CSs and elicit nausea and vomiting—the CRs. Generalization may occur, whereby more and more stimuli become CSs. Theoretically, extinction of the CRs could require visits to the hospital after completion of chemotherapy in order to expose the patient to CSs without additional pairings with the UCS. This is not a practical intervention and, fortunately, there is an effective alternative treatment for conditioned nausea and vomiting, relaxation, which will be discussed later in the chapter.

Respondent Conditioning and the Development of Emotions

From a behavioral perspective, classical or respondent conditioning is the basis for the emotional responses we have to events, objects, situations, or people. John B. Watson (1878–1958) extended application of the model to study the development of emotions in humans.

Watson believed that all learning occurred according to the principles of respondent conditioning, including emotions, which he saw as physiological responses to observable stimuli. He and his assistant experimentally demonstrated that a phobia could be developed by means of respondent conditioning (Watson and Rayner, 1920). In a classic experiment, a 9-month-old named Albert was presented with a white rat and initially showed no indications of fear but rather approached and touched the animal. The child was then presented with the rat as a metal bar was banged loudly, resulting in a startle response. After several conditioning trials, Albert cried at the sight of the rat and would not approach or touch the rat. Additionally, the fear *generalized* to other similar, white furry objects, such as a rabbit, a dog, a fur coat, and a ball of white wool. Unfortunately, Albert's mother left the hospital before Watson could decondition Albert's fear.

Although such an experiment would not be conducted today because of obvious ethical problems, it remains a classic study. It demonstrated that an emotional response and related maladaptive behavior, in this case a phobia, could be acquired through a relatively simple learning process rather than being the result of underlying processes and conflicts that can be neither observed nor studied experimentally.

Conditioned emotional responses (CERs) can be positive or negative depending on the nature of the UCS and the CS and the individual's conditioning history. Albert's fear of white furry objects is an example of a conditioned aversive emotional response. Hearing the voice of one's lover, on the other hand, may elicit pleasurable emotional responses. When dealing with conditioned aversive emotional responses, individuals can engage in avoidance behavior so the CERs do not extinguish. That is, the person avoids pairing the negative CS with a neutral event and extinction cannot occur. Consequently, conditioned aversive emotional responses and avoidance behavior can continue indefinitely. Consider the individual who grows up in a home where his parents have explosive, angry outbursts that terrify him. Throughout life, the person may not only avoid confrontations with others who might get angry with him, but he also avoids confronting his own anger because it is frightening. Continuing avoidance of situations in which he might encounter angry people prevents extinction of the conditioned aversive emotional responses, notably his fear.

In order to understand avoidance behavior and how it is learned, the model formulated by B.F. Skinner and called *operant conditioning* must be considered.

OPERANT CONDITIONING

B. F. Skinner (1904–1991) wrote extensively about the philosophy of science he called *radical behaviorism* (e.g., Skinner, 1953, 1974). This philosophy recognizes private events such as cognitions and emotions as important but also defines these experiences as behaviors that are affected, as are observable behaviors, by environmental events. Private events do not cause other behaviors, according to Skinner; private events are behaviors explained by environmental contingencies. ("Contingencies" refer to the interrelationships among behaviors, antecedents, and consequences.)

Skinner studied discrete and easily measured behavior of the individual subject intensively over time. He designed his own apparatus and recording devices. The "Skinner box" consists of a soundproofed box with a lever and food magazine. Depressing the lever closes a circuit, which automatically records the number of times the lever pressing brought about the delivery of food. The lever press response facilitates investigation of variables and their relationships to behavior. For example, by manipulating the behavioral requirements for delivering food, Skinner could observe reliable, distinctive patterns of behavior specific to the particular contingencies implemented. The methodology he advocated for studying behavior is called the *experimental analysis of behavior.*

Skinner shifted the focus of explanations for behavior to consequences and a type of conditioning he called *operant.* He developed a program of research in *operant conditioning* that resulted in the formulation of basic principles that govern behavior and the extension of these principles, discovered in the animal laboratory, to applications to human behavior.

In operant conditioning, an animal or person "operates" on the environment and produces a change, a consequence for the behavior. As such, the organism is viewed as *active.* In respondent conditioning the subject is passive because responses are *elicited* by stimuli. An operant is *emitted* in the presence of certain stimuli and produces *consequences* that affect the future probability of the behavior. For example, a food-deprived rat in an operant chamber ("Skinner box") depresses a lever, which results in delivery of a food pellet. The animal's response (the lever press) produces a change in its environment—the response closes the circuit and food is delivered. The rat learns that delivery of food is *contingent* (i.e., dependent) on the occurrence of the lever press, which will affect the likelihood of the response occurring again. In the case of respondent conditioning, presentation of the CS produces a CR; it is the *stimulus* that controls the behavior.

Consequences are defined in terms of their effect on behavior. If the effect is to *strengthen* or *increase* behavior, the event is *reinforcing.* When the behavior is *decreased* or *weakened* by the event, it is *punishing* (Table 6—3).

The critical feature of the consequence is not whether it is judged to be "pleasant" or "unpleasant." *It is the effect of the consequences on behavior that is important.* Assume that two different patients, for example, experience the same physiological effects when they take a particular narcotic analgesic. However, one patient may take the medication only once and discard it and another may overuse the medication. The behavior of taking the medication is reinforced or strengthened by the effects of the drug in one case and the same medication effect may *punish* or weaken the behavior in another patient.

Consider as well the typical elementary school classroom. Within a class of 20 to 30 students, some will work quietly for long periods without misbehaving to avoid being scolded by the teacher. Other pupils in the class engage in frequent disruptive behavior because it functions to consistently produce teacher attention, albeit negative (negative attention). In the latter case scolding actually *reinforces* misbehavior (increases the likelihood of recurrence). Without creating disruptions, these children may receive little teacher attention, and *negative* attention may be better than none at all.

Reinforcement

Reinforcement refers to the procedure of increasing the probability of a behavior occurring by the *contingent* delivery of a reinforcing event that follows the behavior. The event that strengthens the behavior is called a *reinforcer.*

Reinforcers may be *positive* or *negative* depending on whether the consequence entails the presentation or removal of some event. For example,

Table 6–3 **Operant Conditioning—Consequences**

TERM	DEFINITION	EXAMPLE
Positive reinforcement	Increasing the probability of a behavior by presenting a positive reinforcer following occurrence of the behavior.	Patient is praised for adhering to diet restriction 1 week and continues to do so for a second week.
Negative reinforcement	Increasing the probability of a behavior by terminating or avoiding an aversive event or the loss of a positive reinforcer following the occurrence of the behavior.	Patient adheres to diet and exercise regimen in order to discontinue daily insulin.
Positive punishment	Decreasing the probability of a behavior by presenting a punisher following occurrence of the behavior.	Patient is reprimanded for smoking and stops for several days.
Negative punishment	Decreasing the probability of a behavior by removing a positive reinforcer or the opportunity for positive reinforcement following occurrence of the behavior.	Patient is not seen for an appointment when he/she arrives more than 15 minutes late, and frequency of tardiness decreases.
Extinction	Decreasing/eliminating a behavior by discontinuing reinforcement that maintained the behavior.	Excessive patient requests for mood-altering medications are decreased by refusing to comply with such requests.

one patient may take medication as ordered because doing so is associated with either improved physical status or attention and praise from family members and the physician. The behavior of taking the medication is *positively reinforced* in this case. Another patient may comply with the physician's order because taking the medication results in the termination or avoidance of unpleasant physical symptoms. In this situation, compliant behavior is *negatively reinforced.* Behavior that is strengthened because it avoids contact with an aversive event is called *avoidance behavior.* When the behavior results in termination or removal of the aversive event, it is referred to as *escape behavior.* Some patients may stop taking the medication once their symptoms have ceased and only resume the regimen when unpleasant effects recur.

There are several different types of reinforcers. The reinforcing properties of *primary reinforcers* seem to be more biologically based rather than being dependent on learning. Examples include food, sex, and water. Other types of reinforcers acquire their reinforcing properties through pairing with other established reinforcers. These are called *conditioned reinforcers*. An example of a conditioned reinforcer is praise, which is frequently paired with other reinforcers. *Generalized reinforcers* are events that acquire and maintain their reinforcer effectiveness through pairing with many other reinforcers. Money, for example, can be exchanged for numerous and diverse objects, events, and so forth, which are reinforcing for the person. Money would cease to be reinforcing if it were no longer paired with other reinforcers. Conditioned and generalized reinforcers can be particularly useful in bridging the time between occurrence of a behavior and delivery of more powerful, but delayed, reinforcers. For example, receiving a letter of acceptance for a manuscript with positive feedback may function to strengthen writing behavior (Table 6–4).

Tokens are a special type of generalized reinforcer that can be exchanged for various objects, events, and so forth, called *backup reinforcers*. They allow for behavior to be immediately reinforced. Token systems have been effectively implemented and used in schools, prisons, and institutions for the mentally retarded. Economic principles are used in setting up these systems.

Several factors influence reinforcer effectiveness. First, the reinforcer must be presented *contingently*. That is, it should be delivered *contingent on the occurrence of desirable behavior*. Second, the most effective procedure is *immediate presentation* of the reinforcer after the behavior has occurred. Third, it is important to consider the difficulty of performing the behavior, how much behavior is required, and the amount of the reinforcer. Although the general rule is "more reinforcer means greater effectiveness," too much reinforcer can result in *satiation* or a *decrease* in reinforcer effectiveness. Generally, the greater the deprivation or limits on contact with the reinforcer, the more effective the reinforcer will be for altering behavior.

Table 6–4 **Types of Reinforcers and Punishers**

TYPE	PROPERTIES	EXAMPLE
Primary	Biologically based; does not require association with other reinforcers or punishers to be effective	
Reinforcer		Food, sex, water
Punisher		Slap, loud noise
Conditioned	Requires association with other reinforcers or punishers to be effective	
Reinforcer		Praise
Punisher		Threat
Generalized	Associated with many other reinforcers or punishers	
Reinforcer		Money
Punisher		Social disapproval

Developing New Behavior

Contingencies of reinforcement can strengthen behaviors once they occur. However, either particular skills may not be in the person's repertoire or the desired behavior may just not occur at all. In such cases there are no opportunities to reinforce the response. The starting point is to identify behavior that is already occurring that resembles the desired behavior and to reinforce it. The behavioral requirement for reinforcer delivery is gradually increased as the behavior becomes more similar to the target behavior. Dissimilar behaviors are extinguished. This is the process of *differential reinforcement* and the result is *response differentiation*. The procedure of differentially reinforcing closer and closer approximations to the final target behavior is called the *method of successive approximations*. Completely new behavior is produced through *shaping*.

Complex behaviors or skills, whether desirable or undesirable, are often developed originally from simple behaviors through the process of shaping, such as learning to play an instrument.

Shaping was an essential component of an intervention to teach toileting behaviors to a 5-year-old child. (Functional encopresis is an elimination disorder [DSM-IV; APA 1994] in which the individual defecates in inappropriate places. Sometimes stool is passed involuntarily because the person retains feces.)

A CASE ILLUSTRATION

An 8-year-old boy was referred for psychological intervention by his pediatric gastroenterologist because of primary functional encopresis. He had never had a consistent period of continence, and his parents requested help for overflow incontinence secondary to functional fecal retention. The child was chronically constipated, retaining stool for a week or more at a time, and causing considerable discomfort and a distended abdomen. Evacuation with enemas was usually necessary. Laxatives were of minimal assistance since he fought to hold back bowel movements brought about by these agents. He had a history of parental criticism and punishment for soiling in his clothes. The youngster refused to sit on a toilet or potty chair at the time the family presented for treatment.

Power struggles between the child and his parents were well entrenched and included, but were not limited to, toileting. Parent training was implemented first with an emphasis on increasing positive consequences for any appropriate behaviors, minimizing aversive controls, and eliminating punishers for soiling. A reinforcement system to shape toileting behaviors was first applied at school. He earned praise and access to a "surprise bag" of small tangible reinforcers at school by sitting, even for a few seconds initially, on the toilet in the classroom after lunch. The duration of time re-

quired to sit on the toilet to earn praise and a trinket was gradually increased. Then the requirement included having a bowel movement, small at first, and then larger to earn the reinforcer. Within 10 weekdays he was sitting on the toilet and having bowel movements with no soiling at school. After 2 additional weeks the program was implemented at home and he began having regular bowel movements there as well. The "surprise bag" was replaced by a token system and, over time, he more and more frequently "forgot" to ask for his tokens. He verbalized pride in his clean clothes and "flat tummy," felt better physically, and was no longer teased by his classmates for "smelling bad," to name but a few of the naturally occurring reinforcers that maintained the child's toileting behaviors after tangible rewards were faded.

Imitation

Obviously all new skills do not require shaping. We acquire a great deal of complex behavior by observing others and imitating their behaviors. *Modeling* is a very powerful means of learning new behavior.

Albert Bandura's classic studies demonstrated very clearly that children can learn behaviors by observing others (Bandura et al, 1963). Modeling has been successfully used to reduce fear and anxiety in children and adults. A filmed model was used by Jay et al (1987) as a component in a cognitive-behavioral program to reduce distress of pediatric oncology patients undergoing bone marrow aspirations and lumbar punctures. The children observed a videotape of another oncology patient successfully using coping techniques during the invasive medical procedures. The treatment "package," which also included breathing, distraction, rehearsal, and reinforcement, was more effective than oral diazepam (Valium), an anxiety suppression medication, in decreasing behavioral distress during the procedures.

Characteristics of the model as well as the consequences of the behavior for the model affect the likelihood of imitation by an observer. Imitative behaviors can become intrinsically reinforcing. The young ballet dancer diligently practices barre exercises such as the *grand battement en avant* so as to "match" the method of the teacher. Performance of the behavior itself is reinforcing. Further discussion of observational learning is presented within the context of social learning theory.

Extinction

In *extinction,* the reinforcer that has maintained a response no longer follows the behavior, and the behavior decreases and is eliminated. Once the response no longer occurs, we say that it has been *extinguished.*

Francis (1988) described a child with obsessive-compulsive disorder with an extinction procedure. The 11-year-old obsessively worried about dying and also engaged in compulsive reassurance-seeking questions. Parents were instructed to withhold their responses and change the conversation when the youngster asked questions seeking reassurance. Francis reported elimination of the behavior within 6 days using extinction.

Chronic pain patients may complain excessively about physical discomfort for which there is no medical cure. Such complaints are frequently maintained, at least in part, by the attention and sympathy they evoke from others. The behavior may be decreased by withholding attention and sympathy when complaining occurs (an extinction procedure) and also socially reinforcing the patient's talk about any subject other than pain (e.g., the weather, how well he or she feels, recent activities, and so forth) with attention and praise.

It is typical to see a *temporary increase* in the intensity, rate, or duration of a behavior when an extinction procedure has been implemented. Emotional behavior intensifies as well, particularly initially. In the case described above, for example, patient complaints would increase at first in intensity and frequency. The patient might become louder, more emotional, and engage in additional nonverbal pain behaviors as well. The time it takes for the behavior to be eliminated depends on the schedule of reinforcement that has maintained the behavior.

Schedules of Reinforcement

The *schedule of reinforcement* is the rule that specifies the time and response requirements for a reinforcer to be delivered. The rate and pattern of the behavior as it is maintained and/or extinguished are determined by the schedule. When there is only one schedule operating in a situation, it is called a *simple schedule.* Such schedules can be *continuous* or *intermittent.*

Continuous reinforcement (CRF) means that every occurrence of the behavior is immediately reinforced. If a behavior is reinforced intermittently, some occurrences will not be reinforced. When establishing new behaviors it is important to reinforce continuously at first. As the behavior is strengthened, the frequency of reinforcement is gradually decreased. The reinforcement program described earlier for the youngster with encopresis included changing the schedule of reinforcement from continuous to intermittent once the target behavior occurred consistently. The frequency of reinforcement was gradually decreased over time.

If a response has been reinforced continuously, then it will extinguish more rapidly than if it has been reinforced on an intermittent basis. Behaviors maintained by intermittent schedules are said to be more *resistant to extinction.* It is easier to discriminate that extinction has begun when every occurrence of the behavior has previously resulted in reinforcement.

A common problem for many new parents is dealing with infant cries at bedtime. The sound of a child crying is distressing to most people, and they will engage in behaviors to terminate the sound (escape behavior that is negatively reinforced for the adult). If crying at bedtime is reinforced quickly and consistently by picking up the baby and, perhaps, rocking her to sleep, it will be easier to extinguish the crying behavior than if the parents let the child cry for relatively longer periods on occasion and then take her from the crib. In the latter case, it is more difficult to discriminate that extinction is occurring. Going to a crying child to check that she is all right (or even to comfort the child briefly) *without removing her from the crib* will not typically reinforce the crying.

Children with chronic or recurrent pain problems may escalate pain complaints when parents respond inconsistently to these behaviors (McGrath, 1991). The same behavior on the part of the child is dealt with differently by the parents on varying occasions. For example, the child may complain of abdominal pain and be taken to school in tears one day only to be allowed on another occasion to stay home with a parent. The intermittent schedule teaches the child to intensify the severity of the complaints and other pain behaviors. These behaviors will also be more difficult to extinguish.

Punishment

We have already discussed the extinction procedure as one way to eliminate behavior. However, it is not always possible to identify the reinforcer(s) maintaining a behavior nor is it always feasible to control reinforcement for some behaviors. For example, a teacher is more likely to ignore misbehavior of a school-age child than are his or her peers. *In order to extinguish a response, any reinforcer maintaining the behavior must be consistently withheld.* There are also situations in which extinction of a particular behavior would be dangerous or unethical. For example, attention may be the reinforcer maintaining self-injurious behavior in a mentally retarded child. However, the child could seriously injure himself or herself if allowed to self-abuse while attention was withheld. Extinction can also be fairly lengthy at times, particularly if the behavior has been maintained on an intermittent schedule of reinforcement. In such cases, it may be more appropriate to use procedures that rapidly suppress behavior.

A *punisher* is an event that decreases the behavior it follows. *Positive punishment* entails the contingent presentation of an event immediately after the occurrence of the behavior with a resulting decrease in the probability of that behavior. *Negative punishment* consists of the contingent removal of a positive reinforcer or the opportunity to have access to freely available positive reinforcers when a behavior occurs, again with a resultant reduction in the future occurrence of the response. Contingent ignoring, restriction of privileges or possessions, and time out from reinforcement are all examples of negative punishment. A simple example of positive punishment is criticism for tardiness to one's job. Negative punishment for this behavior might be losing part of one's wages for the time missed from work (or losing one's job).

We may inadvertently punish adaptive behavior. For example, well-meaning parents may tell their child with a chronic pain problem to stop doing certain activities.

Time out from reinforcement is frequently used as a punisher for child misbehaviors and merits further discussion. The technique includes components of extinction and punishment. *Time out* requires a limited period (usually 1 minute per year of age for the child) of no access to freely available reinforcers or of the opportunity to earn reinforcers. Although children are frequently removed to a specific place devoid of materials to play with or things to do, one can also ignore all behavior for a comparable time period without changing the surroundings.

Sometimes parents send their children to their rooms as punishment and find that it does not suppress the inappropriate behavior. Closer analysis typically reveals that the room provides ready and undisturbed access to an array of positive reinforcers ranging from video games and books to music. Besides, such a practice can establish the room as a negative CS, which can then elicit conditioned aversive emotional responses. This is not a situation conducive to uneventful bedtimes and sleeping through the night in one's own room.

As is the case for reinforcers, there are also different types of punishers. *Primary punishers* do not require association with other punishers to be effective, although effectiveness is diminished through adaptation. *Conditioned punishers* must be paired with other punishers to be effective. Threats of punishment, for example, may deter behavior but only if followed by delivery of the punisher if the behavior is performed. *Generalized punishers,* such as social disapproval, are associated with many other punishers (Table 6–4).

There are several factors that influence the effectiveness of punishment and are essential to consider. First, *it is necessary to reinforce appropriate behavior that is incompatible with the undesired response.* Punishment does not teach *appropriate* behavior; it is a procedure that often rapidly, but only temporarily, suppresses undesirable behavior. Once punishment is terminated, a previously punished behavior will recur unless an appropriate positive alternative is learned and rewarded.

Second, *the punisher should be contingent on occurrence of the behavior and should be delivered immediately.* Delayed consequences, such as punishing a young child at home for behavior that occurred at school, or the use of noncontingent positive or negative punishment are not likely to be effective in changing behavior.

Third, *the person should be deprived with respect to the punisher.* Frequent use of punishers will decrease their effectiveness and result in emotional behavior. There are data indicating, for example, that excessive aversive consequences and noncontingent reinforcement are used by parents of children with conduct disorders (Snyder, 1977). The children learn aggressive behavior through *modeling* and are also taught that there is no relationship between their behavior and consequences. The necessity of frequent administration over time is a good indication that a consequence is not working to reduce a behavior. Using the same consequence for all misbehaviors, whether positive or negative punishment, diminishes effectiveness. An additional consideration here is that the intensity of the punisher often increases as frequency of administration increases. A *habituation effect* occurs over time with greater negative side effects and dimished effectiveness.

Fourth, *behavior that is being punished should not also be reinforced.* If punishment is paired with reinforcement, the procedure will, in all likelihood, not result in a decrease in behavior. For example, someone may frequently criticize another person's behavior and then immediately try to make amends with displays of physical affection. The punisher may actually become a discriminative stimulus for positive reinforcement and not function to decrease the offensive behavior being criticized.

Parents can be taught how to use positive reinforcement, time out, and extinction to change their children's problem behaviors. The following case illustrates application of a parent-training program, modeled after Forehand and associates (Forehand and Long, 1996; Forehand and McMahon, 1982), to address oppositional and noncompliant behavior in a preschool child.

A CASE ILLUSTRATION

A 4-year-old girl was noncompliant with parental requests and frequently cried when her requests were denied. Her parents described her as strong-willed, demanding, and argumentative. It was difficult to complete the most mundane tasks, such as dressing and eating meals, because of the youngster's resistance. Other information provided by the parents strongly pointed to a child with a difficult temperament and frustrated, exhausted parents. The couple inadvertently (positively and negatively) reinforced inappropriate behaviors and had been through a period of escalating frequency and severity of punishment. At the time of initial presentation for behavioral treatment, the parents were admittedly very focused on the child's negative behavior, did not enjoy being with her, and felt helpless and guilty about the situation.

Initially the parents were educated about temperament and the interaction between parenting style and temperament. With additional behavior analysis it was determined that several parenting practices actually exacerbated the child's troublesome behaviors. (Table 6–5 illustrates common mistakes and how to correct them.) Training of each skill entailed: (1) describing the skill and giving a rationale for use; (2) the therapist modeling the behavior while

Table 6–5 **Common Behavior Management Problems and How to Correct Them by Using Rules for Maximizing the Effectiveness of Consequences**

Problem 1: The parents have identified a reinforcer (stickers) to increase the behavior of being dressed on time to catch the schoolbus in the morning for their five-year-old child. They give a sticker to the child when he returns from school each day for his punctuality that morning. However, the behavior of being ready on time continues to occur inconsistently. The youngster earns stickers at school for finishing work on time and has quite a collection. He also gets a new pack of stickers each time he makes the trip to the grocery store with his parents.

Analysis: The reinforcer is presented noncontingently by the parents for going to the store. Moreover, the reinforcer is available for other behaviors. The child has so many stickers there is little motivation to obtain more. Finally, there is a long delay for a 5-year-old between occurrence of the behavior and presentation of the reinforcer.

Rules: 1. Present a reinforcer *contingent* upon occurrence of the behavior.
2. *Limit* contact with the reinforcer.
3. Present the reinforcer *immediately* after the behavior occurs.

Correction: A different reinforcer, which is *not* being used in another situation, is identified to increase the behavior of being dressed on time in the morning. Also, the reinforcer is made available immediately after the child is ready on time each morning and only then.

Problem 2: Time out is used by parents each time their 4-year old-daughter hits her younger brother. The behavior is most likely to occur when the parents are preparing dinner. The parents take turns escorting the youngster to the upstairs hall. The mother or father discusses the daughter's behavior and then leaves the area. At this time, the child leaves too, and for much of the dinner preparation time, one parent is involved in trying to get or keep the daughter in time out. The hitting continues to occur one or more times during the evening.

Analysis: During the time parents are preparing dinner, they are not attending positively to the child and are not reinforcing appropriate interactions with the brother. She engages in negative attention-getting behaviors. The parents talk to the child before time out is completed, during time out, and as they are trying to get and keep the child in the time-out area. All of this interaction reinforces inappropriate behavior the parents want to decrease.

Rules: 1. Reinforce appropriate, incompatible behavior.
2. Do not reinforce behavior that is punished.

Correction: First, the environment is made more reinforcing. The child is given a "task" to perform during dinner and the parents positively attend. If she is "taking care" of her brother, for example, the parents frequently verbally praise her appropriate interactions with him or any behaviors other than hurting him. Second, if hitting does occur, she is told, "No hitting," and is escorted to the time-out area without further discussion. If she tries to leave, the parent takes her back without discussion and increases the length of time required to be in time out. She loses a privilege if she continues to be noncompliant with the time-out routine.

playing with the child as the parents observed; (3) each parent playing with the child and practicing the skill while the therapist watched; (4) the therapist giving feedback to the parent about the skill practiced; (5) the parents practicing the skill daily during 15- to 20-minute play sessions with the child at home; and (6) incorporating the skills into interactions with the child throughout the day.

The first task was to increase positive interactions between parents and child and to break the escalating cycle of negative child behavior and negative parental reaction. Parents were instructed on how to attend to the child without correcting, directing, or questioning. Parental attitudes toward the child began to change within the first week of practicing at home and interactions became more positive.

Next the parents learned how to reinforce appropriate behaviors using praise, affection, activities, and tangible reinforcers. They practiced being very specific and genuine in giving compliments and giving them consistently and immediately after appropriate behaviors. Any activity or tangible reinforcers used to strengthen behaviors were also paired with praise. The parents decided to put a marble in a jar each time she complied with a request. The marbles were traded once or twice a day for one of several specified activities or access to a "grab bag" of trinkets. As compliance improved, the schedule of delivery of tangible rewards was made intermittent but social reinforcers continued to be given frequently.

The third skill entailed ignoring nuisance behaviors that posed no danger to the child or others. It was necessary for the parents to identify behavior they knew they could consistently ignore, even when the behavior increased initially (resistance to extinction). In addition to completely removing their attention from the behavior when it occurred, they were also instructed to reinforce appropriate behavior. Crying and arguing were the first behaviors the parents chose to ignore.

Fourth, parents were given instruction on the appropriate way to give directions so as to increase the likelihood of compliance. Guidelines included making "do" statements that were brief, simple, and very specific once eye contact had been established with the child. Parents were directed to use a firm voice of moderate volume and to use physical gestures as appropriate. Finally, parents were cautioned to be selective and to only make requests they were willing and able to follow through with at the time.

Finally, training in the proper and effective use of time out was provided. The hall was chosen as the place for time out. Parents

*were instructed to present a good direction and if compliance did
not occur within 5 seconds they were allowed to give the child one
warning before implementing time out. They were directed to ignore all child behaviors once the procedure was initiated. The child
was required to be quiet for the last minute of time out in order to
end the time-out procedure. Once it ended, the instruction was
again presented to the child. If compliance occurred, reinforcement
was given; if not, the sequence was repeated. On the two occasions
the child left time out before the interval was over, she lost the privilege of watching a favorite television program.*

*The parents noted changes in the child's behavior the same week
they practiced "attending" and improvement continued over the
next 5 weeks of training. By the end of 6 weeks, the child continued
to test limits but less frequently and with much less persistence.
Compliance with requests and parent-child interactions were signfi-
cantly improved, and the parents verbalized considerable pleasure
in being with their child again. They were encouraged to continue
to use the skills routinely. At 2-month follow-up, the parents reported transient periods of increased power struggles with the child,
most often related to higher levels of parent and/or child stress.
Consistent implementation of the procedures and the parents' successful resistance to falling into "old ways" of interacting helped
prevent significant exacerbations of child misbehavior during these
periods.*

Problems with the Use of Negative Consequences

Although respondent (Pavlovian) and operant (Skinnerian) conditioning
have been discussed separately in this chapter, in reality, the processes are interactive and probably inseparable (Baldwin and Baldwin, 1981). Many of the
problems with using negative means of influencing behavior, such as
punishment and negative reinforcement, relate to the interplay of respondent
and operant conditioning, including the development of aversive emotional responses (Table 6–6). Baldwin and Baldwin (1981) emphasize the use of
positive reinforcement over negative reinforcement or punishment. They
maintain that presenting others with aversive stimuli, as one does with negative reinforcement, such as nagging or criticism, diminishes positive social interactions and, through conditioning, makes the desired behavior an aversive
CS. The person learns to dislike the behavior. For example, if nagging and criticism are used by a child's parents to get the youngster to clean his or her
room, the child will probably learn to dislike cleaning because of the association of cleaning with aversive stimuli. One might also observe emotional behaviors associated with the onset of the aversive stimulation, as in the case of

Table 6–6 **Negative Effects of the Use of Aversive Events to Influence Behavior**

NEGATIVE EFFECT	EXAMPLE
The desired behavior becomes an aversive CS.	A youngster learns to dislike homework because nagging and criticism are used to get and keep the child on task.
Aversive stimuli condition negative emotional responses to people, objects, or situations through association with aversive stimuli.	The child stamps and protests when it is time to do homework.
The punishing agent may model verbal or physical aggression.	A child who is punished with ridicule learns that it is acceptable to ridicule one's peers.
People learn ways to avoid punishment and the punishing agent.	An individual falsely denies committing an act to avoid punishment.
Punishment produces response suppression, which can generalize to other behaviors.	A sensitive child who is severely punished for interrupting adult conversation stops talking when adults are present.

the child who starts to stomp, yell, or cry when told to clean his or her room. The alternative, more effective, strategy is to *positively reinforce* behavior.

Baldwin and Baldwin (1981) recommend minimizing application of punishment, particularly when alternative methods are available, because of several negative effects of using punishment:

The punishing agent often models aggressive behavior, verbally or physically. Severe criticism or ridicule and/or physical punishment teaches the recipient that aggression is an acceptable means of dealing with people. The individual may not aggress against the punishing agent but is more likely to engage in verbally or physically aggressive behavior with peers, especially if male (Bandura, 1973). It is especially counterproductive to punish aggression with aggression. People who use negative punishment procedures (e.g., restriction of privileges, time out from reinforcement) may also apply positive punishers such as criticism or being physically "rough" with a child en route to the time-out area.

Punishment generates emotional behavior and more intense verbal or physical activity. In response to aversive stimulation, a youngster may cry, an adult may threaten, or either may hit depending on the situation. Again, violence is more likely to be directed toward peers, a pattern that, when initiated during childhood, can continue through the adult years, such as the spouse who hits his wife when angry. Application of negative punishment procedures can produce emotional responses as well, such as the child who cries when taken to sit in the corner, the teenager who slams the door and talks back when restricted for the weekend, and the spouse who shouts and storms out of the house in response to the other's refusal to attend or talk.

People learn to avoid punishment and also the punishing agent. Behaviors that avoid punishment are negatively reinforced and are usually undesirable responses. For example, people learn what they can do so as not to get "caught" again for a previously punished behavior. Sometimes this is lying about engaging in a behavior and, when lying is punished, Baldwin and Baldwin (1981) suggest the person learns how to be a better liar. Children may "lose" or "forget" to deliver less-than-satisfactory report cards or notes from teachers about misbehavior to their parents. The adolescent who is prohibited from seeing certain friends or is restricted from all privileges for weeks at a time refines a repertoire of deceptive behavior in order to continue to see friends and engage in activities. When punishment is used frequently or is severe, the recipient also may learn to avoid the punishing agent, thus diminishing the opportunities for the agent to either punish or reinforce other behavior.

Negative emotional responses are conditioned when aversive controls are used. Stimuli present in the situation when punishment is delivered can become conditioned aversive stimuli and elicit negative responses including "anxiety, shame, guilt, or bad feelings about [oneself]" (Baldwin and Baldwin, 1981: 266). As more stimuli elicit the negative CERs, the effects generalize to the point that some individuals' functioning is impaired by symptoms of anxiety or other distress. People also engage in behaviors to avoid negative CERs. For example, children who have experienced little reinforcement and much criticism and other punishers by parents and teachers for academic or behavioral difficulties at school usually say they "hate" school and frequently drop out once they reach legal age to do so.

Response suppression produced by punishment can generalize to other behaviors. The individual's behavioral repertoire generally can be inhibited if punishment is used for many behaviors. Baldwin and Baldwin (1981) indicate that, although severe generalized response suppression is rare, shyness, a milder form, is more common.

Antecedents

So far we have discussed the importance of consequences for operant behavior. The *antecedents* of behavior are also significant variables in explaining behavior (Table 6–7). People behave in the presence of certain stimuli or stimulus situations.

We learn to engage in different behaviors depending on the situation. This is accomplished by means of *discrimination training:* in the presence of some stimuli a particular behavior is *reinforced* and in the presence of different stimuli the behavior is *extinguished.* A young child may learn, for example, that one parent ignores tantrums while the other gives the child what he or she wants and, therefore, will *reinforce* the tantrum. The parent who reinforces the tantrums becomes a *discriminative stimulus* (S^D) for tantrums (i.e., the presence of this parent signals that reinforcement is forthcoming if

Table 6–7 **Operant Conditioning—Antecedents**

TERM	DEFINITION	EXAMPLE
Discrimination training	In the presence of certain stimuli or stimulus situations, a behavior is reinforced, and, in the presence of others, the behavior is extinguished.	A medical student gets credit for labeling an event that increases the behavior it follows a "reinforcer" but not for labeling it anything else.
Discriminative stimulus (S^D)	Signals that reinforcement is forthcoming if the behavior occurs in its presence.	Giving a correct definition in response to the question "What is a positive reinforcer?" results in credit for a correct answer.
S^Δ	Signals that reinforcement is not forthcoming if the behavior occurs in its presence.	Giving the definition for a punisher in response to the question "What is a positive reinforcer?" results in no credit for the answer.
Discriminated behavior	Behavior that is more likely to occur in the presence of the S^D than in its absence.	Giving the definition for positive reinforcer is more likely to occur when asked "What is a positive reinforcer?" than when some other question is asked.
Stimulus control	Achieved for a behavior when it is more likely to occur in the presence of the S^D than in its absence.	The question comes to control the response of the definition.
Fading	Stimulus is gradually removed or faded so that another stimulus presented with it will control the response.	Initially a verbal prompt may be required to facilitate the response of giving the definition but is gradually removed so that the question only controls the response.
Generalization	Behavior occurs in the presence of different and/or novel stimuli or stimulus situations.	Given one example of a positive reinforcer, the student is able to identify others.

the behavior does occur). The other parent is associated with nonreinforcement of tantrums and is called an S^Δ (S-delta) if the behavior occurs less frequently in his or her presence than in the presence of the S^D. When the tantrum is more likely to occur in the presence of the S^D than in its absence, we say that *stimulus control* over the tantrum behavior has been established. The behavior is called *discriminated behavior.*

In clinical medicine, a person with a chronic pain problem may be observed to emit more pain behaviors when another person is present to observe and respond to the behaviors than when no one is near or when someone who does not attend to the pain behavior is present. In this situation, there is stimulus control over the pain behavior. (However, this does not mean that the patient is intentionally or consciously behaving in such a way. One need not necessarily be aware of the contingencies in order for one's behavior to be affected by them.)

In order to facilitate the development of discriminated behavior, two stimuli are sometimes presented together. One stimulus is then gradually removed or *faded* so the other controls the response. For example, modeling initially may be paired with verbal instructions but faded over time.

It is frequently desirable for a behavior to occur in the presence of different and/or novel stimuli or situations. Such an occurrence is called *generalization.* This is accomplished by *generalization training,* which entails reinforcement of the behavior in the presence of other stimuli until all members of a stimulus class are associated with occurrence of the behavior. For example, a person may be working to improve his or her assertiveness skills and begins practicing with one family member. The person practices with more and more family members until eventually he or she is responding assertively with the group (or stimulus class) of family members.

THE PRINCIPLE OF RECIPROCAL INHIBITION

Joseph Wolpe (1993) used an animal model to study the development of emotional reactions or "experimental neuroses" and ways of treating such problems once acquired. Cats were shocked while in cages and sometimes as they approached food. The "experimental neuroses" consisted of behaviors indicative of anxiety associated with the cage and lack of feeding behavior despite severe food deprivation. The behaviors generalized to similar situations and were more intense in situations that more closely resembled the experimental cage, room, and so forth. Wolpe reasoned that since feeding behavior had been inhibited by anxiety, then anxiety might be inhibited by eating. Wolpe subsequently reduced the "neurotic symptoms" in the cats by inducing feeding in the original room or in rooms that resembled the original room. Once the cat fed in the original room without signs of anxiety, it was placed in the cage as well. Wolpe considered the "neurosis" eliminated once the cat ate in the experimental cage without indications of anxiety. He maintained that the animal could not be fearful or anxious and feed simultaneously. That is, anxiety and feeding are *reciprocally inhibiting;* the occurrence of one inhibits the other.

Wolpe extended the treatment procedures based on laboratory work with animals to applications with humans. He developed an abbreviated version of Jacobson's (1938) progressive muscle relaxation procedure and initially used relaxation to inhibit anxiety and fear in the presence of actual anxiety-provoking stimuli. Basically, he sought a method more convenient than gradual *in vivo* (real life) exposure and decided to try imagined scenes. *Systematic desensitization,* as he called it, entails pairing deep muscle relaxation with imaginal scenes in a graded fashion from the least to most anxiety provoking. The responses to anxiety-provoking stimuli are "reconditioned" with relaxation, replacing or "inhibiting" the anxiety. Wolpe also used assertive responses and sexual arousal to inhibit anxiety.

Wolpe's work constituted a bridge between animal experimentation in the laboratory and the development of treatment procedures for human problems. Behavioral techniques developed by Wolpe, such as systematic desensitization, were based on the principle of reciprocal inhibition formulated from experiments. Much research was generated from his work, particularly related to systematic desensitization, and this contributed significantly to the development of behavior therapy.

SOCIAL LEARNING OR SOCIAL COGNITIVE THEORY

The foremost theorist and researcher in the area of social learning is Albert Bandura. He agrees with Skinner that behavior is influenced by contingencies, but he emphasizes cognitive processes such as expectancies and the effects of these processes on the behavior of the person and the environment. Bandura (1986) relabeled *social learning* theory and called it *social cognitive* theory, indicating that as his theoretical approach developed, its scope broadened and extended beyond learning mechanisms alone.

The major principle of social cognitive theory is *triadic reciprocal determinism,* which refers to the mutually causal relationship among *behavior, personal factors,* and *environmental events.* Cognitive capabilities, such as the use of symbols, make it possible for people to process thoughts, communicate with one another, anticipate consequences, and learn by observing others. Individuals are therefore able to motivate themselves and engage in self-directed behavior, including self-evaluation and regulation.

Bandura's conceptualization of causation as the interaction of environmental, behavioral, and personal factors may be illustrated with a discussion of several major contributions of social learning or social cognitive theory—modeling, self-regulation, and self-efficacy.

Modeling

Learning that occurs by observing others and the consequences of their behavior is highly efficient. The survival value of such a process is obvious when compared to trial-and-error learning. For example, acquisition of very complex behaviors, such as driving a car and social skills, are facilitated by observing others.

Modeling is a means by which knowledge, skills, and rules can be learned and represented symbolically. As such, there are a number of functions that modeling can serve with regard to learning, and these may operate concurrently in a given situation (Table 6–8).

1. A new pattern of behavior can be acquired by observing how to combine component behaviors in a different way. For example, dancers have a repertoire of movements and skills that are combined in various ways with each new choreography they learn. Surgical residents learn to apply techniques in specific ways for the type of surgery they are performing by observing the most experienced surgeons.

2. Bandura (1986) also maintains that modeling can function to inhibit or disinhibit performance of behaviors that are part of the individual's repertoire. For example, students may be inhibited from volunteering to answer questions in a particular class because they have observed the instructor consistently finds fault with others' answers. Disinhibition can be facilitated by observing, for example, a model who copes in a difficult situation and is successful. Interventions designed to help children manage the discomfort and fear associated with invasive medical procedures, such as bone marrow aspirations and lumbar punctures, include a coping model component (e.g., Jay et al, 1987).

3. Modeling can facilitate occurrence of, or "induce," appropriate behavior that is already part of the person's repertoire. For example, some people may not give money to a homeless person until they observe someone else do so or they may volunteer to

Table 6–8 **Functions of Modeling**

DESCRIPTION OF FUNCTION	EXAMPLE
Acquire new behavior by observing a model	Surgical resident observes a highly skilled surgeon
Combine component behaviors in a unique way	
Inhibit or disinhibit behaviors in one's repertoire because of consequences observed for other's behavior	Cope with a painful medical procedure after seeing a model similar to oneself use skills and report less distress
Facilitate occurrence of behavior in a person's repertoire (response cueing)	Volunteer for a task after observing others volunteer for the task
Draw attention to cues that make a behavior more likely	See others snacking and then eat even if not hungry
Influence occurrence of an emotional response	Child learns to be anxious by observing an anxious parent

perform certain tasks only after others have first offered their services. Bandura (1986) calls this a *response-cueing* function.

4. The attention of the observer can be directed to certain stimuli or situations by the model's behavior, thus making the observer more likely to perform the behavior in the presence of these cues. For example, some people may snack at a party, even if they are not hungry, because their attention is drawn to the food by the sight of others eating.

5. Finally, Bandura (1986) maintains that modeling can influence occurrences of emotional responses and anticipatory arousal in situations where a model has displayed emotions. Children, for example, can learn to be fearful of situations such as thunderstorms by observing an anxious parent during such events.

According to Bandura (1977), modeling is mediated by a number of component processes (Table 6–9). First, one must attend to the model or modeling stimulus in order for observational learning to occur. There are several aspects of the attentional processes. Characteristics of both the observer and the model affect what will actually be observed. For example, models who are more attractive or pleasing to the observer are more likely to be observed than those without these characteristics. With respect to observer characteristics, the person must have, for example, adequate sensory capacities for attending.

Second, the person must remember the observed behavior by means of retention processes. These include, for example, symbolic coding or having verbal labels or descriptions for the behavior. Symbolic (mental) or motor rehearsal are additional processes that may be used to retain what was observed.

Motor reproduction processes have to do with reproducing the information retained into specific behavior. The physical capabilities of the observer, for example, determine whether the observed behavior can be performed.

Table 6–9 **Component Processes Mediate Modeling**

PROCESS	EXAMPLE
Attention: The model is observed.	An attractive model is more likely to be observed.
Retention: The behavior is remembered.	Rehearsal of the behavior facilitates retention.
Motor reproduction: The behavior is executed.	The observer is physically capable of performing the behavior.
Motivation: There is incentive to perform the behavior.	The observer sees that the model's behavior is reinforced.

Finally, motivational processes determine if the observed behavior will be performed. The processes include, for example, vicarious reinforcement or reinforcement observed for the model's behavior. Bandura posits that individuals who see the model's behavior reinforced will likely expect that their own matching or imitative behavior will also be followed by such consequences. Other motivational processes include the nature of self-evaluation and feedback and self-reinforcement.

Bandura's contributions in the area of observational learning are highly significant. As indicated earlier, his classic studies demonstrated very clearly that children learn aggressive behavior from observing aggressive models (Bandura et al, 1963). Subsequent research has shown that one of the best predictors of aggressive behavior in children is aggressive behavior by the parents (Pfeffer et al, 1983).

Self-regulation

Self-direction is an important aspect of Bandura's social cognitive theory. The capability to regulate one's behavior entails multiple skills. There are three processes involved in self-regulation, according to Bandura (1986): *self-observation, self-evaluation,* and *self-reaction*. This section includes descriptions of the processes and possible behavioral dysfunction related to depression.

Self-observation or Monitoring

In order to obtain information to establish standards of behavior and to judge current behavior relative to these standards, one must observe relevant dimensions of one's behavior with some regularity and accuracy. Self-monitoring is influenced by attentional processes, self-perception, and symbolic representation of information obtained. Dysfunction in this process can be related to a self-perpetuating cycle of depressed mood that adversely affects the way experiences are monitored and processed, and this faulty processing further exacerbates the individual's depressed mood. Bandura (1986) suggests that depressed persons *negatively distort* their perceptions and recollections of events. For example, such individuals may take an important examination and recall more about what they did not know on the test than what they were able to answer. This distorted recollection of the event adversely affects their mood, and they begin to recall other experiences that reflect negatively on their competence.

Judgment or Self-evaluation

This process entails evaluation of behavior in relation to internalized personal standards and other points of reference such as peers or a normative group as well as consideration of the value of the performance. Furthermore, Bandura (1986) indicates that it is important to take into account the causal attributions of the individual with respect to success and failure. Dysfunction in any or all of these subprocesses may be related to depressed mood. The individuals described above negatively appraise their performances either in relation to peers, a normative group, or their own standards and attribute the failure to lack of ability rather than situational factors. Further, these individuals devalue their accomplishments in relation to others.

Self-reaction

The third process in self-regulation is self-reaction, which directs and motivates behavior. Individuals can evaluate their behavior positively or negatively and reward or punish the performance. Depressed persons are less likely to evaluate positively and reward an activity and more likely to punish severely than nondepressed persons, according to Bandura (1986). Repeated negative self-reaction is associated with depressed mood.

It can be adaptive to modify standards and other subprocesses of self-regulation. Consider the case of a 20-year-old college student and musician with a chronic pain problem subsequent to injury in an automobile accident.

A CASE ILLUSTRATION

The patient was a sophomore music student when he was "rear-ended" in a motor vehicle accident. He did not suffer major injury but was left with chronic neck and shoulder pain associated with whiplash some months after the accident. He was an accomplished cellist who was accustomed to practicing 3 to 4 hours each day. He was also an exceptional student who expected to earn As in all of his college classes. After the accident, the patient experienced difficulty in studying for extended periods as well as in sitting for exams because of the strain on his neck and shoulder muscles and the resulting pain. Most attempts to play the cello were followed by significant increases in pain. He was not willing to practice his instrument for only a few minutes on alternating days as his physical therapist advised, and he could not accept less than excellent grades in his courses. He became increasingly depressed and withdrawn, and his pain problem continued to worsen.

Subsequent to his accident, the young man was not able to perform academically or musically according to previous standards. Nevertheless, he continued to apply these standards and to evaluate his performance in reference to them. The result was that he consistently fell short, producing negative and punishing self-reactions and multiple adverse effects, including distorted self-monitoring over time. The patient experienced a sense of failure, self-deprecation, greater physical pain, and depressed mood. He devalued what he was able to accomplish within his limitations and participated in fewer and fewer activities as his depression intensified.

Self-efficacy

Bandura (1986:391) defines the concept of self-efficacy in the following way:

> Perceived self-efficacy is defined as people's judgments of their capabilities to organize and execute courses of action required to attain designated types of performances. It is concerned not with the skills one has but with judgments of what one can do with whatever skills one possesses.

It is Bandura's contention that it is not sufficient that individuals have skills to behave competently; it is also necessary that they have perceived self-efficacy with regard to these skills. People may expect a particular consequence for a behavior (outcome expectation) and have the behavior in their repertoire but not engage in the activity because they judge themselves as deficient in that situation. The greater one's self-efficacy, the more likely it is for the person to persist in the face of difficulty.

According to Bandura (1986), there are four sources of information regarding self-efficacy:

1. *Success experiences* increase self-efficacy and failures decrease appraisals of efficacy. If self-efficacy is strong, occasional failures are more likely to be attributed to situational factors rather than to lack of ability. Bandura also maintains that self-efficacy generalizes to similar situations.
2. *Vicarious experiences* in which others are observed to be capable can facilitate self-efficacy, particularly when the individual lacks information about how to evaluate his or her competence in the situation.
3. *Verbal persuasion* can be a source of information about self-efficacy when the person already has some confidence in his or her capabilities in the situation. When the person then tries and succeeds, self-efficacy is further strengthened.
4. *Physiological state* gives the individual information about susceptibility to failure. A negative cycle of physiological arousal, negative thoughts, and greater arousal can be set into motion. The absence of signs of autonomic arousal is associated with greater likelihood of success.

The concept of self-efficacy is useful from Bandura's perspective in understanding anxiety disorders. He says that expectations regarding outcome and efficacy cause fear and avoidance rather than fear causing avoidance behavior. For example, patients with social phobias may consistently avoid situations that require speaking in front of groups of persons. In such situations they may experience numerous physiological signs of anxiety that intensify their embarrassment and self-consciousness and cause them to further doubt their abilities to speak coherently in front of others. Individuals have expectations about what they would say, how they would say it, and possible consequences (outcome) as well as an expectation about whether they could do what they know how to do (efficacy). From Bandura's viewpoint, experiencing success will increase efficacy and decrease avoidance and fear. Verbal persuasion is less likely to be effective in such a situation.

Turk et al (1992) relate the concept of self-efficacy to coping with chronic pain. They make the case that the strength of the patient's self-efficacy for coping with pain affects the likelihood of the person engaging in coping behaviors and persisting in the face of difficulty. Setting the patient up to succeed with gradual increases in activities and pacing facilitates development of realistic expectancies and, consequently, occurrences of coping behaviors. The authors also suggest that avoidance behaviors are mediated by expectancies about pain. Avoidance of activities persists because the patient believes that performance of the behavior(s) will cause pain, and the expectation is not changed because consequences are avoided and not experienced. Individuals are assisted so that they engage in activities associated with less pain than expected and, through repeated experiences of this type, expectancies are modified to become more realistic and adaptive.

CLINICAL APPLICATIONS: COGNITIVE AND BEHAVIORAL THERAPIES

Behavior therapy or modification entails the application of laboratory-based psychological principles for changing behavior. A great deal of research has been and continues to be generated in evaluation of treatment techniques derived from principles of operant and respondent conditioning. It is also important to note that these procedures are applied in an individualized fashion and that treatment may consist of multiple interventions. Furthermore, an appreciation of the underlying principles of any behavioral treatment is essential to ensure the technique is applied appropriately and efficaciously.

The term *cognitive-behavioral therapy* frequently refers to treatment "packages" (or protocols) that include a number of component procedures. Some of these components may be called "behavioral" such as exposure, relaxation, contingency management, social skills training, or biofeedback. Others are described as "cognitive" because they address factors such as expectancies, self-talk, perceptions, interpretations, self-efficacy, and the like.

Interventions that are intended to modify cognitions usually include behavioral methods such as self-monitoring, rehearsal, or exposure. Historically, studies have not shown clearly that cognitions are altered because of the "cognitive" techniques used or that changes in behavior were due to alterations in cognitions. However, researchers in the field are enthusiastically engaged in treatment comparison studies and component analyses of behavioral and cognitive-behavioral intervention packages for multiple problem areas.

It is beyond the scope of this chapter to review and/or compare cognitive-behavioral and behavioral therapies for psychiatric or medical disorders. This section, however, includes brief presentations of the following: (1) the cognitive or cognitive-behavioral therapies of Meichenbaum, Beck, and Ellis; (2) descriptions/definitions of a sample of therapy techniques and a case study illustration of the application of some of these techniques to treat obsessive–compulsive disorder; (3) behavior therapy applications within behavioral medicine and a case study illustration of the applications of behavior therapy for a health-related problem; and (4) applications of behavior therapy for prevention of illness and disease.

Cognitive Behavior Modification

Meichenbaum (1977) maintains that the same principles that govern observable behavior also can be applied to modify private events, such as cognitions. By altering cognitions such as "self-talk," behavior and emotions can also be changed. Meichenbaum developed two procedures that emphasize the role of self-talk in facilitating behavior change. *Self-instructional training* entails identification of maladaptive thoughts; that is, individuals learn what they say to themselves in situations identified as problematic (e.g., speaking in front of groups of people). Then, the therapist models appropriate self-instructions, positive self-talk, and self-reinforcement for handling the situation successfully. Finally, the person practices, first self-instructing aloud and then silently, and the therapist gives feedback. According to a recent review of cognitive therapy for anxiety disorders by Oakley and Padesky (1990), additional, research is needed to evaluate self-instructional training.

Stress inoculation training focuses on the acquisition of coping skills that can be applied across different situations. According to Meichenbaum (1992), training includes three phases, the first of which is educational. The patient learns about the relationship between maladaptive patterns of thinking and emotions and behavior. Second, coping self-talk is rehearsed for each step of dealing with a stressor, including preparing for it, confronting and handling the stressor, coping with being overwhelmed by the event, and praising oneself for handling the situation. Finally, the skills are applied *in vivo*.

Rational-emotive Therapy (RET)

Ellis (1962) identifies faulty cognitions as the basis for people's distress. *Rational-emotive therapy (RET)* focuses on changing patterns of thinking directly and is based on the assumption that one's interpretation or perception of events produces emotional consequences. In other words, it is not the event itself that causes a person to experience emotions of anxiety, happiness, or fear, but his or her beliefs about the event. Ellis discusses the relationship in terms of an "ABC" model where A is the event, B is the belief about the event, and C is the emotional consequence. Ordinarily, people think their emotions are caused by events but, according to Ellis, they are the result of either rational or irrational beliefs about the situation. Therapy involves disputation of the irrational beliefs. However, Ellis (1979, cited by Oakley and Padesky, 1990) indicates that RET includes many techniques, including numerous behavioral procedures. This makes it difficult to evaluate the effectiveness of RET. The reader is referred to reviews by Kendall et al (1995) and Lyons and Woods (1991). The latter review consists of a meta-analysis of outcome studies. The authors only cautiously conclude that RET is an effective treatment due to significant methodological problems of the studies reviewed.

Beck's Cognitive Therapy

Beck (1967, 1976) proposes a model for conceptualizing and treating anxiety, depression, and other disorders that is based on the premise, similar to Ellis's, that it is the individual's perception or interpretation of events that causes emotional distress. With regard to chronic depression, Beck (1967) suggested that, as a child, the person forms a "negative self-schema" that is characterized by a kind of theme, such as abandonment or criticism, depending on the nature of childhood experiences. Individuals view themselves, the environment, and the future negatively because of the self-schema. When adults have experiences similar to painful childhood experiences, they process the information in ways that are consistent with the negative self-schema (e.g., as abandonment) and feel depressed. The cognitive errors in processing information function to sustain the depression.

Cognitive themes and information-processing errors also apply in anxiety disorders (Beck, 1976). Oakley and Padesky (1990) suggest that once the person judges a situation as dangerous, the entire system is affected—including autonomic arousal, behavior, emotions, and cognitions—and the changes are self-sustaining. A similar scenario also occurs with depression.

Cognitive therapy focuses on the themes of negative self-schemata, but not initially. At first, therapy centers on helping the patient see the relationship among cognitions, emotions, and behaviors through self-monitoring. Behavioral tasks are assigned as "experiments" to have the patient "test out" beliefs about himself or herself against "reality" and, for depressed patients, for activation. As therapy continues, there is more emphasis on evaluating maladaptive thoughts and on "testing" their validity until the person confronts directly the theme of their negative self-schema and works to change it.

Oakley and Padesky's (1990) review includes an excellent description of the application of cognitive therapy for anxiety disorders. The authors' conclusion regarding the effectiveness of Beck's cognitive therapy for anxiety disorders is that it is a "promising approach" but larger, more method-ologically sound studies are needed to draw firmer conclusions regarding efficacy. Hollon et al (1991) reviewed studies comparing cognitive therapy with pharmacotherapy for depression and reached similar conclusions. They indicated that cognitive therapy has not been well established as an alternative to pharmacotherapy for depression because of the limitations of current research. It is often effective to combine cognitive therapy with pharmacotherapy when indicated. Psychotherapy and pharmacotherapy are not mutually exclusive of each other.

THERAPY TECHNIQUES

1. *Contingency management* entails application of the principles of reinforcement and punishment to change behavior, such as increasing compliance with medical treatment or parental requests or decreasing unhealthy or maladaptive behaviors (i.e., overeating, smoking, or physical aggression). Token systems have been implemented to increase medical treatment compliance (Dapcich-Miura and Hovell, 1979).

2. *Parent training* (e.g., Forehand and Long, 1996; Forehand and McMahon, 1982) consists of instruction in contingency management skills including how to: (1) identify specific behaviors to change; (2) increase positive interactions with the child and decrease commands and criticisms; (3) provide positive reinforcers such as praise, affection, and tokens for desirable behavior; (4) extinguish negative attention-getting behaviors; and (5) use time out or *response cost* for inappropriate behaviors. Response cost is a punishment procedure whereby points or tokens are taken away contingent upon occurrences of particular behaviors.

3. Contingencies can be mutually agreed upon and written down in the form of contracts. The *contingency contract* specifies behaviors and their consequences in explicit detail and is most effective when negotiated with all parties having input and agreeing on the contingencies. Taylor and associates (1980), for example, decreased a patient's unnecessary overuse of medical services by making visits to two health professionals contingent on not seeing others without permission.

4. *Social skills training* entails systematic instruction and training in an area of communication using behavioral principles. Global skill areas such as assertiveness or conversational skills are broken down into specific, teachable units of behavior. The

social skills training model consists of: (1) describing the specific behavior to be learned along with a rationale for its acquisition; (2) modeling the behavior; (3) having the person practice the skill by role playing; and (4) giving feedback for the performance. The steps are repeated until each skill is mastered. Chaney (1989) suggests, for example, that training in "drink refusal" for alcoholics is useful as one component of inpatient treatment.

5. *Exposure to fear-provoking stimuli* is the treatment of choice for many anxiety disorders. Table 6–10 includes the disorders for which exposure is the primary intervention or a major component of treatment as concluded by authors of recent reviews of the areas. The procedure can be accomplished in a number of ways. *Gradual in vivo exposure* may be self-paced or arranged by a therapist. An anxiety hierarchy is developed that consists of identifying fear-inducing situations for the person and then quantifying each of these in terms of how much distress the patient experiences (or imagines he or she would experience) if actually in the situation. Typically, the items are quantified by rating "subjective units of distress" (SUDS) on a scale of zero to one hundred. The situations are arranged in the hierarchy, and exposure begins with the least fear-provoking situation. Once the patient experiences minimal to no anxiety in this situation, the next one is faced and so on, until the person can handle the most difficult situations for himself or herself. An example of an anxiety hierarchy for gradual exposure for treatment of a driving phobia is illustrated in Table 6–11.

6. *Systematic desensitization* is basically gradual imaginal exposure. There are occasions when patient anxiety is so severe that treatment with *in vivo* exposure is preceded by

Table 6–10 **Applications of Exposure as a Primary Treatment Component for Anxiety Disorders**

ANXIETY DISORDER	INTERVENTION	REVIEW
Agoraphobia	*In vivo* exposure	Craske et al (1992)
Panic disorder	*In vivo* and interoceptive exposure	Beck and Zebb (1994)
Obsessive–compulsive disorder	*In vivo* exposure with response prevention	Stanley and Turner (1995)
Posttraumatic stress disorder (combat related)	Imaginal exposure with or without *in vivo* cues	Frueh et al (1995)
Simple phobia	Exposure	Borden (1992)
Social phobia	Exposure	Turner et al (1992)

Table 6–11 **Sample Anxiety Hierarchy for a Patient with a Driving Phobia**

100 SUDS	Sitting in traffic on a bridge over a body of water by myself
95 SUDS	Crossing a body of water over a bridge by myself with no traffic in sight
90 SUDS	Sitting in traffic on a bridge over a body of water with someone with me in the car
85 SUDS	Sitting in traffic on a bridge by myself with cars lined up as far as I can see
80 SUDS	Sitting on the expressway by myself with cars backed up as far as I can see
75 SUDS	Sitting in traffic on a bridge with someone with me with cars lined up as far as I can see
70 SUDS	Sitting on the expressway with someone with me with cars lined up as far as I can see
65 SUDS	Driving over a bridge on the expressway by myself in stop-and-go traffic
60 SUDS	Driving on the expressway by myself in stop-and-go traffic
55 SUDS	Driving over a bridge on the expressway with someone with me in stop-and-go traffic
50 SUDS	Driving on the expressway with someone with me in stop-and-go traffic
45 SUDS	Driving over a bridge on the expressway by myself with no traffic in sight
40 SUDS	Driving on the expressway by myself with no traffic in sight
35 SUDS	Driving on surface streets by myself and stopping in a long line of traffic
30 SUDS	Driving on surface streets by myself in stop-and-go traffic
25 SUDS	Driving on surface streets with someone and stopping in a long line of traffic
20 SUDS	Driving on surface streets by myself in stop-and-go traffic
15 SUDS	Driving on surface streets by myself and stopping at a traffic light and not being the first car in the line
10 SUDS	Driving on surface streets by myself and stopping at a traffic light and being the first car in the line
5 SUDS	Driving on a familiar stretch of road that is mildly congested but has no traffic lights
0 SUDS	Driving on a familiar stretch of road that has no traffic lights and very little traffic

systematic desensitization. For example, a homebound ago-raphobic may not be able to venture from the safety of the house at all. Gradual imaginal exposure decreases anxiety and fear sufficiently to make it possible to initiate gradual *in vivo* exposure.

7. *Imaginal flooding* entails indirect exposure in an abrupt and prolonged fashion. The patient is instructed to imagine the anxiety-provoking scenario by the therapist and continues to do so until there is significant reduction in anxiety. Self-re-

port, overt behavior, and physiological responses (e.g., pulse rate and blood pressure) are assessed to evaluate level of anxiety. Imaginal flooding, with and without *in vivo* cues, has been used for treatment of posttraumatic stress disorder associated, for example, with combat experiences (see Frueh et al [1995] for a review of the literature in this area).

Flooding in vivo consists of abrupt, prolonged exposure to the fear-producing stimuli. The patient is accompanied to the situation, as in the case of agoraphobia, or may be presented the stimuli in the office by a therapist. The person stays in the situation until there is a significant reduction in anxiety. The procedure is repeated until the anxiety is eliminated.

There is not a single theory proposed about how exposure works to reduce anxiety. One explanation is that escape and avoidance behaviors as well as anxiety are extinguished because exposure to the situations does not result in aversive consequences. Bandura (1977) suggests that exposure functions to increase self-efficacy, which results in diminished anxiety and additional efforts on the part of the patient to perform such behaviors.

8. *Response prevention* consists of not allowing the patient to engage in behaviors, such as compulsive rituals, that serve an anxiety-reductive function. For example, a compulsive handwasher would not be allowed to wash. The rationale is that performance of the ritual, as in the case of obsessive-compulsive disorder, is negatively reinforced because it terminates or avoids anxiety. The avoidance behavior is extinguished. The behavioral treatment of choice for obsessive-compulsive disorder is a combination of response prevention and exposure (Steketee, 1994).

9. *Relaxation techniques* can be used as a treatment component along with medication for diverse problems such as anticipatory nausea and vomiting associated with cancer chemotherapy, chronic pain, and insomnia, as well as an adjunct to other treatments for stress reduction, hypertension, and anxiety. Some researchers have suggested that patient anxiety may potentiate conditioned responses in chemotherapy, and acquisition and application of relaxation skills can alleviate or even prevent development of anticipatory nausea and vomiting (Burish, et al, 1987). *Progressive muscle relaxation* (PMR) (Jacobson, 1938) entails learning to deeply relax the muscles of the body by systematically tensing each of several muscle groups and abruptly releasing the tension.

This helps increase awareness of the differences in the sensations of tension and relaxation and also how to produce relaxation. Eventually patients are able to induce a state of deep relaxation without the tension-release cycles. *Diaphragmatic breathing,* which typically consists of instruction in how to use one's diaphragm to breath more deeply and slowly, and *imagery or visualization techniques* can also be used to induce relaxation or deepen a relaxed state produced by PMR. Relaxation exercises have applicability across a wide range of psychiatric and medical problems from managing chronic pain to helping prevent recurrences of herpes virus outbreaks cutaneous (Burnette et al, 1991).

10. *Biofeedback* is a tool to promote self-regulation of physiological responses such as heart rate, blood pressure, brain waves, body temperature, penile erections, and muscle activity. Electrical signals from the particular response are measured, amplified, and then converted to visual or auditory information for the patient. This objective, observable feedback about a particular system or function of the body helps the patient learn how to exert control over the response.

    In the area of chronic pain, biofeedback is useful for promoting relaxation as well as for reactivating muscles that have not been used because of the association of movement of those muscles with pain. Other examples of clinical applications include electromyographic (EMG) biofeedback for neuromuscular recovery in cardiovascular disease patients and for fecal incontinence caused by sphincter weakness.

11. *Cognitive restructuring* refers to alterations in patterns of thinking and may include the methods of Ellis, Meichenbaum, Beck, or others. For example, one component of cognitive behavior therapy for binge eating entails identifying, refuting, and changing dysfunctional thoughts about dieting and weight (Smith et al; 1994).

12. *Problem-solving skills training* involves instruction in the use of a model consisting of several steps: (1) define the problem; (2) brainstorm possible solutions; (3) evaluate solutions and implement one; and (4) evaluate the solution implemented. Training can be especially useful for individuals who behave impulsively.

13. *Stress-management training* is frequently based on Meichenbaum's stress inoculation training (Meichenbaum, 1992) and includes educational, rehearsal, and application phases. During the educational phase, the patients learn about their individual responses to stress, sources of stress,

and means of avoiding or coping with stressors. Time management and assertiveness are ways to avoid stress. Relaxation skills training, positive self-talk, and problem solving are examples of coping skills. In the rehearsal phase the patients practice the skills and then actually apply them. Practice may not "make perfect" but dramatically decrease anxiety.

Table 6–12 includes a summary of the techniques and examples of applications.

The following case illustrates application of several interventions for treatment of obsessive-compulsive disorder (OCD) and related problems.

A CASE ILLUSTRATION

At age 32 when she presented for behavioral treatment, the patient had suffered from severe OCD symptoms for approximately 5 years. She was overwhelmed with obsessions and compulsions that were primarily related to an intense fear of hurting others. These included fears of hitting someone with her car or poisoning them. She repeatedly checked any foodstuffs she came into close proximity with and refused to cook food that others were to eat. It was very difficult for her to drive because if she hit a bump of any kind she obsessed about whether she had hit a person. She then checked and rechecked by going around the block, listening for sirens, even listening to the news about a person being injured by a hit-and-run driver. In addition to behavioral rituals, the patient repeated prayers and other thoughts obsessively. She was very tense and distressed and extremely unassertive. A "people pleaser" who neither wanted to hurt nor offend others by telling them how she felt, refusing their requests, or asking them to change their behavior, the patient often felt devalued by others and out of control of her life.

Treatment consisted of exposure and response prevention for obsessions and compulsions and related avoidance behavior (such as not touching others' food or cooking for them), therapist support and reinforcement, stress management, and assertiveness training. Exposure and response prevention were implemented in the areas of handling food and driving with therapist assistance. The patient was also given behavioral assignments between sessions. With respect to poisoning others, exposure first entailed the therapist bringing food to the session and having the client pick it up and hand it to the therapist who then ate it. The task was made more difficult by putting the food in another room and requesting that she bring it into the therapist's office without being watched. Then the therapist placed a bottle of cleanser near the food and the patient was instructed to get the food and bring it to another room without supervision. Over time, the client brought packaged foods and then foods

Table 6–12 **Therapy Techniques**

TECHNIQUE	DESCRIPTION	SAMPLE APPLICATION
Contingency management	Use reinforcers and punishers to change behavior	Compliance with medical treatment
Parent training	Instruct parents in identification of behaviors to change, positive interactions, contingency management, and extinction	Compliance with requests
Contingency contract	Record agreement between parties regarding behavior and consequences	Appropriate use of medical services
Social skills training	Systematically teach skills with verbal instruction, modeling, rehearsal, and feedback	Assertiveness with medical personnel
Gradual *in vivo* exposure	Gradual, real-life contact with a fear-provoking situation until minimal anxiety is experienced in that situation	Agoraphobia
Systematic desensitization	Gradual imaginal exposure to fear-provoking stimuli	Thunderstorm phobia
Imaginal flooding	Abrupt, imaginal exposure to fear-provoking stimuli until anxiety dissipates	Posttraumatic stress disorder
Flooding *in vivo*	Abrupt, prolonged exposure to fear-producing stimuli or situations until anxiety dissipates	Phobia
Response prevention	Prevent occurrence of behavior	Compulsive handwashing, checking
Relaxation techniques	Teach ways of deeply relaxing muscles, diaphragmatic breathing, and imagery	Anticipatory nausea
Biofeedback	Train regulation of physiological responses	Neuromuscular recovery
Cognitive restructuring	Alter patterns of thinking	Binge eating
Problem-solving skills	Use of structured model for defining problems, and generating, evaluating, and implementing solutions	Impulsive behavior
Stress management	Instruction in identifying stressors and individual responses to stressors and skills to avoid and cope with stress	Cardiovascular health

she prepared. Eventually she was able to have the food and a house-hold cleanser on the seat of her car at the same time. Assignments also included taking food to work to share with coworkers and cook-ing for family and friends.

In addition to working on obsessions and compulsions about poi-soning others, exposure and response prevention were used to de-crease anxiety and rituals related to driving and hitting people. The therapist rode with the client in her car around increasingly more populated areas and in parking lots with speed breakers. She was not allowed to circle back to check when she hit a bump or curb and was not permitted to check the rearview mirror more than once. Between-session assignments most often consisted of practicing ex-posure and not performing rituals for situations she had already succeeded with during recent and previous sessions.

The patient participated in assertiveness training that focused on appropriate expression of emotions (positive and negative), refusing requests, and making requests for behavior change. A social skills training model was used to teach specific nonverbal and verbal component behaviors that included the following: (1) make eye con-tact; (2) speak in a normal conversation volume; (3) use "I" state-ments, such as "I feel angry when you make unreasonable requests of me"; (4) say no to the request and offer an alternative, if appro-priate (for example, "I cannot come over at lunch today to take you to the store, Mom, but I can do it after work or on Saturday"); and (5) request behavior change of others, when appropriate. For exam-ple, "I know you are upset, but I would appreciate your not yelling at me. It makes me feel angry, too." Generalization of effects was fa-cilitated with behavioral assignments to practice specific skills, ini-tially in less threatening situations and eventually in more difficult ones.

Stress management consisted of relaxation skills training, Meichenbaum's steps for stress inoculation training, and positive self-instruction and problem solving. The patient practiced all of the techniques and also learned how to praise and reward herself for ef-fort as well as accomplishment.

The patient was very compliant with treatment and within 6 months of the initiation of treatment reported an 80% reduction in obsessions and compulsions and significantly improved mood. Symptoms increased during periods of stress, but she learned to rec-ognize these times, use stress-management, coping, and problem-solving skills, and acknowledge that the temporary exacerbation did not mean total relapse. The patient cooked for others, drove through areas with many pedestrians without checking, and reestablished many activities she had enjoyed prior to onset of severe OCD symp-

toms. She participated in less and less frequent therapy sessions to receive support and assistance with structuring tasks. By the end of 1 year, she came in every 2 to 3 months for follow-up visits.

BEHAVIORAL MEDICINE

Behavioral medicine involves the application of behavior principles and technology to medical or health-related problems. Behavior therapy is useful for treating numerous health-related problems and some of these are listed along with sample interventions in Table 6–13.

The following case study is an example of application of a treatment protocol for tension headaches in a young woman.

A CASE ILLUSTRATION

The patient is a 17-year-old college freshman who lives with her parents and 12-year-old brother. She had weekly tension headaches that could last for a few hours or 1 to 2 days. The patient worried constantly about her appearance, grades, getting a good job, and what her peers and teachers thought of her. All of her classmates and instructors knew about her headaches and greeted her with questions about them. Her family members planned their own activities around how she was feeling and would cancel or postpone family outings if she was not feeling well so they could help her. Because she constantly worried, the patient's family and friends frequently reassured her, telling her not to be so serious and to "take it easy."

Table 6–13 **Examples of Clinical Applications of Behavior Therapy to Health-Related Problems**

HEALTH-RELATED PROBLEM	TECHNIQUES
Anorexia nervosa	Contingency management, cognitive restructuring, family therapy
Bulimia nervosa	Exposure with response prevention, cognitive restructuring
Chronic pain	Contingency management, relaxation, stress management, biofeedback, shaping
Encopresis	Contingency management, biofeedback
Epilepsy	Symptom-contingent relaxation
Headache	Relaxation, biofeedback
Insomnia	Stimulus control, sleep restriction
Irritable bowel syndrome	Relaxation/stress management, hypnosis
Muscular rehabilitation	Biofeedback
Raynaud's disease	Biofeedback

Her younger brother assumed most of her household responsibilities, and her parents tried to protect her from knowing about their stressors.

Multiple behavioral interventions were appropriate for the young woman. Relaxation skills training and other stress-management techniques were taught to her, and she was referred for physical therapy. Her irrational beliefs about herself, including perfectionism, were challenged within sessions, and she was also given less-than-perfect behavior assignments to complete. She was requested to monitor her headaches, including antecedents and consequences. Family responses to the patient's pain were an important part of the intervention. Family members were instructed to continue with their plans even if the patient was not feeling well and to encourage her to perform household tasks and recreational activities even when she did not feel well. Further, they were taught how to ignore her complaints of physical discomfort and to attend and praise efforts to cope with her headaches or to prevent them by engaging in relaxation and/or physical therapy exercises.

The patient reported significant reductions in headache intensity and frequency and benefits of relaxation exercises after 6 weeks of treatment. Further reduction was noted in relation to altered patterns of responding by family members. She also increased leisure activities and reported increased abilities to cope with her discomfort and other problems.

PREVENTION OF ILLNESS AND DISEASE

In addition to treatment of medical problems, behavioral interventions also are useful in primary, secondary, and tertiary prevention of disease and injury as discussed by Oyama and Andrasik (1992). The authors suggest that healthy behaviors can be strengthened and unhealthy ones decreased with the use of behavioral techniques.

Primary prevention includes interventions to prevent onset of illness or injury. For example, Kelly et al (1989) designed a cognitive-behavioral protocol with educational and social skills training components to reduce high-risk sexual behaviors associated with AIDS. Behavioral interventions such as contingency management, modeling, and practice also are useful in preventing child injuries in the home and in automobiles (Roberts et al, 1987).

Compliance with medical treatment and preparation for hospitalization and/or medical procedures are examples of secondary prevention goals of promoting healthy behaviors after an illness has been diagnosed. Newly diagnosed diabetics, for example, must learn how to check their blood glucose levels and administer insulin as well as adhere to particular dietary restrictions. Applicable behavioral strategies to promote such behaviors are behavioral rehearsal, reinforcement, and problem solving (Oyama and Andrasik, 1992).

There is a good deal of empirical support for the benefits of preparing patients for hospitalization or invasive medical procedures. In recent years, behavioral researchers have developed and evaluated interventions designed to provide such preparation in order to reduce the stress associated with the experience and enhance recovery (Ludwick-Rosenthal and Neufield, 1988). For example, Oyama and Andrasik (1992) indicate that preparation for coronary artery bypass graft surgery often consists of provision of information about the procedure, recovery, and postoperative experience, as well as training in relaxation techniques. Intervention packages have been shown to be effective in decreasing behavioral distress of pediatric oncology patients undergoing bone marrow aspirations and lumbar punctures (Jay et al, 1987) and venipunctures (Manne et al, 1990).

COMPARISONS OF THE BEHAVIORAL AND PSYCHOANALYTIC MODELS

A comparison of behavioral and psychoanalytic models for explaining and changing human behavior yields multiple differences (Table 6–14). There is, however, at least one similarity of these two diverse schools of thought, namely *determinism.* Psychoanalysts and behaviorists both posit *causes* for behavior that do not include the notion of free will.

At this point, the two approaches diverge. Major differences have to do with the nature of the causes, the significance of behavior itself, and the focus of interventions to produce change. Psychoanalytic theory proposes that behavior is symbolic of underlying, intrapsychic processes and that neurotic behavior is a symptom of unconscious conflict. The focus of treatment is, therefore, primarily directed toward understanding the underlying processes rather than on the behavior or symptoms. Early experiences are highly significant from a psychoanalytic perspective in which treatment entails bringing unconscious material and conflicts into consciousness.

The behavioral position is that the behavior of the individual is the focus of treatment. Behavior is seen as being determined, not by intrapsychic processes, but by reinforcement history, current contingencies, and genetic endowment. Observable environmental events such as antecedents and consequences, the current contingencies, are analyzed. As such, the behavioral approach emphasizes contemporary rather than historical factors in explaining and changing behavior. Behavioral interventions consist of applying principles of operant and/or classical conditioning to change the behavior itself.

There are also significant differences in the two models from the standpoint of methodology. Psychoanalysis is subjective, and the focus as well as the

Table 6–14 **The Behavioral and Psychoanalytic Models**

BEHAVIORAL MODEL	PSYCHOANALYTIC MODEL
1. Behavior is determined by current contingencies, reinforcement history, and genetic endowment.	Behavior is determined by intrapsychic processes.
2. Problem behavior is the focus of study and treatment.	Behavior is interpreted as a symbol of intrapsychic processes and neurotic symptoms of unconscious conflict. The underlying conflict is the focus of treatment.
3. Contemporary variables, such as contingencies of reinforcement, are the focus of the analysis.	Historical variables, such as childhood experiences, are the focus of the analysis.
4. Treatment entails application of principles of operant and/or classical conditioning.	Treatment consists of bringing unconscious conflicts into consciousness.
5. Objective observation, measurement, and experimentation are the methods used. The focus is on observable behavior and environmental events (antecedents and consequences).	Subjective methods of interpretation of behavior and inference regarding unobservable events (e.g., intrapsychic processes) are used.
6. Theory is based on experimentation.	Theory is predominantly based on case histories.
7. Tenets can be formulated into testable hypotheses and evaluated through experimentation.	Many tenets cannot be formulated into testable hypotheses to be evaluated through experimentation.

mechanisms of change are largely unobservable. Inference and interpretation are used by the therapist. Additionally, psychoanalytic theory was developed from case histories, and tenets of the theory are quite difficult to evaluate empirically and validate.

The behavioral approach, on the other hand, is objective and based on the empirical method. Behavioral theory has been formulated and tested by means of experimentation. Also, the approach entails a commitment to empirical evaluation of behavioral treatment interventions.

CRITICISMS OF THE BEHAVIORAL MODEL

One criticism of the behavioral model is that explanations for human behavior are oversimplified and ignore emotions and cognitions. There are two aspects of the response to such criticism. First, simple principles established in the animal laboratory can be used to account for complex behaviors. Current applications of behavior therapy are often comprehensive and address multiple problems of the person. The second issue raised in this criticism is related to the role of private events in explaining behavior. Although all behaviorists do not ascribe a causal role to internal events in explaining behavior, few deny that thoughts and feelings are important and should be considered. Behavioral, physiological, cognitive, and emotional factors may all be dealt with in treatment depending on the nature of the primary problem. Treatment of anxiety disorders, for example, entails assessment of behavioral, physiological, and self-report indices of fear or anxiety.

A second criticism is based on the assumption that if the person's behavior is determined by principles of operant or respondent conditioning, then the person is passive and does not himself or herself affect the environment. While this may apply in the case of respondent conditioning, in operant conditioning the person operates on the environment and produces a change. There is, therefore, an interactive relationship with the surroundings, not a passive one.

Some critics maintain that changes produced by behavioral procedures are not maintained over time or do not generalize to the natural environment. This is an important issue for all psychological interventions, regardless of theoretical perspective. Maintenance and generalization are aspects of treatment outcome that are addressed in evaluations of behavioral interventions. These data show better results for some types of interventions than others. For example, follow-up data for behavioral treatment of agoraphobia are generally more impressive than the maintenance of weight loss produced by behavioral intervention.

A fourth issue raised by critics of behavioral approaches is that of "symptom substitution." The notion is that elimination of a problem behavior or "symptom," without dealing with the underlying cause, will result in the reappearance of the behavior or the development of another problem behavior (i.e., one symptom will be substituted for another if the intrapsychic conflict is not resolved). The concept is based on assumptions about the nature of maladaptive behavior and inferences regarding unobservable processes that stem largely from psychoanalytic theory and its basis in a "closed hydraulic system" model of psychic energy. It is difficult to investigate symptom substitution empirically due to the lack of specificity by those who propose the argument regarding the nature of the symptoms, the conditions under which it is likely to occur, or the length of time posttreatment that elapses prior to appearance of the "substitute" symptom (Bandura, 1969). Research does not support the argument for symptom substitution. There are situations in which a behavior may be suppressed only temporarily as in the case of punishment for a response without reinforcement for a desirable incompatible behavior. This does not mean that symptom substitution has occurred. It can mean that empirically derived and validated procedures have not been implemented properly.

A related criticism of a behavioral approach by some is that it is superficial and does not focus on promoting insight and self-understanding. From a behavioral perspective, the focus is on changing behavior and setting specific goals that can be objectively defined and assessed. The difficulty in setting similar goals involving insight or self-understanding is apparent. Moreover, behavior change does not necessarily follow insight regarding the causes of the behavior. Self-understanding may, however, be a collateral of behavior change.

Many criticisms are actually misconceptions about behaviorism and behavioral interventions, and some are briefly summarized (and corrected) in Table 6–15. More complete discussions of misconceptions and criticisms about radical behaviorism can be found in Skinner's (1974) *About Behaviorism* and about behaviour therapy in Bellack and Hersen (1980).

CONTRIBUTIONS OF THE BEHAVIORAL APPROACH

Contributions of the behavioral model are related primarily to the major features of the approach, namely objectivity, commitment to experimentation and the empirical method, and an emphasis on learning and environmental

Table 6–15 **Misconceptions about Behaviorism and Behavior Therapy**

MISCONCEPTION	CORRECTION
1. Genetic endowment is ignored in accounting for behavior.	Behavior is explained in terms of current contingencies, reinforcement history, *and* genetic endowment.
2. Individual uniqueness is not considered.	Although principles of behavior are applicable for all persons, the specific contingencies in effect and the learning history are unique for each individual. These factors must be considered for each person. Also, intensive, systematic study of the person over time has been promoted and used by behaviorists as an experimental methodology.
3. The approach is mechanistic and dehumanizing, and behavior therapists are cold and not empathic.	The approach is objective and systematic. The goals are humanistic and include alleviation of human suffering. Research suggests that behavior therapists display warmth and empathy comparable to therapists with different orientations (Sloane et al, 1975).
4. Behavioral techniques are appropriate for only some groups (e.g., children, the mentally retarded) and for very circumscribed problems (e.g., phobias).	Behavioral principles apply across groups and problem behaviors. Research indicates that some treatment procedures are more effective than others for specific problem behaviors or disorders.

contributions to behavior. These features of the approach are important for both clinical practice and research.

The behavioral approach *entails formulation of specific, individualized goals for treatment, which consist of objectively defined and measurable behaviors.* Treatment focuses on current conditions and is also described objectively and precisely so as to allow for reporting and replication by others. Progress toward treatment goals and evaluation of the intervention involve measurement of target behaviors during baseline, treatment, and follow-up periods. Such features of the model are particularly significant from the standpoint of *accountability* in clinical practice as well as the practical utility of specificity in formulating treatment goals and objectivity in assessing progress toward these goals.

Behavior therapy is self-evaluative; *empirical demonstration of the effectiveness and identification of the limits of interventions are a commitment of the field.* Intensive study of the individual allows for investigation of the types of problems and persons for whom a particular intervention is most effective. Important aspects of treatment effectiveness, such as maintenance of effects over time and generalization to other situations and behaviors, are evaluated, and clinical research efforts are increasingly focused on programming and facilitating positive outcomes in these areas. This commitment to evaluation increases the likelihood that the individual patient receives the most appropriate and effective treatment and that the body of knowledge about interventions will continue to grow.

Interventions are often implemented and effectiveness is assessed in the person's natural environment. Because paraprofessionals and nonprofessionals can be trained to implement programs designed by professionals expert in the behavioral approach, the feasibility and cost-effectiveness of intervening in the natural environment are enhanced. This, in turn, enhances generalization and maintenance. *Behavior therapy techniques are frequently less time consuming and less expensive* than other approaches and are as effective or more effective than most of them.

ANNOTATED BIBLIOGRAPHY

Ammerman RT, Hersen M (eds): Handbook of Child Behavior Therapy in the Psychiatric Setting. New York, John Wiley & Sons, 1995

> Readers interested in more information about behavioral applications for diverse problems of children and adolescents may find this a useful resource.

Baldwin JD, Baldwin JI: Behavior Principles in Everyday Life. Englewood Cliffs, NJ, Prentice-Hall, 1981

> This is an excellent resource for information about operant and respondent conditioning with many examples of applications of behavioral principles to day-to-day living.

Bandura A: Social Foundations of Thought and Action: A Social Cognitive Theory. Englewood Cliffs, NJ, Prentice-Hall, 1986

> Social cognitive theory is presented in this source with detailed presentations of observational learning, self-efficacy, and relevance of the theoretical approach for conceptualizing psychiatric disorders such as depression and anxiety.

Craighead LW, Craighead WE, Kazdin AE et al: Cognitive and Behavioral Interventions: An Empirical Approach to Mental Health Problems. Needham Heights, MA, Allyn and Bacon, 1994

> The text presents an overview of behavior therapy and describes the use of behavioral approaches, including cognitive and behavioral perspectives, to multiple problem areas with adults, children, and adolescents.

Kazdin AE: History of Behavior Modification: Experimental Foundations of Contemporary Research. Baltimore, MD, University Park Press, 1978

> Kazdin's presentation of the history of behavior modification is thorough, organized, and readable. A great deal of information about key figures of the behavioral movement and their respective contributions is available in this book.

Maddux JE (ed): Self-efficacy, Adaptation and Adjustment: Theory, Research, and Application. New York, Plenum Press, 1995

> Research regarding various aspects of the relationship between self-efficacy and adaptation and adjustment is reviewed by numerous authors, including Bandura, in this edited text.

Marmor J, Woods JM: The Interface between Psychodynamic and Behavioral Therapies. New York, Plenum Medical Books, 1980

> The authors discuss how behavior therapy can be integrated or used in parallel with psychodynamically oriented approaches.

Skinner BF: About Behaviorism. New York, Vintage Books, 1974

> Skinner presents a lucid, interesting discussion of the philosophy of science called radical behaviorism and addresses numerous misconceptions about radical behaviorism and the experimental analysis of behavior.

Skinner BF: Science and Human Behavior. New York, The Free Press, 1953

> Skinner's discussion of punishment in this book is worthwhile reading. He argues cogently against the use of punishment and for a number of alternative strategies to decrease undesirable behavior.

Tunks E, Bellisimo A: Behavioral Medicine: Concepts and Procedures. New York, Pergamon Press, 1991

> The authors present a practical, readable guide to clinical applications within behavioral medicine.

REFERENCES

American Psychiatric Association: Diagnostic and Statistical Manual of Mental Disorders, 4th ed. Washington, DC, American Psychiatric Association, 1994

Baldwin JD, Baldwin JI: Behavior Principles in Everyday Life. Englewood Cliffs, NJ, Prentice-Hall, 1981

Bandura A: Aggression: A Social Learning Analysis. Englewood Cliffs, NJ, Prentice-Hall, 1973

Bandura A: Principles of Behavior Modification. New York, Holt, Rinehart and Winston, 1969

Bandura A: Social Foundations of Thought and Action: A Social Cognitive Theory. Englewood Cliffs, NJ, Prentice-Hall, 1986

Bandura A: Social Learning Theory. Englewood Cliffs, NJ, Prentice-Hall, 1977

Bandura A, Ross D, Ross S: Imitation of film-mediated aggressive models. J Abnorm Soc Psychol 66:3–11, 1963

Beck AT: Cognitive Therapy and the Emotional Disorders. New York, International Universities Press, 1976

Beck AT: Depression: Clinical, Experimental and Theoretical Aspects. New York, Harper & Row, 1967

Beck JG, Zebb BJ: Behavioral assessment and treatment of panic disorder: Current status, future directions. Behav Therapy 25:581–611, 1994.

Bellack AS, Hersen M: Introduction to Clinical Psychology. New York, Oxford University Press, 1980

Borden JW: Behavioral treatment of social phobia. In Turner SM, Calhoun KS, Adams HE (eds): Handbook of Clinical Behavior Therapy. New York, John Wiley & Sons, 1992

Burish TG, Carey MP, Krozely MG, et al: Conditioned side effects induced by cancer chemotherapy: Prevention through behavioral treatment. J Consult Clin Psychol 55:42–48, 1987

Burnette MM, Koehn KA, Kenyon-Jump R, et al: Control of genital herpes recurrences using progressive muscle relaxation. Behav Therapy 22:237–247, 1991

Chaney EF: Social Skills Training. In Hester RK, Miller WR (eds): Handbook of Alcoholism Treatment Approaches: Effective Alternatives. New York, Pergamon, 1989

Craske MG, Rapee RM, Barlow DH: Cognitive-Behavioral Treatment of Panic Disorder, Agoraphobia and Generalized Anxiety Disorder. In Turner SM, Calhoun KS, Adams HE (eds): Handbook of Clinical Behavior Therapy. New York, John Wiley & Sons, 1992

Dapcich-Miura E, Hovell MF: Contingency management of adherence to a complex medical regimen in an elderly heart patient. Behav Therapy 10:93–201, 1979

Ellis A: On Joseph Wolpe's espousal of cognitive behavior therapy. Am Psychol 34:98–99, 1979

Ellis A: Reason and Emotion in Psychotherapy. New York, Lyle Stuart, 1962

Forehand R, Long N: Parenting the Strong-willed Child. Chicago, Contemporary Books, 1996.

Forehand R, McMahon RJ: Helping the Noncompliant Child: A Clinician's Guide to Parent Training. New York, Guilford Press, 1982

Francis G: Childhood obsessive-compulsive disorder: Extinction of compulsive reassurance-seeking. J Anxiety Disord 2:361–366, 1988

Frueh BC, Turner SM, Beidel DC: Exposure therapy for combat-related PTSD: A critical review. Clin Psychol Rev 15:799–817, 1995.

Hollon SD, Shelton RC, Loosen PT: Cognitive therapy and pharmacotherapy for depression. J Consult Clin Psychol 59:88–99, 1991

Jacobson E: Progressive Relaxation. Chicago, University of Chicago Press, 1938

Jay SM, Elliott CH, Katz E, Siegel SE: Cognitive-behavioral and pharmacologic interventions for children's distress during painful medical procedures. J Consult Clin Psychol 55:860–865, 1987

Kazdin AE: History of Behavior Modification: Experimental Foundations of Contemporary Research. Baltimore, University Park Press, 1978

Kelly JA, St. Lawrence JS, Hood HV, et al: Behavioral intervention to reduce AIDS risk activities. J Consult Clin Psychol 57:60–67, 1989

Kendall PC, Haaga DAF, Ellis A, et al: Rational-emotive therapy in the 1990's and beyond: Current status, recent revisions, and research questions. Clin Psychol Rev 15:169–185, 1995.

Ludwick-Rosenthal R, Neufeld RWJ: Stress management during noxious medical procedures: An evaluative review of outcome studies. Psychol Bull 104:326–342, 1988

Lyons LC, Woods PJ: The efficacy of rational-emotive therapy: A quantitative review of the outcome research. Clin Psychol Rev 11:357–369, 1991

Manne SL, Redd WH, Jacobsen PB, et al: Behavioral intervention to reduce child and parent distress during venipuncture. J Consult Clin Psychol 58:565–572, 1990

Marmor J, Woods JM: The Interface Between Psychodynamic and Behavioral Therapies. New York, Plenum Medical Books, 1980

McGrath PA: Pain in Children: Nature, Assessment and Treatment. New York, Guilford Press, 1991

Meichenbaum D: Stress inoculation training. A twenty year update. In Woolfolk RL, Lehrer PM (eds): Principles and Practices of Stress Management. New York, Guilford Press, 1992.

Meichenbaum DH: Cognitive Behavior Modification. New York, Plenum, 1977

Oakley ME, Padesky CA: Cognitive therapy for anxiety disorders. In Hersen M, Eisler RM, Miller PM (eds): Progress in Behavior Modification, Vol. 25. Newbury Park, CA, Sage Publications, 1990

Oyama O, Andrasik F: Behavioral strategies in the prevention of disease. In Turner SM, Calhoun KS, Adams HE (eds): Handbook of Clinical Behavior Therapy. New York, John Wiley & Sons, 1992

Pfeffer C, Plutchik R, Mizruchi M: Predictors of assaultiveness in latency age children. Am J Psychiatry 140:31–34, 1983

Roberts MC, Fanurik D, Layfield DA: Behavioral approaches to the prevention of childhood injuries, Special issue: Children's injuries: Prevention and public policy. J Soc Issues 43:105–118, 1987

Skinner BF: About Behaviorism. New York, Vintage Books, 1974

Skinner BF: Science and Human Behavior. New York, The Free Press, 1953

Sloane RB, Staples FR, Cristol AH, et al: Psychotherapy Versus Behavior Therapy. Cambridge, Harvard University Press, 1975

Smith DE, Marcus, MD, Eldredge KL: Binge eating syndromes: A review of assessment and treatment with an emphasis on clinical application. Behav Therapy 25:635–658, 1994.

Snyder JJ: Reinforcement and analysis of interaction in problem and nonproblem families. J Abnorm Child Psychol 86:528–535, 1977

Stanley MA, Turner SM: Current status of pharmacological and behavioral treatment of obsessive-compulsive disorder. Behav Therapy 26:163–186, 1995.

Steketee G: Behavioral assessment and treatment planning with obsessive compulsive disorder: A review emphasizing clinical application. Behav Therapy 25:613–633, 1994.

Taylor CB, Pfenninger JL, Candelaria T: The use of treatment contracts to reduce medical costs of a difficult patient. J Behav Therapy Expt Psychiatry 11:77–82, 1980

Turk DC, Rudy TE, Sorkin BA: Chronic pain: Behavioral conceptualizations and interventions. In Turner SM, Calhoun KS, Adams HE (eds): Handbook of Clinical Behavior Therapy. New York, John Wiley & Sons, 1992

Turner SM, Beidel DC, Townsley RM: Behavioral treatment of social phobia. In Turner SM, Calhoun KS, Adams HE (eds): Handbook of Clinical Behavior Therapy. New York, John Wiley & Sons, 1992

Watson JB, Rayner R: Conditioned emotional reactions. J Exp Psychol 3:1–14, 1920

Wolpe J: The Practice of Behavior Therapy, 4th ed. Needham Heights, MA, Allyn and Bacon, 1993.

III Human Development through the Lifecycle

7

Human Sexual Development and Physiology

Judith V. Becker,
Bradley R. Johnson,
and John A. Hunter, Jr.

Because human life begins with procreative activity, it may be appropriate that this section on normal human development begins with an overview of human sexuality. Human sexuality is an integral part of life from birth until death, and concerns about sexuality are an issue throughout the lifecycle. Many factors, such as genetic endowment, biological factors, interpersonal development, and cultural background, can affect sexual development and sexual functioning. Consequently, physicians should be knowledgeable about human sexuality from a variety of perspectives, including biological, psychological, cultural, and behavioral. Physicians are often called on to advise patients regarding sexual matters and assess sexual dysfunction in almost all areas of medical and surgical practice.

Clinicians often report that many patients seen in clinic or hospital settings are uncomfortable discussing issues related to sexuality. Patients tend to rely on physicians and other healthcare professionals to broach the subject first. It is important that the physician be aware of, and sensitive to, the patient's reticence, but it is equally important that physicians be aware of *their own* relative comfort or discomfort in assessing matters of sexuality in their patients. A solid understanding of all aspects of sexual development and physiology will facilitate the clinical skills in this regard and decrease whatever anxiety physicians themselves may experience in dealing with the sexual problems of their patients. This chapter covers basic aspects of human sexuality, including genetic and hormonal factors in determination of genital gender expression, an overview of basic developmental considerations, and the normal human sexual response cycle. Other developmental, biological, and cultural factors as they affect the expression of human sexual behavior are discussed in other chapters of this text. This chapter provides a basic introductory overview of sexuality. Human sexuality and human sexual development are also discussed by Drs. Dell and Dulcan in Chapter 8. Hormonal influences on sexual behavior are discussed by Dr. Pedersen and his colleagues in Chapter 12.

SEXUAL HISTORY INTERVIEW

Several physician guides to sexual history taking are available (see Fagan and Schmidt, 1994). Table 7–1 outlines pertinent areas of inquiry. These interviews should be comprehensive and detailed enough to allow for accurate and reliable diagnosis of common medical conditions that patients experience. However, the physician should be aware that at least as important as the content of the interview is the process by which the physician conducts it.

Given the long-existing cultural prohibitions against open and frank discussion of sexuality in our society, most individuals, including physicians, find such subject matter embarrassing and anxiety provoking. Patient-related reluctance to identify sexual problems can sometimes be unwittingly compounded by the physician's own inhibitions and inner conflicts. Physicians encounter a myriad of human conditions that not only require technical understanding but that also can evoke emotional reactions (i.e., pregnant teenagers, HIV-positive patients, etc.). It is important that physicians acknowledge that they are not immune from such psychological reactions or personal biases and seek to explore with the help of peers and colleagues their own value and belief systems as they relate to sexuality and sexual behavior. This personal exploration can lead to greater professional sensitivity and acumen, such that the physician may simply need to refer some patients elsewhere for professional care or consultation (see discussion of special populations).

Of utmost importance to the gathering of sexual history data is the establishment of an atmosphere of relative patient comfort and confidence. Such interviews should be conducted in private, and the physician should inquire if there are issues that the patient prefers to remain confidential from family or spouse. The physician should be sensitive to the patient's potential embarrassment and anxieties and attempt to convey a nonjudgmental and concerned attitude toward expressed problems. The physician's own body posture and facial gestures can be cues to the patient about the acceptability of the subject matter. A warm smile and gentle nodding of the head can be comforting and reassuring. When the physician informs the patient that he or she has spoken to numerous other patients about sexual issues, the patient not only is reassured but receives the permission and comfort to talk more openly.

In contrast, the avoidance of eye contact or stern inflection by the physician can convey disapproval or give indication that this is a subject that is best

Table 7–1 **Basic Sexual History (modified to age of patient and clinical circumstances)**

Introductory comments about why the interview is being conducted and its routine or special nature given the clinical situation at hand; reassurance about confidentiality

Open-ended questions, to give the patient an opportunity to voice any areas of special worry or concern regarding this part of the interview or sexual concerns in general

Source of information about sex in growing up

Attitudes of the parents toward sex

Age of onset of puberty

Age of menarche and menstrual history in women

Age of first intense romantic or sexually oriented relationship

History of childhood molestation or incest

History of venereal diseases

Attitudes about masturbation and frequency

Age of first intercourse; number of partners

General pattern of attraction to person of the opposite or same sex; general patterns of heterosexuality or homosexuality

Abortions, miscarriages, pregnancies; complications of pregnancies

Method(s) of birth control

Frequency of current sexual activity

Physical discomfort with sexual activity:

Men: Problem with arousal or achieving and maintaining erection, ejaculation control; ability to achieve orgasm; physical comfort with intercourse

Women: Problems with arousal, lubrication, achieving orgasm, physical comfort with intercourse

Conflicts in relationship or marriage over sexual matters: frequency, methods of birth control, sexual dysfunction

Medications or illness that seem to affect negatively sexual desire or functioning

Issues regarding decision to avoid or achieve conception and have children

Risk factors for AIDS or other concerns regarding this disease

---

not discussed. The physician should be aware that it is common for patients, especially adolescents, to be unaware of the technical terminology for various anatomical and physiological functions, and the patients may need to express their concerns using lay terminology. While physicians can help the patient correctly label or describe such functions, physicians should be sensitive to the potential embarrassment of patients and not present information in a pedantic or stilted manner. The extent to which the physician is able to establish good rapport with the patient and serve as a source of information and reassurance will largely determine whether the patient will continue to seek out the physician when concerns arise in the future.

Patients should be reassured that sexual history questions are a confidential routine part of the medical interview and should be given the opportunity to voice any general concerns or questions regarding their sexual life in an open-ended manner before the structured interview questions are asked. For example, the physician may begin the sexual history section of the interview by saying something such as, "Next, I'd like to obtain a sexual history and address any concerns you might have regarding sexuality." Then, one could continue with open-ended questions such as, "Are there any areas of special worry or concern that you have regarding sexuality in general?" Depending on the response to this open-ended question, the clinician might then ask questions about the areas listed in Table 7–1 in a systematic manner.

Asking questions in a manner that assumes the patient has engaged in or been exposed to each area of sexuality being asked about will ease the patient's ability to talk openly about particularly sensitive areas. For example, one might phrase questions in the following manner: "How old were you when you began to masturbate?," "How old were you the first time you engaged in homosexual activity?," or "What type of discomfort do you experience when engaging in intercourse?" Many physicians make the assumption that they know how their patients will answer and, therefore, ask in a manner such as, "You don't engage in homosexual activities, do you?" This not only hints at judgment of sensitive sexual issues but encourages the patient to deny information that would potentially be important to discuss. Additionally, questions should be asked in a way to determine whether the patient currently or has ever engaged in specific sexual activities. Some deny certain sexual activities because they no longer engage in them and do not realize the importance of the historical perspective. Using the phrase "sexual partner" when discussing the patient's sexual history will allow the patient to more easily disclose the gender of his or her sexual partner or partners.

Patients should be reassured that if there are areas they would rather not talk about for any particular reason, certain questions can be deferred to a later date. Likewise, if patients are uncomfortable discussing particular topics, physicians may ask about the nature of their concern. The interview should be modified according to the age of the patient and general clinical circumstances; some areas may be explored in some depth, while others may not be clinically relevant.

SEXUAL DEVELOPMENT

Prenatal

Of the 23 pairs of chromosomes in each cell in the human body, one pair, the sex chromosomes, is responsible for sexual development. The genetic sex of a person is established at conception. The sperm cell contributes either an X or Y chromosome, and the ovum contributes an X chromosome. The outcome of the pairing of chromosomes in the majority of cases is either female (XX) or male (XY). Chromosomal abnormalities can occur, however, and involve either the loss or addition of a chromosome (Table 7–2). For example, when an additional chromosome is added (XXY), the resulting pattern is Klinefelter's syndrome, the most common sex chromosome disorder. Such individuals develop a male body type; during adolescence, sexual development may be delayed because of a testosterone deficiency. The characteristics of Klinefelter's syndrome, namely atrophic testes and infertility, are apparent by adulthood. The XYY genetic pattern is another variation, which on occasion has been associated with impulsive and aggressive behavioral problems.

The absence of a chromosome, such as in Turner's syndrome (XO), produces a female body type and external genitalia; however, ovaries are absent. Short stature and amenorrhea characterize this disorder. Females born with an XXX pattern have diminished fertility.

During the first 6 weeks of life, male and female embryos appear identical; the as yet undifferentiated pair of gonads will differentiate to become either ovaries or testes. If the Y chromosome is present in the embryo, the gonads will differentiate into testes. A substance referred to as the H-Y antigen is responsible for this transformation. In the absence of the Y chromosome or H-Y antigen, the gonads develop into ovaries.

If the gonads differentiate into testes, fetal androgen (testosterone) is secreted and male genitalia (epididymis, vas deferens, ejaculatory ducts, penis, and scrotum) develop. In the absence of fetal androgen, female genitalia (fallopian tubes, uterus, clitoris, and vagina) develop.

Table 7–2 **Summary of Chromosomal Abnormalities In Sex Differentiation**

DISORDER	CHROMOSOMAL PATTERN	PHYSIOLOGICAL–BEHAVIORAL CHARACTERISTICS
Klinefelter's syndrome	47, XXY	Sexual development may be delayed because of testosterone deficiency. Atrophic testes and infertility.
Turner's syndrome	45, XO	Short stature, amenorrhea, ovaries absent.
XYY chromosome syndrome	XYY	Occasionally associated with impulsiveness and aggressive behavioral patterns, retardation, tall stature.
Female adrenogenital syndrome	46, XX	Excessive fetal androgen present and external genitalia masculinized, tomboyishness in childhood.
Androgen insensitivity syndrome	46, XY	Genetically male, however, androgen receptors defective, consequently, external female genitalia develop. Raised as females.

If fetal androgen is present in the body of a genetic female (adrenogenital syndrome), the external genitalia are masculinized. In some cases, the clitoris is enlarged. In others, there is a fully developed penis and scrotal sac (minus the testes). If, in a genetic male, androgen is missing or androgen receptors are defective (androgen insensitivity syndrome), female genitalia will develop.

Sexual Development in the Infant and Young Child

The level of sex hormones in the blood stream of neonates is relatively high for both boys and girls during the first few weeks of life, as the infant adjusts from dependence on the mother to autonomous functioning. These levels typically subside more quickly in females than males but are at prepubertal levels in both sexes by the end of the first year. During the first year of life, males show higher levels of testosterone and luteinizing hormone (LH), whereas females show greater levels of follicular stimulating hormone (FSH).

Upon birth, sexual development and differentiation, which have been controlled *in utero* by genetic and hormonal factors, are then subject to both social and cultural influences. During the first year of life, the child experiences pair bonding. It is important for the infant to be nourished, touched, and held. Because it is usually the mother primarily who meets these needs, the first bond of attachment is to her. The "oral" stage of infant development includes not only the sucking and swallowing reflexes that achieve nourishment but all aspects of bodily contact, including cuddling and touching. (See also Chapter 5 by Drs. Inderbitzen, Furman, and James for psychoanalytic perspectives.)

Male and female children manifest behavioral differences in the first few years of life. In a review of research on sex differences, Maccoby and Jacklin (1974) conclude that males and females differ in four primary areas: (1) girls have greater verbal abilities; (2) boys have greater visual–spatial abilities; (3) boys have greater mathematical abilities; and (4) boys are more aggressive. Both biological and sociocultural factors may be implicated in all of these areas of development and behavior. (Biological and hormonal factors in development in human behavior are discussed at some length in Chapter 12.)

Males and females appear to possess at birth certain neurosensory response capacities associated with later sexual functioning. Male infants frequently exhibit erections during the first few weeks after birth, and female infants may have the capacity for vaginal lubrication. Genital touching or genitopelvic stimulation appear to be relatively common in both males and females during the first year of life, and orgasms have been observed in infants of both sexes before the age of 6 months (Kinsey et al, 1948; Martinson, 1980).

Several investigators (Kolodny et al, 1979; Spitz, 1949) have made distinctions between the more reflective genital play of infants and the volitional and more cognitively driven masturbatory behavior of older youths and adults;

however, genital stimulation-sexual responsiveness is a phenomenon that appears relatively early in life and is observable in young children. Male and female children touch and explore their genitals as early as 6 to 12 months of age. It has been estimated that 32% of males 2 to 12 months of age and 57% of those 2 to 5 years of age have the capacity to achieve an orgasm (Martinson, 1980). Researchers and clinicians agree it is critical that infants be assigned a gender status in accord with their external genital status because gender identity is imprinted during the first 24 to 36 months of life and, once established, is highly resistant to change. In the majority of cases, the physician at delivery observes the genitalia and announces the sex. In those cases where individuals are born with ambiguous genitalia or a defect in the sex organs, there may be a delay in assigning gender status. Parental counseling is imperative to facilitate the assigning of gender status in ambiguous anatomical cases. The decision should be made jointly by the parents and the consulting physician.

Developmentally, by age 3 and sometimes earlier, children develop an awareness of gender identity. Gender identity is typically followed by establishment of sex-role preferences during the preschool and latency years and finally sexual preference (orientation) by puberty (Zucker and Green, 1992). Modeling and reinforcement of sex roles occurs within the family environment and to some extent may be influenced by cultural and social factors. Gender disturbances can occur early in life. Girls appear to be less susceptible to gender disorders than are boys. For example, the ratio of males to females applying for transsexual surgery is four to one. Furthermore, males are more likely to develop paraphilias. Paraphilias are characterized by sexual fantasies or arousal to sexual objects or behaviors that are not considered normative, for example, arousal or sexual urges involving nonhuman objects, children, or nonconsenting partners, and suffering or humiliation (fetishism, pedophilia, exhibitionism or voyeurism, masochism, or sadism). There is evidence to suggest that gender disturbances in children can be linked to early developmental trauma and dysfunctional families (Meyer and Dupkin, 1985).

Sexual interest is displayed during early childhood. Affectionate behavior in children, including hugging, touching, and kissing, can be observed by age 2. Three-year-olds have been shown to evince an awareness of genital differences. By age 4, children may begin to exhibit some sexual play ("show and tell" or "doctor and nurse" games). Four-year-olds also show an interest in learning where babies come from and how they get into or out of their mothers. Also, at age 4, children begin to show the need for privacy in dressing habits and bathroom behavior; however, they continue to be curious about their own bodies and the bathroom behaviors of others.

At age 5, children become more modest about exposing their bodies and, in general, are more self-contained. Six-year-olds display a greater awareness and interest in sex differences. The 6-year-old may also use slang vocabulary and joke about elimination functions. By age 7, children feel more self-conscious about their bodies and body exposure.

The middle (prepubertal) years of childhood have historically been labeled "latency" because it was believed that the sex drive was suppressed; however, later studies of childhood sexuality contradict this belief. Kinsey et al (1953) reported that sex play with peers occurred equally in opposite sex playmates. Furthermore, the number of girls and boys who had experienced orgasm showed a gradual increase in the prepubertal years. Latency also appears often to be a period of intensified romantic interests. Although there is considerable variation in individuals and cultural groups across the country, many prepubertal youths begin dating and engage in kissing and fondling. In some youths, this may involve more intense sexual foreplay or actual intercourse prior to adolescence.

Puberty

Puberty is a period marked by profound anatomical and physiological changes in males and females. These changes are catalyzed by increases in the production of estrogen in females and androgens in males.

In females, the adrenals and maturing ovaries account for the increases in estrogen production. These hormonal increases stimulate bodily changes that include widening of the hips, softening of the skin, and development of secondary sexual characteristics (i.e., breasts, labia, and clitoral growth; the emergence of axillary and pubic hair). Internal sexual structures, including the uterus and vaginal canal, also grow and mature during this period. Menses typically follow the initiation of breast development by a year or two. Endocrine changes that occur during the normal menstrual cycle are seen in Fig. 7–1.

Puberty generally begins later in boys than girls and may occur in a more irregular fashion (Diamond and Diamond, 1986). Fat deposits on the chest and abdomen precede muscular development and are accompanied by growth of the testes, scrotum, and penis. The prostate and seminal vesicles also develop and enlarge during this period. The maturation of the testes results in increased testosterone production, which promotes long-bone growth in addition to sexual changes such as body hair growth.

Both males and females experience growth in height and weight. In general, boys experience a growth spurt about 2 years later than girls. There is a wide variation in the timing of pubertal events that is related to genetic, as well as environmental, factors (Tanner, 1975). For girls, breast budding may begin any time from age 8 to age 13; the onset of menarche usually occurs between the ages of 10 and 16.5. For boys, penile and testicular growth begins between the ages of 10.5 and 14.5 (Marshall and Tanner, 1969, 1970).

In Western societies there has been a decrease in the age of onset of puberty. Over the past 150 years, the age of onset of menarche has dropped from age 17 to 13 (Tanner, 1975). This is probably related to complex changes in nutrition, social conditions, and public health (Meyer-Bahlburg, 1980). Although adolescents become capable of reproduction during puberty, the adolescent

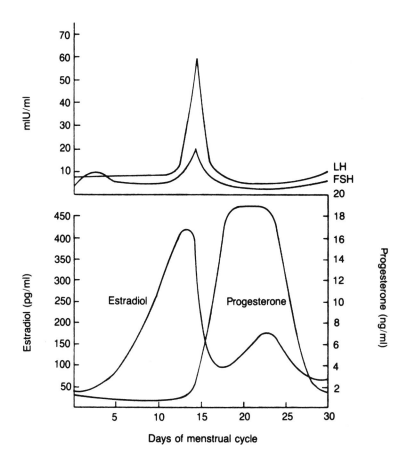

Figure 7–1. *Hormone changes during a typical menstrual cycle. (Reproduced with permission from Benson RC (ed): Current Obstetric and Gynecologic Diagnosis and Treatment, 3rd ed. Copyright 1980 by Lange Medical Publication, Los Altos, CA.)*

girl's first couple of menstrual cycles may not involve ovulation. For male adolescents, ejaculation may occur before sperm are viable. This period of sterility in adolescent males and females is variable.

The physiological events that occur during puberty can extend over a period of 3 to 4 years in females and longer in males. Adolescence represents a critical period of transition between childhood and adulthood and marks major psychological, as well as physiological, changes. Adolescents struggle to develop a sense of identity during this time. The physiological changes that they experience can create considerable anxiety and confusion. These feelings may be accentuated by both intellectual and developmental changes occurring during this period, as well as a greater sense of alienation and separation from parents. Many young adolescents are ignorant of the meaning of the changes they are experiencing, yet they are uncomfortable asking their parents for help. Therefore, they often rely on peers to learn sexual information, which often is flawed or inaccurate.

The physician can be a source of guidance and comfort to young adolescents. For girls, the onset of puberty may mark the first pelvic exam and represent an opportunity for education about the changes they are experiencing. As adolescents are frequently too embarrassed to ask questions directly about these issues, the physician can spontaneously provide relevant information with the simple explanation that it is one of his or her responsibilities to review such matters (Diamond and Diamond, 1986). Common concerns of girls include the rate of development of their breasts, confusion about the length of their menstrual cycle, the timing of ovulation, the variable nature of the menstrual flow, and a lack of understanding as to their internal and external sexual anatomy. Questions may be asked regarding sexual arousal and observed vaginal wetting, as well as the nature of other vaginal discharges. Boys often manifest concerns about penis size and shape, and the development and unevenness of bodily changes and growth (i.e., feet grow before other body parts, etc.). The occurrence of nocturnal emissions also can be a source of concern to young males. Many adolescents bring up questions about relationships with others and normal sexual functioning. As discussed later in this chapter, youths in our society are in need of education regarding birth control and the prevention of sexually transmitted diseases.

During adolescence, males and females may engage in self-stimulatory sexual behavior as well as sexual behavior with their peers. Masturbation to orgasm occurs more frequently in males than females. Leitenberg et al (1993) reported that 30.3% of the males in their study sample had masturbated before age 13, compared to 22.8% of the female sample; however, they also found that 81% of males and 45% of females masturbate at some time in their lives. Hunt (1974) found statistics that were even higher. The frequency of masturbation during adolescence is greater than at any other time during the lifespan for males and may occur several times per day. The psychological and cognitive maturational changes that accompany physiological change during adolescence bring a new meaning to masturbatory behavior in adolescents. No longer is such behavior viewed as simply a physiological outlet for tensions, but it also is considered a mental rehearsal of sexual behavior in the form of sexual fantasies. As such, masturbatory fantasy and behavior can be a step toward the development of sexual identity, sexual preference, and the emerging capacity for sexual intimacy (Weinstein and Rosen, 1991). Even though masturbation is a common practice, it is often a source of embarrassment and guilt and may be against some individuals' parental, cultural, or religious beliefs.

Sex play, including mutual masturbation, may occur during prepuberty and puberty. About 10% of boys and 5% of girls engage in sexual relations with a same sex peer during adolescence, although very few (only 3% of boys and fewer girls) engage in committed homosexual relationships (Chilman, 1983).

Adolescents today engage in intercourse at an earlier age and more frequently than did previous generations of adolescents. According to recent studies, by the age of 15 about 33% of males and up to 25% of females have had sexual intercourse; by the age of 19, 66 to 75% of the females and 79 to 86% of males have had intercourse (Seidman and Rider, 1994). These frequencies vary when race, education, and socioeconomic status are examined. In lower socioeconomic and minority adolescent populations, the age at first intercourse generally is lower, and the rates of youth engaging in nonmarital intercourse are higher, i.e., 88% of black males and 56% of white males were sexually experienced (Seidman and Rieder, 1994). Both males and females tend to engage in first intercourse with older partners (Darling et al, 1992).

Of considerable concern are emerging data indicating that many adolescents who are sexually active have multiple sexual partners and that the majority of juveniles who engage in intercourse do not utilize any form of contraception or protection from sexually transmitted diseases. It has been estimated that only 37 to 44% of females and 33 to 43% of males use a contraceptive during their first sexual experience (Darling et al, 1992). Although one study showed 81.8% of high school students had used a contraceptive method during their most recent sexual intercourse, only 46.2% had used a condom (Kann et al, 1993). The most commonly provided explanation for having unprotected sex for females is that the experience was unplanned. Males cite the lack of availability of a contraceptive as their most frequent explanation, followed by they were intoxicated, "too excited," or that use of a contraceptive was "not their problem" (Darling et al, 1992:99). Some claim they simply do not know how to use a condom properly, cannot find condoms that fit, or complain condoms decrease sexual stimulation. The problem of teenage pregnancy is discussed later in this chapter.

The context of sexual activity and its psychological meaning may be different for adolescent males and females. Females are more likely than males to report that their first sexual experience was in the context of a committed relationship and was an attempt to achieve interpersonal intimacy. Males appear to be slower in evolving toward engaging in relational sexual intimacy than females and more prone in their early developmental years to be motivated by achievement of status, inquisitiveness, and sexual arousal (Weinstein and Rosen, 1991). As a result of the interplay of physical and psychological factors, females are more likely than males to report that their first sexual experience was aversive. In one study, more than 72% of surveyed females reported that they experienced moderate to severe pain during their first intercourse. This experience of pain appeared to be associated with a number of variables, including a lack of physical maturity, conventional attitudes toward sexuality, and unhappiness with the experience and their partners. Adolescent females also are more likely than adolescent males to report feeling exploited during their first intercourse and less physiologically and psychologically satisfied (Darling et al, 1992; Weis, 1985).

The comprehensiveness and complexity of changes that adolescents experience create special vulnerabilities and needs. Because adolescence is a period of sexual maturation, the adolescent may have concerns about his or her changing body and sexual drive. Adolescents often face sexual issues related to masturbation, sexual anatomy, sexual identity, premarital sex, contraception, pregnancy, abortion, and sexually transmitted diseases, including AIDS. For adolescents to resolve these issues successfully, they need to have a knowledgeable, caring, and supportive adult available to listen and provide guidance. The role of the physician is particularly critical because the physician may be the person the adolescent seeks out for assistance with these issues. Consequently, it is important that the physician be nonjudgmental. If, for ethical reasons, the physician feels that he or she cannot be nonjudgmental in regard to some issues (e.g., abortion, contraception), then a referral should be made to other individuals or agencies. In Chapter 8, developmental aspects of human sexuality from infancy through adolescence are discussed further.

Adulthood

Once individuals reach adulthood, they are faced with a plethora of choices in every aspect of life, including marriage, childbearing, and lifestyle. Often brought on by pressure to conform to peer influence and societal and sexual norms, sexual conflict and problems may arise during this period. Individuals may experience problems with pair bonding. For some people, infertility may present a problem; for others, pregnancy may put a stress on their sexual relationship. The presence of a child may reduce the time couples have to spend alone with each other. It is crucial that couples be able to communicate with one another to solve any problems that may arise. It is interesting to note that one study (Ku et al, 1993) showed that as young men enter adulthood, they increased their sexual activity and decreased their condom use. Most adults are sexually experienced, and of those adults sexually active, 18% may engage in unprotected intercourse with multiple partners (Leigh et al, 1993). In fact, only 18% of men and 22% of women always use condoms with their primary partner, and 28% of men and 32% of women always use them with their secondary partners (Dolcini et al, 1993). The 1991 National Survey of Men (Billy et al, 1993) found that 95% of men have had vaginal intercourse, 23% of these men have had 20 or more partners with whom they have engaged in vaginal sex in their lifetime. Twenty percent of men have engaged in anal intercourse, 75% have performed oral sex, and 79% have received oral sex (Billy et el, 1993).

Middle age is a period during which people begin to adapt to the aging process. For some, this period is one of liberation (children leave home, more time for leisure activities); others experience feelings of anxiety and despair. Sexually, physiological changes are seen in both men and women. For women, menopause results from lower levels of sex hormones. As the ovaries age, circulatory levels of estrogen and progesterone gradually decrease. Age of menopause can vary from the late 30s to late 50s. As a result of lowered hormonal levels, a number of changes occur. The vaginal wall, labia, majora, uterus, and fallopian tubes shrink, and the reduction of vaginal lubrication in the expansion of the vagina can make intercourse uncomfortable. If medically safe, estrogen replacement can be considered to treat these problems. However, postmenopausal women typically do not experience significant decreases in their levels of sexual desire or their capacity for orgasm. In women, sexual interest is linked to an interplay of both biological and psychological factors. Biologically, sexual interest is possibly more dependent on the adrenal production of androgens than ovarian production of estrogens. The adrenal production of sex hormones does not appear to diminish significantly with age. Furthermore, there is no evidence of reduced clitoral sensitivity with age. Psychologically, many factors affect a woman's desire for continued sexual activity postmenopause, including issues of self-esteem, a history of having enjoyed sex, and the availability of an interested and emotionally suitable partner. Contrary to popular belief, during menopause there is no evidence of increased psychiatric morbidity (such as depression), although flushing, "hot flashes," and some degree of transient emotional lability may be seen because of fluctuation of estrogen levels.

Physiological changes also occur in males; however, these changes in endocrine and reproduction functions are more gradual and occur somewhat later than in women. Androgen levels, which are relatively constant after puberty, show a gradual decline until the mid-40s, when they drop to 55 to 60% of what they were earlier. By age 65, levels are 30% of what they were at age 30 (Silny, 1980). As the male ages, a number of behavioral changes in sexuality occur. Penile erection is slower, the erectile refractory period following ejaculation increases, morning erections and nocturnal emissions occur less frequently, and there is a decline in ejaculation force and amount of ejaculate (Silny, 1980). Although the male sexual response appears to be more affected by age than the female's, most males remain sexually active throughout middle age.

The Elderly

About 13% of the United States population is over age 65 (U.S. Department of Commerce, 1993). Many men and women have vital, active lives well into their 70s and 80s.

The capacity for sexual enjoyment is present at all ages, as is the need for love and intimacy. Persons who are in good health and have willing and cooperative sexual partners can continue active sex lives until their 90s or older. It is almost a universal phenomenon among physicians to assume that older people are not interested in sex and are generally sexually inactive, or they believe that it is not necessary to inquire about sexual matters in the elderly. To the contrary, there are numerous sexual issues in elderly males and females that can be addressed by the physician. Kinsey's studies showed that 94% of males and 84% of females were still sexually active by age 60 (Kinsey et al, 1948). In fact, sexual activity may remain more stable in middle and late life than previously thought (George and Weiler, 1981); however, advancing age brings on a number of physiological changes that can cause embarrassment and lead to premature withdrawal from sexual activities. In males, androgen levels continue to decrease past age 65 and are only 10 to 15% of the levels during puberty in 75-year-olds. Their testicles seem smaller as compared to younger men's, and they experience less penile tumescence. Thresholds for sexual arousal also appear to increase with age; however, complete erectile impotence does not appear prominent in men until age 75 or older (Silny, 1980).

The number of sperm found in the ejaculate of men decreases with age, but rarely ceases altogether and typically remains at a sufficient level to permit fertilization throughout the lifespan. Medical problems (i.e., diabetes, heart disease, etc.) and many medications (hypoglycemic agents, antihypertensives, vasodilators, cardiac drugs, psychiatric medications, etc.) can lead to problems with erectile function, decreased libido, anorgasmy, delayed ejaculation, and delayed orgasm. The prostate gland tends to increase in size in men as they get older. The result can be troubling symptoms (i.e., frequent urination, leakage, etc.) and impaired sexual function. This is an area where physician counsel and treatment often can be very helpful. Penile implants and the use of certain medications sometimes are helpful to resolve erectile problems arising from medical disease. Changing medication or a reduction in dose can help with drug-induced sexual dysfunction.

As previously discussed, age does not appear to impair sexual capacity in women to the extent that it affects males. Women remain clitorically responsive throughout the lifespan and can be multiorgasmic at an advanced age (Silny, 1980). Unlike males, there appears to be very little change in their refractory period after orgasm (1 minute or less); however, women also face major sexual issues in advanced age, including the scarcity of sexual partners. This problem is accentuated by the generally longer lifespan of women and the greater extent to which the male sexual response is diminished by age. Physician sensitivity to the emotional and physical issues associated with sexuality in the elderly is greatly needed. (See also Chapter 10 by Drs. Wolman and Thompson.)

The physician may need to make practical suggestions to elderly individuals, such as using lubricants to help with vaginal drying, hormone replacement to help with physical discomforts of menopause, use of analgesics prior to sexual activity to decrease pain and help with immobility problems, and alternative sexual positions to decrease excessive weight bearing and discomfort.

SPECIAL PATIENT POPULATIONS

Teenage Pregnancy

The rise of adolescent pregnancy rates in this country is alarming. These rates have risen steadily over the past 20 to 30 years, along with birth rates for unmarried teenage mothers (22.4/1000 to 40.6/1000 between 1970 and 1989) (Bowler et al, 1992; Diamond and Diamond, 1986). It has been estimated that 10% of all female adolescents report being pregnant at least once (Sorenson, 1973), and that there are at least 700,000 adolescent pregnancies each year. These teen pregnancies result in approximately 300,000 abortions, 200,000 out-of-marriage births, 100,000 marriages, and 100,000 miscarriages (Crooks, 1980; Zelnik et al, 1981). The birth rate is up to five times higher for minority teenagers than for white teenagers (Bowler et al, 1992). Because of the relative biological immaturity of adolescent females and possibly other more subtle factors (i.e., less adequate prenatal care, etc.), pregnancy complications are four to five times higher for adolescent females (Crook, 1980; Zelnik et al, 1981). Aside from physical complications, there are a plethora of psychological issues that face teenage parents.

There is a critical need for birth control counseling for sexually active teenagers and support services for pregnant teenagers. Up to 50% of sexually active teenagers report that they did not feel comfortable discussing contraceptive use with their parents, and most do not use contraceptives during their first year of coital experiences (Chilman, 1983; Zelnik et al, 1981). Pregnant teenagers and their parents require not only emotional support, but also help in objectively exploring options of abortion, adoption, marriage, and single parenthood. Teenagers report that support programs provide practical assistance, peer support, a more positive sense of self, and a feeling of being understood (McCullough and Scherman, 1991). Physician involvement is needed in the direct provision of these services and in their planning and development.

Homosexual Patients

It is estimated that there are at least 20 million homosexual persons living in the United States today, comprising approximately 10% of the total population (Caulkins, 1981). Seidman and Rieder (1995) suggest that 12 to 25% of men have had homosexual contact during their lifetime. Gay men and lesbian women face innumerable social, psychological, and health-related issues and concerns. Because of societal prejudices and discrimination, they often have been denied access to basic services, including health care. Homosexual men and women who do seek out physicians are often uncomfortable confiding in their physician the nature of their sexual orientation. The absence of such identification may hinder accurate diagnosis, proper counseling, medical treatment and basic trust in the doctor–patient relationship.

Sexually active gay men, in particular, encounter a number of risks and special health concerns. The number of cases of AIDS in the United States in gay and other high-risk populations is a matter of national concern (see discussion on treatment of HIV-positive patients). Their healthcare needs may extend beyond what is normally provided to heterosexual individuals (i.e., genital, oropharyngeal and rectal cultures, periodic HIV testing, etc.) and cannot be adequately met unless they are afforded a physician–patient relationship based upon respect, acceptance, and understanding (Caulkins, 1981). Physicians must explore their own personal feelings as they relate to the treatment of homosexual patients. To the extent that the physician's personal beliefs engender emotional discomfort or disdain for homosexual individuals, ethics dictate that he or she should make referrals to other treatment providers.

The origins and determinants of homosexual orientation is an area of current study and debate. Research has been conducted to look at hormonal, brain structure, and genetic differences when comparing homosexual and heterosexual populations. Hormone theories, including hormone levels in adults compared to sexual orientation, as well as prenatal hormone exposure compared to later development of sexual orientation, have not been proven as a cause and effect relation in studies thus far (Byne and Parsons, 1993). Recently, attention has been paid to brain structure differences in homosexual versus heterosexual persons, but studies have been contradictory and flawed (Bancroft, 1994). The most convincing biological evidence thus far shows a possible genetic inheritance of homosexual orientation, possibly linked to the X chromosome (Hamer et al, 1993); however, the issue of nature and nurture regarding homosexual orientation will likely need to be studied for years to come. Regardless, it is now clear that biological and genetic variables play a major role in homosexual orientation.

HIV-positive Patients

The number of HIV-positive individuals continues to increase each year in this country, with AIDS representing a health threat not only to homosexuals but also to heterosexuals, youths, and older adults. Given this rise in incidence, nearly all physicians will encounter HIV-positive patients. This phenomenon presents the physician with medical issues of proper diagnosis, treatment, and psychological issues related to patient care and feelings of personal safety and comfort.

No longer is risk of HIV infection limited to populations of gay men or intravenous drug users. An alarming number of adolescents and young adults appear to be at risk. As discussed by Bowler et al (1992), the number of AIDS cases in adolescents and young adults increased 53% between the end of 1988 and 1990. AIDS is now the seventh leading cause of death in the 15- to 24-year-old age group. Given the several years of "incubation" typically seen before the onset of AIDS symptoms, many young adults with AIDS are presumed to have become infected during adolescence. African Americans and Hispanics are disproportionally represented in both adolescent and adult groups. Although males are generally at greater risk than females in all age groups, this difference is considerably diminished in the adolescent population (10:1 male to female ratio in adults; 3:1 in adolescents). The greater risk for female adolescents may be the result of several factors, including the high incidence of unprotected sex in adolescence, apparently higher rates of engaging in anal intercourse, particularly among some urban minority youths, and perhaps greater physiological vulnerability to infections (Bowler et al, 1992).

It is imperative that physicians feel comfortable addressing the risk of HIV infection with their patients, particularly with those from populations that are at highest risk for contracting it. Often the patient may be concerned about it but too embarrassed to make inquiries. Physicians need to provide information to their patients in an open and candid manner and with a sensitivity to the complexity of the emotional issues involved. Those physicians who treat AIDS patients not only need to be able to provide these individuals with appropriate medical treatment, but also deliver these services in the context of an emotionally supportive relationship. Physicians must show understanding of and empathy for their patients, regardless of the manner in which the individual contracted the disease. As with other emotionally laden issues, the physician must first explore his or her own personal values and areas of emotional sensitivity. To the extent that the physician's own beliefs conflict with those of the patient, or the patient's condition creates significant emotional discomfort or vulnerability that cannot be resolved, the physician should consider a referral to another healthcare provider.

Impact of Life Events on Sexuality

Persons at any age may undergo a life experience that can affect their sexual functioning. It is important that physicians be aware of these events; they include sexual assault, illness, trauma (spinal cord injuries), surgical procedures (mastectomy, hysterectomy, enterostomy), medication (antihypertensives, psychotropics), and sexually transmitted diseases (HIV infection, herpes, and so forth). The effects of medical illness on sexual functioning has been reviewed elsewhere (Fagan and Schmidt, 1993).

HUMAN SEXUAL RESPONSE

Human sexual response represents a complex interaction of the nervous, vascular, and endocrine systems, which interact to produce sexual desire, arousal, and orgasm. In order to understand the sexual response cycle, it is necessary to have an understanding of its anatomical and physiological determinants.

Male Genital Anatomy

Male sexual anatomy consists of external organs (the penis, scrotum, and testes) and internal organs (the prostate, vas deferens, seminal vesicles, and Cowper's glands).

The penis consists of the glans penis, corona, corpora cavernosa, and corpus spongiosum (which also contains the urethra). The corpora spongiosum and cavernosa contain erectile tissue. The corpora cavernosa diverge at the base of the penis to form the crura, which are attached to the pelvic bone (Figs. 7–2 and 7–3).

The testes are located within the scrotum. The principal functions of the testes are production of sperm and testosterone. Sperm are produced within the seminiferous tubules.

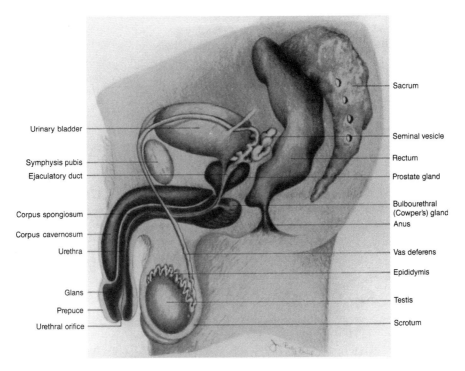

Figure 7–2. *Internal side view of the male reproductive system.*

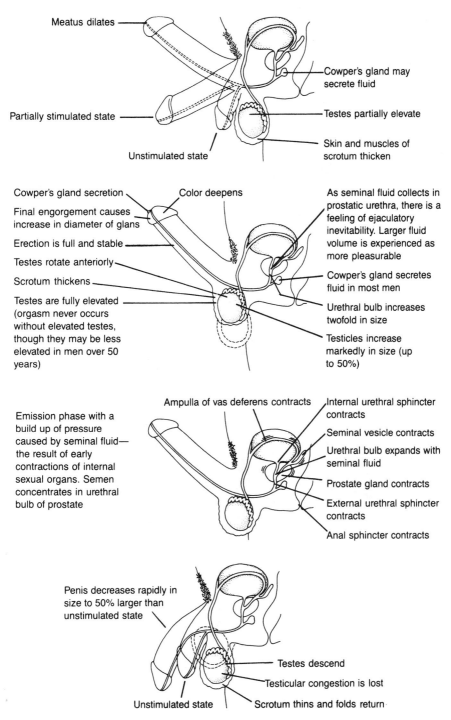

Meatus dilates

Partially stimulated state

Unstimulated state

Cowper's gland may secrete fluid

Testes partially elevate

Skin and muscles of scrotum thicken

Cowper's gland secretion

Final engorgement causes increase in diameter of glans

Erection is full and stable

Testes rotate anteriorly

Scrotum thickens

Testes are fully elevated (orgasm never occurs without elevated testes, though they may be less elevated in men over 50 years)

Color deepens

As seminal fluid collects in prostatic urethra, there is a feeling of ejaculatory inevitability. Larger fluid volume is experienced as more pleasurable

Cowper's gland secretes fluid in most men

Urethral bulb increases twofold in size

Testicles increase markedly in size (up to 50%)

Emission phase with a build up of pressure caused by seminal fluid— the result of early contractions of internal sexual organs. Semen concentrates in urethral bulb of prostate

Ampulla of vas deferens contracts

Internal urethral sphincter contracts

Seminal vesicle contracts

Urethral bulb expands with seminal fluid

Prostate gland contracts

External urethral sphincter contracts

Anal sphincter contracts

Penis decreases rapidly in size to 50% larger than unstimulated state

Testes descend

Testicular congestion is lost

Unstimulated state

Scrotum thins and folds return

Figure 7–3. *External and internal changes in the male sexual response cycle.*

Female Genital Anatomy

As in the male, the female sexual anatomy consists of external organs, including the mons, labia, clitoris, and perineum, and the internal organs, which consist of the vagina, cervix, uterus, ovaries, and fallopian tubes. The mons is the area of fatty tissue and hair that covers the pubic bone. From the bottom of the mons extend the labia majora, which merge with the perineum. Within the labia majora are the labia minora. The labia minora enclose the clitoris, urethral opening, and vaginal opening (Figs. 7–4 and 7–5).

The clitoris, which consists of the glans and shaft, is covered by the clitoral hood. The clitoral shaft, like the penis, contains the corpora cavernosa

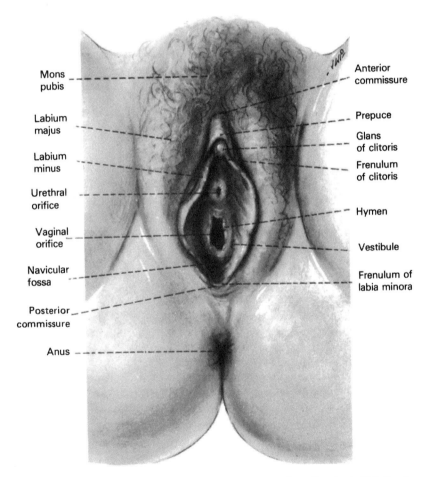

Figure 7–4. *The vulva. (Reprinted with permission from Danforth DN, Scott JR: Obstetrics and Gynecology, 5th ed. Philadelphia, JB Lippincott, 1986).*

Figure 7–5. *Internal changes in female sexual response cycle. (A) Excitement stage; (B) plateau stage; (C) orgasm stage; and (D) resolution stage. (Reprinted with permission from Reeder JR, Martin LL: Maternity Nursing, 16th ed. Philadelphia, JB Lippincott, 1987.)*

and the corpus spongiosum. The base of the shaft forms the crura, which are attached to the pelvic bone. The perineum is the area between the posterior boundary of the labia and the anus.

The vagina has been described as a "potential space." The vagina has the capacity to contract and expand and is lined with squamous epithelium cells, which are responsible for vaginal lubrication. At the top of the vagina is the cervix, which is a passageway between the vagina and uterus. The uterus is a muscular structure comprised of three layers. The ovaries are located on either side of the uterus. The ovaries secrete the hormones progesterone and estrogen and release ova, which are transported from the ovary to the uterus by the fallopian tubes.

Human Sexual Physiology

Sexual response is not limited to the functions of the genitalia. To fully understand sexual response, the role of sexual stimuli and the response of the nervous system also must be examined.

Weiss (1972) suggests that sexual stimuli can be divided into two categories: reflexogenic (direct, tactile stimulation of erogenous zones) and psychogenic (thoughts, images, fantasies, sights, smells, sounds, tastes, and so forth). The source of sexual stimulation in many instances is a combination of both. There is tremendous variability in what serves as sexual stimulation for people. Learning and conditioning play a major role in determining what a particular person will find arousing.

The nervous system serves as the communication system to the body to facilitate the sexual response. In this interaction both the central nervous system and the peripheral nervous system are involved. When a person is exposed to sexual stimuli, a message is sent from the brain or spinal cord through the peripheral nervous system (to either the autonomic or somatic branches). Stimulation of the somatic branch is responsible for the muscle tension that occurs during sexual stimulation. Stimulation by the autonomic system is responsible for penile erection and vaginal lubrication.

The autonomic nervous system has two branches, the parasympathetic and sympathetic. These two branches are seen as antagonistic, in that the parasympathetic branch releases acetylcholine and is dominant during periods of relaxation, whereas the sympathetic branch releases adrenaline and nonadrenaline and responds during periods of stress. These systems work in concert during sexual arousal. The *parasympathetic* nervous system is responsible for the expansion of the arterial blood vessels and the concomitant erection of the penis in males and vaginal lubrication in females. As arousal increases, the sympathetic nervous system plays a greater role, as evidenced by an increase in heart rate and blood pressure. Ejaculation is triggered by discharge of the sympathetic branch. This discharge creates an imbalance in the autonomic nervous system and is compensated by the release of acetylcholine from the parasympathetic branch. With this release comes the sensation of relaxation and warmth after orgasm in both men and women.

As mentioned previously, sexual experience can vary tremendously from individual to individual. Responses to sexual stimulation can be influenced by a number of factors. Byrne and Byrne (1977) describe three components that serve to influence a person's response to sexual stimulation; these are informational, emotional, and imaginal. The *informational* component represents a person's beliefs and expectations regarding sexuality. The *emotional* component consists of perceptions and feelings about sexual stimuli. For example, a person may experience happiness, joy, anxiety, or guilt in response to sexual stimuli. The *imaginal* component refers to the images or fantasies a person experiences when faced with sexual stimuli.

The endocrine system plays a crucial role in sexual response. The hormones responsible for sexual and reproductive functions are produced by the endocrine glands under the supervision of the hypothalamus. The hypothalamus is responsible for sending messages to the autonomic nervous system and regulating hormone levels. The endocrine glands involved in sexual functioning include the anterior pituitary, adrenal glands, and gonads (testes or ovaries). The sexual hormones secreted by the anterior pituitary include follicle-stimulating hormone (FSH), lutenizing hormone (LH), and prolactin. These hormones, called gonadotropins, stimulate the gonads to produce hormones. Estrogen and progesterone are produced and secreted by the ovaries, testosterone by the testes. Prolactin is responsible for progesterone production and the stimulation of the mammary glands to produce milk after childbirth.

The role of the vascular system is equally as important. In males, penile erection is achieved through vascular engorgement of erectile tissue in the cavernosa and spongy corpora of the penis. There is controversy, however, over the specific neurovascular mechanisms involved. There is also controversy over the role nervous mechanisms and arteriovenous shunts play in the control of tumescence.

In females, data suggest that precapillary arterial dilation accompanies the early phases of vasocongestion and shifts to arterialized blood flow, and increased venous output occurs as arousal increases (Wagner and Ottesen, 1980).

The Sexual Response Cycle

A number of models of the sexual response cycle, ranging from a two-stage model to a four-stage model, have been proposed. Ellis (1906) proposed a two-stage model, which involved the processes of tumescence and detumescence. Kaplan (1979) described a three-stage model, including *desire,* produced by activation of a specific neural system in the brain, *excitement,* produced by reflex dilation of blood vessels, and *orgasm,* reflex contractions of certain genital muscles.

Masters and Johnson (1966), based on their psychophysiological laboratory studies, describe a four-stage model. The four stages are *excitement, plateau, orgasm,* and *resolution* (Fig. 7–6).

Excitement is characterized by the onset of sexual feelings. During this stage, blood pressure and heart rate increase, breathing becomes faster and deeper, and skin "mottling" occurs. In males, erection is experienced, the scrotum thickens, the scrotal sac flattens, and the testes begin to elevate. In females, the breasts begin to swell, nipples become erect, and vaginal lubrication occurs. Some women experience vasocongestion of the clitoris. The uterus enlarges and begins to rise from the pelvic floor. The vagina begins to enlarge.

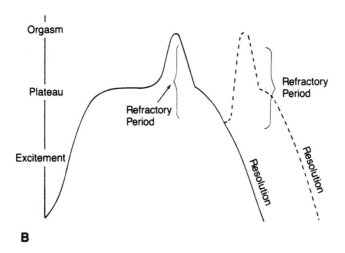

FIGURE 7–6. *The sexual response cycle.* **A.** *Three representative variations of female sexual response. Pattern 1 shows multiple orgasm; pattern 2 shows arousal that reaches the plateau level without going on to orgasm (note that resolution occurs very slowly); and pattern 3 show several brief drops in the excitement phase followed by an even more rapid resolution phase.* **B.** *The most typical pattern of male sexual response. The dotted line shows one possible variation: a second orgasm and ejaculation occurring after the refractory period is over. Numerous other variations are possible, including patterns that would match 2 and 3 of the female response cycle. (Masters WH, Johnson VE: Human Sexual Response. Boston, Little, Brown & Co, 1966. Copyright 1966 by Williams H. Masters and Virginia E. Johnson.)*

The *plateau* stage is characterized by a more advanced stage of arousal. The penis is distended, and the testicles have thickened and elevated. Reflex contraction of the cremasteric muscles cause the testes to move upward toward the body. The testes may increase as much as 50% from their basal size.

Females experience a marked vasocongestion of the outer third of the vagina during the plateau stage. Masters and Johnson have labeled this the *orgasmic platform.* The vasocongestion causes the labia minora to become larger and thicker, and they may change in color to dark red or purple. During the plateau stage, the uterus has ascended from the pelvic floor.

Orgasm is a reflex brought about by the vasocongestion and myotonia that occur during arousal. The buildup of muscle tension during sexual arousal is a major factor in triggering the orgasmic response. In the male, ejaculation occurs. During the first stage (emission) of ejaculation, semen is moved to the urethra. Masters and Johnson have labeled the sensations that occur during the emission phase as the period of "ejaculatory inevitability." The ejaculatory phase (expulsion) is characterized by semen being expelled from the urethra. The contractions of the bulbocavernosus muscles create the expulsion. Following ejaculation the male experiences a refractory period (a certain length of time must elapse before he can ejaculate again). The length of the refractory period varies from male to male. In general, it is correlated with age in that the older the person, the longer the refractory period.

For the female, orgasm is characterized by rhythmic contractions of the perineal, bulbar, and pubococcygeal muscles, and the muscles of the perineal floor. Females do not experience a refractory period; thus, multiple orgasms are possible within a relatively short period of time.

The final stage, *resolution,* is characterized by the body's return to its basal state.

Commenting on these various models, Rosen and Beck (1988) note that, while it is important to formulate and specify sexual arousal in terms of a model, the existing models are incomplete and potentially biased. These authors further propose that the three- and four-stage models are little more than elaborations of the biphasic model. Further research addressing the key psychophysiological concepts is necessary. As noted in Fig. 7–6, multiple patterns of sexual response may occur, particularly in women. About 5 to 10% of women may rarely or never experience orgasm, yet experience marked sexual pleasure during sexual activity. Most women usually require direct clitoral, noncoital stimulation (i.e., by manual or oral methods) to achieve orgasm during sexual activity.

DISCUSSION

The overview that has been presented relates to sexual functioning in an intact individual. Sexual dysfunctions occur when there are disruptions in the psychological, physiological, or anatomical processes involved in the process. It is important for physicians to be aware that sexual problems can arise in both heterosexual and homosexual relationships. The physician should not assume that the patient is in a heterosexual relationship. When taking a sexual history, use the phrase "sexual partner" so that the patient is free to disclose, if she or he chooses, whether the partner or partners are male, female, or both. It is important when providing good patient care that physicians be aware of their own attitudes regarding sexuality and sexual preference and are nonjudgmental in providing services to patients whose sexual preferences are different from their own.

A discussion of the specific types of sexual dysfunction and their treatments is beyond the scope of this chapter and is discussed in the companion text to this volume on clinical psychiatry (Fagen and Schmidt, 1994).

It should be emphasized, however, that sexual concerns and dysfunction occur quite commonly in the general population, especially in the context of medical illness.

Physicians have an essential, educational, and therapeutic role in helping patients with sexual matters, and, therefore, the importance of a sound knowledge for physicians in both normal and abnormal sexual functioning cannot be overemphasized.

Finally, it should be emphasized again that sexuality must always be understood and assessed in the context of each individual patient's psychological, physical, and social matrix. The approach to assessing a patient's sexual functioning or dysfunction will be determined by the patient's developmental stage, age, social situation, sexual orientation and preferences, medical status, and cultural, religious, and ethical considerations. In an era during which sexual behavior and attitudes toward sex have undergone profound changes in all areas of society—including the healthcare sector—special challenges are presented for physicians in providing medical care, education, counseling, and treatment for their patients.

The techniques and format for taking a medically oriented sexual history from a patient have been briefly reviewed. Table 7–1 lists the essential areas that should be covered in this type of interview, whether it is taken as a separate examination or as part of a comprehensive medical history. Of equal importance as *what* is asked is *how* the interview is conducted. For more details regarding sexual development, physiology, the diagnosis and treatment of specific sexual dysfunctions, see selected articles in the Annotated Bibliography.

ANNOTATED BIBLIOGRAPHY

Becker JV, Kavoussi RJ: Sexual disorders. In Talbott J, Hales R, Yudofsky S (eds): Textbook of Psychiatry. Washington DC, American Psychiatric Press, 1987

  An overview of sexuality and sexual dysfunction from the standpoint of clinical psychiatry.

Fagan PJ, Schmidt CW: Sexual dysfunction in the medically ill. In Stoudemire A, Fogel BS (eds): Psychiatric Care of the Medical Patient. New York, Oxford University Press, 1993

Excellent overview chapters for medical students of basic approaches to assessing and treating sexual dysfunctions most commonly encountered in general medical practice.

LoPiccolo J, Stock WE: Treatment of sexual dysfunction. J Consult Clin Psychol 54:158–167, 1986
> A review of current knowledge on treatment of sexual dysfunctions.

Masters WH, Johnson VE, Kolodny RC: Human Sexuality. Boston, Little, Brown & Co, 1982
> Good introductory-level text on topic of human sexuality.

Money J, Ehrhardt A: Man and Woman, Boy & Girl. Baltimore, John Hopkins Press, 1974
> Comprehensive presentation of the differentiation and dimorphism of gender identity from conception to maturity.

REFERENCES

Bancroft J: Homosexual orientation: The search for a biological basis. Br J Psychiatry 164:417–440, 1994

Billy JOG, Tanfer K, Grady WR, et al: The sexual behaviors of men in the United States. Family Planning Perspectives 25:52–60, 1993

Bowler S, Sheon AR, D'Angelo LJ, et al: HIV and AIDS among adolescents in the United States: Increasing risk in the 1990s. J Adolescence 15:345–371, 1992

Byne W, Parsons B: Human sexual orientation: The biologic theories reappraised. Arch Gen Psychiatry 50:228–239, 1993

Byrne D, Byrne L: Exploring Human Sexuality. New York, Thomas Crowell, 1977

Caulkins S: The male homosexual client. Issues Health Care Women 3:321–340, 1981

Chilman CS: The development of adolescent sexuality. J Res Dev Ed 16:17–25, 1983

Crooks R: Our Sexuality. Menlo Park, CA, Benjamin/Cummings Publishing Co., 1980

Darling CA, Davidson JK, Passarello LC: The mystique of first intercourse among college youth: The role of partners, contraceptive practices, and psychological reactions. J Youth Adolescence 21:97–118, 1992

Diamond M, Diamond GH: Adolescent sexuality: Biosocial aspects and intervention strategies. J Soc Work Human Sex 5:3–13, 1986

Dolcini MM, Catania JA, Coates TJ, et al: Multiple partners: The National AIDS Behavioral Surveys. Family Planning Perspectives 25:208–214, 1993

Ellis H: Studies in the Psychology of Sex. New York, Random House, 1906

Fagan PJ, Schmidt CW Jr: Sexual dysfunction in the medically ill. In Stoudemire A, Fogel BS (eds): Psychiatric Care of the Medical Patient. New York, Oxford University Press, 1993

Fagan PJ, Schmidt CW: Psychosexual disorders. In Stoudemire A (ed): Clinical Psychiatry for Medical Students, 2nd ed. Philadelphia, JB Lippincott, 1994

George LK, Weiler SJ: Sexuality in middle and late life. Arch Gen Psychiatry 38:919–923, 1981

Hamer DH, Hu S, Magnuson VL, et al: A linkage between DNA markers on the X chromosome and male sexual orientation. Science 261:321–327, 1993

Hunt M: Sexual Behavior in the 70s. New York, Dell, 1974

Kann L, Warren W, Collins JL, et al: Results from the National School-Based 1991 Youth Risk Behavior Survey and Progress Toward Achieving Related Health Objectives for the Nation. Public Health Reports 108(Suppl 1):47–55, 1993

Kaplan HS: Disorders of Sexual Desire. New York, Bruner/Mazel, 1979

Kinsey AC, Pomeroy WB, Martin CE: Sexual Behavior in the Human Male. Philadelphia, WB Saunders, 1948

Kinsey AC, Pomeroy WB, Martin CE, et al: Sexual Behavior in the Human Female. Philadelphia, WB Saunders, 1953

Kolodny RC, Masters WH, Johnson VE: Textbook of Sexual Medicine. Boston, Little, Brown & Co., 1979

Ku L, Sonnenstein FL, Pleck JH: Young men's risk behaviors for HIV infection and sexually transmitted diseases, 1988 through 1991. Am J Public Health 83:1609–1615, 1993

Leigh BC, Temple MT, Trocki KF: The sexual behavior of U.S. adults: Results from a National Survey. Am J Public Health 83:1400–1408, 1993

Leitenberg H, Detzer M, Srebnik D: Gender differences in masturbation and the relation of masturbation experienced in pre-adolescence and/or early adolescent to sexual behavior and sexual adjustment in young adulthood. Arch Sex Behav 22:87–98, 1993

Maccoby E, Jacklin C: The Psychology of Sex Differences. Stanford, CA, Stanford University Press, 1974

Marshall WA, Tanner JM: Variations in the patterns of pubertal changes in boys. Arch Dis Child 44:291–303, 1969

Marshall WA, Tanner JM: Variations in patterns of pubertal changes in girls. Arch Dis Child 44:291–303, 1970

Martinson FM: Childhood sexuality. In Women BB, Money J (eds): Handbook of Human Sexuality. Englewood Cliffs, NJ, Prentice-Hall, 1980

Masters WH, Johnson VE: Human Sexual Response. Boston, Little Brown & Co, 1966

McCullough M, Scherman A: Adolescent pregnancy: Contributing factors and strategies for prevention. Adolescence 26:809–816, 1991

Meyer JK, Dupkin C: Gender disturbance in children. Bull Menninger Clin 49:236–269, 1985

Meyer-Bahlburg H: Sexuality in early adolescence. In Wolman BB, Money J (eds): Handbook of Human Sexuality. Englewood Cliffs, NJ, Prentice-Hall, 1980

Rosen RC, Beck JG: Patterns of Sexual Arousal. New York, Guilford Press, 1988

Seidman SN, Rieder RO: A review of sexual behavior in the United States. Am J Psychiatry 151:330–341, 1994

Seidman SN, Rieder RO: Sexual behavior through the life cycle: An empirical approach. In Olham JM, Riba M (eds): Review of Psychiatry 14:639–676, 1995

Silny AJ: Sexuality and aging. In Wolman BB, Money J (eds): Handbook of Human Sexuality. Englewood Cliffs, NJ, Prentice-Hall, 1980

Sorenson R: Adolescent Sexuality in Contemporary America. New York, World Publishing, 1973

Spitz RA: Autoerotism: Some empirical findings and hypothesis on three of its manifestations in the first year of life. In Spitz RA (ed): The Psychanalytic Study of the Child. New York, International Universities Press, 1949

Tanner JM: Growth and endocrinology of the adolescent. In Gardner LI (ed): Endocrine and Genetic Diseases of Childhood and Adolescence. Philadelphia, WB Saunders, 1975

U.S. Department of Commerce: Statistical abstracts of the United States (Table 17, 17). Washington DC, 1993

Wagner G, Ottesen B: Vaginal blood flow during sexual stimulation. Obstet Gynecol 56:621–624, 1980

Weinstein E, Rosen E: The development of adolescent sexual intimacy: Implications for counseling. Adolescence 26:331–339, 1991

Weis DL: The experience of pain during women's first sexual intercourse. Cultural mythology about female sexual initiation. Arch Sex Behav 14:421–437, 1985

Weiss HD: The physiology of human erection. Ann Intern Med 76:793–799, 1972

Zelnik MD, Kanther JF, Ford K: Sex and Pregnancy in Adolescence. Beverly Hills, CA, Sage Publications, 1981

Zucker KJ, Green R: Psychosexual disorders in children and adolescents. J Child Psychol Psychiatry 33:107–151, 1992

8 *Childhood and Adolescent Development*

Mary Lynn Dell
and Mina K. Dulcan

This chapter reviews the basic principles and theories of normal human development from conception through adolescence. Significant milestones in physical, cognitive, language, emotional, and social growth are covered. In the discussion that follows, roughly 20 years of development are divided into pre-natal, infant (the first year), toddler (1 to 3 years), early childhood (3 to 6 years), school age (6 to 12 years), and adolescent periods. At each stage, development in physical, cognitive, language, affective, and social domains is described, as well as special topics applicable to that age group. Interactions between physical illness or hospitalization and developmental status and important aspects of family functioning and development are covered in the last two sections of the chapter.

WHY STUDY DEVELOPMENT?

Within the context of the biopsychosocial model, knowledge of the normal development of children and adolescents provides an essential framework for the understanding of adult development and of both child and adult psychopathology. Developmental factors may influence the pathogenesis and symptoms of mental illness at any age. Knowledge of the developmental process also facilitates the medical care of young persons and adults and their families by making understandable their phase-specific emotional reactions to illness at each stage of the lifecycle.

Different Views of Development

There are two fundamental ways of discussing development. One may take a *cross-sectional view,* describing all aspects of a particular stage, or describe each developmental domain *longitudinally,* using one or more theoretical perspectives. This chapter takes the cross-sectional option in an attempt to integrate the various developmental theories and capabilities at each developmental stage, because this is the way patients present in the clinical setting.

What Is Normality?

Although this may seem like a question with an obvious answer, there are widely discrepant definitions of what constitutes "normality." The term may be used to describe data that fit a normal or gaussian frequency distribution, with a symmetrical distribution of scores and a mean that coincides with the median. In this case, the mean plus or minus two standard deviations encloses 95% of the contents. The term "normal" is then applied to individuals who score within this 95% range on a particular measure. For example, "normal" height and weight are typically determined in this way. A related use of the term "normal" refers to a statistical norm or average that, of course, is tied to the original population from which the data were gathered.

Alternatively, "normal" may refer to what is socially or culturally acceptable (to a particular group). Cultural aspects of normality and psychopathology are discussed in Chapter 4 by Dr. Brown and colleagues. "Normal" also may be used to describe individual-specific response patterns (i.e., what is normal or usual for a given person), in an attempt to distinguish unusual but stable characteristics from those that represent a change or deviation.

"Normal" also may be used to mean healthy, without pathology, or ideal. In the context of preventive medicine and psychiatry, normality implies that the individual or group carries no excess risk of future disease or psychopathology.

Development has many aspects, including physical, cognitive, and emotional, with finer subdivisions in each of these three areas. It is important not only to assess in which areas a person's development is normal or abnormal but also to evaluate the evenness or synchrony of development across different domains.

Developmental Models

This chapter presents multiple theories of development, because at present no single theory is sufficiently comprehensive. Multiple perspectives, all with some degree of inherent value, must be invoked to provide an integrated and balanced view of the many factors that affect human development.

Each developmental theory identifies stages that unfold in an orderly progression, each phase building on the previous one, becoming more complex and differentiated, and then launching the next phase. Developmental theories identify the maximum expectable capabilities at each stage. A profile can be constructed for each person, noting progress compared to expected norms in each developmental area. In both normal children and in those with psychopathology, development may progress at different rates in different areas. For an individual, development rarely proceeds at a constant rate. Periods of apparent stagnation alternate with rapid growth. There are even times when regression to an earlier stage of development is not only normal but facilitates subsequent growth.

Psychoanalytic, object relations, and behavioral and learning theories of development are described in Section II of this text, and psychosocial (Eriksonian) theory is discussed in Chapter 10. Current knowledge about the biological underpinnings of behavior is summarized in Section IV of this text.

This chapter focuses primarily on observable developmental milestones or landmarks, physiological and neurological aspects of development, cognitive development, and interactions between the child and the family as development proceeds. Findings from clinical observations and research in developmental psychology are applied to the child, adolescent, and family as they are likely to present in the medical setting.

Temperament

Temperament, the "how" or style of behavior, is a concept that cuts across developmental stages. The concept was developed by Thomas and Chess (1986) from the findings of their New York Longitudinal Study, which followed 133 children from 85 middle-class families from infancy through young adulthood. The nine relatively stable dimensions or traits identified in infancy are listed in Table 8–1.

Many of the children studied were found to demonstrate clusters of these variables (see Table 8–2). The *easy* child is a delight to parents and has a relatively low risk of emotional or behavior problems. *Difficult* children are at the highest risk (70%) of developing behavior problems. In the New York

Table 8–1 **Dimensions of Temperament**

1. Activity level
2. Rhythmicity (regularity and predictability of biological functions)
3. Approach or withdrawal to novel stimuli
4. Adaptability to environmental change
5. Intensity of reaction
6. Threshold of responsiveness (intensity of stimulation required to evoke a response)
7. Quality of mood (positive, neutral, or negative)
8. Distractibility
9. Attention span and persistence

Table 8–2 **Temperamental Clusters**

EASY
Positive mood
Regular biological rhythms
Adaptable
Low Intensity
Positive approach to novelty
DIFFICULT
Negative mood
Irregular biological rhythms
Slow to adapt
Intense reactions
Negative response to novelty
SLOW TO WARM UP
Negative responses to new stimuli
Mild intensity
Gradual adaptation after repeated contact

(Adapted from Thomas A, Chess S: Temperament in Clinical Practice. New York, Guilford Press, 1986)

Longitudinal Study, difficult children were 10% of the total sample, but constituted 23% of the children with behavior problems. Children characterized as *slow to warm up* are also at risk, but the risk can be significantly reduced by sensitive management by parents and teachers.

A crucial predictor of outcome is the temperamental match or "goodness of fit" between the child and the parents' own temperament, expectations, and child-rearing style. Parent–child interactions, cultural expectations, and the child's own characteristics (e.g., sex, IQ) can reinforce inborn temperamental characteristics or change them for the better or the worse. Anticipatory guidance to parents from pediatricians can facilitate understanding of, and adaptation to, children's individual differences.

Thomas and Chess's work has inspired additional research on the measurement and properties of temperament characteristics. Twin studies suggest a substantial genetic contribution to temperament and other personality variables. Children demonstrating "behavioral inhibition to the unfamiliar" have been studied extensively. At age 2 years, these children are extremely inhibited, quiet, shy, and fearful in unfamiliar situations. The majority tend to remain shy and socially avoidant at age 7. Consistently inhibited children have greater sympathetic reactivity than more outgoing children, as measured by heart rate acceleration and early-morning salivary cortisol levels. These children are at risk to develop anxiety disorders. Their parents have an increased prevalence of both childhood anxiety and adult anxiety disorders (Hirshfeld et al, 1992). In contrast, 2-year-olds who are uninhibited tend to remain fearless and outgoing.

Developmental Milestones

Pediatrician Arnold Gesell and his colleagues at the Yale Clinic of Child Development made a major contribution to pediatrics and child development with their objective observation of behaviors and capabilities in large numbers of children at various ages. Their data identified "milestones" by which to measure the intactness of the child's abilities, resulting from the interaction between biological endowment and environment. Areas assessed include motor, personal-social, adaptive (use of motor abilities to interact with the environment), and language domains (Gesell et al, 1940). There is a range of normal for the age at which each milestone appears, and times presented in this chapter are averages. The Denver II (Fig. 8–1), a recent revision and restandardization of the widely used Denver Developmental Screening Test, graphically displays the age at which each milestone is attained by 25%, 50%, 75%, and 90% of normal infants and children (up to 6 years of age). This test can be easily used by a physician or nurse to estimate a child's developmental status and to determine whether additional evaluation is needed.

Piagetian Cognitive Development

Jean Piaget, a Swiss cognitive psychologist, became intrigued by the *wrong* answers given to questions on intelligence tests by children of different ages. He devoted his career to the study of *epistemology,* or how thought is transformed into a body of knowledge. Unlike Freud, whose theories were developed primarily by retrospective extrapolation from neurotic adults, Piaget's conception of cognitive development was based on the direct observation of his own three children, starting in their infancy. He viewed children as active participants in learning, rather than as passive recipients. He believed that intelligence and knowledge of the world must be discovered and structured by the child's own activities.

Piaget believed that four factors influence cognitive behavior:

1. Maturation of the nervous system.
2. Experience.
3. Social transmission of information, or teaching.
4. *Equilibration:* The innate tendency for mental growth to progress toward increasingly complex and stable levels of organization.

Piaget defined four major stages of cognitive development: *sensorimotor, preoperational, concrete operations,* and *formal operations.* These are not uniformly attained but appear within a rather wide range of ages (see Figs. 8–2 and 8–3). Each child's rate of development is determined by his or her intelligence and the above factors.

Certain definitions are essential to understanding Piaget (Piaget and Inhelder, 1969). A *scheme* is an organized pattern of behavior that is repeatable and generalizable (e.g., sucking, reaching for a mobile hanging in the

Figure 8–1.

Figure 8–1.

Figure 8–2. *Correspondence of stages of development—birth to 2 years.*

Age-Years	Milestones	Freud	Erickson	Mahler	Piaget
2	Solitary play / Toilet Trained				
3	Copy Circle Parallel Play / Know First and Last Names	Anal	Autonomy vs.		
4	Copy Cross Know Primary / Colors Cooperative Play	Urethral / Phallic	Shame & Doubt	Firm Object Constancy	Preoperational
5	Draw 3 part Man / Copy Square		Initiative		
6	Draw 6 part Man / Print Name	Oedipal	vs.		
7	Copy Diamond / No Longer reverse Letters		Guilt		
8	Jump Rope, Tie Shoes / Ride 2 Wheel Bike		Industry		
9	Define abstract words		vs.		Concrete
10		Latency	Inferiority		Operations
11	Puberty-Girls				
12			Identity		
13	Puberty-Boys		vs.		Formal
14			Diffusion		Operations
15	Repeat 6 digits forward / and 5 digits backward	Adolescence			
16					
17					

Figure 8–3.

crib). Development proceeds through certain processes that represent basic tendencies in human beings:

1. Active seeking of stimulation.
2. *Organization:* The tendency to arrange processes into coherent systems.
3. *Adaptation:* A dynamic process combining *assimilation* and *accommodation.*
   Assimilation: The tendency to use current schemes to deal with the environment, in both familiar and new situations.
   Accommodation: The modification of the child's cognitive structures in response to environmental pressures.
4. The need for action to precede intellect.

Despite his small and select database and methods that would be considered primitive by today's standards, Piaget's theories have been highly influential in the study of child development. Although subsequent research has found that children can solve problems much earlier, and developmental stages are far more flexible, less discrete, and more responsive to context and affect than Piaget believed, his notion that thought and reasoning change qualitatively as well as quantitatively with development has remained important in our understanding of intellectual development.

Intelligence

Evaluation

The ability of "intelligence" testing in infancy to predict IQ test results at school age is controversial. Changes in IQ estimates can be attributed to both the remarkable resiliency of the central nervous system of the human infant and the marked differences in types of abilities able to be tested at different ages. At best, scores on specific tests in infancy account for 50% of the variation among children in specific cognitive and language abilities at age 2 years (Siegel, 1981). The accuracy of predicted IQ decreases as the time interval increases, in part because the caretaking environment can powerfully exacerbate or ameliorate early damage.

Mental Retardation

Mental retardation is a condition of childhood onset defined by a score on a standardized intelligence test (see Table 8–3) that is significantly below average (i.e., IQ score below approximately 70), together with significant impairment in adaptive functioning (measured by a test such as the Vineland Adaptive Behavior Scales). It is important to remember that scores on standardized IQ tests can be significantly affected by cultural, motivational, and attentional factors.

Mental retardation has a wide variety of causes; the more common are listed in Table 8–4. Mild mental retardation (IQ from 50–55 to 70), by far the

Table 8–3 **Tests of Intelligence**

STANDARD IQ TESTS

Kaufman Assessment Battery for Children (K-ABC)
    Age 2½ to 12½ years
    Less dependent on culturally based information and schooling
Stanford-Binet Intelligence Scale (4th Edition)
    Age 2 years to adulthood
    Heavily language based
Wechsler Preschool and Primary Scale of Intelligence Revised (WPPSI-R)
    Age 4 to 6½ years
Wechsler Intelligence Scale for Children, 3rd Edition (WISC-III)
    Age 6 to 16 years
Wechsler Adult Intelligence Scale-Revised (WAIS-R)
    Age 16 years through adulthood

TESTS FOR SPECIALIZED USES

Adaptive Behavior Scale (American Association on Mental Retardation)
    Age 3 years to adult
    Assesses self-help competence, maladaptive behavior
Bayley Scales of Infant Development–Revised
    Age 3 to 30 months
    Estimates cognitive developmental level in very young children
Leiter International Performance Scale
    Nonverbal test for use with children who are deaf, autistic, or do not speak
        English
    Not as well standardized as other IQ tests
Peabody Picture Vocabulary Test (PPVT-R)
    Brief test of receptive language abilities, often used as screening test of IQ
Vineland Adaptive Behavior Scales
    Measure of behavioral capabilities, based on interview with primary caretaker
    Birth to adulthood
    Especially useful for developmentally handicapped individuals
Wechsler Individual Achievement Test (WIAT)
    Age 5 to 20 years
    Linked with Wechsler Intelligence Scales
    Covers learning disabilities specified in PL 94–142 (1975)
Wide Range Assessment of Memory and Learning (WRAML)
    Ages 5 to 17 years
    Assesses active learning and memory

most common category, is not usually attributable to a known medical cause but rather to a combination of factors including inheritance from parents whose genetic endowment is below average, lack of cognitive stimulation, malnutrition of mother and child, inadequate prenatal and pediatric medical care, environmental toxins such as lead, and illicit drug use. There is considerable diversity among retarded children, even when matched for IQ. Typical patterns of cognitive abilities, social and affective characteristics, and behavioral symptoms differ according to etiology (e.g., Down's syndrome versus fragile-X syn-

Table 8–4 **Significant Causes of Mental Retardation**

GENETIC FACTORS

Chromosomal abnormalities
  Fragile-X syndrome
  Down's syndrome
  Cri-du-chat syndrome
  Many other rare, named syndromes
Single gene abnormalities—inborn
  errors of metabolism
  Phenylketonuria (PKU)*
  Maple syrup urine disease*
  Homocystinuria*
  Tyrosinemia*
  Galactosemia*
  Hypothyroidism*
  Lipid storage diseases
  Glycogen storage diseases
  Lesch-Nyhan syndrome
  Wilson's disease

Neurocutaneous disorders
  Sturge-Weber syndrome
  Tuberous scierosis
  von Recklinghausen's disease
  Craniofacial anomalies
Genetic endowment at the
  lower end of the distribution

PRENATAL FACTORS

Maternal chronic illness
  Diabetes mellitus
  Anemia
  Emphysema
  Hypertension
  Malnutrition
Maternal infection passed to fetus
  Rubella (German measles)
  Cytomegalic inclusion disease
  Syphilis
  Toxoplasmosis
  Herpes simplex
  AIDS

Maternal ingestion of toxic substances
  Alcohol
  Narcotics
  Cocaine

OBSTETRIC COMPLICATIONS

ACQUIRED COGNITIVE DEFICIT IN INFANCY OR CHILDHOOD

Severe malnutrition
Infection
  Encephalitis
  Meningitis
Head trauma
Lead intoxication
Asphyxia
Brain tumors

ENVIRONMENTAL AND SOCIOCULTURAL INFLUENCES

* *Note:* Newborn screening techniques are available to permit early identification and treatment, which prevents or reduces sequelae of these disorders.

drome) (Bregman and Hodapp, 1991). Among the mildly retarded, these characteristics, along with family resources and educational and vocational interventions, contribute more to adult adaptation than does IQ.

Other categories of mental retardation fortunately are less common. Moderate retardation (IQ from 35–40 to 50–55) accounts for 10% of this population. Significant academic limitations exist, but these individuals can learn to communicate in social settings, attend to personal hygiene, and perform simple tasks in highly supervised settings. Three to four percent of retarded persons fall into the severe range (IQ 20–25 to 35–40). Attainable goals include simple speech, basic physical self-care abilities, and recognition and understanding of "survival" words. When these young people reach adulthood, the nurture and supervision of family or group homes is usually required. Profound retardation (IQ below 20–25) exists in 1 to 2% of the retarded population and is often accompanied by serious neurological impairment. These individuals require virtually constant, often specialized, care and supervision (American Psychiatric Association, 1994; Harris et al, 1996).

Primary prevention (reduction in the numbers of retarded children) includes efforts such as improved family planning and prenatal care, education of mothers, and larger societal efforts to reduce poverty. Immunization against rubella, genetic counseling, prenatal diagnosis through techniques such as ultrasound and amniocentesis, and newborn screening for disorders such as phenylketonuria (PKU) can reduce the incidence of some of the more severe forms of mental retardation.

Secondary prevention focuses on early identification and intervention to reverse or minimize developmental delays. *Tertiary prevention,* minimizing complications and maximizing adaptive functioning, requires specialized treatment and rehabilitative services.

PRENATAL DEVELOPMENT

The prenatal period is an important one for both parents and fetus. The child's endowment depends on both genetic makeup and the prenatal environment. Subsequent influences include the timing and nature of the birth process, medical interventions, and later social, emotional, and physical factors in the environment of the child.

Risks to the Fetus

Low Birth Weight

Low birth weight predisposes a child to numerous developmental, medical, and behavioral problems in infancy, childhood, and adolescence. Two chief reasons for low birth weight are prematurity and intrauterine growth retardation. Causes of prematurity include multiple pregnancy, fetal abnormalities, anatomical or endocrine abnormalities in the mother, and substance abuse, particularly cocaine. Infants who have experienced intrauterine growth retardation are small for their gestational age. Contributing factors include maternal malnutrition, maternal drug abuse, placental abnormalities, infection, and maternal illnesses such as hypertension. Obstetricians and neonatologists increasingly are able to prevent and treat the sequelae of intrauterine growth retardation and prematurity. However, very low birth weight children (1250 grams or less) have a greater frequency of motor and learning problems that become increasingly apparent in the preschool and school-age years (Marlow et al, 1993).

Genetic Abnormality

Genetic counseling prior to pregnancy or use of new methods of prenatal diagnosis can reduce the incidence of babies born with a chromosomal aberration (e.g., Down's syndrome) or inherited abnormality of a single gene (e.g., Tay–Sachs disease). Neonatal screening with subsequent dietary treatment has significantly reduced the sequelae of other genetic disorders such as PKU.

Maternal Disease

Early and thorough prenatal care reduces the risk to the fetus by identification and medical management of maternal diabetes, hypertension, or other disorders.

Immunization of potential mothers protects babies from the often-devastating effects of maternal rubella infection. Intrauterine infection with the AIDS virus, transmitted across the placenta from an infected mother, is a rapidly increasing problem.

Adolescent Pregnancy

Infants of mothers less than 15 years old are at increased risk for low birth weight and neonatal death, in part because teenage mothers are less likely to obtain prenatal care. Injuries, illnesses, and sudden infant death syndrome (SIDS) have an increased incidence in the children of mothers less than 17 years old (McAnarney and Hendee, 1989).

Maternal Ingestion of Substances
Harmful to the Fetus

Fetal alcohol syndrome (FAS) is characterized by varying degrees of prenatal and postnatal growth retardation, dysmorphic features, other physical malformations, below-normal intellect, and attentional and learning disabilities (Steinhausen and Spohr, 1986). At similar quantities of maternal alcohol consumption, FAS is more prevalent and more pronounced in children of lower socioeconomic status.

Cigarette smoking during pregnancy leads to increased risk for the child of hyperactivity, short attention span, impulsiveness, hypersensitivity to sensory stimuli, and delays in the development of language and academic skills (Naeye, 1992).

Babies born to mothers addicted to narcotics have a low birth weight and show a neonatal abstinence syndrome consisting of extreme irritability, emotional liability, and intense reactions to environmental stimuli. Evidence is increasing of long-term effects on behavior and intelligence. As cocaine and "crack" abuse have reached epidemic proportions, the number of infants affected *in utero* continues to increase. The effect of cocaine is mediated primarily through lack of prenatal care, malnutrition, prematurity, intrauterine growth retardation, and microcephaly. Although "crack babies" are at high risk, the media have exaggerated their disabilities and made them appear more impaired and untreatable than they are. It is also crucial to recognize the effects of poverty and of inadequate parenting, rather than to attribute all of these children's problems to intrauterine "crack" exposure.

Emotional Factors

Emotional stress during pregnancy has been implicated in the genesis of birth defects and complications of pregnancy and delivery as well as in later abnormalities. Animal data suggest a possible mechanism via alterations in levels of steroid hormones.

Complications in the Newborn Period

Sophisticated medical care in the newborn period can avert or moderate the harmful effects of birth injury, prematurity, hypoxia, hyperbilirubinemia, hypothyroidism, and infection.

Outcome

Although problems during pregnancy, birth, and the neonatal period may have physical, cognitive, and/or emotional sequelae, many high-risk infants, especially those with uncomplicated premature birth, improve with time and eventually demonstrate far less impairment than originally expected. Social risk factors such as single parents, poverty, and limited maternal education are powerful predictors of poor outcome. Early intervention with children, accompanied by family support services, can significantly improve outcome, even in infants with very low birth weight (less than 1.5 kg).

Communication

Even *in utero* the fetus's heart rate responds to chemical, auditory, and emotional stimuli to the mother and habituates to repeated exposure to these stimuli. At 7 months' gestation, the fetus perceives, discriminates, and responds to sounds.

INFANCY: THE FIRST YEAR

The neonate is much more competent than previously thought, although there is considerable variation among normal infants. Historically, the infant was viewed as passive. In the earliest psychoanalytic models, the child was seen as acted upon by instinctual drives. Classical behaviorists view the baby as a *tabula rasa,* shaped by external stimuli and contingencies or consequences. It is now recognized that babies are active participants in developing relationships and in influencing their environment. Heterogeneity in abilities and temperament leads to a variety of developmental paths.

Even in the first days of life, the newborn has considerable sensory, motor, intellectual, communicative, and affective abilities, which progress rapidly in the next 12 months (see Fig. 8–2).

Physical Development in Infancy

Neurological
As neurons sprout multiple and branching dendrites, cortical synapses develop rapidly in the first year of life, to a number greater than that in adults. Excess synapses are subsequently "pruned" to reach adult numbers.

Newborns have remarkable sensory abilities. Visual fixation is possible within a few hours after birth. Infants seem to be genetically programmed to pay attention to complex patterns such as the human face. Infants less than 1 day old preferentially follow with their eyes and head a drawing that resembles a human face. By 2 days of age, infants look longer at their mothers' faces than those of unknown women. The 1-week-old infant can distinguish and prefers complex visual patterns and movement. Within the first month of life, the infant can use visual information to modulate motor responses such as reaching and grasping. Four-month-old babies are able to accommodate visually as well as an adult can.

Neonates can search with their eyes for the source of an interesting sound, especially speech. Within a week of birth, infants can distinguish their mother's voice and the smell of her breast milk from those of another woman. The pattern of the infant's sucking indicates a preference for sweet liquids.

The senses of proprioception, pressure, and touch are all functional at birth. Even premature infants are at least as sensitive to pain as adults. This evidence is ending the unfortunately common practice of performing circumcision or even major surgery on infants without anesthesia.

Gross Motor
At birth the neonate is unable to purposefully reach or grasp and has primitive motor reflexes. By 16 weeks of age, the infant can hold up his or her head. The child sits with support at 28 weeks, and sits alone, creeps, and pulls to stand at 40 weeks. Standing alone is achieved around 48 weeks. By 12 months of age, the ability to walk with support ("cruising") appears.

Sleep

Most infants sleep through the night (or at least do not fuss when they awaken) by 6 to 9 months of age. Up to half of all infants, however, have irregular sleep patterns and occasional or persistent night awakening throughout the first year.

Growth

The first year is a period of rapid physical growth, with an increase in weight of approximately 300%.

Cognitive Development in Infancy

Piaget's first stage, the *sensorimotor,* covers approximately the first 2 years of life. In the first 4 months of age, the infant demonstrates *primary circular reactions:* motor reflexes or habits centered upon his or her own body. These are initially quite simple (e.g., putting the thumb in the mouth and sucking), but they become increasingly complex as the baby uses trial and error to attempt to repeat an interesting but accidental result. At this stage children are able to turn toward sounds, to engage in mutual imitation of sounds, and to visually follow a moving object.

Secondary circular reactions emerge in the 4- to 10-month-old as schemes are extended to the external environment to reproduce interesting chance events (e.g., shaking the legs makes the crib mobile jiggle). The baby is able to follow the expected path of a moving object that disappears and to recognize an object, even if parts of it are hidden. By 10 to 12 months, babies begin purposefully to combine secondary schemes to reach a goal. At this age the infant can overcome simple obstacles, perceive a connection between events, and anticipate the next object in a familiar series. The child learns that a thing continues to exist even when out of sight (*object permanence*) and searches actively for an object that has disappeared. This progress is facilitated by the rapid enhancement of memory between 8 and 12 months of age.

Communication in Infancy

In the baby's first month of life, most parents learn to decipher their infant's cries as differentiated signals of fatigue, pain, hunger, fear, discomfort, anger, or wish for contact. In addition, babies engage in apparently noncommunicative crying that seems to serve the function of discharge of tension. This type of crying occurs at discrete, regular periods of the day, most often in the late afternoon and evening, for up to 2 to 3 hours. It can be distinguished from other crying, and the usual means of comfort are unsuccessful. It is most noticeable from 3 to 10 weeks, corresponding to "3-month colic." All normal babies demonstrate this type of crying to some extent, although there is wide variation in duration and intensity. Anticipatory guidance can help parents deal with the anxiety and tension these fussy periods cause, and avert the development of more serious problems.

The young child also has a repertoire of nonverbal techniques (e.g., smiling, reaching, looking toward or away from a person or object) for engaging with and eliciting behavior from adults.

Between 5 and 10 months, the infant begins to babble and to play with sounds, both alone and in interaction with an adult. At 1 year of age, most children use 2 or more words besides "mama" and "dada" and understand simple commands.

Affective Development in Infancy

Early Attachment

In the study of the development of the infant's relationship with the mother, it has become increasingly clear how powerfully the infant can influence adult behavior. The term *attachment* is used to describe the infant's behaviors, feelings, and cognitions directed toward the mother (or mothering figure). Attachment is an affectional or emotional tie formed between one person and another that endures over time and leads to seeking physical closeness to the important figure. Attachments are highly specific, although the infant may form an attachment to more than one person. Attachments are formed to both mother and father at about the same time. *Attachment behavior* promotes proximity or contact. Babies demonstrate this behavior toward both parents. When in distress, however, infants less than 2 years of age preferentially seek out the mother. The term *bonding* (unfortunately used rather indiscriminately) should be reserved for the parent's positive feelings and behaviors toward the infant.

John Bowlby and his colleague James Robertson became interested in attachment via their work with children separated from their parents by World War II, or for briefer periods by hospitalization or foster care. Bowlby (1969) drew from his own observations as well as from ethology (the study of the naturalistic behavior of animals), evolutionary theory, psychoanalysis, cognitive-developmental theory, and systems theory in his conceptualization of the purpose and mechanisms of attachment formation. He took a Darwinian view that the inborn behavioral systems characteristic of a species enhance survival, and proposed that the biological function of attachment behavior is protection from environmental danger because it ensures parental interest and proximity. In the human infant, he observed behaviors that are initially reflexive, such as following with the eyes, clinging, sucking, and smiling. These behaviors, maintained and promoted by cognitions and feelings, are used increasingly in a social interactive context with the parent.

As early as the first hours of life, the parents and child can engage in a reciprocal interaction that initiates the development of attachment. At 6 to 8 weeks of age, the infant selectively recognizes the mother's smile and smiles in response. This is the true *social smile,* and it produces a powerful affective response in the mother. The strength of these tendencies, their likely neuro-biological underpinnings, and the remarkable adaptability of the human infant can be seen in blind babies, who show a specific smiling response to their mother's voice. Other infant behaviors that signify and strengthen attachment include crying, vocalizing, looking, greeting, and clinging, which are selectively directed at the mother (or other primary attachment figure).

Although the attachment process begins soon after birth, it is not instantaneous but develops over time. In order to develop a stable attachment, the infant must have sufficient contact with a mothering person, the ability to distinguish the mother figure from other people, and at least the beginning of the conception that another person has an independent existence even when not present. Once the first attachment has formed, the infant can generalize to a small number of other people. Illness or handicap in the child, physical or emotional illness in the parent, or parental lack of sensitivity to the needs of the baby can all impair attachment formation. Abuse or neglect of the infant can prevent the formation of attachments, with catastrophic consequences for future personality development and the ability to form meaningful relationships.

The realization that attachment and bonding can begin immediately after birth has been influential in humanizing hospital maternity procedures and in increasing opportunities for parental contact with premature and ill newborns. In many circles, however, there has been an unfortunate overemphasis on a "critical period," a very brief period of time immediately following birth after which formation of attachments and parenting ability are said to be impaired. This notion has added to the stresses on adoptive parents and parents of ill babies. Objective data do not support this "sensitive period" in the *first hours* of life or the necessity for extended immediate contact with the *neonate* in order to establish a secure, affective relationship between the baby and either the mother or father.

Goldberg (1983:1379) summarizes the evidence and its implications:

> Even among those who feel that early contact has been overrated, there are few who would argue that it is unimportant. Initial contacts are one phase in an ongoing process, and parents should be supported in this phase as well as others. Therefore, when not medically contraindicated, the opportunity for early interaction in the delivery or recovery room should be offered in order to make the experience of birth more humane, more positive, and more rewarding for parents.
>
> Second, individual differences in enthusiasm for immediate or even extended contact are normal. Insofar as possible, it is desirable to offer or allow contacts to occur when comfortable and convenient for the parents. The mother who wants or needs time to rest before

holding her baby should not be made to feel that she is abnormal for not wanting to do so immediately. The mother who does not prefer rooming in or who does not keep the baby in her room as much as possible should also be made to feel comfortable with her decision.

Finally, the notion of early contact as critical rather than potentially beneficial needs to be dispelled. The emphasis on 'early bonding' has already created an expectation on the part of many parents that if they do not have this experience they have somehow failed and will never be fine parents.

Erikson identified the establishment of *basic trust* as the primary affective task of this developmental period (see Chapter 10). This period also roughly corresponds to the Freudian *oral stage* of development described in Chapter 5.

Attachment Behavior and the Effects of Maternal Deprivation in Infancy

Mary Ainsworth pioneered in identifying and measuring attachment behaviors as indicators of the strength and security of attachment. She and others have found that insecure, anxious, or weak attachment may predict developmental problems later in childhood. A *securely attached* infant experiences separation anxiety when left by the mother. The baby seeks proximity and contact with the mother, especially when frightened or in a new situation. When with the mother, the child is able to play and to explore comfortably. When left, the infant protests or follows.

There are several types of *insecure attachment,* which are believed to have negative implications for the development of trust and healthy relationships, even into adulthood. A phenomenon that Ainsworth called *anxious resistant attachment* is believed to be promoted by parental inconsistency. The parent is available and helpful at some times but not at others. There are frequent separations. Threats of abandonment are used to control the child, leading to feelings of uncertainty and excessive separation anxiety. Children demonstrating what Ainsworth calls *anxious avoidant attachment* expect to be rejected by others. This pattern is believed to result from constant rebuffs when the mother is approached for comfort or protection. This is most extreme in the case of severe abuse, neglect, or prolonged institutionalization. Mothers of insecurely attached infants have been observed to be less attuned to the baby's needs, often not giving assistance when needed, or intruding with help when the child does not need it. Others discourage the infant's efforts at exploration and autonomy. The pattern of attachment seen in the first year has been correlated with observations at ages 3½ and 6 years (see pages 287–292) (Bowlby, 1988).

Attachment behavior is most discriminating between the ages of 6 and 12 months. By 10 months infants are capable of selective attachments to 3 or 4 people.

Stranger anxiety develops between 9 and 18 months, not only in response to strangers, but to anyone other than the mothering adult(s). At this age the infant can remember the mother's face, compare it with the stranger's, and realize the difference and the absence of the mother.

It is clear that the first year is a crucial time for forming the first attachment, and that afterwards the process is much more difficult. This has important implications for the care of infants who must be placed outside of the home.

Although some infants who are subjected to extreme stressors show remarkable resistance to developmental problems related to attachment, probably due to the child's genetic endowment and compensating factors in the family or support network, developmental trauma in this period may have lasting effects on the personality and vulnerability to childhood and adult psychiatric illness. Problems in developing secure attachments may be manifested clinically in later childhood, adolescence, and adulthood by persons who have difficulty in forming close, lasting, emotionally intimate relationships. Such persons may have "learned" from the inconsistency of the mother to anticipate rejection and the emotional distress and pain that accompanies it. Hence, closeness with other people may be viewed as an inherently risky emotional proposition where the threat of rejection or disappointment is always present. The anxiety resulting from expecting rejection or emotional abandonment may lead to a defensive posture of maintaining emotional distance and avoiding intimacy and commitment. In Chapter 11, Dr. van der Kolk discusses the scientific evidence for the lifelong consequences of developmental trauma during this stage of life.

Attachment behavior is exaggerated under stress from physical discomfort, fear, or separation from the mother. When separated from the mother, a baby older than 6 months of age shows a predictable sequence of emotions: first *protest,* with acute distress and crying; then misery and grief, or *despair;* followed by apparent apathy and disinterest, or *detachment* (Bowlby, 1975). Brief separations are benign, but as separations become longer, repeated, and/or accompanied by other stressors, the likelihood of emotional sequelae increases. Traumatic, prolonged separation can result in *anaclitic depression* (a state in which the child becomes withdrawn and relatively mute, and will not eat) or even death. Later sequelae may include an inability to form meaningful relationships or experience empathy for others, or the symptoms of posttraumatic stress disorder.

A favorite baby game, peek-a-boo, demonstrates how the child's egocentric cognitive perspective (if I can't see something, it isn't there) is used in the practicing of separation from the parent. By covering and uncovering the eyes, the infant is making the adult come and go, thereby gaining control of the experience and of the anxiety about being left alone.

Many of the details of attachment theory need to be rethought in view of the current rarity of "traditional" families (two married parents, with the mother as full-time homemaker and the almost exclusive caretaker of the baby). One-year-old infants of mothers who work full-time or part-time in the first year of life are as likely to be securely attached to their mothers as infants whose mothers do not work outside the home (Zimmerman and Bernstein, 1983).

Rene Spitz's pioneering work on *hospitalism* and *anaclitic depression* identified the devastating effects on infants of separation from their mother when compounded by lack of stimulation (Spitz, 1945, 1946). Absence of a suitable mothering figure prevents or disrupts the formation of attachments. Severe maternal deprivation can lead to a decrease in intelligence, impaired ability to trust or to form meaningful interpersonal relationships, and even death. The syndrome of *failure to thrive,* characterized by lack of growth despite adequate access to food, listlessness, and delayed cognitive, social, and motor development, has been attributed to insufficient or inappropriate mothering, although subtle physiological factors often contribute.

Separation-Individuation
Mahler's model of the process of the infant's separation and individuation from the parent is covered in detail in Chapter 5 by Drs. Inderbitzen, Furman, and James. Drs. Wolman and Thompson, in Chapter 10, describe how the thematic paradigm of separation-individuation can be repeated throughout the lifecycle. However, observational data about infant behavior and capabilities have called into question some of the details of this theory, particularly the stage of so-called normal autism.

The Transitional Object
By the end of the first year, many children have chosen what Winnicott calls a *transitional object:* a toy, blanket, pillow, or piece of clothing, usually soft, to which the child is very attached, and that is used for comfort, most often at times of separation or when going to sleep. It represents both the child and the mother. Whether or not a child has an identifiable transitional object has not been found to have prognostic significance.

THE TODDLER: AGES ONE TO THREE (1–3)

Figures 8–2 and 8–3 summarize development in this period along multiple lines of development.

Physical Development of the Toddler

Gross Motor
By 30 months of age the child not only stands, but walks and runs with ease.

Fine Motor–Adaptive

During this period there is a rapid increase in fine motor abilities, such as using a crayon, and in eye–hand coordination.

Sleep

Parents are frequently concerned about their toddler's sleep habits. Among middle-class 1- to 3-year-olds, daily sleep time averaged a total of 12 hours, including a 2-hour nap. In 1 week, 10% of the children reported a nightmare, and 7% experienced a *night terror (pavor nocturnus;* see later under Early Childhood). Twenty-one percent of 18- to 23-month-olds awakened during the night. Thirty-one percent of the 24- to 29-month-olds took more than 30 minutes to fall asleep on more than 3 nights in a week. Children aged 30 to 36 months were the most likely to have difficulty settling (16%) and to express fears of the dark (24%) (Crowell et al, 1987). Another survey of 1- to 3-year-old children found that 42% resisted going to bed. Thirty-five percent woke and cried during the night (Johnson, 1991). The use of a nightlight is almost universal at this age.

Growth and Feeding

Young toddlers show increasing interest in feeding themselves, first with their fingers, then using utensils. The child's reduced nutritional needs, resulting from much slower physical growth than in the first year and compounded by increasing interest in activity and in the environment, lead to dramatic decreases in appetite. The parent who views this with alarm and focuses excessively on eating can promote a feeding problem. It is important to avoid turning mealtime into a power struggle. The child who consumes excessive quantities of milk or juice or other "empty-calorie foods" can develop serious deficiencies in iron or other essential nutrients. Overindulgence in highly sweetened foods can result in obesity and/or tooth decay.

Toilet Training

Toilet training typically begins between ages 18 and 30 months. Prerequisites include regularity of bowel and bladder function, the ability to sense bladder and rectal fullness, the ability to control the sphincter muscles, the psychological ability to delay, the wish to imitate adults and to please the parents, the ability to communicate the need to use the toilet, and sufficient motor control to walk, stoop, stand, and remove clothing easily. A child reported to have been trained earlier than this is usually a very regular child whom the parent has learned to "catch," by putting him or her on the potty at predictable times of elimination. When toilet training is started too early, the resulting learning process is longer and often more difficult. Capitalizing on the child's wish to imitate adults and using rewards such as praise and small treats can facilitate learning in a positive manner. Punitive or threatening methods of training should not be used under any circumstances. Most children establish control of urination during the day by age 2 ½ and at night by age 3 ½ to 4 years. Approximately 10% of 6-year-olds (predominantly boys) still wet the bed, however. Late attainment of nocturnal control tends to be familial. Almost all children have achieved bowel control by age 4.

Cognitive Development of the Toddler

Piaget's Stages

The *sensorimotor stage* continues. In the first half of the second year the *tertiary circular reaction* develops. This is the attempt to produce novelty for its own sake by extending existing schemes to a variety of objects. The *preoperational stage* begins in the third year (see section entitled "Early Childhood" for description).

Object permanence, the conviction that something continues to exist even when out of sight, solidifies around 18 to 20 months of age, but begins to develop as early as age 4 months. Children understand this about people, especially their parents, before they understand it about things.

Milestones

Eighteen-month-olds can recognize themselves in mirrors and pictures. By the latter half of the second year, the child is able to retain and use mental symbols, a necessary precursor to the use of language.

Increased interest in the environment and ability to explore, in the absence of judgment or understanding of consequences, put toddlers at extremely high risk for accidents. Parents must ensure safety but avoid overly restricting the child's exploration or responding punitively to inadvertent damage of objects. Systematically "child proofing" the house and using tactics that redirect the child into other activities can reduce both danger and parent–child power struggles.

Speech and Language Development of the Toddler

Over the first 6 months of this period, toddlers make extensive use of *jargon* (sounds that resemble speech, but are unintelligible). Most 2-year-olds have a 300-word vocabulary, use phrases and two-word sentences, and can point to body parts when named. Around 30 months of age, most children can use pronouns correctly. In all children, comprehension precedes expressive abilities.

Private speech, which has a social intent but fails to communicate specific meaning, precedes true social speech. The child still has idiosyncratic meanings for some words. Toddlers often use pronouns without referents, as if the listener knew to whom the pronoun referred without being told.

Some *echolalia* (repetition of overheard words or phrases) is normal into the third year. Developmental dysfluency or repetition of words or phrases is normal between ages 2 and 4. This should be differentiated from *stuttering,* a symptom that includes blocking and repeating of sounds, with motor and subsequent emotional tension, and eventual severe anxiety about speech.

Although normal children vary widely in their rate and style of language acquisition, a hearing test and a language assessment are indicated if an 18-month-old uses no words or just "mama" and "dada," and does not point to what he or she wants. An evaluation is warranted if a 2-year-old is not putting two words together, has a vocabulary less than 20 words, has speech that is unintelligible to the parents, or does not understand commands or questions without gestures (Allen et al, 1988). Although a few normal children are simply late talkers, such a delay could be caused by deafness, aphasia, mental retardation, autistic disorder, or developmental language disorder. The Early Language Milestone Scale can be used by primary care practitioners to screen for speech and language delay (up to 48 months of age) (Coplan and Gleason, 1990). Hearing sensitivity can be tested using brain stem auditory evoked response audiometry on even the least cooperative child. Gross indications that the child hears sounds do not eliminate the possibility of a hearing impairment sufficient to limit the development of speech and language.

Affective Development of the Toddler

Object Relations

In the first half of the second year, a phenomenon that Emde and colleagues have called *social referencing* appears, in which the infant looks to the parent for emotional cues about a novel event.

Mahler's description of this period is discussed in detail in Chapter 5. To briefly recapitulate, as the *practicing subphase* continues (12 to 18 months), the toddler moves away from the parent to explore. The child returns frequently to the parent to "refuel" (to establish emotional contact and to refresh the internal image of the mother). A securely attached child is able to use the mother as a base from which to investigate the environment. In the *rapprochement subphase* (16 to 24 months), children's growing realization of their separateness, physical ability to move away from the parent, and their own helplessness leads to intense ambivalence about their attachment and dependency needs. Many toddlers increase clinging to parents, tantrums, thumb or finger sucking, and need for their transitional object. The child's third year sees *consolidation* and resolution, as the child becomes comfortable with brief separations. In later stages of development, such as adolescence and young adulthood, portions of the separation–individuation process may be repeated (see Chapter 10).

The third year is marked by the child's struggle for psychological autonomy and separateness from the parents. This may be seen in the form of negativity and tantrums as children practice making decisions and asserting themselves, but then become overwhelmed by feelings that they cannot yet express verbally. The middle of this year is the height of "the terrible twos." Although the duration and intensity vary greatly among children, some degree of negativism is essential in the child's development of a sense of independence and individuality. Children benefit from consistent, firm, but sympathetic limits. Tantrums should be ignored and *never* rewarded, to prevent transforming an expression of frustration into a device for manipulating adults. Whenever possible, direct confrontations should be avoided. It is helpful if parents can resist the temptation to interpret the toddler's obstinate behavior as a personal affront. Taking a punitive or rigidly controlling approach can be destructive to the child's development and to the parent-child relationship. The most effective means of handling defiant behavior is usually by brief periods of "time out" or in the case of tantrums, by ignoring them (see Chapter 6 by Dr. Dorsett.) Physical punishment should not be used. Often, the adult can ease the process by presenting the child with choices, both of which are acceptable to the parent.

Emotions and Mechanisms of Defense

In the third year of life, a sense of empathy for others begins to emerge. The child also has a growing understanding of emotions and an ability to label them verbally. *Reaction formation* is a defense mechanism that typically appears in this period, as seen in children who have recently been toilet trained and become excessively upset by messiness. This defense is presumed to protect the child against wishes to urinate and defecate at will. The development of defense mechanisms is discussed in a psychoanalytic framework in Chapter 5.

Fears

The toddler's lack of experience, small size, and helplessness compared to adults foster the development of fears such as of loud noises, animals, the dark, and separation from parents. Fears of the bathtub or toilet are common, exacerbated by toddlers' inability to judge relative sizes and determine that they could *not* actually fit down the drain.

Gender-related Issues

Core morphological or *gender identity* is the usually unshakable conviction of being a male or a female, which develops through a complex interaction of physiological and environmental factors (Money, 1987). It can be seen around 18 months, or even earlier, and is often established by 24 to 30 months. Absolute integration of gender identity can be expected by age 3. While psychological and sociocultural factors play an important role in shaping gender identity, for most persons, biological gender determines psychological identity as a male or female.

As discussed in the preceding chapter by Drs. Becker, Johnson, and Hunter, *in utero,* sexual differentiation proceeds in the female direction in the absence of masculinizing hormones (androgens). Androgens alter the development of the central nervous system as well as of the genitalia. Normally, all of the child's gender-related characteristics are consistent: chromosomes, prenatal hormones, gonads (ovaries and testes), internal and external genitalia, postnatal hormones, and secondary sex characteristics (developing at puberty).

Cultural factors are extremely important in the development of *gender role behavior,* that is, behavior that is considered by society to be appropriate for one sex or another. Examples for children include tone of voice, physical mannerisms, gait, clothing, play activities, and playmates. Adults treat boys and girls differently from infancy (Shepherd-Look, 1982). Boys are picked up more as newborns, handled more roughly than girls, and more frequently engaged in rough-and-tumble play. Mothers talk more to girls than to boys. Adults offer different toys to boys and to girls, and by age 1 year, toy preference along stereotypical gender lines is established. Beginning in the second year, fathers pay significantly more attention to boys than to girls. By age 2, boys show a clear preference for their fathers over their mothers (Hodapp and Mueller, 1982). Differential treatment and expectations continue throughout the course of development. Extrafamilial influences are also important. Sex differences have been found in children's response to social reinforcement of specific behaviors. Girls respond to both male and female teachers and to other girls, but ignore reinforcement from boys. Boys, on the other hand, respond to reinforcement from male peers, but are unresponsive to reinforcement from girls or from teachers (Fagot, 1985). The peer group is a powerful determinant of gender role behavior, as are adult figures popularized by the media.

It has now been recognized that masculinity and femininity are not polar opposites, each being found in varying amounts in both males and females. The interaction of physical and environmental factors in the development of gender identity and role behavior is complex.

Genetic females with congenital adrenal hyperplasia, a defect in cortisol synthesis that leads to prenatal and postnatal excess of androgenic hormone precursor, are born with masculinized external genitalia and normal female internal organs. Clear, early gender assignment with consistent medical and surgical treatment can result in stable gender identity as *either* a male or a female, depending on initial assignment. Reassignment attempts fail if carried out after 18 months to 3 years.

Androgen-insensitivity syndrome (testicular feminization) in XY genetic males is characterized by insensitivity of all body cells to testosterone, leading to female-appearing external genitalia. These children are usually reared as females. Histologically normal but nonfunctional testes are removed to avoid virilization and increased risk of malignancy. If the child is treated as a normal girl, she usually develops female gender identity, stereotypically feminine role behavior, and, in adolescence, sexual interest in males.

Tentative evidence from children prenatally exposed to treatment with estrogen and progestogen (to avoid loss of the pregnancy) shows behavioral demasculinization of males and increased feminization of females.

Social Development of Toddlers

Early in this period, children are curious about other children. The first half of the third year sees the development of *parallel play:* solitary, unrelated play conducted in pairs. Over the next 6 months, children begin to engage in *associative play,* in pairs or small groups, doing the same thing side by side, but not really interacting. Toddler play is based on sensorimotor activity—opening and shutting, emptying and filing—with more interest in the process than the product.

EARLY CHILDHOOD: AGES THREE TO SIX (3–6)

Physical Development in Early Childhood

Gross Motor

Most 3-year-olds can stand on one foot, jump, run smoothly, and climb stairs using alternating feet. They are beginning to show hand preference and to be able to ride a tricycle. Four-year-olds should be able to ride a tricycle well, to climb on a jungle gym, and to throw a ball overhand. By age 5, balance is better, and the child should be able to skip smoothly.

Fine Motor-Adaptive

The 3-year-old can build a tower of 9 or 10 blocks. By age 4, most children can button and lace, feed themselves neatly, pour from a pitcher, and dress and wash themselves. Drawing ability progresses from copying a circle (3 years), to copying a cross and drawing a simple man with head, eyes, and legs (4 years). The 5-year-old can copy a square and a triangle and draw a recognizable man with basic body parts (eyes, nose, mouth, body, arms, legs, and feet). The 5-year-old plans pictures in advance and may include elaborate scenes or complex events.

Sleep

Many 3-year-olds still take an afternoon nap, but give it up by age 4 or 5 years. A phenomenon that is often confused with nightmares is the *night terror* or *pavor nocturnus.* Unlike nightmares, which occur during rapid eye movement (REM) sleep, and are often remembered, the night terror occurs during the deep *non-REM* sleep stages 3 and 4. The child appears terrified, screaming, confused; has dilated pupils, sweating, rapid pulse, and hyperventilation; and does not respond to comforting. Once alert, the child rapidly returns to sleep. There is no memory of the episode in the morning. This phenomenon is most common in children ages 3 to 6 and does not indicate psychopathology. It is usually much more upsetting to parents than to the child!

Toilet Training

Most children are dry at night by the latter half of the fourth year. They are able to use the toilet independently in the daytime, at least in familiar places.

Cognitive Development in Early Childhood

Piaget's Stages

The *preoperational stage* of intellectual development extends from approximately 2 to 7 years of age, including both the toddler period and early childhood. The child learns to classify, to place objects in order (by trial and error), and to construct sets equivalent in number by matching one to one. Piaget believed that the preoperational child is unable to deal with more than one dimension (e.g., height and width) at a time, or to recognize that a person or thing conserves its identity when it undergoes minor variations in appearance. Problem solving is by trial and error, rather than by planned strategies.

The use of nonverbal mental symbols, followed by language, gives the child the ability to transcend space and time. This ability can be seen in the child's deferred imitation of actions, drawing of scenes clearly based on memory, and meaningful use of words. *Symbolic play* appears, consisting of pretend, or imaginative play with toys or dramatizing roles and stories in which toys and roles symbolize real objects and real persons.

Preoperational children are normally *egocentric,* relating everything to themselves. Piaget believed that the child was unaware of the point of view of the listener or even that the listener may have another point of view or different knowledge. More recent work has shown that 4-year-olds do speak differently to adults than they do to 2-year-olds, indicating an awareness of the listener's ability to understand. The 4-year-old is able to show some understanding of another's perspective, if the task is carefully designed.

Children this age often have difficulty understanding cause and effect. Thinking tends to be *concrete,* with explanations often based on past experience, whether or not it is relevant. Reasoning is often *transductive* (attributing causality to juxtaposition in time or space) rather than *inductive* (from the particular to the general) or *deductive* (from the general to the particular). Piaget called this *phenomenalistic causality.*

Young children are *animistic,* believing that all events can be explained by the action of some humanlike agency or force that wills things to happen for its own purposes. Words and actions are not fully differentiated. *Magical thinking,* the belief that words, thoughts, and wishes can cause events in the external world, is typical of the child in the preoperational stage. Older children, or even adults, may regress to magical thinking under stress.

Four-year-olds have difficulty distinguishing truth from fiction. Even at age 7, strong wishes may distort the perception of reality. Adults may misinterpret this as deliberate lying. A child who desperately wishes he had not broken his mother's vase may actually convince himself that he did not. This phenomenon may be seen in older children and even adolescents who are cognitively or emotionally immature or under stress.

Moral development in the 3- to 6-year-old is characterized by *moral realism:* the belief in immanent justice, and the inevitability of punishment. Physical misfortunes and accidents may be seen as direct punishment for wrongdoing (present at some time in all children, at least in thought). Piaget termed the morality of this stage *objective,* by which he meant that guilt is determined solely by the amount of damage, not the intent or motivation. A child who spills a whole bottle of ink while trying to help set the table is judged more guilty than a child who spills a drop of ink while playing with a pen that he has been forbidden to touch. Young children are absolute in their judgment of right and wrong. The inability to see simultaneous positive and negative aspects of the same person or event, considered pathological *splitting* in adults, is normal in early childhood (see Chapter 5).

Preoperational children do not know or follow rules of games, but insist that they do. They believe that rules are originated by a godlike absolute authority and are unchangeable. Children are more likely to follow parents' rules if they are highly identified with their parents (admire them, believe they take after them, and want to grow up to be like them). Hence, the ethical examples set by loving, fair, and honorable parents are far more important than the prohibitions and punishments imposed in an effort to train children in moral behavior.

Milestones

Four-year-olds have little understanding of past and future. By age 5, there is a better understanding of the concepts of yesterday and tomorrow, and an ability to carry over play activities from one day to the next. There is a beginning understanding of clock and calendar time. Five-year-olds can identify simple similarities among and differences between objects. Children at this age believe that death is reversible, like sleep.

Speech and Language in Early Childhood

Language permits the mastery of negative feelings by putting them into words instead of acting upon them, yielding improved impulse control and ability to delay gratification.

During this period, vocabulary typically develops at the amazing rate of nine new words per day until the age of 6. Three-year-olds ask constant questions, just for the sake of talking. They play with words, and use and understand prepositions like *in, on,* and *under.* Four-year-olds' articulation is still somewhat immature, but their speech should be largely intelligible in context. Word play includes crude puns. Complex parts of speech, such as adverbs, and more difficult prepositions and conjunctions appear. By the age of 5 years, articulation should be clear and correct, answers to questions more succinct and relevant, and questions fewer, more direct, and more meaningful. Correct, finished sentences can be constructed, including hypothetical and conditional clauses. In this period, language development is ahead of the ability to understand concepts. Adults must be cautious not to assume that children understand more than they actually do.

Affective Development in Early Childhood

Object Relations

Mahler proposed that firm emotional *object constancy,* the ability to maintain a positive inner image of an important person despite the level of need or satisfaction, is established by around 36 months (see discussion of object relations theory in Chapter 5). The timing varies, however, depending on the child's previous experience and the character of the mother–child relationship. Under stress, previously attained object constancy can be temporarily lost.

Fears

Normal fears include the dark, animals, bodily harm, monsters, ghosts, and death. Cognitive development at this age does not permit the use of sophisticated psychological defenses to control anxiety in the face of perceived danger.

Gender-related Issues

The learning of gender roles and societally determined gender role behavior starts in the toddler period. By age 3, children can identify tasks and possessions as masculine or feminine. Culturally determined gender role behaviors are so strong that they can override parental determination to encourage androgyny. Even kindergarten children know the sex-role stereotypes of Western culture, aspire to stereotypical sex-appropriate occupations, choose same-sex friends, and evaluate the work of same-sex adults and children more highly than those of the opposite sex. Each child has an individual balance of masculine and feminine characteristics, influenced by temperamental factors and parental modeling and expectations.

Cross-gender behavior is normal in boys until age 5 years. Cultural expectations for gender role behavior in girls are much more flexible, so tomboyish behavior is generally not considered abnormal at any age, unless it is accompanied by a rigid avoidance of all feminine clothes and activities. Boys are more aggressive than girls as early as age 2 years, continuing through adolescence.

Sexuality

Three-year-olds are aware of sex differences but are prone to primitive theories regarding sexuality and pregnancy. Boys are increasingly aware of sensations in the penis. The fear of loss of, or damage to, the genitals may be accentuated by viewing female genitals and by punitive threats made by parents attempting to stop a child from masturbating. Detumescence of the penis after an erection may reinforce fears of castration.

Belief in oral impregnation (encouraged by jokes about swallowed watermelon seeds turning into babies) may lead to irrational attitudes toward food. Children begin to demonstrate behavior that suggests fantasies about, observation of, or hearing sounds associated with parental sexual intercourse, which may be confused with some form of physical attack, fighting, or wrestling. Sex education geared to the level of the child's curiosity and understanding is important. Preoccupation with, or detailed knowledge about, sexual behavior suggests inappropriate exposure to adult sexual activity or even sexual abuse.

Imaginary Companions

Up to one-fifth of 3- to 6-year-olds have an imaginary companion, a fantasy person or animal to whom the child gives a name, an appearance, and a character. Children may or may not tell their parents about their imaginary friends. The phenomenon most often is seen in creative children of above-average intelligence. At various times the companion serves as scapegoat, playmate, and protector. By 10 years of age, the imaginary companion is usually given up.

Dreams

Until about 5 years of age, the child believes that dreams are real events. Children frightened by their angry or aggressive feelings toward their parents may project them onto monsters, who then appear in nightmares.

Family Relationships

Toward the end of this period, children begin to recognize the discrepancy between reality and their idealized image of their parents. This leads to the "family romance," the fantasy that the child has other, real parents, who are far wiser, kinder, and more successful than those with whom he or she lives. This stage may be particularly difficult for adopted children and their parents.

Even those who do not accept Freudian developmental theory and the concept of the Oedipus complex (see Chapter 5), observe that many 3 to 6-year-olds show exaggerated "romantic" behavior toward the parent of the opposite sex, coupled with disinterest in, or even rivalry with, the parent of the same sex. As this stage passes, the child moves from a dyadic (one-to-one) preoccupation with the parent of the opposite sex to a more balanced relationship and identification with both parents, and a readiness to invest energy outside of the family into friendships and schoolwork.

Social Development in Early Childhood

Three-year-olds are able to play alone in parallel with another child for longer periods of time than is the toddler. Fours-year-olds are more able to engage in *cooperative* or small group play. They are beginning to be able to share, but are often bossy and have difficulty understanding the feelings of other children. By age 5, most children can engage in the planning and execution of group projects and participate in elaborate dramatic play. Empathy and leadership begin to appear. Children who are friendly and helpful tend to be popular with peers, while aggressive and disruptive children are rejected. Rejection by peers is a powerful predictor of later psychopathology.

Play serves a critical defensive function, enabling children to regain a sense of control by playing out scenarios in which they have been passively acted upon (e.g., during a medical procedure) by taking an active role in the play. Libidinal and aggressive impulses can be discharged through symbolic or fantasy play. Play also is used to develop mastery of both skills and emotions and to prepare for adult roles. Play and recreation continue to fill a useful role throughout life.

Television

Preschool children watch an average of 3 to 4 hours of television per day, and in the vast majority of homes viewing is completely unsupervised. Research has shown that regular viewing of action/adventure programs leads to increased aggressive behavior in young children. Heavy television viewing also interferes with learning to read (Singer and Benton, 1989). The cognitive limitations of children in the Piagetian preoperational stage of development make it difficult for them to distinguish fantasy from reality, especially with the realistic special effects of today's television programs.

Starting School

The period from ages 3 to 6 is often called the preschool period because the child who has been cared for at home by the parent(s) often has the first experience with major separation at entry to nursery school (age 3 or 4) or kindergarten (age 5). A temporary regression manifested by crying, clinging to the parent, wetting or soiling, refusal to eat, or sleep disturbance is not unusual. In an otherwise well-adjusted child, if the separation is handled sensitively by teacher and parent, the child soon returns to his or her previous level of functioning, or even makes a jump ahead. For children who have not mastered previous stages of separation-individuation, are temperamentally inclined to avoid new situations, or have parents reluctant to separate from them, the first signs of separation anxiety disorder or school phobia may be seen at this stage. Children whose prior exposure to peers has been limited may have more difficulty adjusting to the preschool experience. This is also the age at which oppositional defiant disorder or attention-deficit hyperactivity disorder may first become apparent, because the child is expected to function as a member of a group and follow rules, and is observed by the teacher, who has a wider experience with normative child behavior than the parents.

MIDDLE CHILDHOOD: AGES SIX TO TWELVE (6–12)

This period of development is often called *latency,* a term derived from the psychoanalytic developmental model. Most children attend elementary school during these years. The age of 7 (plus or minus 1 year) represents a significant developmental milestone in virtually all present and past cultures (Shapiro and Perry, 1976). This is the age at which the child is considered to be ready for formal schooling, apprenticeship, or more active learning of adult skills and roles. For example, the Roman Catholic Church has established the age of 7 as "the age of reason" and, therefore, the time for First Communion. Other religions and cultures have similar rituals to mark this developmental stage. The child's increasing cognitive and motor capacities allow for gradual independence from the family.

Physical Development in Middle Childhood

Neurological

Changes in the child's abilities, interests, and role in society coincide with significant maturation of the central nervous system (Shapiro and Perry, 1976). By age 7, the brain has attained about 90% of its adult weight. The cerebral cortex is completely myelinated, and the electroencephalogram (EEG) is better synchronized, with a stable alpha wave pattern. Structural and functional changes at the microscopic level can be documented in the frontal lobe, perhaps facilitating verbal regulation of behavior. Children are able to perceive and to understand increasingly complex sensory stimuli. Their ability to integrate and to coordinate various sensory and motor capacities improves dramatically. They attain the ability to distinguish right from left, first in themselves, and then in others. Handedness is established around age 7, followed by dominance of one eye and one foot.

Gross Motor

Between the ages of 7 and 10, balance, equilibrium, control of large muscles, and timing improve dramatically. Children are able to learn a variety of sports, including skating, jumping rope, swimming, diving, riding a two-wheel bicycle, and the beginnings of team sports such as soccer.

Fine Motor–Adaptive

Small muscle control improves, and average 8-year-olds can tie their shoes easily, wink, snap their fingers, and whistle. Games such as jacks are mastered. In drawings, the 8-year-old can use perspective and correct body proportions.

Sleep

At age 8 years, sleep averages 10 hours, decreasing to 8 to 9 hours by age 10.

Growth and Pubertal Changes

At age 10, girls and boys are approximately equal in size and sexual maturity. Girls are the first to show subtle signs of puberty. The growth spurt begins at 9 or 10 years, with the growth rate peaking at 12. Hip rounding, nipple projection, waist accentuation, and early pubic hair follow the growth spurt. Puberty begins, on average, 2 years later in boys. A slight increase in the size of the penis and the testes, and the beginnings of pubic hair appear at age 10 or 11, with the growth spurt beginning at 11 or 12 years. Appetite tends to increase around age 10, especially in boys. (Pubertal development is also discussed in Chapter 7 by Drs. Becker, Johnson, and Hunter.)

Cognitive Development in Middle Childhood

Piaget's Stages

In the stage of *concrete operations* (7 to 11 years) the child acquires the ability to *decentrate,* that is, to consider more than one dimension simultaneously (e.g., height and width). Ability to take the perspective of another person improves. Children become able to reverse operations mentally, a skill essential to comfort with addition and subtraction. They develop the ability to *conserve,* first quantity (6 to 7 years), then weight (9 to 10 years), and finally volume (11 to 12 years). In other words, they come to understand that these properties of a substance are not changed by alterations in shape or size. Their explanations of conservation progress from negation or reversibility (you could just make it the way it was before), through identity (it's the same, none was added or taken away) to compensation or reciprocity (a short wide glass holds the same amount as a tall narrow one).

As moral development progresses, children are able to take motivation into account in judging right and wrong. Morality becomes *subjective* as the child is increasingly able to understand the feelings of other people and the influence of their own actions on others.

Milestones

Perceptual-integrative abilities improve dramatically during this developmental period. School placement is crucial. If the work is too easy, it leads to boredom and poor study habits. If too hard, failure, loss of motivation, feelings of incompetence, and/or behavior problems result. Around 3% of school children are mentally retarded and need a special class or school. Approximately 10 to 25% of children are slow learners, with borderline or low normal IQ, 40 to 50% are average, 20 to 25% are bright or above average, and about 10% are gifted. Expectations vary from school to school. For example, a child with an average IQ may have difficulty getting good grades in a competitive suburban or private school. In general, girls tend to be better students than boys.

By age 7, accurate comprehension of time and calendar organization leads to a better understanding of the past and the future and an increased ability to delay gratification. Most 8-year-olds are able to read for pleasure, but their ideas still exceed their writing ability. Nine-year-olds, typically in the fourth grade, should have an improved ability to set and to finish a task. Most find school enjoyable but may fear failure. Some previously immature children show a rapid growth in learning at this time. Alternatively, increased demands for using reading and math skills may uncover a learning disability that was not previously noticed.

Most 10-year-olds memorize well but still have difficulty with abstraction. They can count forward indefinitely by ones, twos, fives, and tens, and backward by ones. They are also able to identify similarities and differences between objects, define concrete words, and add and subtract with ease.

By age 11, children should be able to interpret simple proverbs and perform multiplication and division. They are, however, usually unable to understand irony or sarcasm.

A more realistic concept of death is developing in children aged 10 to 11. Most understand that death is universal, especially those who have reached the Piagetian stage of concrete operations, but more than half of fourth graders do not yet clearly understand the irreversibility of death. Elementary-school-age children continue to view death as a punishment for bad behavior (White et al, 1978).

Five-year-olds literally think out loud, with a running description of their activities. By age 6 to 8, thinking becomes more covert or private, and takes on a self-regulatory and then problem-solving function. Private speech also takes on a role in academic performance. By age 10 or 12, children have developed *metacognitive* abilities (i.e., they understand something about what they know and how they learn) and are able to consciously develop strategies for learning. Impulsive children with learning, conduct, or attentional problems either do not develop these skills or do not use them when appropriate. Specific interventions have been developed to teach them, with variable degrees of success.

Affective Development in Middle Childhood

Superego and Conscience

New cognitive abilities permit better inhibition and control of drives, and postponement of action and gratification. Freudian developmental theory (described in Chapter 5) proposes that the *superego,* which emerges as the Oedipal crisis is resolved, is divided into the prohibiting and punitive *conscience,* and the *ego-ideal* or idealized model to which one aspires. The child identifies with the parents, and gives these identifications authority, facilitating obedience to parental instructions even without parental presence. Satisfying the ego-ideal leads to increased self-esteem, comfort, and well-being. Major discrepancy between the child's ego-ideal and actual abilities may lead to demoralization and low self-esteem, or to a defiant refusal to even attempt to succeed. Early in this period the newly developed superego is alternatively punitive and ineffective. Guilt may be handled by projection or by provoking punishment. When children misbehave, or believe that they have misbehaved, without parental awareness, they may then engage in further mischief until finally punished. A parent may say, "I don't understand it, Johnny was *asking* for it!" Under stress, children may be prone to regression, with loss of superego control. Emotions are often fluid, intense, and rapidly changing.

By ages 8 to 10, the superego is more firmly established, and the ego is stronger and more firmly consolidated. Children should be able to distinguish right from wrong and to be honest and truthful. Behavior is generally based on internalized values rather than on seeking rewards or avoiding punishment. More mature obsessional defenses and sublimation can facilitate improved school performance. Normal compulsive traits are seen in the strong interest typical of this phase in establishing and organizing collections (e.g., stamps, rocks, dolls, baseball cards). If pronounced, these defenses, along with increased repression, may lead to a decrease in creativity and spontaneity.

Sexuality

Although this period has been termed latency in psychoanalytic developmental theory, it is only sexual wishes toward, and fantasies directly concerning, *parents* that are typically latent. Sexual exploration, comparing of genitals, and group or mutual masturbation are common among boys. Prepubertal boys show a renewed interest in anal or fecal humor and in using sexual or excretory terms as expletives. Sex education begun in early childhood should be continued, although children of this age may not be willing to confess ignorance by asking questions. As puberty approaches, academic tasks may no longer provide adequate gratification and excitement or bind youthful energy. Interest is transferred to sports and teenage activities, and in dysfunctional social and family environments to "gangs."

Fears

Some fears, such as those related to body integrity, may be dealt with by counterphobic defenses and risk-taking behavior. Many children worry about their competence or appearance. Nightmares are usually related to daytime events, and children are easily calmed when awakened.

Social Development in Middle Childhood

Eight-year-olds should have a firm grasp of basic rules and an ability to cooperate well when playing games. By age 9 or 10, they should be able to both cooperate and compete, although games may still be interrupted by disagreements about the rules. By age 11 or 12, a legalistic fascination with making, changing, and negotiating rules emerges. An entire afternoon may be spent setting up teams, choosing leaders, making rules, and devising punishments for breaking rules (addressing all possible contingencies), without disappointment at never playing the actual game. Children come to understand that rules have been invented by human beings and are maintained by mutual consent. Rules may be altered if the change is fair and if all agree. Rules serve to promote social interaction, to define socially unacceptable behavior, and to strengthen the barrier against regression. Children who are generally helpful and who follow rules tend to be more popular with peers, although athletic and academic competence contribute more to popularity than they do for younger children. Bossy, aggressive, disruptive, hyperactive children (especially boys) are likely to be rejected by peers. Peer judgments tend to be long lasting, even after a child's behavior changes (for example, methylphenidate [Ritalin] treatment of a hyperactive boy improves his behavior but he is still unpopular).

Both boys and girls generally prefer single-sex groupings for play, sports, and social events. There is extreme peer pressure, especially on boys, for culturally appropriate gender role behavior and the exclusion of girls or even effeminate boys. Boys and girls both harbor rigid sexual stereotypes, even in families in which parents have equivalent roles at home and at work.

Girls have more intense friendships than boys do, with one or two peers, and may develop "crushes" on older adolescent or young adult women, who concretely represent their ego-ideal. These feelings should not be regarded as signs of homosexuality.

Compared to earlier stages, the school-age child is far more exposed to and influenced by the environment outside of the home. Childhood has its own subculture, passed from child to child by word of mouth, without adult intervention. This includes rhymes, chants, superstitions, rituals, jokes, riddles, and secret codes. Both boys and girls engage in hero worship of sports, music, television, or movie stars; coaches; or even teachers.

The ubiquitous sex and violence in the media exert a powerful influence. Viewing television violence has been demonstrated to increase aggression in children and adolescents (Pearl et al, 1982). Television, movies, and music videos probably provide a significant amount of sexual overstimulation and often present poor role models of precocious, promiscuous, or violent sexuality.

Informal groups and clubs are increasingly important, often with little purpose other than to include some children and exclude others. Organizations such as the Boy Scouts and Girl Scouts also are popular. To be accepted by peers, children must learn to be loyal, to be able to compromise, to be good sports, and not to "tattle." Social competence and peer acceptance result from specific skills and characteristics, such as the ability to size up a social situation and adapt to it, to respond positively to approach by peers, and to take a gradual, indirect, process-oriented approach to social goals (Asher, 1983).

Unfortunately, group behavior is not always positive. Teasing is often cruel and persistent. Peer pressure may lead to dangerous or immoral behavior. Boys are especially vulnerable to dares or to suggestions of cowardice.

Even prior to adolescence, girls are acutely aware of cultural concepts of physical attractiveness. Many express unrealistic concern about obesity and try to diet, despite normal weight. In vulnerable girls, this may be accentuated at the beginning of puberty, with the normal increase in body fat, and may lead to the development of anorexia or bulimia nervosa.

ADOLESCENCE

The major tasks of adolescence are the development of a secure personal and sexual identity, an occupational choice, and personal values. For many youth, prolonged education and the resulting economic dependence on the family extend the period of adolescent development well into their middle and late 20s.

Physical Development in Adolescence

Neurological
Dendritic connections attain their adult level, which is a reduction from earlier proliferation. By age 14 the EEG shows mature alpha rhythms.

Endocrine
Puberty is the attainment of reproductive capacity. There is wide diversity in timing among youth of both sexes. On average, boys attain sexual maturity 2 years later than girls, typically at age 15 in girls and at age 17 in boys. Early maturation is generally an advantage for boys but a disadvantage for girls. As a result of improved nutrition and fewer serious childhood diseases, the average age of menarche in girls has declined from 15 to 16 years in the 1880s to 12 years. Combined with the prolongation of the adolescent stage for economic and educational reasons, the result is a long period of sexual maturity before it is culturally appropriate to marry and to start a new family.

Pubertal changes focus the adolescent's attention on his or her body. Many teenagers are extremely concerned about their physical appearance. Hormonal changes accompanying puberty, along with social and cultural factors, lead to an increased interest in sexuality and sexual experimentation. In addition, the pervasive sexuality in television, movies, music, and advertising may lead to overstimulation and pressure to engage in sexual activity.

Cognitive Development in Adolescence

Piaget's Stages
At the level of *formal operations,* the youth is able to use abstract thought, to consider theoretical notions, and to devise hypotheses and ways of

testing them. The late adolescent becomes able to understand metaphor and complex, abstract subjects such as algebra and calculus. A few children reach the stage of formal operations as early as the age of 12 years. It is attained by only 35% of 16- to 17-year-olds. *Many adults never reach this stage, and have a limited ability to deal in a flexible and rational manner with such abstract concepts as religion, ethics, morality, philosophy, and politics.* Even when the stage of formal operations is attained, emotional pressure may cause temporary regression to functioning at the level of concrete operations.

Affective Development in Adolescence

Adolescent Turmoil

Adolescents in American society are beset by multiple stressors and pressures. The move from a smaller elementary school to a larger middle school or high school results in less supervision, more impersonal relationships with teachers, and a larger, more diverse peer group. Academic work is increasingly demanding, and there is a pressing need to make decisions regarding work or further education after high school.

Early psychoanalytic and Eriksonian theories propose that *adolescent turmoil* (psychological upheaval leading to significant disruption in personality organization, disequilibrium, and disturbances in mood and behavior) is not only ubiquitous but necessary for successful separation from parents and formation of adult identity. Studies conducted in the 1960s and 1970s by Offer et al (1981) of normal adolescents and those with a variety of emotional and physical illnesses found that serious emotional or behavioral problems are *not* normal in adolescents. Most teenagers cope reasonably effectively, without undue disruption of school or family life, with the tasks of adolescence. About 20% of youths experience tumult or diagnosable psychopathology in their teen years, most often those from less stable backgrounds and with more family conflict. About one-quarter of adolescents, most often those who experience few stressors and have parents who encourage independence, demonstrate essentially continuous growth and good interpersonal relationships. The remainder are characterized by developmental spurts alternating with periods of conflict. These youths, often "late bloomers," report more disagreements with their parents and more feelings of depression and anxiety.

It is normal, particularly in early adolescence, to experience a transient disturbance of self-esteem, increased feelings of anxiety and depression, and oversensitivity to shame and humiliation that do not reach a clinical level and are usually related to particular stressful situations. Interestingly, the 1970s cohort of adolescents surveyed by Offer et al (1981) reported feeling less self-confident, controlled, and trusting of others than the teenagers studied in the 1960s.

Prior to adolescence, behavioral and emotional disorders are more common in boys than in girls. In adolescence, the girls catch up, and even exceed boys in the prevalence of eating disorders and depression.

Critical Developmental Challenges
and Issues of Adolescence

Shapiro and Hertzig (1988) identify eight issues that must be resolved in the course of adolescent development:

1. Dependence versus independence from the nuclear family.
2. Behavioral license versus intellectualized control.
3. Loyalty to family versus to peer group.
4. Normalizing function of sharing thoughts and feelings with peers versus need for privacy.
5. Idealization versus devaluation of peers and adults.
6. Formation of identity, role, and character.
7. Consolidation of sexual role and sexual object choice.
8. Reshuffling of defenses and the consolidation of style of functioning.

Mechanisms of Defense

Adolescents may show a temporary increase in less mature mechanisms such as *projection, externalization, denial, reaction formation,* and *repression,* as well as development of the more advanced defenses of *rationalization, identification,* and *sublimation.* On balance, adolescents have an improved ability to use mature defenses, to tolerate frustration, and to delay gratification. (See Chapter 5 for more specific definitions of these defense mechanisms.)

Risk-taking Behavior

Unfortunately, feelings of entitlement and the belief in their omnipotence and invulnerability common in adolescents may lead to dangerous experimentation and risk-taking behavior. The three leading causes of death in adolescents are accidents, homicide, and suicide. The 1990 national Youth Risk Behavior Survey found that almost 1 in 5 high school students had carried a gun, knife, or club at least once in the past month (Centers for Disease Control, 1991). Although adolescents cognitively understand the meaning of death, they do not accept that this is a real possibility for them. Some teenagers have a mental image of "surviving in fantasy," imagining how their parents and peers would react to their death, classically portrayed in Tom Sawyer's attendance at his own "funeral."

Adolescents commonly fluctuate between unrealistically positive and negative views of themselves. Compared to adults, they are more likely to attribute responsibility for their failures to others. They are generally able to take appropriate credit for success. In later adolescence, normal youth are able to give up their fantasies of omnipotence and recognize that some hardship is inevitable in life.

Adolescence is the critical period for initiation of drug abuse. Adult onset of drug use is rare. Interference with normal developmental tasks puts young adolescent drug users at greatest risk for serious substance abuse and its medical, cognitive, and emotional sequelae. Youth who are rebellious, place a low value on achievement, are alienated from their parents, are influenced by peers with behavior problems, and live in a chaotic environment without clear discipline are at especially high risk. Experimentation with substances proceeds in a predictable sequence, beginning with tobacco and alcohol and progressing to marijuana. A smaller number of youth move on to abuse sedatives, stimulants, and psychedelics, with even fewer subsequently using cocaine or narcotics.

The high prevalence of adolescent substance abuse seen in the late 1960s and 1970s showed trends of decline until the early 1990s. An average of 35% of high school seniors smoked cigarettes regularly from 1975 to 1990, with approximately 10% of all youth smoking daily. By 1993, 19% of seniors identified themselves as daily cigarette smokers. In 1994, 14.5% of eighth graders, 24% of tenth graders, and 28% of high school seniors endorsed heavy drinking, defined as five drinks during one sitting in the 2 weeks preceding the survey.

Marijuana, the most commonly abused illegal substance, was used daily by 2.4% of high school seniors in 1993, and less regularly by 26% of youths from 1991 to 1993. Although experts generally agree that the use of most forms of cocaine among high school students has declined during the 1990s, the recent increases and resurgences in the use of nicotine, cannabis, stimulants, and heroin are of grave concern. These trends are made meaningful by the recent increase in adolescents who do not believe substance abuse presents as much, if any, threat to their physical and psychiatric health as medical and public health authorities claim (Chatlos, 1996; Johnston et al, 1991, 1994).

Sexuality

Masturbation is normal and (especially in early adolescence) serves a generalized function of reducing anxiety and discharging tension. Teens often experiment with a variety of masturbation fantasies, and transient homosexual fantasies and activities are relatively common.

As noted in the preceding chapter, sexual activity during adolescence is becoming the norm rather than the exception. The 1990 school-based Youth Risk Behavior Survey found that 61% of males and 48% of females in grades 9 through 12 reported ever having had sexual intercourse. Of sexually active students, only 49% of males and 40% of females reported having used a condom during the most recent sexual intercourse (Centers for Disease Control, 1992). Risk factors for early sexual activity include lack of parental support and structure, less religious affiliation, early and frequent dating, and lack of educational ambition (McAnarney and Hendee, 1989). Adolescents who engage in unprotected and/or indiscriminate sexual activity run the risk not only of pregnancy but of AIDS and other sexually transmitted diseases. The United States has the highest rate of teenage pregnancy of any industrialized nation. In the 1980s, nearly one-quarter of all adolescent girls became pregnant by the time they were 18 years old, with about half of the pregnancies resulting in a live birth (Brooks-Gunn and Chase-Lansdale, 1991). The high physical, psychological, and socioeconomic morbidity for both mother and child create a major public health problem.

Although demonstration projects have been successful in decreasing the rate of teenage pregnancy in local areas (Vincent et al, 1987), these proven strategies have not been widely implemented. The relationship with the pediatrician is often ruptured in adolescence, stemming from resistance from both physicians and teens. There is an urgent need for pediatricians and family physicians to become more comfortable with and skilled in providing anticipatory guidance, ongoing counseling, and medical care related to sexuality, birth control, and sexually transmitted diseases.

Adolescence is a particularly painful time for teenagers who are becoming aware that they have a gay or lesbian sexual identity. Adolescent peers are even more homophobic than adults and are more likely to reject, tease, or even become physically aggressive toward schoolmates who are perceived or identified as homosexual. Parents are typically unsupportive and may even reject their child completely, extending the rejection to expulsion from home. Gay and lesbian adolescents are at increased risk for suicidal thoughts and attempts.

Family Relationships

The adolescent should experience gradual independence and autonomy from the nuclear family. There is a normal increase in parent–child arguing around the time of puberty. Young adolescents are increasingly critical of their parents, oppositional, and deliberately provocative. This may represent evolutionarily determined preparation for leaving home. In American culture, however, young adolescents are not emotionally or financially prepared to leave home, although they may be biologically ready.

Social Development of Adolescents

The psychiatrist Harry Stack Sullivan described early adolescent *chumship,* an intense friendship with a youth of the same sex. Adolescents are acutely interested in their peers. The need for absolute peer conformity is more important to younger than to older adolescents. There is a new interest in establishing heterosexual relationships.

Renewed egocentrism leads to the belief that others are similarly obsessed with the teenager's own behavior and appearance, leading to a feeling of being under constant scrutiny. Painful self-consciousness peaks in early adolescence.

THE ROLE OF THE FAMILY IN DEVELOPMENT

Cultural Influences

While family systems theory and therapy are dealt with in detail in Chapter 9 by Drs. Kaslow, Gilman, Aronson, and Wootten and also discussed in the context of overall adult development by Drs. Wolman and Thompson in

Chapter 10, the role of the family is briefly introduced here within a child and adolescent developmental context. Societal expectations of families and their members vary widely in different cultures. Even within the United States, regional and ethnic differences in families can be identified. The changing role of women, the increasing prevalence of divorce, and the growing number of two-career families have significantly changed roles and functions in many American families. However, certain tasks and functions must be carried out in some way by every healthy family or family group.

Family Tasks

Fleck (1966) has identified seven essential tasks for families with children:

1. To form and maintain a *marital coalition* between the adults that meets their emotional needs.
2. To form and maintain a *parental coalition* between the adults who function as parents to assure support and consistency when dealing with the children. In joint custody arrangements following divorce, maintenance of the parental coalition, despite dissolution of the marital coalition, is essential for successful adaptation of the children.
3. To *nurture* the children, physically and emotionally.
4. To create and maintain appropriate *boundaries* between generations and individuals within the family and between the family and the community. Families may have difficulties if the boundaries are too strong and rigid or too weak and permeable.
5. To *enculturate* the younger generation, instilling the values of the family and the culture.
6. To promote *independence* and then emancipation of the children.
7. To deal with *crises*.

Insufficient material or psychological resources, parental psychopathology, and/or severe stressors can interfere with a family's accomplishment of these tasks, resulting in developmental difficulties or even psychopathology in the child.

Parenting Styles

Research in child development has identified patterns of parenting that correlate with, although by no means inevitably lead to, certain outcomes in children (see Table 8–5).

Discipline characteristics that have been associated with aggressive and delinquent children include inconsistency, parental response based on the par-

Table 8–5 **Parenting Styles**

STYLE	CHARACTERISTICS	POSSIBLE OUTCOMES
Authoritarian	Firm rules and edicts No bargaining or discussion with children	Weak conscience Low self-esteem Social withdrawal Unhappiness
Indulgent–permissive	Few controls or restrictions Accept children's demands Unpredictable parental harshness	Low self-reliance Poor impulse control Aggression
Authoritative–reciprocal	Firm rules Shared decision making Discuss children's demands	Social responsibility Self-reliance Self-esteem Low aggression
Indifferent–neglectful	Uninvolved	Aggression Low self-esteem Low self-control Poor parent–child relationship

(Data from Rutter M, Cox A: Other family influences. In Rutter M, Hersov L (eds): Child and Adolescent Psychiatry: Modern Approaches, 2nd ed. Oxford, Blackwell Scientific Publications, 1985)

ent's own mood rather than the child's behavior, expression of dislike for the child, and lack of positive direction (Patterson, 1982).

Stages of Family Development

The First Baby

Parents of an infant must integrate a new, very demanding, and totally dependent person into their lives, which requires major readjustments in their previous relationship. Parenting of infants is accompanied by fatigue and anxiety. Fathers at times may jealously resent the attention given to the baby.

The Toddler

The child at this stage requires close supervision while he or she makes increasing demands for autonomy. Parents must be able to let the child go without pushing him or her away. Parents with a strong need to control may have great difficulty with the 2-year-old.

The Child Aged 3 to 6 Years

As children pass through the Oedipal stage, they may be quite overtly seductive to the parent of the opposite sex. Parents may be flattered and respond in an overstimulating way, particularly if the relationship with the spouse is not emotionally or physically gratifying. The child's wish for an exclusive relationship with the opposite-sex parent may lead to jealousy and marital discord, if not understood and handled sensitively by the parents. Alternatively, parents may become guilty about their own fantasies elicited by the child's attentions, and they may become overly punitive or withdraw from the child. Parents who were sexually abused as children may be especially sensitive to these difficulties. The child may find a divorce particularly difficult at this time.

Sibling Rivalry

During these years, parents may express concerns about the onset of sibling rivalry. For the most part, this form of conflict is extremely common, provides practice in compromise and coexisting with others, and alternates with calmer periods of pleasant interaction. Research shows that, in most households, the peaceful minutes outnumber the conflictual ones, and children acknowledge predominately positive feelings about their sisters and brothers (Newman, 1994).

The School-Age Child

With the beginning of mandatory education, the child is no longer the exclusive possession of the parents. School and peers become increasingly important. Parents may view a teacher's complaints about their child as a criticism of their parenting ability. On the more positive side, parents now have more time and energy for their own interests. Previously isolated parents may benefit from participation in their child's school, church, or recreational activities.

The Adolescent

The family of an adolescent needs to provide more privacy and to tolerate the teenager's increasing autonomy. Parents should permit and encourage the degree of separation and independence that is appropriate for the youth's age and emotional development. They should be able to understand and tolerate frequent shifts between apparent maturity and behavior typical of a much younger child. In many ways, it is reminiscent of parenting a toddler, but with a child who has much wider freedom of movement and is heavily influenced by peers. Parents must be flexible and tread carefully between the dangers of holding too tightly and precipitously letting go.

Parents who find their loss of power and the adolescent's challenges to their authority intolerable may have difficulties with this stage of emancipation. Other parents may compete with their teenager in an effort to avoid recognition of their own aging. The most successful parents minimize power struggles and emphasize important rules and values, while being tolerant of many details of behavior, particularly with respect to clothing and hair styles. A style of collaborative negotiation and problem solving, begun prior to puberty, facilitates discipline and decision making.

Working Parents

As changing societal expectations for women and economic necessity lead to ever-increasing numbers of working mothers, the issue of day care becomes more crucial. Mothers of young infants are the fastest growing segment of the labor market. In 1986, 7.8 million preschool children in the United States had mothers working outside the home (U.S. Bureau of the Census, 1987). By 1989, half of all infants in the United States had mothers who were employed. An estimated 75% of all American mothers with children at home are in the work force (Zigler and Hall, 1988).

The effects of day care are difficult to study because of the inability to form appropriate control groups by randomly assigning children to care by their mother or various forms of day care. Mothers who choose (or are able) to stay home are different in many ways from those who are employed outside of the home. Many families with two working parents compensate for the mother's absence by increased involvement of the father in childrearing and by increased intensity of interaction with the child during the time the mother is in the home. Mothers who work outside the home place greater emphasis on independence training than do full-time homemakers. Families may experience more difficulties when the mother works more than 40 hours per week.

For young children, outcome is related to the amount of time spent in day care and the quality of the day care setting, especially the staff-to-child ratio and stability of caretakers. Other important factors are the mother's feelings about working and about her job, maternal stress, family financial status, parental absence, stability in the home, the quality of the child's attachment, and the child's temperament (Zigler and Hall, 1988). Children are *not* more likely to become primarily attached to the day care provider instead of the parent. There is no evidence of general maladjustment as a result of day care. Individual children vary in their response to day care. Some studies have found children who have been in group day care to be more social, assertive, and aggressive (especially boys). A few children may become more anxious when placed in a group day care setting. There are suggestions that children in out-of-home care prior to the age of 1 year are slightly more likely to show behavior in the laboratory (on the Ainsworth Strange Situation Test) characteristic of insecure attachment to their mothers, and to be more active, oppositional, and noncompliant at age 2. It is important to note that the findings from the Strange Situation Test may indicate greater independence or greater familiarity with unknown caretakers, rather than insecure attachment. Daughters may be more likely than sons to benefit from the greater independence and less stereotyped sex roles fostered by mothers who are employed.

School-age children who are on their own after school and during the summer when their parents work ("latchkey children") may be at risk for higher levels of fear and anxiety, as well as for poorer social skills, juvenile delinquency, and accidents (Zigler and Hall, 1988). The negative effects appear primarily when the child associates with peers during these times and may be more related to variables leading to their self-care status (e.g., poverty, single working parent without a support network) than to the lack of adult supervision *per se*. Children who are immature or impulsive may have more difficulty.

Nontraditional Families

The "typical" nuclear family, including a husband and wife and their biological children, continues to decline in frequency. Only about 60% of children live with both biological parents. The number who will continue to do so throughout childhood and adolescence is even smaller. As noted above, the full-time mother is vanishing. Divorced parents and step-families are discussed in the next section of this chapter. Increasing numbers of children are born to single mothers.

Increasing attention has been paid to the children of gay and lesbian parents (Patterson, 1992). Most of these children were born in the context of a heterosexual relationship between the biological parents. Typically, divorce is associated with one or both parents' acknowledgment of a homosexual orientation, although some of these couples decide not to divorce even after a parent has come out. The gay or lesbian parent (alone or with a same-sex partner) may be custodial or not, or custody may be shared. More recently, children have been reared entirely by a gay or lesbian single parent or couple, following adoption or artificial insemination. Although courts and social agencies have often been hostile to gay men and lesbians who seek parental rights, currently available research has not found any indications that homosexuality *per se* impairs parenting ability. There is no existing evidence that having a homosexual or even a transsexual parent leads to homosexuality, disturbance of gender identity or gender role behavior, or psychopathology in the child. Interestingly, children being raised by lesbians are more likely to have contact with their fathers and with other adult males than are the children of divorced heterosexual women. Younger adolescents have more difficulty learning for the first time of a parent's homosexual orientation than do younger children or older adolescents.

CHILDREN AT RISK

Attempts to understand and prevent pathology in children and adolescents have led to an interest in children who may be vulnerable. The risk or liability of a particular outcome is determined by a complex interaction of *diathesis* (negative genetic factors), environmental stressors, and assets or protective factors.

Divorce

The number of children affected by divorce continues to climb (see Chapter 9). The effects of a divorce differ between boys and girls, and at different developmental stages. The likelihood of a negative outcome is increased by the degree of family conflict preceding and following the divorce as well as by associated stressors such as economic hardship, loss of extended family, need to move from familiar home, neighborhood, and school, or decreased emotional support from an angry or grieving parent. Children commonly blame themselves for the divorce and internalize the experience as their failure to keep the parents together. Most children wish for their parents to be reunited, and many believe they have the responsibility and/or power to bring about a reconciliation. Adolescents are more likely to have difficulty following a divorce if they feel caught between hostile parents (Buchanan et al, 1991).

Most children of divorced parents spend a period of time in a single-parent home, but the frequency of remarriage is high. Marriage of a single parent with children creates what is known as a *reconstituted family.* An estimated one in every six American children under the age of 18 lives with a step-parent. The parents must simultaneously form new marital and parental coalitions while dealing with the behavior and emotional adjustment of children of various ages, who have their own feelings about the divorce and remarriage. Teenagers may be particularly resistant to developing a positive relationship with the step-parent. Children may fear being disloyal to the other parent if they accept a step-parent.

Children of Alcoholic Parents

Children whose parents drink excessively are at increased risk of both emotional and physical abuse as well as neglect. Children of mothers who are "problem drinkers" are at twice the risk of serious physical injury as children of mothers who are nondrinkers. The risk is further increased if the father is also a moderate or heavy drinker (Bijur et al, 1992). A significant minority of children of alcoholic parents have behavioral problems, especially conduct problems, restlessness, inattention, poor academic performance, dropping out of school, and alcohol abuse, as well as emotional symptoms such as anxiety and depression. Probable mediating factors include marital conflict, divorce, disrupted family routine, inadequate parental nurturance and supervision, economic hardship, and modeling of maladaptive coping styles (West and Prinz, 1987). Genetic contributions (especially for conduct disorder in males), as well as the teratological effects of a mother who drinks during pregnancy (see the section in this chapter on prenatal development), may add to the risk. Impairment is by no means inescapable, however, and many of these children and adolescents appear to cope reasonably well. The preservation of family activities is a protective factor. Special self-help groups have evolved for adolescent children of alcoholics (Alateen) as well as for adults (ACOA).

Children of Mentally Ill Parents

Both genetic factors and the effect of mental illness on parenting skills and family environment increase risk. When abuse and neglect are present in a family with a mentally ill parent, the risk of child behavior problems increases. Children whose parents have a mood disorder have an increased (but not inevitable) incidence of depression and suicide as well as nonspecific behavioral and emotional disturbance (LaRoche, 1989). Maternal depression results in impaired mothering skills and marital discord, both related to psychopathology in the children (Gelfand and Teti, 1990). Anxiety disorders are commonly shared by parents and children, probably due to a combination of genetic risk and learned behavior. Children of parents with major depression and/or panic disorder and agoraphobia have an increased frequency of "behavioral inhibition to the unfamiliar" (Rosenbaum et al, 1988), a marker for increased risk of subsequent anxiety disorder (Hirshfeld et al, 1992). Children of schizophrenic parents are more likely to demonstrate abnormalities in attention and information processing and poor social competence, even before emergence of any overt symptoms (Dworkin et al, 1991; Masten and Garmezy, 1985). They are at risk for a variety of psychopathology in addition to schizophrenia and related disorders.

Resilient Children and Adolescents

Graduated stressors or challenges that can be mastered may promote the development of flexible, diverse, and successful coping strategies and positive outcome. Children from high-risk groups who do not appear to suffer negative consequences have been called *resilient* or "invulnerable." There is great interest in elucidating how some children not only resist and cope with unusual stress but thrive and succeed despite adversity. Identified *protective factors* include a cohesive and emotionally supportive family environment, as well as external support systems, such as caring extended family members or other adults, and/or institutional supports. Characteristics of resilient children include intelligence, hardiness, autonomy, positive social orientation, and self-esteem (Masten and Garmezy, 1985). Strong genetic endowment also probably plays a role in the ability of such children to survive and adapt to developmental stress and trauma.

Prevention and Early Intervention

Intervention programs for young children and their parents aim to counteract the effects of prenatal and neonatal insults, compounded by poverty and deprivation, which lead to impaired performance in school and eventually in adult life. The most prominent example is Project Head Start, an ambitious preschool program for disadvantaged children aged 3 to 6, established with federal funding in 1965. While the Head Start program itself has been difficult to evaluate due to political controversy, wide disparity among local programs, and lack of appropriate control groups, long-term follow-up of children enrolled in preschool prevention and intervention projects finds that children show gains in IQ and other cognitive measures during the first year of the program, with cognitively structured curricula producing greater change than play-oriented programs. Some programs also produce improvement in adjustment to school and in social skills. Unless intervention, including parent involvement, continues after the child's entry into regular school, IQ declines to the lower 90s and below, especially in the most deprived children. Programs that focus simultaneously on parent and child, especially those beginning with 1- and 2-year-olds, yield substantial gains in IQ for both the target child and younger sibling, and these gains are maintained at least through the first grade. For the most severely intellectually and economically disadvantaged families, intensive and personalized family support programs that include day care, health care, nutrition, housing, advocacy for the family, and vocational training for parents are required if children are to show or maintain improvement (Bronfenbrenner, 1974; Ryan, 1974). At long-term follow-up, success may be measured in maternal variables (employment, education, smaller family size) and such child measures as school attendance and reduced need for special education (Seitz et al, 1985).

DEVELOPMENTAL CONSIDERATIONS IN MEDICALLY ILL CHILDREN, ADOLESCENTS, AND FAMILIES

Few medical students will ultimately become child and adolescent psychiatrists, but all students will care for physically ill children and their families at some point in their training and many in their practice. A thorough understanding of the developmental principles and risk factors discussed in this chapter is crucial to appreciating the reactions of children and families to the real and perceived threats of acute and chronic illnesses and life-threatening accidents.

Parental Response to Physical Illness or Handicap in a Newborn

The parents of an ill or handicapped infant are faced with the task of mourning the loss of their expected healthy child. The stages are similar to those following a death: anger, denial, and grief (see also Chapters 10 and 14). Parents must resign themselves to the loss of their fantasies of an ideal child and begin to adapt their expectations to the child's realistic potential. Parents (and others) may view an infant's medical problems as a negative reflection on the parents. Parental guilt adds to the burden, especially for genetic diseases or complications that may be attributed (rightly or wrongly) to maternal behavior. The parents' anger, resentment, guilt, and/or denial may interfere with their ability to work with the pediatric team. Parents may find it difficult to relate to an infant with medical problems, especially if the baby's survival is in question.

Realistic additional care-taking and financial burdens may add stress to parents beyond their ability to cope. Parents with unresolved negative feelings, overwhelming stressors, insufficient emotional or material support, and/or inadequate understanding of the medical situation may be unable to comply with medical regimens after they take the baby home. Marriages may break down under the stress of the multiple demands of caring for a physically or mentally handicapped child. The importance of the primary physician in providing ongoing emotional support and assistance in obtaining appropriate services cannot be overemphasized.

Response of Child and Family to Physical Illness in Infancy

When infants less than 6 months old are hospitalized, they are most upset by change in the usual routine. It is helpful to have the parents provide as much of the care as possible and to arrange for consistent nurses. For the older infant who has formed strong, differential attachments, separation is traumatic, especially in the alien hospital environment and when accompanied by physical discomfort and frightening and painful medical procedures. Stranger anxiety adds to the baby's distress. The infant's immature cognitive development exacerbates the problem, because explanations are not understood. The constant presence of a parent is extremely important. In the absence of an attachment figure, the baby's thrashing, refusal to eat, and inability to sleep may have serious medical consequences. Fortunately, most pediatric hospital settings not only permit but encourage parents to room in while their young child is hospitalized.

Response to Illness and Hospitalization During the Toddler Phase

Hospitalized toddlers react primarily to separation from their parents. They may react by rejecting parents when they visit, being aggressive toward parent surrogates (e.g., nurses), regressing in toilet training, and/or refusing to eat. If parents are absent, children may develop depression, sleep disturbance, diarrhea, or vomiting. Fortunately, virtually all hospitals allow and encourage parents to stay with young children. The presence of a transitional object (e.g., a favorite teddy bear or blankie) or other familiar items from home may be helpful.

Children with pre-existing problems in development or in the parent–child relationship have more sustained difficulty, although a child who is weakly attached may show less immediate distress on separation. A child who has been neglected may be indiscriminately eager for adult attention and stimulation.

Toddlers are concerned about the intactness of their bodies, as seen in their great interest in stick-on bandages. Some children believe that body contents can leak out through a cut in the skin.

Response to Physical Illness in Early Childhood

Separation from parents due to hospitalization remains difficult, even for a child who is comfortably able to separate under other circumstances. Anxiety about castration, mutilation, and the belief in immanent justice increase the child's fears. When possible, preparation by simple explanations and a visit to the hospital may help. Regression is common, manifested by such behavior as whining, clinging, and loss of toilet training. Interestingly, even adults may regress and demonstrate similar types of immature childlike behavior under the strain of illness and hospitalization or another major life stress.

Response to Physical Illness in Middle Childhood

School-age children usually tolerate acute illness and hospitalization relatively well, especially if they are prepared, parents visit daily for substantial periods, and preceding development was on course. Children this age may still have irrational explanations of illness. Oppositional or immature behavior is common. Unfortunately, nursing staff have limited tolerance for a child of this age who whines, cries, clings, or refuses to cooperate with medical procedures. Loss of recently acquired skills due to illness or injury is a major blow to the child. Chronic illness interferes increasingly with developmental tasks, especially those related to school and to peer relationships.

Response to Physical Illness in Adolescence

Adolescents are increasingly able to take pride in being responsible for their own body and medical care. When ill or injured, their fears are more realistic than those of younger children. Loss of autonomy and privacy is especially painful for teenagers.

For chronically ill or handicapped adolescents, concern with physical appearance often leads to a view of their bodies, and therefore themselves, as defective. Low self-esteem may decrease adolescents' belief in their own ability to control their fate, resulting in hopelessness, impaired ability to resist peer pressure, and noncompliance with medical regimens.

Both individual adolescents and the peer group are intolerant of differences in appearance or behavior. Adolescents with a handicap or chronic illness may be embarrassed about their condition. Compliance with medical treatment may be avoided, because it exposes the teen as different. Peers may even encourage the violation of restrictions on diet or activities.

Chronically ill adolescents may use a variety of defense mechanisms, including denial, intellectualization, projection, displacement, regression, development of rituals, and identification with the aggressor (sometimes perceived as the physician). It is important to note, however, that psychopathology is not inevitable in chronically ill adolescents.

Possible contributing factors to medical noncompliance include the following: denial or lack of acceptance of the disorder; frustration with the outcome or nature of treatment; lack of knowledge or skills; miscommunication or lack of relationship with medical caregivers; rebellion against parents; inability to resist peer pressure; and psychopathology in the adolescent.

Family Responses to Physical Illness

Physical handicap or chronic or life-threatening illness places significant stress on both parents and siblings. Factors that may hamper a family's ability to function and to comply with medical regimens include an inability to encourage and foster independence as the child matures; unresolved parental guilt, denial, anger, or fear; poor family communication skills; lack of an adequate family and social support system; insufficient financial resources; other stressors on family members; and problems originating in other relationships (e.g., marital discord) being acted out in conflict over the child.

Green and Solnit (1964) have described a *vulnerable child syndrome,* which occurs after a child survives a potentially fatal illness. The family may have completed anticipatory mourning and have difficulty reintegrating the child. Alternatively, the child may subsequently be overprotected and underdisciplined, with resulting immaturity and difficulty with age-appropriate separation and development.

Canam (1993) has identified eight tasks that families must address in their efforts to cope with a member child's chronic illness. These include:

1. Accepting the condition.
2. Managing the condition daily.
3. Meeting the normal developmental needs of the chronically ill child.
4. Meeting the normal developmental needs of other family members.
5. Coping with ongoing stress and acute crises.
6. Helping family members deal with feelings.
7. Educating others about the illness.
8. Establishing a support system.

The emphasis given to any specific task will vary with the age, temperament, and strengths of the child, the nature of the illness, the family form and psychodynamics, and available medical and community support services (Canam, 1993; Clawson, 1996).

SUMMARY

This chapter has been, of necessity, a dense, compressed, and abbreviated summary of the wealth of current theory and knowledge regarding human development from conception through adolescence. An understanding of the major concepts and principles of development stands the physician in good stead, no matter what the ultimate specialty choice. In all spheres, normal development proceeds in certain predictable sequences, although the rate varies considerably among healthy individuals. There is a constant reciprocal interaction between children and adolescents and their environment, with each shaping the other. Developmental outcome is not simple to predict, but is the result of multiple factors within the child, the family, the school, and the larger culture. Developmental considerations beyond adolescence and into early adulthood are discussed in Chapter 10.

ANNOTATED BIBLIOGRAPHY

DeAngelis CD: Ambulatory pediatrics. In Oski FA (ed): Principles and Practice of Pediatrics, 2nd ed. Philadelphia, JB Lippincott Co., 1994

> Thorough yet understandable review of common pediatric concerns in the developmentally normal, generally healthy child and adolescent.

Dulcan MK, Martini DR: Concise Guide to Child and Adolescent Psychiatry. Washington, DC, American Psychiatric Press, 1998

> A compact handbook on the evaluation and treatment of psychopathology in children and adolescents, targeted to students and residents beginning clinical work with children.

Gemelli R: Normal Child and Adolescent Development. Washington, DC, American Psychiatric Press, 1996

> Comprehensive, very accessible textbook for students and residents describing major aspects and leading theories at each stage of development.

Konner M: Childhood. Boston, Little, Brown and Co., 1991

> An easily readable narrative about child and family development in many different cultures, written by an anthropologist with medical training.

Levine MD, Carey WB, Crocker AC (eds): Developmental-Behavioral Pediatrics, 2nd ed. Philadelphia, WB Saunders, 1992

> A comprehensive text directed toward pediatricians. An excellent reference for medical and developmental problems in children.

Lewis M, Vokmar F: Clinical Aspects of Child and Adolescent Development, 3rd ed. Philadelphia, Lea & Febiger, 1990

> The best comprehensive summary of normal development. Written especially for medical students.

Sugar M (ed): Female Adolescent Development, 2nd ed. New York, Brunner/Mazel Publishers, 1993

> Comprehensive overview of biological, psychological, and social development of young females.

Zeahnah CH (ed): Handbook of Infant Mental Health. New York, The Guilford Press, 1993

> A thorough authoritative treatment of all areas of infant mental health, including the family and social contexts, risk and protective factors, assessment, disorders, and interventions.

REFERENCES

Allen DA, Rapin L, Wiznitzer M: Communication disorders of preschool children: The physician's responsibility. Dev Behav Pediatr 9:164–170, 1988

American Psychiatric Association: Diagnostic and Statistical Manual of Mental Disorders, 4th ed. Washington, DC, American Psychiatric Association, 1994

Asher SR: Social competence and peer status: Recent advances and future directions. Child Dev 54:1427–1434, 1983

Bijur PE, Kurzon M, Overpeck MD, et al: Parental alcohol use, problem drinking, and children's injuries. JAMA 267:3166–3171, 1992

Bowlby J: Attachment. In: Attachment and Loss, Vol 2. New York, Basic Books, 1969

Bowlby J: Developmental psychiatry comes of age. Am J Psychiatry 145:1–10, 1988

Bowlby J: Separation: Anxiety and anger. In Attachment and Loss, Vol. 2. New York, Basic Books, 1975

Bregman JD, Hodapp RM: Current developments in the understanding of mental retardation, part I: Biological and phenomenological perspectives. J Am Acad Child Adolesc Psychiatry 30:707–719, 1991

Bronfenbrenner U: A Report on Longitudinal Evaluations of Preschool Programs, Vol. 11: Is Early Intervention Effective? Washington, DC, Office of Human Development, USDHEW, 1974

Brooks-Gunn J, Chase-Lansdale PL: Children having children: Effects on the family system. Pediatr Ann 20:467–481, 1991

Buchanan CM, Maccoby EE, Dornsbusch SM: Caught between parents: Adolescents' experience in divorced homes. Child Dev 62:1008–1029, 1991

Canam C: Common adaptive tasks facing parents of children with chronic conditions. J Adv Nursing 18:46–53, 1993

Centers for Disease Control: Weapon-carrying among high school students. JAMA 266:2342, 1991

Centers for Disease Control: Sexual behavior among high school students. JAMA 267:628, 1992

Chatlos JC: Recent trends and a developmental approach to substance abuse in adolescents. Child Adolescent Psychiatric Clin North Am 5:1–27, 1996

Clawson JA: A child with chronic illness and the process of family adaptation. J Pediatr Nursing 11:52–61, 1996

Coplan J, Gleason JR: Quantifying language development from birth to 3 years using the Early Language Milestone Scale. Pediatrics 86:963–971, 1990

Crowell J, Keener M, Ginsburg N, et al: Sleep habits in toddlers 18 to 36 months old. J Am Acad Child Adolesc Psychiatry 26:510–515, 1987

Dworkin RH, Bernstein G, Kaplansky LM, et al: Social competence and positive and negative symptoms: A longitudinal study of children and adolescents at risk for schizophrenia and affective disorder. Am J Psychiatry 148:1182–1188, 1991

Fagot BI: Beyond the reinforcement principle: Another step toward understanding sex role development. Dev Psychol 21:1097–1104, 1985

Fleck S: An approach to family pathology. Compr Psychiatry 7:307–320, 1966

Gefland DM, Teti DM: The effects of maternal depression on children. Clin Psychol Rev 10:329–353, 1990

Gesell A, Halverson HM, Thompson H: The First Five Years of Life: A Guide to the Study of the Preschool Child. New York, Harper and Row, 1940

Goldberg S: Parent-infant bonding: Another look. Child Dev 54:1355–1382, 1983

Green M, Solnit AJ: Reactions to the threatened loss of a child: A vulnerable child syndrome. Pediatrics 34:58–66, 1964

Harris SL, Delmolino L, Glasberg BA: Psychological and behavioral assessment in mental retardation. Child Adolescent Clin North Am 5:797–808, 1996

Hirshfeld DR, Rosenbaum JF, Biederman J, et al: Stable behavioral inhibition and its association with anxdety disorder. J Am Acad Child Adolesc Psychiatry 31:103–111, 1992

Hodapp RM, Mueller E: Early social development. In Wolman B (ed): Handbook of Developmental Psychology. Englewood Cliffs, NJ, Prentice-Hall, 1982

Johnson CM: Infant and toddler sleep: A telephone survey of parents in one community. Dev Behav Pediatr 12:108–114, 1991

Johnston LD, Bachman JG, O'Malley PM: Reporting on the 1993 results of the 19th annual National Survey of American High School Seniors and their 3rd annual survey of eighth and tenth grades. University of Michigan, News and Information Services, January 31, 1994

Johnston LD, O'Malley PM, Bachman JG: U.S. Department of Health and Human Services: Drug Use Among American High School Seniors, College Students, and Young Adults, 1975–1990, Vol. 1, NIDA, Department of Health and Human Services Publication No. (ADM) 91–1813, 1991

LaRoche C: Children of parents with major affective disorders: A review of the past 5 years. Psychiatric Clin North Am 12:919–933, 1989

Marlow N, Roberts L, Cooke R: Outcome at 8 years for children with birth weights of 1250 g or less. Arch Dis Child 68(3 Spec No):286–290, 1993

Masten AS, Garmezy N: Risk, vulnerability, and protective factors in developmental psychopathology. In Lahey BB, Kazdin AE (eds): Advances in Clinical Child Psychology, Vol. 8. New York, Plenum Press, 1985

McAnarney ER, Hendee WR: Adolescent pregnancy and its consequences. JAMA 262:74–82, 1989

Money J: Sin, sickness, or status: Homosexual gender identity and psychoneuroendocrinology. Am Psychol 42:384–399, 1987

Naeye RL: Cognitive and behavioral abnormalities in children whose mothers smoked cigarettes during pregnancy. J Dev Behav Pediatr 13:425–428, 1992

Newman J: Conflict and friendship in sibling relationships: A review. Child Study J 24:119–152, 1994

Offer D, Ostrov E, Howard KI: The Adolescent: A Psychological Self-Portrait. New York, Basic Books, 1981

Patterson CJ: Children of lesbian and gay parents. Child Dev 63:1025–1042, 1992

Patterson GR: Coercive Family Process. Eugene, OR, Castalia, 1982

Pearl D, Bouthilet L, Lazar J (eds): Television and Behavior: Ten Years of Scientific Progress and Implications for the Eighties. Washington, DC, US Government Printing Office, 1982

Piaget J, Inhelder B: The Psychology of the Child. New York, Basic Books, 1969

Rosenbaum JF, Biederman J, Gersten M, et al: Behavioral inhibition in children of parents with panic disorder and agoraphobia. Arch Gen Psychiatry 45:463–470, 1988

Ryan S: A Report on Longitudinal Evaluations of Preschool Programs, Vol. 1: Longitudinal Evaluations. Washington DC, Office of Human Development, USDHEW, 1974

Seitz V, Rosenbaum LK, Apfel NH: Effects of family support intervention: A ten-year follow-up. Child Dev 56:376–391, 1985

Shapiro T, Hertzig M: Normal child and adolescent development. In Talbott JA, Hales RE, Yudofsky SC (eds): American Psychiatric Press Textbook of Psychiatry. Washington, DC, American Psychiatric Press, 1988

Shapiro T, Perry R: Latency revisited: The age 7 plus or minus 1. Psychoanal Study Child 31:79–105, 1976

Shepherd-Look DL: Sex differentiation and the development of sex roles. In Wolman B (ed): Handbook of Developmental Psychology. Englewood Cliffs, NJ, Prentice-Hall, 1982

Siegel LS: Infant tests as predictors of cognitive and language development at two years. Child Dev 53:545–557, 1981

Singer, DG, Benton W: Caution: Television may be hazardous to a child's mental health. Dev Behav Pediatr 10:259–261, 1989

Spitz RA: Hospitalism: An inquiry into the genesis of psychiatric conditions in early childhood. Psychoanal Study Child 1:53–74, 1945

Spitz RA: Anaclitic depression. Psychoanal Study Child 2:313–342, 1946

Steinhausen HC, Spohr HL: Fetal alcohol syndrome. In Lahey BB, Kazdin AE (eds): Advances in Clinical Child Psychology, Vol. 9. New York, Plenum Press, 1986

Thomas A, Chess S: Temperament in Clinical Practice. New York, Guilford Press, 1986

U.S. Bureau of the Census, Statistical Abstract of the United States: 1987. Washington, DC, US Government Printing Office, 1987

Vincent ML, Clearie AF, Schlüchter MD: Reducing adolescent pregnancy through school and community-based education. JAMA 257:3382–3386, 1987

West MO, Prinz RJ: Parental alcoholism and childhood psychopathology. Psychol Bull 102:204–218, 1987

White E, Elsom B, Prawat R: Children's conceptions of death. Child Dev 49:307–310, 1978

Zigler E, Hall NW: Day care and its effect on children: An overview for pediatric health professionals. Dev Behav Pediatr 9:38–46, 1988

Zimmerman IL, Bernstein M: Parental work patterns in alternative families: Influence on child development. Am J Orthopsychiatry 53:418–425, 1983

9 Medicine and the Family

Nadine J. Kaslow,
Sari Gilman Aronson,
and Jennifer P. Wootten

Luis and Julia, who were of Cuban descent, were still trying to come to terms with their 3-year-old daughter Margarita's recent diagnosis of insulin-dependent diabetes mellitus (IDDM). They had met with the pediatrician, diabetes nurse, and dietician, but refused to talk with the social worker. Julia testily said to Luis, "How can she possibly know how we feel." Julia's parents, who were often critical of their daughter's child-rearing techniques, intimated that poor feeding practices had caused Margarita's problem. Julia and Luis did their best to take care of Margarita, and the healthcare team thought the little girl was doing well. However, on the most recent visit, Margarita told the doctor that she was "a bad girl" and then began to cry. Julia scooped her up into her lap and then looked down. The pediatrician saw Julia's eyes brim with tears when she told him that her mother had scolded Margarita yesterday about eating two cookies. When he asked whether Julia's parents understood Margarita's IDDM, she said curtly that "they have their own ideas about things." She said that Luis could deal with them better than she, as "they listen to him because he's a man." The physician offered to meet with the entire family, and Julia refused. He also suggested that Luis come to the next appointment so that they could discuss how this illness affected family relationships.

An illness[1] not only affects the individual but also impacts profoundly the person's family of origin (e.g., parents, grandparents, siblings) and family of creation (e.g., partner, children). Conversely, a family's beliefs, feelings, and actions affect a family member's view of health and sickness, capacity to cope with medical problems, decision to seek care, and adherence to a medical regimen (Ramsey, 1989). Further, the doctor–patient relationship occurs within the context of the family systems of both doctor and patient. Thus, the doctor, patient, and family dynamics and interactions are inextricably interwoven. Therefore, it is imperative that physicians be interested in the families of their patients. *Family systems medicine, which combines psychiatry and behavioral sciences, primary care medicine, and family therapy, provides a framework for physicians to work collaboratively with patients, their families, and other healthcare professionals.* Such collaboration places the needs of patients and families at the heart of medical care.

A family-oriented approach to medicine focuses on the role of illness in the interpersonal relationships of the family as well as on the personal life of the patient (McDaniel et al, 1992). This approach integrates the biopsychosocial and family systems perspectives with patients, families, healthcare professionals, community groups, and agencies (McDaniel et al, 1992). A family systems medicine perspective focuses on individual and family strengths and coping processes, rather than on medical pathology. The primary goals of medical family therapy are to strengthen the patient and family's sense of control, enhance their capacity to make adaptive choices, and increase their sense of connection with one another and other supportive people. This approach ensures that the family collaborates in the care and decision making regarding their loved one who is ill (McDaniel et al, 1992). A family perspective on health care, which is multidisciplinary in nature, is consistent with the growing emphasis on ecosystemic approaches that unite psyche and soma and consider people in their social environments (Rolland, 1994).

This chapter offers an historical perspective on family systems medicine, followed by a definition of the family, a description of family theory, and a review of family therapies. Subsequent sections cover the physician's role with the family, with attention to levels of physician involvement, countertransference reactions, and consultation or referral for family intervention. *Our goals are to highlight the need to bring the family to the foreground of medical practice and to encourage physicians to engage in collaborative family health care.*

HISTORICAL PERSPECTIVE

Family systems medicine has been influenced most by the biopsychosocial model and family systems theory, both of which emphasize the individual within

[1] For purposes of brevity, the terms *illness* and *medical problem* will refer to both disease and disability.

a social context. Engel's (1977) biopsychosocial model, much of which is based on Adolph Meyer's approach to patient assessment, set the stage with its emphasis on the family as the key aspect of the social component of medical treatment. Family systems approaches, which undergird the practice of family therapy, share two basic assumptions: (1) if the individual is to change, his or her social context must change; and (2) an individual's problems impact all family members, and the family's reaction affects the individual (Kaslow and Celano, 1995).

The first systemic model regarding families with an ill member was the *psychosomatic* view (Minuchin et al, 1975). From the psychosomatic perspective, children with certain medical conditions (e.g., anorexia nervosa, asthma, poorly controlled juvenile insulin-dependent diabetes) reside in families that are *enmeshed* (overinvolved, too much togetherness), *overprotective,* and *rigid* (inflexibility in roles and rules), and either have problems with conflict resolution or are *conflict avoidant.* This model represented for the first time an acknowledgment of the importance of bidirectional influences of illness. Unfortunately, this model implicitly suggested that family dynamics played an etiological role in the development of certain illnesses, and thus was perceived by many as blaming families for the illness. Though not the original intent of this view, the biological aspects of disease were minimized compared to family dynamics on the development and maintenance of the illness.

The past decade has witnessed efforts to integrate the biopsychosocial view with an emphasis on comprehensive assessment and intervention of patient and family. These efforts, broadly referred to as *family systems medicine,* underscore the need for the physician to attend to the ways in which the patient's illness and its sequelae create family stress (e.g., emotional, financial, practical), how a family's history of illness and loss impacts their coping, and how the family's health beliefs influence the illness course and outcome (Rolland, 1994). The mental health application of family systems medicine is *medical family therapy,* the biopsychosocial treatment of individuals and families dealing with illnesses (McDaniel et al, 1992).

WHAT IS FAMILY?

The normative societal expectation of a family is two parents, 2.2 children, and a pet living in a single home. A physician, however, rarely will see such a family, as the nontraditional family unit has almost become the norm. In the United States today, the intact, two-generation family has been joined by single-parent homes, blended families, cohabiting heterosexual or gay couples, multigenerational families, young adults returning home to live with their parents (i.e., boomerang families), foster families, commuter marriages, and group living with or without sexual intimacy. Thus, as can be seen from the example below, a family is a group of people united by marriage, blood, residence sharing, and/or adoption, whose main function is the mutual exchange and nurturance among family members to meet the physical, emotional, and social needs of each individual (Kaslow and Celano, 1995).

> *Samantha and Susan, devoted partners for 12 years, decided to have a child. Since Samantha's job as a self-employed business consultant offered her more flexibility than Susan's job as an attorney, the couple decided that Samantha would carry the child. Their closest male friends, Thomas and Edward, who had been a couple for 10 years, were extremely supportive of this plan, and Thomas agreed to donate his sperm. The pregnancy has gone smoothly, with all four attending the visits to the obstetrician and the ultrasound appointments. The four are in agreement that the baby will live with Samantha and Susan, with Thomas and Edward serving as loving "daddy uncles."*

Epidemiological data reveal that two-income, single-parent, step-families, and childless couples characterize the majority of American families, and the traditional family (father, nonworking mother, and children) accounts for only 8% of American families. Fewer than 30% of adolescents live in a continuously intact family, as divorce rates skyrocketed in the 1980s, with one of every two marriages ending in divorce (Goldenberg and Goldenberg, 1994). The divorce rate has reached a plateau and may be declining (Guyer et al, 1996). Single-parent families, most of which are headed by women, represent more than 20% of families with children (Goldenberg and Goldenberg, 1994). The proportion of children born to unmarried women is high (approximately one of three children); these rates seem to be declining (Guyer et al, 1996). Other recent trends also have influenced the American family: (1) family functions are being shared by schools, businesses, and government agencies; (2) increased life expectancy has resulted in more stress on families for more long-term care of the elderly; and (3) increased isolation of family members from one another, as individuals are more involved in extrafamilial relationships, work, and technology. Further, the following economic changes have altered family structure and process: (1) women are older when they marry and have their first child; (2) the increase in the number of two-income households has led to the need for more negotiation about roles, responsibilities, and commitment to family and community; and (3) the greater emphasis on material goods, decreased time availability, and increased need for expedience has led to greater reliance on modern day conveniences (e.g., fast food, catalogue shopping) and an associated decrease in family time. It has been suggested that all of these changes taken together may be associated with family stress evidenced by poor communication, family violence, and substance abuse. While it is unclear if these family problems actually are more prevalent, they have been seen as signals of significant family fragmentation.

FAMILY THEORY

Table 9–1 provides definitions for the major family theory concepts.

General systems theory, which emerged from the biological sciences, provides the underpinnings for family systems theory. A *system* is a group of elements interacting with one another. The balance between stability and change enables the family to function adaptively. Families seek to maintain homeostasis (stability); change, whether negative or positive, is stressful. For

Table 9–1 **Key Family Theory Concepts**

CONCEPTS	DEFINITIONS
System	Group of elements interacting with one another
Homeostasis	The maintenance of a relatively stable environment
Feedback loops	Circular patterns of response in which there is a return flow of information within the system
Circular causality	Single events are viewed as both cause and effect
Structure	Family organization and the way in which subsystems are arranged
Function	The suitability of behavior for achieving common goals
Hierarchy	Organization of a system based on power and decision-making ability
Wholeness	A key structural property where the whole is greater than the sum of the parts
Subsystems	A person or group of people who are themselves a system, but who also play a specific role in the functioning of the family
Boundaries	Invisible lines drawn within and among family members that form subsystems
Rigid	Boundaries that are inflexible
Diffuse	Boundaries that are highly permeable and that allow for too much flow of communication between subsystems
Closed system	A family system in which all members are expected to share similar views, and self-expression is not valued
Open system	A family system encouraging and supporting honest self-expression by all members
Disengagement	Extreme family type in which each family member is cut off emotionally from one another and each functions without regard for the other
Enmeshment	Extreme family type in which family members are overly involved in one another's lives, and family relationships are undifferentiated, closed, and diffuse
Alignment	The ways in which family members join together or oppose one another in an effort to maintain homeostasis
Triangulation	Detouring conflict between two people by involving a third person, thus stabilizing the relationship of the first two people
Rules	Operating principles for the tasks of daily living
Roles	Expected behaviors of family members
Family life cycle	Family stages that are defined by developmental tasks

example, marriage, while a positive event, is associated with change, leading to stress for each member of the marital dyad and each person's family.

Family systems continuously exchange information via *feedback loops,* circular response patterns characterized by a return flow of information within the system. Family interactions reflect circular causality; single events are both cause and effect (reciprocally related) with no beginning or end to the sequence of events. For example, when one partner behaves passively, the other may become aggressive, triggering increased inhibition, which then leads to further hostility and control.

The following example of a family currently in family therapy is provided to illustrate some of the major tenets of family theory. After the vignette, key points of family theory will be presented using examples from the Broadway family.

The Broadway family, a low-income Caucasian family, had sought family therapy about 2 years after the death of the father at age 42 from a myocardial infarction. Mother, who has relapsing, remitting multiple sclerosis, has tried her best to raise Dennis (age 10) and Dominique (age 17), both of whom have gotten into trouble at school. A family evaluation revealed that Dominique has had primary responsibility for household chores, the raising of Dennis, and caring for her mother whenever her mother is ill. As a result, Dominique does not feel that she needs to mind her mother and resents any efforts that her mother makes to set and enforce rules for either of the children. Dominique also gets into frequent verbal altercations, both with her mother and her mother's on-again-off-again boyfriend, Charles. Family therapy efforts were geared to helping each family member assume more age-appropriate responsibilities. Although initially the family reported improved communication and decreased tension, Dominique could not stand living at home and moved in with her 30-year-old boyfriend, Joe. Joe was adamant that he wanted Dominique to prove her love to him by having as little contact as possible with her mother. The mother was concerned about her daughter's actions, and Dennis felt abandoned by his sister, yet he became upset whenever his mother badmouthed her. The mother felt powerless to get her daughter to alter the situation. A few months later, mother was hospitalized with pneumonia, which responded well to treatment. During her hospital stay, Dennis went to live with Dominique and Joe, both of whom took good care of him. Mother's boyfriend, Charles, had no interest in helping out. When Mother went home, Dominique "disappeared" rather than coming home to help out as she had promised her mother in front of the hospital social worker. As a result, Mother told Dennis to stay home from school for 2 days to take care of her until Grandmother could come. At the first family session after Mother's

*hospitalization, the family therapists encouraged the family to dis-
cuss their feelings and reactions to Mother's medical problems and
any memories her hospitalization elicited about their father's
death. It was clear from their silence that talking about illness and
death was taboo and that expressing one's fears and pain regarding
sickness was unacceptable.*

Families can be conceptualized in terms of *structure* and *function.* Structure refers to the family organization, the way in which the subsystems are arranged and the power *hierarchy* (chain of command). In the Broadway family, the power hierarchy is unclear and under contention, as Mother has difficulty assuming the parental role and often depends on her children for her own caretaking. The key structural property of the family unit is its *wholeness:* that is, the whole is greater than the sum of its parts. The family unit is comprised of interdependent *subsystems* that carry out distinctive functions to maintain themselves and sustain the system as a whole. Each individual is his or her own subsystem. Each family member belongs to several other subsystems, based on generation (parental or sibling subsystems), gender (grandfather–father–son triad), interest (love of sports or the arts), and/or function (caretaking or domestic duties). These subsystems provide the basis for different kinds of relationships between family members. Family systems maintain a power hierarchy, which distinguishes different subsystems from each other, particularly parents and children. The family unit also is a subsystem, as it interacts with the extended family, larger community, and outside world.

Subsystems are delineated by *boundaries,* which protect the subsystem's integrity while allowing interaction among subsystems, the family unit, and the outside world. Boundaries can be more or less permeable and adaptable to the changing needs of the family system. Impaired functioning occurs if boundaries are too *rigid (closed system)*, not allowing adequate communication between subsystems, or too *diffuse,* allowing too much communication between other subsystems. In the Broadway family, boundaries are too diffuse, as evidenced by the lack of clarity in the role of the mother's boyfriend and the adolescent daughter's moving in with her much older boyfriend. In an extreme form, rigid boundaries lead to *disengagement,* where family members are isolated from one another and function autonomously, whereas diffuse boundaries are associated with *enmeshment,* where family members are overly involved in one another's lives. The Broadway family's functioning is indicative of both disengagement and enmeshment. For example, the adolescent daughter's unwillingness to help out once her mother returns home from the hospital is consistent with her being disengaged in certain ways from the family unit, whereas the son's remaining home from school to care for his mother is suggestive of enmeshment. Healthy families are characterized by boundaries that are relatively permeable (*open system*), allowing developmentally appropriate interactions within the family and between family members and the outside world in a manner that supports each person's integrity.

Alignment refers to the ways in which family members join together or oppose one another to maintain familiar family functioning. For example, in the Broadway family, the mother attempts to disrupt the bond between her children by making critical comments about the daughter in front of the son and expecting the son to concur with her negative feelings toward her daughter. Boundaries and alignments depend on power or force. Dysfunctional family alignments require at least three participants. *Triangulation* occurs when two opposing family members each insist that a third member side with him or her against the other. The third person, often a child, is caught in this conflict and often will show signs of stress. There are a number of triangles evident in the Broadway family, such as the daughter being triangled between mother and daughter's boyfriend (Joe), as well as between mother and mother's boyfriend (Charles).

To maintain their structure, family systems have *rules,* operating principles enabling them to perform the tasks of daily living. Some rules are openly negotiated and overt; other rules are unspoken and covert. For example, in the Broadway family, it is understood implicitly that no one in the family can discuss openly their feelings about illness and death. Healthy families have consistent, clearly stated, and fairly enforced rules that can be adapted to the changing developmental needs of the family as well as to the special needs of someone who becomes ill. For example, when a family member is undergoing chemotherapy, his or her expected responsibilities around the house are reduced, and he or she is only expected to do those chores that are realistic.

Each family member plays a number of *roles* (i.e., a predicable set of behaviors associated with their social position) that may include that of spouse, parent, child, sibling, grandparent, breadwinner, caretaker, martyr, scapegoat, and hero. In the Broadway family, the daughter was initially the caretaker, a role then relegated to her younger brother. Role behavior is influenced by family of origin, birth order, gender, and generation. Optimally, roles are negotiated to accommodate the developmental stages and health status of the participants and to eliminate dysfunctional roles (e.g., scapegoat). A preadolescent with a sibling with cerebral palsy may be expected to assume more caretaking responsibilities for himself and his older sister than would typically occur. Parental sensitivity to the preadolescent's desire for more peer contact should lead to decreased caretaking duties.

Analogous to the stages describing the life cycle for individuals, *family life cycle* stages are defined by developmental tasks: (1) leaving home: single young adults; (2) joining of families through marriage: the new couple; (3) families with young children; (4) families with adolescents; (5) launching children and moving on; and (6) families in later life (Carter and McGoldrick, 1989). Difficulties negotiating the tasks associated with a given stage result in increased problems for the family in resolving later family life cycle stages.

Often, family events (e.g., divorce, remarriage, death), individual members' personal choices (e.g., deciding to remain single, selecting a parent without a partner, or to not have children), and cultural background (e.g., immigrant families) increase the complexity of the tasks related to each family life cycle stage or alter the family life cycle. As is the case of the Broadway family, untimely illness or death of a parent when the family is in stage 3, 4, or 5 can exacerbate structure and function problems already existing in the family system.

There are divergent views regarding healthy, midrange, and dysfunctional family dynamics and interactional processes (Walsh, 1993). The various portraits of healthy families indicate that normal family functioning depends on the family's life cycle stage and sociocultural context. Key dimensions of family functioning include cohesion, change, and communication. Optimal families are cohesive, with a clear, yet flexible structure, allowing for both closeness and age-appropriate autonomy. They adapt their power structure, role relationships, and rules in response to situational and developmental demands and new information from the environment. Relatively equal power is the norm for the marital dyad, and a clear power hierarchy exists between the parental subsystem and the children that is modified based on the children's developmental stages. There is ample opportunity to alter standards for behavior control using negotiation and problem solving. All family functions are performed so that members are not overburdened with too many roles, and there is flexibility in the roles played. Communication is clear, effective, and consistent. Even "healthy" or "normal" families can experience enough stress (e.g., prolonged illness or untimely death of a member, trauma) that their coping strategies are insufficient to help them function effectively. At such times, these families may appear dysfunctional, when in actuality their difficulties are almost normative under the circumstances (Rolland, 1994).

FAMILY THERAPIES

Family therapy is designed to help families function more effectively. The family learns to alter its view of reality, develop alternative understandings of the problem, and practice better communication and problem solving. During the past four decades, many family therapy models have been proposed (Kaslow and Celano, 1995). This section reviews two influential models, structural and multigenerational, and then describes an integrative treatment for families dealing with illness.

Structural Family Therapy

The structural model, which serves as the basis for much of the family therapy practiced today (Minuchin, 1974), identifies a number of aspects of structure, communication, and affect expression to explain family organization, coping patterns, and adaptation to developmental changes. This brief therapy typically includes family members who interact daily. The primary goal is the resolution of the presenting problem through the restructuring of family inter-actions. The family is presumed to have the capacity to adopt new patterns, and, therefore, structural therapists look for competence within the family, rather than uncover the roots of dysfunctional behavior.

This approach incorporates *joining, assessing,* and *restructuring.* The therapist joins the family rapidly and as a leader to collect data and understand the problem. The therapist must learn how the family experiences reality in order to discern family rules, myths, and themes. The presenting problem initially is accepted as the real problem, and interventions are designed to re-lieve the symptom and improve family functioning. During the assessment, the therapist evaluates the family structure, boundary quality, capacity for change, subsystem interaction patterns, role of the patient in maintaining family homeo-stasis, context of the presenting problem, and developmental stage of individual members and the family as a whole. Such an assessment gives rise to a family map and conceptualization of the association between structural problems and current symptoms. The restructuring phase reviews the structural difficulties identified. The stance is taken that parents have the power in the family system and are supported by the therapist to use such power wisely. How the family in-teracts both verbally and nonverbally (process), rather than what is said (con-tent), is the key to therapy. A number of techniques are associated with restructuring. Spatial interventions (rearranging seating in a session; removing members temporarily) facilitate change in interpersonal boundaries and alter family members' perspectives. Enactments, in which the family is asked to demonstrate in the session habitual and dysfunctional interactions, provide the therapist opportunities to intervene directly to facilitate structural change. For example, in the Broadway family, the therapist might prolong the mother-daughter disagreement to increase stress, which would force them to interact differently. To change family members' views of the presenting problem, the therapist tries to shift the family from using a simple cause and effect model (Dominique is a bad person and therefore does not help out enough) to one in which family members appreciate the complex origins and effects of family pat-terns on the development and maintenance of a symptom (due to the intense demands for caretaking that had been placed upon Dominique, she did not have enough time to play or to be nurtured by Mother and was pushed into a rela-tionship with Joe, precipitating her move out of her mother's house). Education may be provided in an effort to restructure the family. The therapist may sug-gest homework, which serves to assess the family's openness to change *and* to alter maladaptive family structure and communication. Appropriate homework might include mother's arranging for a home healthcare nurse for herself and then her spending pleasurable time separately with each child doing something that they enjoy.

Multigenerational Family Therapy

Multigenerational therapy, or family of origin therapy, views psychological symptoms as a product of disturbed interpersonal relationships (Bowen, 1988). A person's level of anxiety and ability to maintain an identity separate from one's family of origin (*differentiation*) influence one's relationships. Bowen asserted that chronic anxiety is the primary source of psychological dysfunction, which can be improved through differentiation (Friedman, 1991). Bowen (1988) offered a number of interlocking constructs to elucidate his theory (Friedman, 1991), which are presented in Table 9–2.

Multigenerational family therapy is generally structured and long term with a marital dyad or an individual adult. Greater *differentiation of self* within one's family of origin is the core objective. A second goal is to *detriangulate* three-party systems (*triangles*) by helping the individual to become emotionally disentangled while original two-party tensions are addressed and resolved. Family of origin sessions encourage each person to speak rationally to decrease emotionality. This goal is accomplished by the therapist alternately asking each partner about themselves, their responses to each others' comments, about the presenting problem, and their nuclear and extended family history (gathering multigenerational history). The therapist educates

Table 9–2 **Key Constructs of Multigenerational Family Theory**

CONCEPTS	DEFINITIONS
Differentiation of self	Extent to which one separates emotions and intellect and maintains a sense of self (i.e., people whose intellectual functioning is dominated by feelings and who depend on others are poorly differentiated)
Emotional cutoff	A process whereby a person withdraws or denies the importance of their family (geographic separation)
Family emotional system	Emotionally interdependent people who form a system organized by their individual and collective thoughts, feelings, and relationship history; these systems are formed by people with similar levels of differentiation
Family projection process	Parents project their difficulties onto the child with the lowest level of differentiation (i.e., the most vulnerable child)
Triangles	Triangles are the smallest stable relationship; triangulation is a mechanism by which two people try to stabilize the tensions due to anxiety in their relationship by involving a third party
Multigenerational transmission process	Severe dysfunction is transmitted over generations
Sibling position	Birth order is an important influence on interactional style and role in the family
Societal regression	Chronic anxiety, external pressures, and stresses lower the society's functional differentiation

them about multigenerational theory and encourages visits to the family of origin to work through unresolved attachments and foster increased differentiation. Presenting problems are interpreted in the context of degree of *fusion* (merging of the intellectual and emotional aspects of a person, paralleling the degree to which that person loses the sense of being an individual in relationships) and differentiation. Problems are reframed, needs and desires are clarified, increased reciprocity and cooperation are fostered, and nonfunctional relational system rules are modified.

A major technique to facilitate multigenerational work is the construction of a *genogram,* a visual depiction of a family tree (McGoldrick and Gerson, 1985). Genograms provide information about individual family members, the family's structure, and relationships over generations. Information important in constructing a genogram includes: demographic data; dates of significant life events (e.g., births, deaths, marriages, divorces, diagnosis of illnesses); psychiatric, substance abuse, and medical histories; key personality characteristics; and description of relationships (e.g., disengaged, enmeshed, conflictual), roles, and family functioning. Genograms are useful in engaging the family and suggest hypotheses about behavior, beliefs, and legacies inherent in a family's functioning. They also may be used to help the therapist reframe and detoxify current and past family problems to improve interpersonal interactions and enhance differentiation. As genograms are not driven by a given theoretical approach, they are used by clinicians from diverse theoretical orientations.

Figure 9–1 is a genogram of the Broadway family.

Integrative Model for Families and Illness

A number of models offer a framework for understanding and helping families with ill members (Kazak and Simms, 1996; Wood, 1995), one of the most influential of which is Rolland's (1987, 1994) Family Systems–Illness model. Rolland distinguishes two dimensions key to working with families in the medical setting. The first dimension, *time phases of the illness,* refers to a view of the illness as a process over time (rather than a point in time) with "landmarks, transition points, and changing demands" (Rolland, 1994:54). The three major time phases are crisis, chronic, and terminal. The primary task of the crisis phase, which may begin prior to diagnosis, is for family members to come together to cope with various aspects of the initial and often acute phases of the illness (diagnosis, uncertainty, encounters with healthcare system). The core tasks of the chronic phase are to accept permanent change, grieve over the illness-related changes and impairments, develop new care taking roles, find a balance in meeting family members' needs, and strive to normalize one's life to the degree possible given the adverse conditions. During this phase, families actively and competently care for their loved one. In the terminal phase, which is marked by the patient's impending death, families

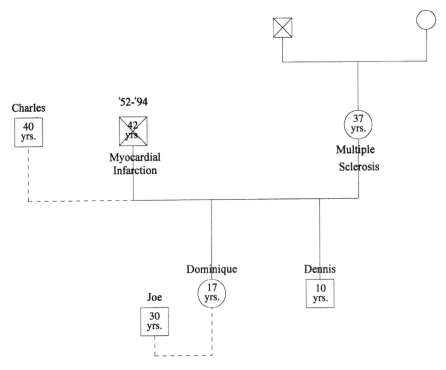

Figure 9–1. *Genogram of the Broadway family.*

must say goodbye, resolve unfinished business, grieve their loss, and facilitate these processes for the dying family member.

The second dimension refers to the *disease classification,* a construct that incorporates the onset, course, outcome, and degree of incapacitation associated with the illness. Onset may be acute (myocardial infarction) or gradual (osteoporosis); course may be progressive (acute leukemia), relapsing (sickle cell disease), or constant (phenylketonuria); outcome may be fatal (pancreatic cancer), associated with a shortened lifespan (insulin-dependent diabetes mellitus) or nonfatal (psoriasis); and degree of disability may be incapacitating (significant spinal cord injury) or nonincapacitating (treated hypothyroidism).

Time phase of the illness and disease classification have different effects on patients and families. Of interest, diseases that differ in terms of their etiology and presentation may have similar psychosocial effects on the family. Interventions are most effective if they are based on the time phase and disease classification and acknowledge the individual and family life cycle stages. The therapist must know about the natural history of the illness in order to help the family predict and cope with transitions and to identify warning signs of need for intervention.

LEVELS OF PHYSICIAN INVOLVEMENT WITH FAMILIES

While all physicians need to develop skills in working with families, the level of involvement depends on the nature of medical practice (specialty, setting), degree of interest in psychological and family matters, level of expertise in working with families, and degree of personal maturation (Doherty and Baird, 1987). One's level of involvement with a family determines the components of medical family therapy (McDaniel et al, 1992) that are incorporated into the doctor–patient–family interactions. A physician may engage with patients' families in a number of different ways, depending on knowledge base, personal development, and clinical skills. This section describes five levels of increasingly sophisticated involvement, each of which builds upon and incorporates the previous set of skills and modes of interaction (Doherty and Baird, 1987).

Minimal Emphasis on Family

Physicians may become involved with families only for practical or medical reasons. In such cases, no value is placed on the role of the family in an individual's care. Reliance on a strict biomedical model leads to a significant percentage of doctor–patient interchanges at this level. Thus, there may be many missed opportunities for improving patient care and compliance and enhancing both patient and physician satisfaction.

Ongoing Medical Information and Advice

Physicians may form an alliance with the family (joining) and use an educational approach. This includes gathering the family's perspective on the history of present illness (i.e., disease-related material) and social history (e.g., financial considerations, transportation), providing the family with ongoing medical information and advice, responding to basic medical questions and concerns posed by the family, and discussing lifestyle issues that impact the illness (e.g., secondary smoke, necessary household dietary adjustments). To function effectively at this level, a stance consistent with a biopsychosocial framework, the physician needs the requisite medical knowledge and an appreciation that the doctor–patient relationship is embedded in a social context. This stage of involvement requires that the physician communicate medical findings and intervention options and elicit relevant information, questions, and concerns from the family. The physician tends to channel most of this communication through one or two key family members.

Feelings and Support

Increasingly, physicians involve families in the care and decision making regarding their loved ones using a psychoeducational approach. They sensitively provide information about the illness and its psychological sequelae, showing more appreciation for the importance of including families in a biopsychosocial approach to care. A physician is more likely to interact with families in this more in-depth manner when there is a comfort with emotions, a willingness to maintain an open stance about the illness and possible biological change, an awareness of normal family development and reactions to stress, and a sensitivity to the feelings and concerns associated with coping with a loved one's illness or with death and dying. At this level, physicians support each family member and the family unit as a whole, facilitate the expression of feelings and concerns related to the patient's physical well-being and its influence on the family system, normalize negative and often unpredictable feelings (e.g., anger, resentment, sadness, guilt, shame, fear), and help the patient and family to accept their painful emotions, foster an awareness of the social factors that may heighten (e.g., intense interpersonal conflict) medical difficulties, and help the family identify those social variables that may diminish strain on the family and alleviate some of the patient's distress (e.g., organize a system to provide ongoing patient care, food, transportation, child care, emotional support). Similarly, delivery of health care in a supportive and collaborative fashion can reduce some of the stress associated with caring for the patient (Hobbs et al, 1985).

To provide medical information, advice, and recommendations, as well as support and empathy in a manner consistent with the style, needs, and level of functioning of the family, the physician must solicit the *illness story* and gather historical data using a genogram. The illness story refers to the patient's and family's perspectives on the experience and meaning of having and living with a disease (Kleinman, 1988). To gather such information, the physician must ask about the: (1) experience of the illness and its evaluation and treatment; (2) beliefs about the etiology, course, and appropriate treatment for the condition; (3) thoughts about how the illness impacts the family with regard to changes in family roles and responsibilities; and (4) plan of action for coping with and managing the illness over time.

It also is useful to construct a genogram (McGoldrick and Gerson, 1985) with attention to the family's multigenerational history with illness, loss, and crisis, family patterns for coping with illness, and the health beliefs of the family. The genogram allows for the identification of illness-related themes in the family history and places the patient's and family's illness in an historical context (McDaniel et al, 1992). Data from the illness story and genogram enable the physician to develop a basic plan for working in a manner that capitalizes on the family's strengths and coping abilities, to empathize with the family's reactions to illness, to accept the varying types and levels of denial manifested in the family, and to normalize the effects of the illness on the family.

Systematic Assessment and Planned Intervention

The most sophisticated level of involvement that physicians not trained as family therapists attain is systematic assessment and planned intervention. Skills required for this level of involvement include the capacity to reflect about one's role in interpersonal relationships and systems (own family, patient's family, larger community), an awareness of common family patterns of response to different illnesses, and attention to the family's sociocultural context and developmental stage (Kaslow and Brown, 1995; Rolland, 1994; Wood, 1995). Effective engagement in systematic assessment and intervention also requires that the physician be able to work with families who communicate poorly (e.g., carry out a family conference in which the members verbalize feelings and concerns in a manner in which they feel supported and not ostracized); reframe the definition of the problem to help the family gain a more realistic and nonblaming view of the illness in order to increase the likelihood that family members will work together to solve the problem(s); and know when a referral to a family therapist is required. Physicians with this level of personal and professional development are able to work with all individuals and families, even the most challenging.

Family Therapy

The most involved patient–family interaction is family therapy, which requires expertise on the part of the physician in family systems theory and practice and effective ways to address interactions between various types of dysfunctional families and healthcare providers. A family therapist is skilled at maintaining perspective; using diplomatic skills to address conflicting and often intensely emotional pressures from family members, healthcare providers, and oneself; and facilitating changes in family structure and function that foster adaptive growth and development of each individual member and the unit as a whole.

Effective medical family therapy is sensitive to developmental, cultural, and gender considerations. Attending to developmental issues includes understanding: (1) the longitudinal course of the illness including its psychological and social sequelae; (2) the reciprocal influences of the illness type and phase, states of individual development, and family life cycle stage; and (3) the need to help the family negotiate both the demands of the illness and the developmental tasks of all family members and the family unit as a whole (McDaniel et al, 1992; Rolland, 1994). To provide culturally informed interventions, the family therapist considers disease parameters, the patient and family's ethnic group and socioeconomic background, and the sociodemographics of the therapist, as ethnicity, race, religion, and socioeconomic status impact family members' and therapists' beliefs and behaviors regarding illness and health (Kaslow and Brown, 1995; McGoldrick et al, 1996). The practice of family systems medicine in a gender-sensitive manner requires that the therapist acknowledge gender considerations as they affect roles, responsibilities, and responses to illness. For families who behave according to stereotypical gender roles and in which one or more family members is dissatisfied with role expectations and demands, the therapist must facilitate renegotiation of family members' roles and responsibilities.

A number of basic principles guide medical family therapy: (1) education—the role and potential value of family therapy is described and therapy is framed as an ongoing process that may be required only during times of crisis management and resolution (e.g., initial diagnosis, relapse, death, family stress not directly related to the illness); (2) empowerment—families are encouraged to communicate honestly with healthcare providers, participate actively in care and decision making, and resume control of their own lives in relation to the illness, while accepting factors that they cannot control; (3) emotional support—the emotional needs of the patient, the family, and all those affected by the patient's illness are attended to, with respect for different styles of coping; (4) use of illness story—the family is helped to achieve a level of acceptance of the illness without blaming anyone; (5) identification and mobilization of social support—the family is encouraged to identify sources of support within their extended family, social network, and larger community (e.g., support groups, church or synagogue, Compassionate Friends), and to participate in multiple-family discussion groups (Gonzalez et al, 1989; Meyerstein, 1992); and (6) future planning—families are supported in developing a future plan, whether that be life with an ill member, living with a loved one whose condition is either deteriorating or unpredictable, or preparing for the future after one's death. Family therapists strive to both support the family's capacity to make good decisions and manage effectively without the help of the therapist *and* underscore their availability for short- or long-term consultation when needed.

COUNTERTRANSFERENCE TO THE FAMILY

The interpersonal relationships among the physician, patient, and family can be challenging when the patient's medical condition or the family situation is inherently difficult or the physician has strong emotions. Emotional responses are even more difficult to untangle when dealing with a family rather than an individual, as the likelihood of conflicting needs and concerns is greater. Impaired doctor–patient–family communication is associated with poor clinical outcomes, patient and family dissatisfaction with medical care, and physician stress. Circumstances that can be associated with a breakdown in communication are discussion of death, do not resuscitate orders, living will issues, family or patient requests for physician-assisted suicide, family-assisted suicide, child abuse, domestic violence, refusal of or noncompliance with medically accepted or life-sustaining treatments, or psychiatric problems (e.g., somatization disorders). When a physician is a family member of a patient, role ambiguities (being both a family member and a doctor) may lead to medical care that is erratic, inappropriate, or confused, in addition to causing stress in all relevant parties, including the treating doctor.

The first thing that a physician needs to do when involved in one of these complex family situations is to step back and identify his or her own emotional reactions (e.g., anger, fear, sadness, helplessness). Second, it is helpful to articulate for oneself the circumstances of the patient's family dynamics eliciting such responses. It is important to be sensitive to precipitating factors arising from the patient, family, treatment team, and medical system, or the physician's personal background (e.g., family of origin dynamics, cultural and religious background, current family life circumstances). The third task is to pay attention to how one's own emotions lead to patterns of behaviors that impact one's interactions with the family and the overall nature of the health care delivered. Typical physician responses to families that warrant attention include: avoiding the patient and family out of discomfort or fear, acting in a controlling manner, trying to placate the family, or inappropriately expressing one's negative (e.g., disgust, disdain, frustration, disinterest) or positive (e.g., engaging in inappropriate sexual behavior) reactions. When such responses occur, it is imperative that the physician recognize and address the personal and interpersonal origins of these reactions. This may require consultation with colleagues, seeking personal therapy, and/or seeking a consultation for the doctor–patient–family–healthcare team system with a skilled medical family therapist. The physician also may find it useful to discuss certain issues directly with the family, but such a discussion should be persued only after careful thought and planning.

SEEKING CONSULTATION AND MAKING REFERRALS

A 40-year-old Caucasian woman, Emma, consulted her internist for fatigue and poor sleep. After a thorough evaluation, the diagnosis of clinical depression was the most likely etiology of her symptoms. Emma wanted only medication for her problems and refused psychotherapy for her depression. Despite her insistence that she was "really trying," the patient stopped taking 3 medications in 3 months. Feeling puzzled, Dr. Shen asked more questions about Emma's personal life. Hesitantly, she acknowledged that her husband, Brad, was suspicious and critical of the treatment. In pursuing this further, Emma revealed Brad and she were having frequent disagreements about the etiology and treatment of her symptoms. He called her a "fat, lazy cow" and said that she was just feeling sorry for herself. She was afraid that if she contradicted him, he might hurt her.

As indicated throughout this chapter, there are specific areas encountered when dealing with families that are usually beyond the scope of the primary care physician, as in the case with Emma and Brad. Once these issues have been identified by the physician, a referral for family therapy can be made. When the following factors are revealed in the course of obtaining the psychosocial history, or if such factors emerge during the course of a person's medical treatment, the physician should consider a referral for family intervention (Doherty and Baird, 1987): (1) psychopathology in a family member (e.g., significant alcohol or drug problems, psychiatric and personality disorders, acute emotional reactions) that interferes with the care of the patient; (2) longstanding family dysfunction (e.g., communication and/or problem-solving difficulties, significant family conflict) that impedes the family's capacity to respond flexibly to the patient's illness; and (3) emotional, physical, and/or sexual abuse by one family member toward another (e.g., parent–child, spousal), which also requires a referral to the appropriate authorities as mandated by state law.

Once a family is identified as needing further help, there are various steps to take to ensure an effective referral. First, make the referral as easy as possible for the family. This involves offering to make the appointment for the family before they leave the office or giving them the requisite telephone numbers and addresses. Appropriate releases of information that enable the referring physician to communicate with the family therapist should be obtained. In addition, it is useful if the primary care physician can provide the family with some education about the purpose and value of therapy, as well as offer reasonable expectations about family therapy. Further, it is essential to convey to the family that therapy is an important part of medical care. The physician must reassure the family of his or her intentions to provide ongoing medical treatment and to remain interested in the family's emotional well-being. Some families may feel that they are being "dumped," and thus it is crucial to communicate the importance of family-oriented medical care. All of these steps are accomplished most effectively when the primary care physician has a positive attitude about family therapy. Taken together, these steps should facilitate the process of making a successful referral and increase the family's ability to cope effectively with the patient's condition. However, despite a physician's careful planning and hard work, families may refuse much needed family treatment. In these difficult circumstances, physicians must determine if such refusal interferes significantly with the medical care of the patient. If so, the physician may need to meet with the patient and family, reiterate the necessity of family therapy for the optimal medical care of the patient, and try to understand with the family the nature of their reluctance. In some situations, it may be possible and desirable to invite a medical family therapist to conduct such a meeting with the physician, patient, family, and other key individuals present.

CONCLUDING COMMENTS

Given the recent empirical support for the efficacy of family interventions in treating physical illness, there is an increasingly important role for medical family therapy in the evolving healthcare delivery system (Campbell and Patterson, 1995). A family systems approach to health care has as its primary goal the management of acute and chronic illness, health promotion, and disease prevention within a family systems framework (Saba et al, 1996). The possibility of offering medical care using such an approach is most likely when an effective and mutually beneficial family/patient and physician/team alliance is formed. Such a relationship entails the development of trust, effective communication, and clearly defined and comfortable roles for all participants. As a consequence, all members of the family unit and the healthcare team can work together in a collaborative fashion with the goal of health promotion and effective disease management.

A comprehensive understanding of the patient and family requires that the physician be attuned to sociocultural factors (e.g., culture, class and economic status, gender, race/ethnicity, politics, and spiritual beliefs), inter- and intrapersonal variables that affect issues of health and illness (e.g., lifecycle, family roles and rules, family structure), and health and illness beliefs and behaviors (Saba et al, 1996). For the physician to collaborate with the patient and family, the physician's own continual professional development (e.g., role as a physician, personal growth) must be focal. In addition, awareness of the healthcare delivery setting (e.g., level of managed care penetration, hospital versus outpatient clinic, training versus nontraining facility) and the collegial relationships that inform one's learning and delivery of care (Saba et al, 1996) will allow the physician to be a more effective member of the healthcare team, which leads to improved patient and family care. The awareness on the part of the physician of multiple influences on the patient, family, healthcare team members, and physician him or herself enables the physician to form a strong and trusting relationship with the patient and family. Such a relationship provides the context within which optimal health care can occur.

ANNOTATED BIBLIOGRAPHY

Gurman AS, Kniskern DP (eds): Handbook of Family Therapy, Vols. 1 and 2. New York, Brunner/Mazel, 1991

> This is a two-volume comprehensive text that addresses all the major theories of family therapy. The approaches are presented in an established format that allows for comparison and integration.

McDaniel SH, Hepworth J, Doherty WJ: Medical Family Therapy. New York, Basic Books, 1992

> This book utilizes the biopsychosocial approach to dealing with families with health problems. It offers techniques and guidance for the general practitioner, as well as the family therapist, through numerous case examples.

Ramsey CN (ed): Family Systems Medicine. New York, Guilford Press, 1989

> This book provides a closer look at the science of family medicine, as well as its influences. The book then goes on to examine in a more detailed way the family impact on the process of medical care.

Roberts MC, Wallander JL (eds): Family Issues in Pediatric Psychology. Hillsdale, NJ, Lawrence Erlbaum Associates, 1992

> This book looks at family issues pertinent to individual illnesses as well as in terms of the more general adaptation necessary in dealing with chronically ill children.

Rolland JS: Families, Illness, and Disability: An Integrative Treatment Model. New York, Basic Books, 1994

> This book is a useful guide when dealing with families. It offers many practical techniques and interventions that aid the clinician in working with families under stress. The author shows that the variables of the course, outcome, onset, and degree of incapacity influence the stress on the families.

REFERENCES

Bowen M: Family Therapy in Clinical Practice. Northvale, Jason Aronson, 1988

Campbell TL, Patterson JM: The effectiveness of family interventions in the treatment of physical illness. J Marital Fam Ther 21:545–583, 1995

Carter B, McGoldrick M (eds): The Changing Family Life Cycle: A Framework for Family Therapy. Boston, Allyn and Bacon, 1989

Doherty WJ, Baird M (eds): Family-Centered Medical Care: A Clinical Casebook. New York, Guilford Press, 1987

Engel GL: The need for new medical model: A challenge for biomedicine. Science 196:129–136, 1977

Friedman EH: Bowen theory and therapy. In Gurman AS, Kniskern DP (eds): Handbook of Family Therapy, Vol. 2. New York, Brunner/Mazel, 1991

Goldenberg H, Goldenberg I: Counseling Today's Families. Pacific Grove, CA, Brooks/Cole, 1994

Gonzalez S, Steinglass P, Reiss D: Putting the illness in its place: Discussion groups for families with chronic medical illnesses. Fam Process 28:69–87, 1989

Guyer B, Strobino D, Ventura S, et al: Annual summary of vital statistics—1995. Pediatrics 98:1007–1019, 1996

Hobbs N, Perrin JM, Ireys HT: Chronically Ill Children and Their Families: Problems, Prospects, and Proposals for the Vanderbilt Study. San Francisco, Jossey-Bass, 1985

Kaslow NJ, Brown F: Culturally sensitive family interventions for chronically ill youth: Sickle cell disease as an example. Fam Syst Med 13:201–213, 1995

Kaslow NJ, Celano MP: The family therapies. In Gurman AS, Messer SB (eds): Essential Psychotherapies: Theory and Practice. New York, Guilford Press, 1995

Kazak AE, Simms S: Children with life threatening illnesses: Psychological difficulties in interpersonal relationships. In Kaslow FW (ed): Handbook of Relational Diagnosis and Dysfunctional Family Patterns. New York, John Wiley and Sons Inc., 1996

Kleinman A: The Illness Narratives: Suffering, Healing, and the Human Condition. New York: Basic Books, 1988

McDaniel SH, Hepworth J, Doherty WJ: Medical Family Therapy: A Biopsychosocial Approach to Families with Health Problems. New York, Basic Books, 1992

McGoldrick M, Gerson R: Genograms in Family Assessment. New York, W.W. Norton, 1985

McGoldrick M, Giordano J, Pearce JK (eds): Ethnicity and Family Therapy. New York, Guilford Press, 1996

Meyerstein I: Creating a network of volunteer resources in a psychoeducational family asthma program. Fam Syst Med 10:99–110, 1992

Minuchin S: Families and Family Therapy. Cambridge, Harvard University Press, 1974

Minuchin S, Baker L, Rosman BL, et al: A conceptual model of psychosomatic illness in children: Family organization and family therapy. Arch Gen Psychiatry 32:1031–1038, 1975

Minuchin S, Rosman B, Baker L: Psychosomatic Families: Anorexia Nervosa in Context. Cambridge, Harvard University Press, 1978

Rolland JS: Families, Illness, and Disability: An Integrative Treatment Model. New York, Guilford Press, 1994

Rolland JS: Chronic illness and the life cycle: a conceptual framework. Family Process 26: 203–221, 1987

Saba GW, Shore WB, Sommers PS, et al: Teaching a systems approach to family practice residents: The "2-on-2" curriculum. Fam Syst Health 14:151–165, 1996

Walsh F (ed): Normal Family Processes. New York, Guilford Press, 1993

Wood BL: A developmental biopsychosocial approach to the treatment of chronic illness in children and adolescents. In Mikesell RH, Lusterman DD, McDaniel SH (eds): Integrating Family Therapy: Handbook of Family Psychology and Systems Theory. Washington, DC, American Psychological Association, 1995

10 *Adult and Later-Life Development*

Thomas Wolman and
Troy L. Thompson II

In the recent past, adulthood was seen not as potentially a new beginning but as an endpoint to development; however, a healthy lifecycle is, in large part, synonymous with growth and development, and someone who has ceased growing has, in a sense, stopped living optimally. Therefore, one may define mental health as the capacity to adapt to the various developmental tasks that a person encounters over the lifespan. Adult development has been one of the most understudied areas of human behavior and, therefore, receives special attention in this text.

The purpose of this chapter is to discuss the adult lifecycle in a manner that is relevant and practical to physicians in the practice of medicine. The events of the adult lifecycle are related to health and illness, with particular focus on the vulnerable transition points (e.g., choices about marriage, parenthood) where problems are more likely to occur. Bereavement, dying, and death are also discussed in the context of the adult lifecycle. If an individual is not able to successfully negotiate, or becomes "stuck" or chronically symptomatic (anxious, depressed, phobic, etc.) at any of these phases, he or she should be referred for psychiatric evaluation, and probably receive psychotherapy and possibly a psychotropic medication (at least for the short term).

THE LIFECYCLE

Personal development is the unique path that each person takes through that sequence of milestones called the lifecycle. The lifecycle is a universal template whose features appear to remain generally constant for all people, cultures, and eras. Stages of infancy, childhood, adolescence, courtship, adulthood, marriage, parenting, and old age are universal. All have phase-specific developmental challenges and opportunities. Traditionally, knowledge about the usual lifecycle patterns has resided in the folk wisdom of each culture. Great literature of all eras, from the Bible to Shakespeare to modern authors, has reflected this knowledge.

In recent times, people have often looked to physicians for advice about problems encountered in lifecycle phases. Until recently, however, physicians were hampered in their patient education and counseling in these areas due to spotty and unsystematized research and knowledge of the specific biological, psychological, and social complexities of each developmental phase. At the turn of the century, even childhood was unknown territory as far as systematic and scientifically based knowledge of development was concerned. Freud (1958) and his followers began the exploration of childhood stages of psychological development, and interest in this area has greatly expanded. In the 1960s, researchers like Mahler (1975) produced the first detailed glimpse into the first 2 years of life. (See Chapter 8 by Drs. Dell and Dulcan and Chapter 5 by Drs. Inderbitzen, Furman, and James). Adolescence also became the subject of much interest, thanks to the pioneering work of psychoanalytic clinicians and researchers such as Anna Freud. Nevertheless, Erik Erikson (1963) in his "eight ages of man" paradigm (which is discussed later in this chapter) was the first to view the total lifecycle as a continuum (Table 10–1).

Table 10–1 **Erikson's Psychological Stages of the Lifecycle**

	USUAL AGE RANGE	**FUNDAMENTAL ISSUES**	**ROUGH EQUIVALENT**	**STRENGTHS BASED ON FAVORABLE OUTCOME RATIOS**
Stage 1	0–18 mo	Basic trust vs mistrust	Infancy	Drive and hope
Stage 2	18 mo– 3½ yr	Autonomy vs shame and doubt	Toddler stage	Self-control and will power
Stage 3	3½ yr–5 yr	Initiative vs guilt	Oedipal stage	Direction and purpose
Stage 4	5 yr–12 yr	Industry vs inferiority	Latency	Method and competence
Stage 5	12 yr–20 yr	Identity vs role confusion	Adolescence	Devotion and fidelity
Stage 6	20 yr–35 yr	Intimacy vs isolation	Young adulthood	Affiliation and love
Stage 7	35 yr–65 yr	Generativity vs stagnation	Maturity	Production and care
Stage 8	65 yr and up	Ego integrity vs despair	Old age	Reconciliation and sense of integrity

(Adapted from Erikson EH: Childhood and Society. New York, WW Norton, 1963)

As was mentioned earlier, study of the lifecycle has been skewed toward the early years, mostly encapsulated by infancy on one hand and adolescence on the other. In part, this is a legacy of Freud's hypothesis that the personality is largely "fixed" by the age of 6. Yet recent autobiographical studies of Freud himself (Anzieu, 1986) underscore the importance of his own midlife crisis in setting him on a course toward the discovery of psychoanalysis. This "distortion toward the young" has been partly overcome by recent studies of aging and adult development (Colarusso and Nemiroff, 1981; Gould, 1972; Levinson et al, 1978; Vaillant, 1977). More research, however, is needed in many developmental areas and processes. For example, differences between males and females, heterosexuals and homosexuals, socioeconomic groups, and many other groups would be important information to use in patient care.

NEW DEVELOPMENTAL CONCEPTS

The Triad of Stage, Transition, and Normative Crisis

Life change may unfold through a typical sequence of preparation (a transitional period), rapid change (such as may occur with a normal developmental step or normative crisis), consolidation (the achievement of a new life stage), and "plateauing." Such a formula helps to organize an approach to the lifecycle, provided it is not taken too literally. For example, adolescence (or any other period) may be viewed in part as a *normative crisis,* as a *transition,* and as a *stage.* One of the important discoveries of recent years is that healthy psychological change and development may proceed on different paths and at variable rates (Table 10–2).

Stages

From Erikson onward, most research on the human lifecycle divides the developmental continuum into discrete *stages.* Each stage is characterized by its own specific tasks, conflicts, and viewpoints. Some stages, such as those of childhood, maturity, and old age, are universal; others, such as those of the age 30 and age 40 transition, are more culturally dependent. Stages indicate periods of relative developmental stability in which considerable time is spent on age-specific tasks; these are periods of *consolidation of skills* rather than of rapid change.

Transitions

A more specialized period of transition is needed to bridge the wide gulf between the demands of successive stages (Levinson et al, 1978). People require time to get used to new demands, challenges, and outlooks. At the same time, they need the time to consider what to relish and what to relinquish from earlier periods. Most people make a transition of a different type every

Table 10–2 **Psychological Developmental Concepts**

CONCEPT	BRIEF DEFINITION	EXAMPLES
Transition	Bridge or junction between successive stages	Late adolescence Courtship Midlife transition
"Limbo state"	A "sticking" point in development, usually at the transition between two stages	Pseudo-adulthood (prolonged adolescence) Prolonged courtship
Rite of passage	Social ritual that facilitates a transition	Graduation Marriage Funerals
Normative crisis	Period of rapid change and/or turmoil that strains person's adaptive capacity	Childbirth Midlife crisis Marital crisis
"Normal illness"	Hybrid state with features of both an illness and a normative crisis	Pregnancy Maternal preoccupation Bereavement
Stage	Period of consolidation of skills and capacities	Early adulthood Mature adulthood
Plateau	Period of developmental stability	Adulthood up to midlife
Developmental lines	Independent course of development of a particular skill or capacity	Love Work Play
Delay/precocity	Variations in the timing of developmental lines	Precocious adulthood "Late bloomer"
Regression	Temporary retrograde vector in development	Revival of adolescence or childhood attitudes and behaviors in midlife
Repetition	Reworking and reliving all or part of previous stage(s)	The second separation–individuation crisis of young adulthood/late adolescence

evening as they prepare themselves for sleep. Reverie and hypnagogic imagery are transitional states between conscious thinking and sleeping and dreaming.

Transitional states are like vehicles that carry the person from one stage to another. Rites of passage (or rituals), such as cadaver dissection and dog laboratories for medical students and internship for house staff officers, perform the same function in a social context (Van Gennep, 1960). They help to concretize the change, give it a sort of external scaffolding and make it feel more real to the participants. In addition, transitional states act to allay the anxiety of the person and of the group, for whom change always represents some degree of threat.

The Normative Crisis

The rate of change may vary considerably throughout life. Almost everyone is familiar with the experience of overwhelming changes that strain their capacity to adapt. One can define a normative crisis as any period in the lifecycle whose chief characteristic is *turmoil.* This turmoil can result from external factors, such as illness or misfortune, or it can result from internal conflicts between opposing alternatives: self versus others, freedom versus bondage, and living versus dying. In many "crises," childbirth, for example, external and internal factors coexist.

The Normative Crisis in Health and Illness

In our culture, individuals sometimes tend to define a normative crisis as a symptom of an illness. In the past, physicians have contributed to this trend, most notably in their attitudes toward pregnancy. An important task of today's physicians is in helping their patients reinterpret what is normative versus what is truly pathological. At times, this may mean revision of some physicians' attitudes toward developmental blocks, obstacles, plateaus, doldrums, and even reversals.

It may even be a good exercise to try to reinterpret the "obviously" pathological as if it were a normative crisis. Doing so serves to place the illness inside the more manageable framework of the lifecycle, thus allowing greater adaptation and assimilation of what seems alien. For example, symptoms of anxiety in young adults may be interpreted in the context of some expected difficulties in leaving the parental home. Promiscuity in a middle-aged man may be a sign of the midlife crisis. Some mild depression in parents would be considered normal after their children's departure for college (the so-called empty nest syndrome).

On the other hand, the physician also needs to be knowledgeable about particularly vulnerable points in the lifecycle, those points that can more easily trigger actual illness. The transitional periods are particularly important in this regard. Adolescence frequently has been associated with the onset of schizophrenia and the midlife period with severe depression. Transitions can sometimes become prolonged into "limbo states," where people languish indefinitely, postponing the process of further growth.

Lines

Development is not a unilateral process. It is less like a single, uniform mass and more like an army advancing along a broad front in a series of uneven "columns" or "lines." Each developmental line (love, work, play) acts like an independent unit and proceeds at its own pace (Freud, 1963). Consequently, any line(s) may be considerably out of phase with others. The same person can be advancing rapidly in some areas, retreating in others, and remaining stationary in still others.

Timing

This implies that development proceeds according to a person's own timetable. There is a certain fixed order to the stages and general age ranges for each, but these must not be interpreted too literally. There is an innate rhythm to each person's development that, unless extreme, should usually not be hurried or imposed upon by external factors. Each new stage is a challenge and a potential obstacle. It is best to reject fixed notions of the course of development as largely illusory. *Normal development is not synonymous with uniform forward progress, nor does it reach a peak at some predetermined point, followed by a rapid downhill course or shift toward another stage.*

There is considerable variation in rate of normal development. *Delay* and *precocity* (precocious behavior) are typical examples. Normative bias may prompt one to ask what is wrong in all cases of delay, but, in many cases, delay is simply a function of the unique rhythm of that person's growth curve. Folk wisdom recognizes this in the expression "late bloomer." For example, some people have a desire to "settle down" and have children in their 20s; others may not have this focus until their 30s, and still others may not resolve the issue about whether to have children until their 40s. This may be more of an issue for some women since the "biological clock" and menopause limit how long they can delay becoming pregnant.

Similarly, there is a tendency to view precocity as superiority, yet cases are known in which precocity is followed by later failure. Precocity may mean that a particular stage or line of development has been shortchanged and needs to be reworked at a future time. The child who functions with adult maturity may be masking childhood needs that will resurface in some form at a later date.

Regression

During development, the person may appear to take "two steps forward and then one step backward" (i.e., regress in some area). *Regression refers to the revival of earlier and more childlike behavior and coping strategies in response to stress.* It is an expected feature of most normative crises and transitions. For example, most people are familiar with the child who begins to act more like a baby after the arrival of a new sibling; yet they sometimes forget that parents tend to regress under the same circumstances. The father, for example, may be secretly nursing a jealous grudge against the new baby for monopolizing his wife's attention, as he also may have done *vis-à-vis* his own mother when one of his younger siblings was born. The mother herself may also have increased dependency needs to be cared for and nurtured as she nurtures her own baby.

Behavioral regression often occurs in adults if they develop a severe or chronic illness. Accepting their mortality and adapting to feeling like "damaged goods" may lead to grief and mourning of their previous image of themselves as "invulnerable" and "immortal."

Repetition
People tend to underestimate the extent to which repetition is built into the lifecycle. Also, periodic "lulls and plateaus" may be as intrinsic to the life-cycle as rapid spurts of development, but to the person caught in one of these doldrums, the reality is that "he or she is not getting anywhere." Only careful assessment can determine whether the complaint indicates a normal degree of pause or if it represents a "sticking point" requiring mental health intervention.

One adaptive aspect of repetition is the opportunity it affords to rework tasks and conflicts of earlier eras, particularly those of separation–individuation. In optimal cases, this amounts to a second chance at development through greater mastery of previously highly conflicted issues. Psychotherapy attempts to facilitate this "second chance." Because it is stressful to talk about and thereby partially reexperience and focus upon conflicted issues, psychotherapy generally is also associated with some transient regression.

During transitional periods, people, in a sense, look backward as well as forward, in a kind of Janus, or double-faced, posture. *Transitions reflect the developmental need to reassess, rethink, reexperience, and rework the past* while planning for the future. Only in retrospect can one generally see the positive aspects of a lull or get a new perspective on a period of rapid life change that seemed to be a blur at the time. Perhaps this is why adult stages of development have been relatively neglected until recently. Most of those doing scholarly research on the lifecycle are immersed themselves in a middle age, lifestage plateau, and it is generally much more difficult to look carefully and critically at one's self than at others.

Erikson's Eight Ages of Man

Erik Erikson's model of human development (Erikson, 1963) laid the foundation for later lifecycle studies. Erikson divided the lifecycle into eight discrete, well-defined stages. Each stage is characterized by a specific task, usually a fundamental one that affects multiple life sectors. His "eight ages of man" (see Table 10–1) shows an underlying order in the lifecycle in a simple format, and its simplicity makes it a valuable tool for organizing life experience. For example, the first stage, *basic trust*, applies to all human relationships, self-confidence, and even religious faith. The pairing of each task fulfillment with its potential failure, or problems remaining within it, circumscribes a range of possible outcomes.

Each stage is a link in the chain of life. This has been called the *epigenetic* approach (i.e., the initiation and success of a new stage is partly dependent on the degree of successful negotiation of previous stages). The image of the chain emphasizes the continuity of life. *Failure* is defined as development of a weak link or a break in the chain. Consequently, it implies that childhood lays the foundation for adulthood; however, success with basic mastery of childhood stages carries proportionately more weight in determining the probability of later successful development. Also, failure or major problems early on tend to be less reversible and to cause broader-ranging difficulties than problems that develop later in life.

The merits of Erikson's approach also determine its limitations. It is a sketch of development, not a detailed blueprint. His divisions are too broad to do total justice to the subtleties of an individual's life. They also may be too uniform to suggest the markedly different paths, lines of development, and rates of change that frequently occur in people's lives. The adult stages also seem relatively meager in number and in substance. Occupation, for example, is not mentioned at all. Many of these "deficiencies" can be mitigated by viewing the adult stages as *midpoints* of the multiple other stages of development. By taking into account all related stages, each adult stage appears more comprehensive. Each adult stage also takes on added significance when it is viewed in the light of the quest for an individual's personal identity.

Identity and the Lifecycle

Erikson (1959) saw the lifecycle as a lifelong quest to achieve a coherent *personal identity.* By identity, he meant an inner sense of "sameness" or developing continuity of a "solid core sense of your goals and values" in the midst of change. Erikson was the first to affirm the importance of a sense of identity for success and happiness as a human being. A stable sense of identity is both a prerequisite for and an outcome of successful development, but even with a strong foundation in the early years, the sense of a stable personal identity can never be taken for granted. It is always a precarious achievement, liable to be upset or even overturned by the vicissitudes of change, such as a personal illness or external circumstances. Every normative crisis threatens to disrupt the ongoing sense of identity. The successful negotiation of adult stages requires extensive psychological reworking, adaptation, and integration. Everyone is periodically challenged to rework, revise, and reorient former ideas of whom he or she was, is, and wants to become; those who are able to do so as needed and to adapt accordingly have the highest degree of mental health and happiness. (The development of personal identity in the context of overall family development is also discussed by Drs. Kaslow, Aronson, and Wootten in Chapter 9.)

The childhood stages contribute to people's first sketch of their own identity and sense of self. *Basic trust* gives children the conviction that they belong in this world and have a right to exist in their own right. It forms the fundamental basis of how one responds to others and expects others to respond. The stage of *autonomy* works in the other direction by helping the child learn that it is acceptable at times to say "no" to others' wishes and demands, and that, in part, *people define themselves by what they oppose, as well as by what they value and support.* The stage of *initiative* fixes the first blueprint of identity through the activities with which each person selects to be involved and often relates to the parental ideals. *Industry* helps to consolidate and expand the new sense of self by learning that hard work tends to pay off and that identification with a peer group is important, both by being supportive and pleasurable.

The transition to young adulthood (Erikson's stage of *identity consolidation versus role diffusion*) poses the first major challenge to identity for some people. The range and intensity of life changes during young adulthood may peak and severely strain the established psychological structure. Also, the biological vulnerability to onset of schizophrenia appears to peak in late adolescence and the early 20s. Therefore, during this time, a person becomes more vulnerable to more severe breakdowns in identity, including the extreme of psychosis. But given some measure of success in the early stages, the person may be able to tolerate or postpone aspects of the chaos of multiple changes long enough for reintegrative psychological forces to "catch up." Erikson calls the postponement of adult commitments to allow more time to rethink and gradually address changes a *moratorium.*

Early adulthood initiates the process of forging a new adult identity from the fragments of adolescent flux. Accomplishing this goal often amounts to a major reorientation, a revolution, if you will, in the self-concept. The new structure must reconcile the competing claims of dependency, craving for autonomy, sexuality, and body image changes. Old attachments must be relinquished or preserved with modifications. New commitments have to be entered into, at first tentatively, and later definitively, in the stage of intimacy.

The stage of *generativity* ushers in a further modification and expansion of adult identity. The life space widens to include the next generation; there is an identification with the parental role in the broadest sense. Individuals redefine their own contributions as a "passing of the torch" to their potential heirs. The need for bold self-assertion usually lessens. Occasionally, this new orientation is incorporated into a "mission" or life's work that results in an increased focus and enhanced productivity, optimally produced from a playful creativity and a renewed partnership with others. In the full sense, generativity connotes a confluence of love, work, play, and identity.

The completion of one's identity is the task of late life. Erikson labeled this the stage of *ego integrity versus despair.* Integrity implies a feeling of self-worth associated with a final self-reconciliation. Seeing one's life as a whole highlights a person's achievements as well as disappointments and failures. Integrity is based on an awareness of the limits of any human life. It is often hard to face these limits and to let go of one's omnipotence once and for all, but this final work of "delimitation" can also bring about a sense of underlying meaning, order, and uniqueness to the person's life. A process of reworking issues associated with each earlier stage occurs during each life stage in the context of the demands, opportunities, and limitations of the new stage, including the ultimate limitation of death (see Table 10–2).

THE STAGES OF ADULTHOOD

The Transition to Adulthood

After the initial period of adolescent flux, young people initiate their first tentative movement toward adulthood (Table 10–3). The transitional identity of student or apprentice teaches them the background skills, without committing them to full responsibility (Levinson and Goodeneh, 1985; Levinson et al, 1978). In this guise, they can allow themselves the freedom to be experimental, to try out various roles. Such playful exploration is normative for a transitional stage and does not necessarily imply a lack of ability to focus or persevere.

The tasks of young adults are consistent with their transitional role of "novice" or learner. Several of these tasks merit consideration:

1. The relationship to the parents must undergo substantial modification. The old childhood dependence on the parents must be given up and replaced by a more mature partnership with them. One is not free to make strong future attachments while old ones are still totally in place. Moreover, one cannot feel truly independent while holding on to the idea that a parental figure will always be there to help put things right. Such magical expectations undermine the motivation to accept personal responsibility and to develop adult initiative.

2. The identity of "student" or "novice" serves as a helpful transition to mature mutuality (i.e., two adults interacting as each other's equals). The relationship of mentor to pupil includes some of the old parent-child dependent qualities. Some of the issues can be seen in the personal and professional development of medical students. Medical students understandably often complain of their passive position in the learning process: the long lectures, the hours of memorizing, the examinations; in short, their relative lack of control. On the other hand, the professor or mentor hopefully helps to model a more active and independent stance. Students may be progressively more encouraged to take their own positions and ask their own questions, as in small group discussions, to develop their own approaches to situations, to design their own projects, and to be responsible for their own learning.

3. Identification with the mentor both fuels and modifies young people's idealism. In this context, they elaborate this identification into dreams for their future and later into more articulated adult aspirations (Levinson et al, 1978). Idealism helps to bridge the gap between childhood fantasies and adult hopes and aspirations. Early childhood fantasies are modified and, in

Table 10–3 **Some Postinfancy Aspects of Psychological Stages in the Lifecycle**

STAGE	TRANSITIONAL ISSUES	RITE OF PASSAGE	SYMPTOMS OF CRISIS	PATHOLOGICAL OUTCOME
Transitions before adulthood	Novice, student, apprentice	School matriculation	School or work phobia	Agoraphobia
Consolidation of adulthood	New title	Graduation	Repeated career changes	"Pseudo-adult"
Courtship	Experimentation	Dating, "trial marriage"	Premature or delayed commitment	Schizoid character, precocious adult
Transition to marriage	"Contract" with spouse	Marriage ceremony	Boredom or constant warfare	Separation or divorce
Pregnancy	Physical changes, "new space"	Baby "shower," childbirth education classes	Hypochondriasis, detachment	Denial or pseudocyesis
Childbirth	Pregnancy	Labor and delivery	Excessive anxiety: prepartum and during labor	Postpartum depression
Parenting	Primary maternal pre-occupation, "holding"	Naming ceremony	Marital unrest, developmental delay in child	Parental deprivation or overstimulation of child
Midlife transition	Mourning, loss of youth	"40th birthday," midlife crisis	Withdrawal, sudden life change	Depression, substance abuse
Transition to old age	Repository of cultural values	Retirement, illness, death of spouse and friends	Regression, "King Lear" complex	Depression, pseudo-dementia

part, incorporated into the new adult identity. Continuity is thus maintained between past and future. Keeping this in mind guards against the tendency of some adults to discourage or dismiss youthful idealism merely because it is unrealistic or rebellious in tone.

4. Studenthood is more specifically the transition to an occupation. It is a time of intense preparatory learning, during which students are protected from the full weight of responsibility for their performance. They can "try out" the work under supervision and in progressively larger doses. Normally, there is an atmosphere of tolerance of student's needs to experiment with different styles, techniques, and roles, regardless of the inconsistencies these shifts may appear to entail. Possibly more disruptive, but still under the rubric of experimentation, is the tendency to go from one job to another, or one passionate interest to another.

5. The same bent for experimentation often rules the attempts to establish intimate relationships. There may be a prolonged period of "playing the field" or a series of "trial relationships." It must be borne in mind that success and happiness in relationships requires a period of learning as well. The peer group, as well as knowledge and fantasies about what the parents' early relationship was like, may provide the equivalence of mentorship in this area. Notions about the ideal mate must be tested against reality. Views about sexuality and love must be explored in the "laboratory" of a real relationship.

"Sticking Points" and Failures in Early Adult Development

Problems in early adulthood are often associated with delay in initiating adult tasks, and by far the most frequent cause for these delays is the failure to relinquish and separate from the parents. Such failures are often brought to the attention of the physician in the form of anxiety or depressive symptoms. Virtually all college students in their first year away from home are grappling to some degree with separation–individuation issues. This process recapitulates many aspects of separation–individuation discussed in Chapters 5 and 8 that are part of early childhood development. For example, a student's "school phobia" may screen a more profound yearning for the parental home and grief and mourning over losing the daily contact and support from parents, siblings, and home. The physician often can be helpful in bringing out the underlying depression and grief and in helping students adjust to their separation from home. Sometimes a period of regression is necessary, during which the student may move back home for a while; frequent, but brief, trips back and forth from school to home also can be recommended to permit emotional "refueling," to decrease the strain of abrupt separation, and to allow more time for the individuation process to progress.

The young person who fails entirely to leave home may present physicians with a somewhat more difficult problem. Such persons also may have failed to initiate dating or job seeking. Their school phobia may have worsened into agoraphobia. Paradoxically, an escalation of their symptoms may also signal the alarm they increasingly feel in being isolated and removed from the mainstream of others their age. Often, it is the parents who bring these young people to medical attention out of concern that the symptom is exacerbating and perpetuating the young person's dependency, which, of course, it is designed to do. The literal fact of living at home is less important than the inner emotional attachment to the parents. An occasional young person can be living in the parental home past the age of 30 and still possess a clear sense of personal independence. In contrast, others may live thousands of miles away, yet be very tied to their parents and locked in unresolved, conflicted relationships with them. In the latter case, geographic distance becomes an attempted substitute for the emotional distance that cannot be achieved by other means.

The "Pseudo-Adult"

At times, the attachment to the parents and to the world of childhood in general leads to a kind of temporal dissociation, instead of to delay. Such persons feel that they can "have their cake and eat it, too." They may fabricate an adult "false self," while still maintaining their true internal identity as a child who never grows up. This condition has been dubbed the Peter Pan syndrome (Kiley, 1983) from the popular childhood story of a mythical boy who never wanted to grow up. In terms of the lifecycle, the pseudo-adult is stuck in a limbo, a "never, neverland," if you will, between childhood and adulthood. This syndrome often first becomes apparent in individuals in their 30s.

A CASE STUDY

Mr. N., a charming and moderately successful artist in his mid-30s presented to a psychiatrist with symptoms of dissatisfaction with his marriage. Although talented, he had a formidable psychological block against advancing his career. His Peter Pan identity allowed him to work well under conditions of play, but he rebelled when it came to keeping a regular work schedule and to attending to the bookkeeping and business aspects of his work. He loved to think up new ideas but hated the work necessary to implement them. The same basic problem plagued him in his marriage. He could not stand the idea of having to work and compromise with his spouse to resolve the inevitable conflicts associated with a long-term, intimate relationship. In effect, he was going through the motions of being an adult without putting his heart and soul into it. He found that he could easily fool others with his act; many mar-

veled at his "togetherness." This reinforced his secret wish to have it both ways: success in the adult world without ever having to grow up.

Precocious Adulthood

For some, the problem is not one of attachment but rather of precocious autonomy and independence. As children, these persons typically detached themselves from dependence on their parents at a relatively young age. In some instances, they may have resorted to "self-parenting" as a result of parental deprivation, including having parents who were not able to play joyfully with the child to teach the child the pleasure of relationships and that fun and playing are not just for kids. Others may have had workaholic parents and felt deprived of a parent's loving and playful attention. In other cases, they may have been allocated the role of "parental child" and been delegated the task of taking care of younger siblings, grandparents, or others. Regardless of etiology, their precocity would seem to obviate any need for a transition to adulthood. They are already there. What is missing is their childhood "roots." They are often perceived by others as highly competent and responsible, but at the same time, as stilted and as lifeless as robots. Their resemblance to automatons is based on an early identification with an ideal of total self-reliance and a lack of ability to be relaxed and playful.

Some of these individuals exhibit a pressured and almost manic pursuit of their goals and ideals, to the exclusion of any reflection or self-awareness. So immersed are they in life's materialistic externals that their inner life is stillborn; they never developed an appreciation of relaxation and playfulness as a catalytic aspect of being creatively alive. They often become adult workaholics who perpetuate this pattern by treating their own children as they were treated when they themselves were small. This flight into constant activity may carry them along for a surprising length of time, but they are at risk of a traumatic midlife crisis, including ultimate alienation from their children and friends, and an old age filled with loneliness, regret, and despair.

Others with this type of precocity develop a schizoid indifference to interpersonal life. One such patient presented at the age of 34 with the chief complaint of never having been physical or emotionally intimate with a single person, man or woman. In a way, he was bothered more by what other people thought about this than by personal distress, yet he had some degree of awareness that an important sector of life that is meaningful and enjoyable for many others was passing him by.

The Consolidation of Adulthood

In favorable circumstances, young adults reach a point when they can say, "Now I am a man (or woman)" (Blos, 1967). This stage of consolidation of adult personal and occupational identity usually occurs around the age of 30

(Vaillant, 1977) and may be associated with the so-called age 30 crisis (Gould, 1972). It may have gradually evolved out of a variety of components, or it may have "crystallized" with some degree of abruptness. In some cases, the crisis does not come without some measure of inner struggle over the new "fixity" of adulthood, its associated commitments, and the loss of other options.

Recently, the term "consolidation" has become almost synonymous with the consolidation of occupational or professional identity; this is due, in part, to the central role that work plays in modern life (Simons, 1985). Increasingly, some have come to see work not as something they *do,* but as something they *are.* For many, it has become more of "a calling" than "a job." Conversely, people whose work is "only a job" may feel a need to find their "real life's work." People who are failures at their work are sometimes considered failures in life. Accordingly, work has become a kind of microcosm of life. In addition to income, some look to work to provide them with their sense of status, self-esteem, productivity, creative outlet, as well as social life, friendly collaborations, and even their "subculture" (the corporate or professional culture). Many workaholic physicians fall into this category. Recent realities of the work place, such as "rightsizing," require reserves of flexibility and adaptiveness in the new tasks of retraining, relinquishing old ties, and entry into new work environments. Retirement, especially if forced, may be a major stress for such individuals. If a person is not able to disengage from his or her work without a major, ongoing loss of self-esteem, it may be wiser to slow down gradually or shift to volunteer or other activities.

The rite of passage into true adulthood sometimes involves a type of graduation or certification *ritual.* This confers upon students a new title or name, which formalizes their new identity as well as cancels their old student identity. While important in this regard, graduation also has become more of a public recognition of a *fait accompli.* It is intended to give official, public recognition to what has already been accomplished, sometimes largely in private.

Medical students may provide an example in this regard. If one asks medical students at the beginning of their second or third year how they prefer to be addressed, the majority will answer, as a medical student, "Mr., Ms.," and so forth. If one asks them the same question again in the fourth year, many will say, "Student Doctor" and some will say, "Doctor." At some point in the fourth year, the student will start "living up" to that title. They will start thinking and acting much more like a physician than like an earlier-year medical student. And the moment these students start making their own patient care decisions, the less they will need others to tell them what to do, and they will begin to view others more as consultants. Their newfound feelings of basic competence as a physician may produce a sense of euphoria and power. At this time, they can begin to expand their sense of their work to include a sense of playfulness and relaxation at appropriate times, and a sense of mastery.

A CASE STUDY

Dr. G. a young resident physician, presented to a psychiatrist with complaints of extreme anxiety over the performance of medical procedures. Lately, he had started to ask consultants to do this type of work for him. He felt so ashamed over this state of affairs that he actively considered abandoning his medical career. After a period of psychotherapeutic work, Dr. G. related this fear to the image of a punishing father. His father had often been quite critical of and detached from him, while his mother had been more understanding and supportive. He vividly recalled making rounds with his father, who was a veterinarian, and witnessing procedures, often castration, performed in a cold, detached manner on numerous farm animals. In effect, he had integrated the "maternal" aspects of being a doctor, but not the "paternal," as those were represented in his family. He was a responsible physician who cared for his patients and worked hard on their behalf; however, his inability to integrate the degree of "intrusiveness and aggressiveness" that is needed to complete some medical tasks into his image of himself was holding up his adult consolidation as a comprehensive physician. The resolution of his "age 30 crisis" involved some rapprochement between aspects of both parents.

The Triad of Courtship, Marriage, and Marital Crisis

Courtship

Courtship is part of the transition to a committed partnership, often signified by marriage, in the same sense that student status is part of the transition to an adult occupation. In the former, the focus is "pair identity," while in the latter, it may relate to joining an organizational or professional "family" (sometimes referred to as a "brotherhood" or "union"). Temporally, the stages of early adulthood and courtship usually parallel each other, and issues of intimacy occupy both. In courtship, its achievement is defined as the formation of a couple.

In American culture, dating functions as a rite of passage into the courtship stage. Recent concerns about AIDS and other sexually transmitted diseases have fostered new customs, such as group dating, in some cases. The function of dating is to bring the young person into contact with the pool of possible marital partners. Complaining of the artificiality of the rituals involved, young adults sometimes express the wish to bypass this process. Nevertheless, some artificiality is a facet of all rituals and must be borne to some degree. The absence of dating in an adult's life history is virtually always significant. It may signal a delay in the courtship phase, or it may indicate that those stages were skipped, as in premature marriage.

In recent decades, it has become more common to have the stereotypical "honeymoon" precede the marriage. "Trial marriage" or "living together" has become an accepted part of courtship in most Western industrial societies. Optimally, living together might function as a laboratory for the exploration of what the realities of marriage would be for the couple. In practice, however, this does not always occur. When the "honeymoon" precedes the marriage, there is sometimes lack of recognition or postponement of consideration of the more contractual aspects of couplehood until after marriage.

Courtship in American society sometimes progresses into a kind of "limbo" that does not lead to the transition to marriage. For some couples, courtship may then become a prolonged honeymoon or an indefinite extension of dating. Other couples choose to live together like roommates, out of convenience or friendship, and to keep their romantic liaisons outside the relationship. A tendency to progressively split the romantic from the contractual aspects of the relationship may continue into or develop into marriage, and sometimes results in stress and possibly divorce despite years of preparatory living together.

Marriage

Naturally, the psychological formation of a "couple" does not always coincide with the marriage ceremony. Some couples form a solid partnership well in advance of their marriage; other couples do not crystallize until some time after their marriage; still others are effectively "divorced" before they are married. Nevertheless, most couples go through some type of postcourtship transition to the married state.

Marriage takes for granted a certain degree of personal maturity in both partners. Ideally, each of them should be capable of seeing the other as a whole, separate person with his or her own life and viewpoints. Each must be able to tolerate the good and the bad in the other, as reflected in the phrase "for better or for worse" that is frequently used in marital vows. Each must be able to empathize with (and not be overly threatened or annoyed by) the other's positions, even when they conflict with his or her own. In short, the partners ideally will have acquired a sense of their own identity and self-worth as separate persons and the capacity to appreciate the same characteristics in others.

Some couples start married life before the partners have consolidated their own adult identities. They may unconsciously decide to continue some model of infantile or adolescent dependence on each other. This kind of symbiosis can be mutually reinforcing in a way that may prevent an evolution of the relationship to more mature levels. Other couples feel so threatened by the new level of intimacy of their married state that their precarious coalition is vulnerable to decompose into two warring individuals.

Both the symbiotic couple and the "warring couple" lack clear boundaries between the partners. In the symbiotic couple, the partners function as "auxiliaries" for undeveloped aspects of each other. The warring couples are so threatened by defusion of boundaries that they must resort to opposition to reinforce and clarify those boundaries. The more exaggerated the differences in their positions, the easier it is to see and to grasp their separate identities. The partners in the latter type of couple may have too much privacy, just as in the symbiotic type, the partners may not have enough to facilitate further growth. Neither type possesses the basis for a mature partnership between equals.

The marriage ceremony is a rite of passage to transform two separate people into a new couple. The device that unites the pair is a simple contract in that *marriage is a formal arrangement imposed on the couple by society.* The contractual features are evident in *legal* trappings: an official representative of society (e.g., priest, rabbi, judge), the exchange of explicit vows, the presence of witnesses, and the finality of a signed document.

An especially thorny issue may be the question of the household division of labor. Traditionally, this matter was decided along the lines of stereotypical sexual roles. Now the couple must first decide where they stand on the sex role continuum before task allocation *per se.* Some successful marriages opt for a complete reversal of traditional sex roles, while others stay with the more traditional arrangement; still others occupy a middle ground.

At some point in the process of working out these issues, the partners may recognize a renewed sense of mutuality based on working together as equals. They may see that working together validates their separateness at the same time that it draws them closer together. The partnership is now the property of the couple and no longer something imposed by society. The framework of the contract helped them to discover a new mode of creative collaboration in which their different perspectives may play off each other with creative and novel results. Several of these may be an enriched sexual experience, a readiness for new ventures, and a vital miniculture of shared history and values.

Marital Crisis

It is quite common for physicians to encounter patients whose hidden or overt agenda is a marital crisis or a failing marriage. The patient may want the physician's permission to exit a moribund marriage. He or she may want the spouse to be "treated"—in other words, "brought into line." It may be the spouse who wants the patient "treated." The clue to the underlying situation is often revealed when, inevitably, the spouse is drawn into the discussions. If physicians fail to see the hidden agenda, they may unwittingly develop with the patient an unfruitful alliance that supports a bad marriage. (Family systems theory, family therapy techniques, and the physician's role in the referral process are also discussed in Chapter 9.)

We have discussed several ways in which the transition to the married state may result in turmoil for the couple; the forces of individuation may threaten to tear apart a fragile alliance. A crisis may occur whenever new conditions place excessive strain on the old arrangements, so a crisis most likely will occur during a transitional period, such as childbirth, parenting, and the "empty nest syndrome." A crisis is more likely if the development of the marriage is out of synchrony with that of the partners. Many marriages have lasted 7 to 10 years before one or both of the partners has reached maturity as adults and has become established in occupations or professions. When individuals go beyond their spouse's sphere of understanding and experience, they may begin to feel bored and constrained within an outmoded arrangement. For example, occupational success can throw the previous "contract" out of kilter.

A crisis may be preceded by a prodromal period during which signs of trouble are ignored. The increasing turmoil may make itself felt as tension and fighting or the reverse: excessive calm, boredom, and withdrawal. Sometimes a full-blown crisis is necessary as a "wake-up call" that something is wrong. When the problem is recognized, the partners may be able to spell out their dissatisfactions to each other and begin a process of reformulation of their marriage contract.

Such a reconciliation process, however, is often complicated by the tendency toward regression that marks any crisis. In the context of the couple, this usually means a return to "nonpair" ways of relating. The prototypic example is a reversion to mutual blaming. In the first round of many marital squabbles, each partner wants to blame the other for the problem. Instead of viewing the problem in pair terms, he or she sees it primarily as the other person's responsibility. Frequently, there follows an escalation of blaming during which the pair revives many of their past conflicts and shortcomings.

Couples who already have an established pattern of fighting may be especially vulnerable at this point. Such a couple is usually unable to resolve a major crisis without professional help because they have great difficulty recovering their "pair perspective." Spouse abuse is an ominous sign of such a deteriorating situation in "fighting" couples. If they can recover their couple perspective, they face the task of reassessing and then restructuring their marriage. They may have to renegotiate the old agreements from scratch. At best, they will have to substantially modify past agreements.

Although marital crises often occur at fairly specific points in the adult lifecycle, such as after childbirth, at midlife, and during the "empty nest" phase, it would be erroneous to view the developmental line of most marriages as a long period of stagnation due to latent conflict followed by an explosive climax. There is a unique evolution of every latent conflict, but in a healthy marriage, there is usually a dynamic sequence of growth, plateauing, stagnation, reassessment, and new growth. The time frame for some of these phases may be years, months, or occasionally, just weeks.

The Role of Counseling and Psychotherapy

Even a normative crisis may carry significant risks. For example, the high rate of divorce (about half of all marriages) reflects the inherent instability associated with marital crises as much as it does the pathological aspects of a marriage and the changing mores of society. Thus, it is quite natural and wise for an individual or a couple to look for outside professional help when they see no other way out of their difficulties. When the couple can no longer mediate effectively between themselves, society can provide them with an outside mediator. The external mediator is, in a sense, a new version of society's official representative who married them in the first place. This role can be filled by any person in authority: a religious leader, physician (ultimately, often a psychiatrist), other mental health counselor, or even lawyers and a divorce court judge.

If the couple has never really learned how to negotiate, the psychiatrist or other psychotherapist may begin teaching them this art. One entire style of marriage therapy, aptly called "contract therapy," does just this (Sholevar, 1981); however, with most couples, it is more a question of restarting a stalled negotiation. The first step may be a search for a new area of compromise. Each partner may need help in articulating his or her position, or in refraining from attack and counterattack. Most of all, they need encouragement to keep talking. In acting as a mediator, the psychotherapist must be careful to remain neutral. The partners will usually try to draw him or her to their side as an ally, or to do their talking for them. (This phenomenon is also known as "triangulation" and is discussed in Chapter 9.) The psychotherapist gently deflects all such invitations away from himself or herself and back into discussion between the partners. Similarly, the psychotherapist discourages them from using other people, including children and relative in-laws, for the same purpose. The psychotherapist thus tries to stabilize the couple's coalition by decreasing use of outside coalitions that may undermine it.

Alternatives to Traditional Marriage and Parenting

The previous section discussed the fact that collaborative partnerships are not an invariable outcome of marriage. Many marriages endure despite the absence of any true alliance, and many viable partnerships develop outside the confines of traditional marriages into stable, long-term relationships. Also, nonmarital types of collaborative partnerships in our society include working partnerships, the psychotherapeutic alliance between therapist and patient, and community and religious networks.

Hence, there is some justification for the reverse assumption that the establishment of a collaborative partnership produces a "marriage." Increasingly, our society has come to recognize a relationship as "binding" when there is public evidence of the existence of a partnership. This broader definition might include common-law marriages and homosexual marriages. In this context, "marriage" is a metaphor for any dedicated, supraindividual relationship; however, the "other party" to this relationship is not necessarily limited to one special person. Emotionally, a person may feel "married" to a collection of persons, a group/organization, a life's work, a political cause, or even God, as exemplified in some religious rituals and communities.

Parenting may sometimes also supply the reason for existence for such a "marriage." In examining the wide variations in parenting at all levels of society, many family studies have demonstrated the importance of collaboration for family development. They have defined collaboration according to three criteria: (1) a division of parental function between the role of a "mother"- and a "father"-type figure; (2) some degree of recognition and representation of differences in the parental roles; and (3) a barrier against cross-generational alliances, and of incest, in particular (Sholevar, 1981). (See also Chapter 9.)

According to these criteria, many situations that were previously considered exceptions to the traditional model of parenting may prove quite capable of raising healthy families. Many successful families make effective use of surrogate parents, and in single-parent families, the role of surrogate may be played by grandparents, uncles, aunts, or friends. Other families distribute the roles of mother and father among several people; this method is present in the Israeli kibbutz and is typical of extended families and of postdivorce merged families. In homosexual parenting arrangements, the parental roles are divided between persons of the same sex. Such arrangements may be successful, and usually there will be some differentiation between the roles of the two parents. A third method uses the institutions of day care, professional babysitters, and neighborhood networks to provide "auxiliary parents." It is common for single-parent families to call on all three methods at various times and settings; this is reflected in the saying, "It takes a village to raise a child." Even in so-called "matriarchal" families, the place of the "missing" parent is often occupied by a symbolic figure, such as a socially positive influence (e.g., the local minister, principal, benevolent TV parental figure) or, unfortunately at times, an antisocial figure (e.g., neighborhood criminal, drug dealer).

It is this view of marriage (i.e., the formation of a collaborative partnership), and this point cannot be emphasized too strongly, that constitutes the true developmental task; however, there are some persons for whom traditional marriage is contraindicated for a variety of reasons. For instance, the prototypic unmarried professional person may find deep satisfaction in dedication to (and partially feel "married" to) career, patients, clients, students, etc., and thereby arrive via a different path to "generativity" and a healthy validation of his or her self-worth.

Childlessness

The "ticking of the biological clock" is more than just a clicheé. For many women it is a major crisis that influences their decisions about work and marriage. It is not unusual for single women in their late 30s (or older) to feel a sense of panic over childbearing issues. They may seek out a man who will agree to have children and use this as a major criterion for marrying him. They may consider becoming a single parent through artificial insemination, adoption, or other means. Other women may wrestle with a sense of guilt or question their female identity if they decide they do not want children.

Some couples consciously decide not to have children, and there are a multitude of reasons for such a decision. As long as the decision is mutual, the couple may work out a deeply satisfying relationship in which other activities occupy the time and energy commitment that children would have filled.

Problems may arise, however, when one partner wants a child or when both wish to become parents, but the couple is infertile. Both situations may lead to tremendous discord and possible divorce. The second situation may represent a growing problem in the United States. As many as 20% of couples who wish to conceive cannot do so, and women who have waited to have children sometimes find they are infertile, sometimes possibly due to age-associated physiological changes or complications from venereal diseases. Couples who cannot conceive may spend enormous time and money at infertility clinics and may subsequently turn to adoption. Many couples who want children do not succeed in having them, and the divorce rate is quite high in these couples.

The Triad of Pregnancy, Childbirth, and Parenting

Pregnancy

Nature usually offers expectant parents a 9-month "grace period" before the travails of childbirth and parenting begin. Pregnancy gives the couple time to make room for a new person in their lives and to realign their relationship and duties accordingly. Conception has the secondary meaning of a "new idea," the idea of a child and new family member. Conception brings the idea of a child to life in the minds of the parents. The child becomes a subject of fantasy in both mother and father. The specific content of the fantasy will indicate to some degree the hopes, wishes, and fears concerning the new arrival.

The gradual physical changes in the mother-to-be give another support to the creation of a new "space" in the family. At first, they are the only evidence of the "reality" of the child. Most mothers cannot ignore what is happening to their own body, but the father is, of course, somewhat more removed from that process. He can avoid a tendency toward denial by actively discussing with the mother what she is feeling and by feeling the abdominal area for signs of fetal movement (quickening).

Bodily changes also direct the mother's attention inward to a growing identification with the living child inside her (Bibring et al, 1961; Winnicott, 1965). It is normal for her to become relatively more preoccupied with herself during pregnancy, to the relative neglect of externals. Her early attachment to the new baby is dependent on her undergoing this "normal illness," known as primary maternal preoccupation. The father can help by making arrangements and taking on some duties so that the mother need not be overly distracted from this state of mind. In recent years, some women have gone to the other extreme in believing all expectant mothers should continue with their lives as if nothing new were happening until actual labor begins.

Mothers who cannot enter this preparatory state of mind to some degree often have trouble forming a strong initial bond to their infant. In contrast, there are mothers who become excessively caught up in bodily sensations to the point of hypochondriasis. Fathers also may identify with the mother and become anxious; some develop a wide range of physical symptoms (e.g., nausea) and bodily changes (e.g., weight gain) during the pregnancy. This phenomenon is called the *couvade syndrome.* One can see that pregnancy creates some very real demands on the mother's and father's sense of adult identity. The new space for the child may be experienced as a kind of incursion. Mothers and fathers with a poorly formed sense of themselves and with strong ambivalence about parenthood may be more vulnerable to some forms of postpartum depression and other psychiatric reactions.

For both parents, the baby in the womb is a metaphor for a new growing space in their lives and marriage. The first fantasies about the baby are often elaborated into plans for the future. Usually an infant's room is decorated and furnished. Some account is taken of the parent's feelings about one sex or the other. Universal fears about the health of the child and mother are usually aired, a process that helps to make the responsibility of parenting more concrete. The preparation also involves the choice of names for the baby. The name selection helps create a new place in the family network that hopefully will someday be filled by a healthy human being. The names selected (e.g., the meaning of the names, history of the names in the family and new parents' lives) can indicate a great deal about the hopes, expectations, and even concerns regarding the baby. Sometimes the naming is celebrated in a *bris,* in which males are circumcised, or other ceremony shortly after birth.

Childbirth and Early Postpartum Period

The first challenge is posed by the tendency of labor pains to cause some degree of anxiety and sometimes even panic in the mother and father. Extreme pain of any kind signals the possibility of catastrophy for the organism (Simons, 1985). Somehow, a context must be found in which this pain is perceived as normative and indicative of work being done. In a sense, childbirth classes facilitate making labor and delivery a rite of passage into parenthood. One of their main goals is to remove the alarm that accompanies labor pain by reinterpreting it in a new context. Toward this end, childbirth classes teach basic physiology, as well as specific techniques for labor pain management, and place labor and delivery at the endpoint of the preparation process started in pregnancy. They stimulate the couple's anticipatory planning for the future in tandem with the working through of anxiety. They help lay the foundation for parenting by encouraging the couple to act as a team. Giving the father the role of "coach" helps to counter his sense of helplessness in the face of his wife's labor-related activities and possible suffering. The multiple-couple, group context of these classes provides support as well as a circle of initiates on the threshold of parenthood.

On the other hand, it is important that the ideological underpinnings of these classes not foster magic expectations. Some pain is still a fact of life for most deliveries; however, it is important to educate the parents-to-be that epidural injections and other techniques can assure that discomfort remains at a mild and manageable level. The expectant mother also should be told to ask for analgesia when the pain begins to become unpleasant, rather than unbearable, so that less overall medication will be needed to control it. Not all fathers can deal with the actual physical and medical aspects of birth. Most couples know instinctively what goes beyond the limits of their endurance. Their feelings should be assessed and honored by the physician.

Even with 9 months of active preparation, childbirth is virtually always a normative crisis in the lives of the new parents. This is because the rate of change in their lives due to childbirth and the immediate postpartum period is tremendous. The experience often leaves couples in a state of at least mild emotional shock and physical exhaustion. It is not uncommon for new parents to experience feelings of depersonalization, derealization, and a distortion of time sense. At times, the shock can be masked or delayed by feelings of exhilaration after a healthy birth. Weeks or even months may go by before the full reality of the event begins to sink in. During this phase of normal "letdown," the new parents may start to recognize the automatic nature of their responses and the postponement of their affective reactions until well after the fact. Indeed, these patterns of automatic behavior and postponement of responses often continue well into the first year.

This period may be particularly difficult for the woman who has the perception, due to recent social pressures, that she should "do it all," must "do it all" for financial reasons, or wants to "do it all" simultaneously. These women may have to come to terms with how they will function as a new mother, a wife, and previously full-time member of the work force. Some women have compromised by saying, "I can do it all, but do not want to do it all at the same time." During this period, some women cut back to part-time or no work outside the home if finances permit. They reason that their children will be young only once and so they want to have the opportunity for positive early experiences with them, whereas the work world will always exist. Others return to full-time work outside the home almost immediately and make arrangements for child care.

Parenting

The skills of parenting lean heavily on the established partnership of the couple and on the individual health and background of each parent, including the experiences each had with his or her parents. The demands of a new baby challenge the couple to improve their teamwork even further. Usually, this involves some modification and reallocation of roles and tasks; however, the new task orientation may present a danger to the intimacy of the couple and make previous marital problems worse. The partners may be tempted to communicate through issues involving the new "third party," instead of with each other directly; therefore, parents may need to work to preserve and protect their private relationship in the service of teamwork. They thus ensure from the start that parenting will not undermine the marriage that supports it. Some couples use parenting as a way of hiding or avoiding facing the issues in a bad marriage; these couples are most vulnerable to emotional problems. This period is often more stressful for a parent who has not worked outside the home and whose primary identity and self-esteem has been related to being a parent.

The couple's teamwork forms the basis of a "holding environment" for the new baby (Winnicott, 1965). "Holding" refers in a general way to all their efforts to adapt to the baby's needs, both psychological and physiological. It takes into account the literal holding of the child, as well as the monitoring of the early physical environment, of which the establishment of a stable home life is an important part. Also important is the protection of the child from stimuli and outside impingements that are beyond the child's capacity to assimilate. The earliest holding environment builds on the mother's growing empathy with her infant, itself founded on primary maternal preoccupation. The father's primary parental role in the beginning is to "hold" the mother and child "couple," so they can devote themselves much of the time to each other. This requires maturity and sensitivity in the father. He may need to act as a substitute mother, thus allowing the mother some time to recover her "individual" identity.

Beyond the stage of facilitating intimacy between the mother and child, the father helps the child later to begin separating emotionally from the mother (Greenspan, 1982). In this new role, he can allow himself to be seen as someone different from the mother, someone who represents a limit or even sometimes an interference in the mother–child relationship. At the same time, he is also supporting the child's growing independence.

With the passage of time, these roles may be distributed freely between the parents. Some role reversals may help to solidify the partnership by defusing stress. For example, it permits the parents to alternate in the role of disciplinarian, which makes discipline a joint effort rather than the duty of one parent alone.

Raising children places a variety of stresses on the parental partnership. Even if both parents have achieved emotional adulthood, which is often not the case, they will be prone to some regression during the absolute dependency stage of a newborn. Such extreme dependency may evoke a range of reactions from stoic counterdependency (the feeling they do not need help from anyone else) to childish resentment. After weathering this phase, they must adjust to strains in the opposite direction when the child begins to separate. With the onset of the rapprochement crisis (Mahler, 1972), at about 21 months of age, children alternate between intense clinging to and pushing away of the parents. Unless this is understood as a normal developmental struggle, it is often enough to drive the family into a minicrisis.

The holding environment must continue to be strong and flexible enough to assimilate later developments, such as sibling rivalry, children learning to try to play one parent against the other, and adolescent rebellion. The parents must resist any action that threatens to drive a wedge between them, such as taking sides repeatedly in a "sibling war."

Nothing poses a greater challenge to parental teamwork than behavioral "acting out" by their children. Temper tantrums or an adolescent's breaking of curfew both require the setting of limits. Discipline is limit setting in action. The idea is not so much to punish as it is to contain behavior that threatens the holding environment. Children usually react positively to thoughtful limit setting that is explained because they accurately interpret it as a sign of love and concern, and reflective of parental interest in facilitating the children's learning to set healthy limits for themselves.

As noted in Chapter 6 by Dr. Dorsett, discipline should not be confused with punishment. Physical or corporal punishment is ultimately ineffective in developing an internal sense of right and wrong and is indicative of parental ignorance about effective methods of disciplining. Physical punishment basically molds behavior around fear of retaliation, teaches children to hurt others (including possibly their future children) when they do not like what they do, and motivates children to focus on avoiding being caught rather than "doing the right thing." A goal of healthy development is to enable children to internalize self-regulatory behavior, appreciate the effects of their actions on others, develop empathy and consideration for the feelings of others, and solidify the substrate of a moral, ethical, and social conscience. Therefore, corporal or physical punishment should be condemned by physicians, and parents should be educated and counseled about other methods of limit setting and disciplining, such as brief periods of time out and withdrawal of rewards. These issues are discussed in detail by Dr. Dorsett in Chapter 6 and by Drs. Dell and Dulcan in Chapter 8.

By challenging the parents to strengthen their internal cohesion as a couple, children act as a catalyst to further adult development. The experience of being a parent emphasizes to adults the importance of reliability and consistency, which are essential to any position of responsibility. It also affords parents an opportunity to reexperience and rework some of their childhood stages. Thus, parents retain a vital connection with the world of childhood at the very time when they are detaching themselves further from it.

The Single Parent

The single parent (usually female) often faces additional challenges in parenting because he or she may not have a partner with whom to share the burdens of parenting. Some choose to be single parents. Others may feel this situation was forced upon them by divorce or an unplanned pregnancy. These differences often have an impact on how they see their role as a parent and how they view their children. Minor crises can more frequently become major issues. What does the single parent do with the sick child when he or she needs to go to work? What about their needs for adult companionship when their primary relationship and time involvement is with one or more children?

Many single parents meet these challenges with success, but few do so without additional stress. Those who do well find ways to get their own needs met without sacrificing the needs of their children. Creative solutions include support networks and alternative childcare arrangements.

Those who do less well may become bitter and resentful toward their children and may view them as adult surrogates (i.e., may overburden the children with their adult concerns and needs). Additionally, they may find it difficult to let their children become independent if the children have been their main source of emotional support. Others may be so overwhelmed by life stresses that they have little emotional support and guidance to offer their children.

The Effects of Separation and Divorce

Children often react to their parents as a couple in two contradictory ways. On the one hand, they want to drive a wedge between the parents to try to dominate and to control them. On the other hand, they have a deep need to get or keep their parents together in a productive relationship.

When parents separate or divorce, the partial wish to split up the parental couple becomes a reality. This wish explains one reason many children see themselves as the cause of the separation and react with guilt. This may be so painful to children that they may attempt to deny the reality of the situation. If they accept the threat as real, they may engage in frantic reparative efforts to get the parents back together. Some may try to become "perfect" children and not share their concerns and stresses with their parents, thereby possibly short-circuiting some of their own developments and an open, honest relationship with their parents. If the parents themselves are vascillating on the issue of separation, children may discover that they alone are holding their parents together; such a sense of responsibility may only add to their burden of guilt, fear, and anger.

Separation and divorce are almost always traumatic to some degree to children and parents. Naturally, the child's capacity to cope is influenced by the family context. If the marriage has violence or has been a cold, barren desert, separation and divorce may be anticipated with something approaching relief. In some cases, the parents' capacity for parental collaboration may improve when living apart. In any case, the outcome is likely to depend on the parents' being able to sustain some degree of collaboration. The use of a child as a pawn in the parents' "games," sometimes played out in a courtroom, jeopardizes the holding environment needed for children's development. Some form of escape, such as regressing to acting much younger or attempting premature independence by the child may be the only way out of such an intolerable situation. Some form of psychotherapy for parents and children is often indicated to minimize the deleterious effects of separation and divorce on both.

The Midlife Transition

Some time between the ages of 35 and 55, most adults realize that they have reached the midpoint of their lifespan. This realization often has a special psychological significance. Beyond the midpoint, one can no longer say that most of one's life lies ahead. The end is now visible, as well as the beginning. It may be like stepping outside of the stream of life and seeing its horizon for the first time. From this perspective, one may grasp life as a whole, along with its boundaries and limits. The confrontation with these limits may form the basis of a thorough readjustment of the adult self.

Before the midpoint of life, many adults are basking in the mild euphoria of "consolidation." They are often continuing to make steady progress toward their professional and personal goals and are so immersed in various engagements that little time is taken for introspection. Indeed, they may wish to postpone indefinitely any such self-assessment. It is much easier to be carried along on the tide of youthful dreams than to realize one will not live forever.

It often takes some life crisis or trauma before this mild illusory state is interrupted. New realities make their appearance in midlife: signs of physical aging, including the onset of menopause in women and the first diminution of sexual desire in some men, the "sandwiching" produced by the simultaneous responsibilities for their children and for their aging parents, and plateauing of advancement at work. Menopause may trigger in some women the feeling of being less attractive. This feeling may be more pronounced if they did not have the children they desired. Menopause has recently received more attention, as in Gail Sheehy's (1991)book *The Silent Passage,* and also in medical discussions on the pros and cons of hormone replacement therapy. Not infrequently, a first major medical illness, such as a myocardial infarction, begins to drive home the idea that death is inevitable, or the reality may dawn when a peer dies in the prime of life.

Some experience of disillusionment of more youthful fantasies seems to be necessary in making the transition to mature adulthood. Coming face to face with what psychoanalysts have called "narcissistic blows" may help people to give up the universal fantasy of unlimited possibilities (Jaques, 1965; Kernberg, 1980; Viorst, 1986). They may be motivated to undergo a comprehensive life review, in which the past and present are reassessed (Levinson et al, 1978). Each aspect of life will have to be measured against the new limits associated with the confrontation of one's own mortality. The ultimate goal of this quest is a new integration of self, in which a number of conflicting polarities such as love–hate, self–other, male–female, success–failure, are partially reconciled (Levinson and Goodeneh, 1985; Levinson et al, 1978; Settlage et al, 1988). Although largely internal, such a readjustment is bound to influence relationships with others. Some have formulated this change as one of new "tragic" awareness replacing an earlier romanticism (Schafer, 1970).

The term "midlife crisis" is sometimes used to describe a block or maladaptive response to the midlife transition. For example, Mr. C. presented to a psychiatrist with apprehension about an extramarital affair. In many ways, Mr. C.'s feelings about the affair resembled his passionate attachment to flying an airplane, an experience he described as "better than sex." Flying represented his last stand against the limits of earthbound mortal life. Up in the sky, nothing could stop him, nothing could pull him down, nothing could get in his way. The controls were in his hands. He was initially quite oblivious to the fact that his marriage was already in a "nosedive" and that he could "crash" if he were not careful.

Bereavement

Loss plays a necessary role in every life transition. Every step forward in development implies the letting go of an important piece of one's past life. Thus, every developmental gain requires the working through of reactions to some loss, both real and imagined (Viorst, 1986); however, it may be helpful to distinguish between reaction to loss, which is a function of all transitions, and the more specific reaction to the loss of a person to whom one has been attached, referred to in this chapter as bereavement. In overcoming any major loss, whether it be of a spouse, parent, child, relative, or even a body part, the person must commit his or her psychological resources in part to the task of reviewing and reliving his lost relationship (Freud, 1958). Such a task is necessarily somewhat painful and also may be painstaking, protracted, and time consuming. Therefore, bereavement may be viewed as a largely self-limited psychological process that unfolds through a series of stages from initiation to resolution.

The initial reaction to sudden loss is often some form of denial. People are likely to react to any catastrophic event with exclamations like, "No, it can't be," or "You've got to be kidding." Some people react to loss with an almost total absence of emotion. They are the ones on whom others may initially rely for support and, for example, the smooth execution of funeral arrangements. For many, the apparent absence of emotion is due to shock or psychic numbing. They may continue to go about their business in a kind of altered state of consciousness, as if on autopilot. In any case, the effect of such denial is that their actual grief experience is postponed or never reached.

Everyone recognizes the signs of true grieving, which is characterized by intense emotion that includes admixtures of sadness, tearfulness, and sometimes rage. Grieving people are usually preoccupied with their feelings and inner experiences. Quasihallucinatory phenomena, such as hearing the voice of the departed relative or believing they saw the person in a fleeting manner, are considered within the normal range of acute bereavement. Many of these feelings are worked through and reexperienced in private because some subcultures in our society discourage public displays of grief. Other subcultures encourage public displays of grief and mourning.

An important task in grief is the coming to terms with *ambivalence;* every meaningful relationship has some mixed feelings of caring and frustration. Bereavement tends to exaggerate normal ambivalence but may short circuit the working through of negative feelings by such injunctions as considering it wrong "to speak ill of the dead." Hence, some degree of guilt feelings is a normal aftermath of grief. For example, bereaved persons may chastise themselves for even tiny sins of omission, such as some slight or error years ago, not being present at the moment of death, not trying some experimental treatment, or not prolonging an inevitable death through every conceivable mechanical medical means.

Some bereaved people may feel that any degree of ambivalence is unacceptable. They may tend to split their ambivalence by *overidealizing* the image of the lost person and by setting up scapegoats, whom they can blame for their loss. It is not uncommon in recent years for physicians to be placed increasingly in this role, particularly if he or she has been guilty of some perceived error or oversight in management of the case. Many malpractice suits have their origin in this emotionally charged response; such a legal battle may prolong or prevent resolution of grief and mourning. In the ordinary course of events, however, the bereaved are able to pull together their feelings of love and disappointment, annoyance, or hate concerning the lost individual into a more integrated, internalized picture. If they can begin to see the lost person for what she or he was, both good and bad, they often find they can cherish her or his memory in a more meaningful and realistic way.

This task concluded, the stage is set for the final detachment from the lost person and the resultant freeing up of emotional energy for new emotional investments. Such detachment is facilitated by the reality testing that takes place every time the bereaved person falls back into the illusion that the dead person is still alive and then must remember that he or she is no longer to be found. Some have particular difficulty accepting the finality of losses. Some of these people are particularly attracted to stories that JFK, Elvis Presley, and others are still secretly alive. Only with gradual detachment can one truly "bury the dead" and go on with the business of living. For people whose grieving has been incomplete, the dead still "live" in another world or as ghosts, which haunt the survivors, refusing to let them go. Others conceptualize the dead as their guardian angel, looking over them from another world and awaiting a joyful reunion after the grieving individual dies (thereby also lessening the person's fears of death).

The whole grieving process is also marked by rites of passage that include funerals, eulogies, vigils, fasts, condolence rituals, wakes, and burial rites (Van Gennep, 1960). The erosion and weakening of some public mourning rituals may place a greater burden on the person's private means and resources. Wherever possible, public mourning provides a valuable support for many individuals' solitary efforts. For example, viewing the body may help some persons to accept the death as an undeniable reality (Simons, 1985). A funeral also helps the bereaved to remember the dead and to begin to relinquish their attachments in the presence of a group of others who also had attachments to the deceased. It emphasizes the continuity of life (the community of mourners and their link with the transcendent) as it dramatizes its transience.

To some extent, public mourning has been transferred from religious to medical settings. The physician now may often take the role formerly occupied by the clergy. Within this setting, the physician can be of great help in assisting the bereaved. Physicians can use their position and skills to guide bereaved people through the stages of grief. Simply by allowing patients and family members to grieve openly, physicians lend support to the legitimacy of grief, a legitimacy that is sometimes undermined by society's at times phobic attitude toward bereavement in general. More specifically, the physician's presence works to counteract bereaved individuals' fears that something is wrong with them ("Doctor, am I depressed?") and their guilt that they are overreacting emotionally.

Thus, bereavement is treated as a kind of "normal illness," analogous to puberty, pregnancy, menopause, and so forth. As a potential illness in the strict sense, it is up to the physician to diagnose and treat pathological complications of grief and mourning. In pathological bereavement, one or more features of the grieving process become exaggerated and/or fixated. Examples include absent grief, chronic bereavement, excessive guilt, and the loss of reality (psychosis). These and associated conditions, such as depression, mania, and psychosomatic illness, may be triggered by the stress of grief and must be treated in their own right because, once triggered, these conditions tend to take on "a life of their own," regardless of what initially triggered them.

Psychotherapy for the bereaved can serve as a catalyst to the grieving process and as a means of unearthing blocks in the search for a healthier degree of resolution. The extent to which psychotherapy deals with issues of "stillborn," or inadequately resolved, grief reactions has probably been underestimated. For example, a 33-year-old cabinetmaker consulted a psychiatrist for frequent outbreaks of panic and depression. In the course of psychotherapy, he revealed that his father had died about 10 years ago, suddenly and unexpectedly. For several years preceding his death, the patient had noticed a certain reserve in his otherwise cordial relations with his father. Now, it seemed as if a cruel fate had made any considerations of experiencing his sad feelings irrelevant. Instead of grieving in the manner of his distraught mother, he said to himself, "Now you are the man of the family, so you better act like one," which to him meant to be a stoic. Ever since then, he had resolved to suppress all evidence of emotion and to "face reality" in a cool, detached manner. His recent decision to start psychotherapy was his way of keeping the appointment with this postponed grief and of owning up to it for the first time. This enabled him to begin to integrate his grief into his overall sense of his life experiences.

A CASE STUDY

Mrs B., a 62-year-old woman, was brought to see a psychiatrist by her son and daughter. They were concerned that she had "not gone on with her life" after the death of her husband 6 years earlier and of her mother 2 years later. Her children observed that she had become more bitter, withdrawn, and covertly angry at them for "not understanding what she is going through." In psychotherapy, the patient was able to talk about her sense of self-sacrifice and her feeling that she had devoted her life to her husband and mother, who had then deserted her. Her fear was that if she gave up her "grief," she would lose the last remnants of the people who gave her life meaning. The work of psychotherapy with this patient was multifaceted. She needed support for her role as a "giver to others." At the same time, she needed to begin to deal with her ambivalence about the demands placed on her by her husband and mother and her anger about those demands and her anger at them for leaving her. She also needed encouragement to make new attachments in which she was again able to see herself as important and helpful to others.

The Transition to Late Life

Our society's recently improving enlightened attitudes toward late life sometimes may tend to obscure its realities. An older person might say with a sense of humor that old age is not exactly what he or she had in mind. The sacrifices of this life stage in terms of illness, physical decline, and the death of loved ones are very real, yet many older persons respond to these losses as challenges to imbue their lives with new depth of meaning. One sign of increasing recognition of this challenge, as well as of many older person's capacity to meet it, is the resurgence of interest in psychotherapy and psychoanalysis for the elderly.

A major task of old age is to enhance and maintain a sense of inner emotional integrity in the face of increasing external threats to health, financial status, and support systems. Throughout the lifecycle, the sense of identity is often propped up by a variety of external supports, including an attractive and healthy body, a social network and family, some authority in the work place, and demonstrable productivity. Even a generally healthy person in the prime of life may suffer from identity defusion when deprived of these supports, as may occur during a hospitalization, imprisonment, or other prolonged separations from family and friends. Such stresses call on a person's inner resources in combating depersonalization and identity confusion.

Luckily, one usually does not have to endure such trials all at once in the transition to old age, and each potential threat to a person's emotional integrity may be met and conquered using a variety of techniques. Among these are a search for new external supports, experiments with new methods of self-validation, and psychotherapy. These developmental issues are often discussed under the headings of retirement and the challenge to establish a sense of integrity.

The relinquishing of power and authority must stimulate a search for new sources of productivity and creativity (Levinson and Goodeneh, 1985); retirement often marks this transition. Less tied to the demands of the work place, the older person may become freer to explore new interests and to deepen old ones. Adult education, travel, and the like present popular means to this end.

A renewed student status may reflect a basic change in older people's engagement with the world. Regardless of the specific activity, they may re-engage society from a different angle. What they have to offer others, whether as grandparent, teacher, employee, or adviser, is the sum of the wisdom gained from their experiences. They are experienced experts on the human lifecycle and a vital link with the traditions of the past. Therefore, one social role for the elderly is to embody those traditions and to serve as a kind of archivist and transmitter of cultural values and history.

What the elderly may lose in actuality, they often can regain in symbolic forms; however, they may need to get used to the idea of being a "figurehead," at least to some degree. Yet, even when they have to delegate many duties, they still have worth as the embodiment of societal, business, professional, and family values. Society's general attitude—veneration or vilification of their elderly members—makes a difference in this regard; symbolism works better if society lends weight to it. Ironically, society's veneration may be most visible in the political arena, where older persons sometimes have been able to parlay the role of elder statesman into increased power and influence.

The older age transition usually requires the construction of new social networks to replace the previous ones, which were centered in the nuclear family and the work place. Grandparenting may offer a new connectedness to family members. New peer relationships are made possible by the increasing number of people surviving into old age and the proliferation of institutions that focus on the needs of senior citizens.

Not everyone succeeds, however, in the readjustment to older age. Some are seduced into a fantasy that retirement means an end to work, growth, and development. Of course, such beliefs often produce a self-fulfilling prophecy. These are the people who may go through a "honeymoon" phase after retirement, followed by disenchantment. Others approach retirement with great reluctance and refuse to give up the reins of power and authority. Some express their ambivalence by making a show of handing over the responsibility, while still holding on to the ultimate authority, as occurs in *King Lear.* Some inner opposition to the "passing of the scepter" is probably inevitable; however, a pronounced or prolonged conflict in this area is an indication for a psychiatric consultation and psychotherapy.

A CASE STUDY

Mr. H., a 65-year-old hospital administrator, consulted a psychiatrist with the complaint of excessive anger at the prospect of being replaced by a younger person. He noted that his whole life had been a search for new challenges that would confirm his identity as an effective person. What made stepping down particularly distasteful

was the fact that, in his eyes, the replacement lacked even the basic
qualifications for his position; yet, despite this lack of respect, he felt
guilty at begrudging a "child" figure the chance to make good.
Verbalizing these feelings helped him overcome this obstacle to his
retirement and to go on with his life in a fulfilling manner and to be
able to collaborate in a supportive and constructive manner with
his successor during a transition period.

The Battle for Integrity

Isolation remains the most common threat to the sense of integrity of older persons. The elderly are especially vulnerable to the stimulus deprivation that results from decreasing sensory acuity (e.g., vision, hearing, smell, taste). As inner resources decline, the importance of external supports increases. Surrounded by familiar people and objects, even a person with mild-to-moderate visual and hearing impairment and dementia may be able to maintain a sense of positive personal identity for a long time. Physicians may be helpful in correcting or partly reversing the insidious combination of the effects of aging and by teaching compensatory mechanisms for those disabilities. Physicians also may be helpful by being aware of the loss of external supports, such as lower income, illness or death of a spouse, and family relocation. Physicians can support the family of an ill or demented older person by providing education and referral to assistance groups in the management of the home environment. In addition to medical treatment, such measures include recommending frequent family and friend visits; regular orientation to time, place, and person, and a routine daily schedule; family photographs on the wall; the use of a nightlight; and providing updates on current events through television news, newspapers and new magazines, and magazines and books focusing on their career and hobby interests.

In more optimal circumstances, older people may feel challenged to view sickness and death as a test of their personal integrity and inner resources. The near-universality of some type of illness during this stage of life may make illness a kind of "normative crisis" that the elderly recognize as a rite of passage into old age. By finding ways of overcoming the passivity and the helplessness often associated with a major illness, the elderly may learn to see illness and even death as experiences that underscore their basic humanity; the major "battle" between integrity and despair is often fought in this arena.

Religion provides solace and comfort to its believers, and as a coping mechanism may shield medically ill individuals from depression, possibly by counterbalancing feelings of inadequacy and improving feelings of being in control. Religious affiliations also may facilitate the individual's social support network (Koenig et al, 1992).

With improved medical technologies, illness and recovery are becoming common experiences of mid and late life. Such illness may play a key role in the midlife crisis and acts as a challenge to personal integrity and self-esteem.

Physicians need to sensitize themselves to patients' varying needs to participate in the process of recovery, and to use their own adaptive measures to maintain a sense of autonomy and control. Physicians at times may not oppose eccentric and unorthodox approaches to self-treatment by a patient if they do no harm and add to the patient's feeling of being more in control.

Death and Dying

The approach of death paradoxically may open up new avenues for feelings of inner continuity. When the future is foreclosed, there may be a greater intensity to the present moment and a greater depth of self-awareness. At the end of their lifecycle, individuals may feel nearer to the beginning, nearer to the cycle of the generations of which they are a part. Having come full circle, the end of life may be approached with a heightened sense of mystery and an enriched interest in the transcendent, often expressed through an increased involvement with religious concerns and other larger social issues.

The encounter with one's own impending death, however, is obviously unique among life's transitions. The idea of death, especially when it will occur before the expected end of the lifespan, is anticipated by most people as a very emotionally traumatic event whose impact often exceeds even that of bereavement. (For the purposes of this section, the dying patient will be assumed to be conscious and aware; situations when this is not the case are addressed more under the section on Bereavement).

The disturbing quality of impending death is often due to three factors. First, death represents a threat to the part of our minds that seeks to place us in control of our destiny. At one time or another, almost everyone harbors the fantasy and wish of immortality. We find it difficult, even as adults, to grasp the idea of our own nonexistence. Second, the primitive fears and fantasies that death stirs in us may transform death into a horrifying specter, like the ghosts and monsters of our childhood. The ghouls, vampires, and other varieties of the dead who turn out to be "undead" personify these fears and are the characters of the "slasher movies," so popular with some adolescents. The image of the dead returning to take revenge on the living, implied by the adage mentioned in the section on Bereavement "not to speak ill of the dead," is but one of many fantasies reflecting archaic vestiges of thought about death from childhood. Death evokes, almost universally, a series of infantile emotional danger situations (Freud, 1963), including loss of the self and of the loved person (or "object"), loss of the object's love, castration and other forms of physical mutilation, and abandonment by parental caretakers (often symbolized as God) or fate. Third, Western culture of the past 100 years has produced a massive denial of death. This is not meant to imply that some degree of denial of one's own death is inherently abnormal. In a study of the Hiroshima survivors, Robert Jay Lifton (1967) showed how an excessive exposure to death may undermine and destroy much of the meaningfulness of life. A certain degree of adaptive denial may actually improve life expectancy in male patients with myocardial infarction (Levenson et al, 1984). This same denial-based attitude of "nothing bad can happen to me" undoubtedly proves helpful to some soldiers in the heat of battle and lethal to others. The effect of *societal* denial, however, is to place death *outside* the realm of the normal lifecycle, and thus to try to exclude it from everyday awareness. How else can death appear then, except as an alien unwelcome intruder?

Death, however, was not always viewed as such an extraordinary event in Western society (Ariès 1973). During the Middle Ages, many people met their deaths with a sense of resignation and acceptance. Part of this attitude probably was due to the near-universality of religious faith and frequent exposure to death on a day-to-day basis. On the other hand, another part of it often arose from the belief that death was not some extraordinary event, but rather an expected, if unwelcome, "guest" in this life. In the arts of that era, death often was personified as a mysterious stranger with whom one could have a conversation. Such a "dialogue with death" is dramatized in Ingmar Bergman's film, *The Seventh Seal,* in which the protagonist plays a game of chess with Death.

The revived interest in death and dying in medical settings, partly catalyzed by the studies of Elizabeth Kübler-Ross (1969) in the 1960s, led to a rediscovery of the latter attitude. Kübler-Ross conceived of the encounter with death as a developmental process not unlike other life transitions. Indeed, Leo Tolstoy (1981), in his classic short novel, *The Death of Ivan Ilych,* demonstrated that the encounter with death in a 45-year-old man contained most of the elements of a midlife crisis. In that novel, Ivan's encounter with death involves a lengthy and painful task of self-reassessment and realignment. It is interesting that the acceptance of death-related tasks described by Kübler-Ross—denial and isolation, anger, bargaining, depression, and acceptance—are roughly analogous to the stages of bereavement. This should not be surprising, since much of the pain of loss in bereavement is due to the emotional investment in the lost person, which makes it similar to the loss of one's self.

The first death of a patient is usually a painful experience in the professional life of medical students, and it puts to the test one's attitudes toward death. That first death may reveal that they, too, were motivated in part to become physicians by altruistic "rescue fantasies" (a somewhat heroically tinged desire to correct the wrongs of the world, including illness, disability, and death), which they have measured primarily by the saving of life. Subsequently, some physicians align with society's recent prevailing attitude of denial, which is sometimes translated as "life at any cost." Most, however, ideally will expand their definition of medical "success" to include helping dying patients and their families come to terms with and to achieve a dignified, painless, and peaceful death.

Physicians' attitudes toward death often are revealed also in the way in which they approach the task of informing their patients of a terminal prognosis. Sensitive handling of this juncture can go a long way toward helping patients face their own death with more equanimity. A goal of the physician is to respect and enhance the patient's freedom to define this task in his or her own way. To reach this objective, the physician must avoid any preestablished or "prescribed" policy in this regard. Physicians who never inform their patients of their specific medical situation, as well as those who sometimes bluntly inform *all* of their terminal patients of all the details, may interfere with freedom of choice for some patients.

Some patients indicate through their speech and behaviors that they do not want to know the specific prognosis of their illness. Some patients may not even want to know their diagnosis, or if they do, will prefer to discuss it in vague terms (i.e., a growth or tumor, rather than a malignancy or cancer). These patients seldom ask the physician, "Am I going to die?" or "How long do I have to live?" While this attitude certainly shows some denial, it also indicates a certain choice of how to approach death. These patients, in effect, approach death as an invisible horizon, always just beyond their range of vision. They remain fully focused on the practical tasks of improving their situation and often wish for some palliative improvement and discovery of a miracle cure, which allows them to maintain their denial, to live with more hope, and to bolster their optimism. Lest one judge this attitude as naive or representative of unrealistic denial, it is well to remember that this degree of denial comes close to the normal day-to-day attitude of healthy individuals toward their own death, which is just as inevitable as that of the dying person. The point is that the physician is not in a position to know *beforehand* what path will be chosen by an individual patient.

Extreme denial may place a burden on the patient's family and business by resulting in lack of preparation of a will and of other planning for the future. Sometimes a patient can be persuaded to make a will and to see to related matters in the name of "covering all contingencies." A will commits individuals to the serious consideration of their own death and its consequences for others. Physicians usually are able to determine when patients are ready to discuss this task. Some patients will ask the physician directly whether they are going to die from their condition and how much time they probably have left. At this point, the physician, besides answering such questions, can promise assistance to the patient in whatever tasks lie ahead.

For many, death in the abstract is not the main source of anxiety. There are, of course, individuals who tend to brood and ruminate over the meaning of death. When faced with the actuality of one's death, however, the concerns and fears are usually more mundane and circumscribed, hence also more manageable for the physician. Such patients may want reassurance, not that the physician will save them, but that he or she will stay with them as an ally, partner, and consultant right to the end. Often, the dying patient's most haunting fear is of being left alone. In the same vein, patients want reassurance from their physician that they will not allow the patient to be overwhelmed by pain and physical suffering.

Several of these points are illustrated in the following hospital consultation.

A CASE STUDY

The staff of a medical-surgical unit suggested the surgeon request a psychiatric consultation on Mr. R., a 50-year-old man with terminal metastatic colon cancer. Mr. R. was aware of his diagnosis and prognosis and was tearful and despondent at times. The staff, however, was mainly concerned about oddities in Mr. R's behavior. For the past few weeks, he had been asking his wife to bring him huge quantities of his favorite, nutritious foods (many dating back to his childhood), which he ate with relish several times a day. In addition, he had told the nurses that he sometimes felt as though they were trying to poison him through the intravenous (IV) lines.

After talking with the patient, the consulting psychiatrist began to see these behaviors and concerns as due to partial psychological regression. For most of the time, Mr. R. acted like a mature man trying to work through his feelings about his impending death. His tearfulness was mostly due to the mourning process he was going through for the life he had to give up. In this area his reality testing was relatively intact, and the meals he was eating became like a kind of "last supper." In order to deal with the inescapable ending of his life, Mr. R. had shrunk his temporal horizon to encompass only his next meal. Instead of thinking of the frightening future, he would instead substitute the prospect of his next meal, which he could anticipate with pleasure.

Mr. R. was relating to his caregivers—his wife and the staff nurses (both male and female)—as all-powerful "mother" figures who held the power of life and death over him. He simultaneously felt as though they could keep him alive with magical, lifesaving food, or they could kill him with poison introduced into his IV line. The latter fantasy was amplified by the fact that his pain was being controlled by fairly large doses of analgesia, which also somewhat blunted his rational thought processes. Thus, according to this fantasy, it was they—the "mothers" (to whom he could relate)—who decided his fate and not the inevitable progression of his disease.

In the case of Mr. R., the psychiatrist only had to support and encourage the staff to accept the patient's unique approach to death. The psychiatrist encouraged Mr. R. to speak openly about his feelings and, at the same time, tolerated his partial behavioral regressions without criticism. Discussion with the staff also helped them to take a more permissive attitude toward the regressions and to see his tearfulness as evidence of an ongoing mourning process.

In the course of this developmental process, many patients come to conceive of their relationship to death in terms of some overriding metaphor. Death may be conceived of as a fight that has been lost, a journey, a culminating closure of one's life, a return to the beginning of the lifecycle (mentioned in the section on old age), a profound rest that is akin to sleep, and even as a reward for religious faithfulness during life. Interestingly, many patients come to think of death as a transition of sorts, different only in degree from other life transitions. One patient, for example, dreamed about his death as a move from his old house to a new one; in the process of this move, the old house was completely divested of all its furniture and decorations, leaving it bare and empty, a mere shell or skeleton.

Perhaps the one aspect of psychological death work that sets it apart from other developmental tasks is the obvious need for a more thoroughgoing divestment from all of life's attachments. The dying person must, in effect, bid farewell to every person and thing that has held meaning in his or her life; and finally, one must bid farewell to something that almost everyone is quite attached to, namely one's "self."

As has been alluded to earlier, it cannot be emphasized enough that the most fundamental fear of patients is not necessarily death itself, but the fear of being alone, abandoned, in pain, and helpless *in the process of dying.* In this respect, the physician may play a powerful supportive role for the patient with terminal illness in a number of ways. First, the physician should reassure patients that they will not be abandoned and that the physician will be available to them "no matter what happens." This assurance of help and support markedly decreases fears of dying alone. Physicians who withdraw from patients because they cannot emotionally tolerate the idea of death, or who react to the patient's terminal illness as a failure of their own to "save" the patient, are abandoning not only the patient but one of the most essential duties and obligations of being a physician. Emotional withdrawal and avoidance of the dying patient by the physician may derive from a variety of factors: the physician's own fear of death, discomfort with dealing with the emotional pain of bereavement, or, as noted above, a sense of helplessness and failure in the physician. It is important, therefore, for physicians to be aware of their own feelings toward death and the dying process and to possess the ability to self-analyze their own avoidance or detachment from patients if this occurs in the context of terminal illness.

The second major fear of patients is the fear of feeling helpless in the process of dying. Again, physicians may provide comforting reassurance that everything will be done to assist patients in their care to ensure as much autonomy as possible, and that they will be allowed to participate in any medical decisions regarding their care.

Finally, physicians may provide powerful reassurance that the patient will not be allowed to be in significant pain. Terminal illness is not the situation in which to demonstrate conservatism in the use of narcotics. Patients should be reassured that adequate pain relief will be provided for them, as needed.

Hence, far from being helpless, the physician may provide powerful emotional and practical intervention in the care of dying patients and their families in order to relieve their fears and suffering during the dying process.

Choice in Adult Development: The Transitions as Crossroads

In the patient examples used in this chapter, each individual was confronted with a fateful choice. Mr. N., the artist in his mid-30s, had to decide whether to continue as an artist or to pursue a more business-oriented career. Dr. G., the resident physician, found himself at a crossroads of his professional life. He had to decide between continuing his career as a primary caregiver or switching to a consulting practice. Mr. H., the 65-year-old hospital administrator, eventually chose a constructive path of retirement over the options of holding on to his job or seeking another position, which had previously been his typical life pattern.

In these patient examples, decisions in the lifecycle about relationships (e.g., marriage, parenthood, divorce) are as important as those involving job and career. Mr. N. and Dr. G. both were considering separating from their wives. In the case of Mr. N., who had a 5-year-old son, this choice also was about being a part-time or full-time father. In the course of treatment, the 34-year-old schizoid man finally took the plunge and successfully asked and took a woman on a date. His decision was, in part, a conscious effort to break out of his self-imposed prison of isolation. And finally, Mr. C., the man who loved to fly, found himself caught between his devotion to his wife of 20 years and his recent infatuation for an attractive female colleague. For Mr. C., the hardest task was acknowledging that he had to make a choice, that it was either one or the other. As he put it to his psychiatrist; "I know I can't have my cake and eat it, too."

Ultimately, however, it is not just a question of "this job or that job," or this relationship or that relationship, but of this or that life path. The individual must choose among various "lifelines." Committing oneself to one choice often means changing the direction of an entire life, and in some cases, altering one's destiny and sense of identity. From this viewpoint, adult transitions involve more than just a change from one stage to another. They also may be viewed as crossroads in the lifecycle, an opportunity for choice against the background of inevitable biological and psychosocial change.

The range of choices in adult life are wide, but most midlife and later choices do not necessarily involve dramatic changes in behavior. In fact, radical changes in lifestyle in the midlife transition are more the exception than the rule. Some individuals do, however, make major changes in midlife, such as career shifts, geographic relocations, divorce, remarriage, becoming a parent again, and step-parenting. For others, the changes may be more symbolic and on a smaller scale, such as the resolution to change one's eating, smoking, and drinking habits, to get a regular physician and physical checkup, to start attending church and visiting family more often, to take a different kind of vacation, and to take an adult education course or develop a hobby in an area unrelated to professional concerns. Some important choices may involve no changes whatsoever in outward behavior. It is important to remember that the act of choosing does not require change for the sake of change. An individual may opt to "stay the course," or, in other words, continue in her or his habitual modes of behavior. As the result of a process of reflection and the exercise of choice, the option of no change may be as valid as any other.

Initially, it may seem strange, however, to have "refocusing on life choices" as part of the lifecycle stage, which also includes accepting the absolute inevitability of death, yet even in the face of death, a wide range of human choice is not lacking, including the option of rejecting or accepting the finality of death; that is, Kübler-Ross's stages do not imply universal progression leading inevitably to "acceptance." Many patients, without denying their own deaths, consciously choose to fight against death to the end. After all, such a combative stance follows a well-established tradition in Western society, summed up in the famous line about death from a Dylan Thomas poem, "Rage, rage against the dying of the light." On the other hand, the alternative of "acceptance" should not be viewed as passive capitulation. In true "acceptance," the individual reaches a position where he or she, in effect, "chooses" to die, as if dying were somehow their decision (although to some degree the "when and how" may be). For such a patient, death may be thereby changed from an impersonal event into "my death." As implied in the section in this chapter on Death and Dying, reaching such a position with a sense of equanimity and grace is an extraordinary human accomplishment.

In later life, some individuals feel robbed of the idealized life they fantasize they would have had "if only they had made different choices." They are part of the group of adults who feel that their lives have been the product of situations and forces outside of their control. The midlife and late-life transition offers many of these people real or symbolic second chances; however, some adults are blocked from doing so by an ideology that "failure is my fate," which they have developed to justify their condition. These individuals may present to a psychiatrist or other physician with a complaint like "Nothing ever goes right for me," "I'm jinxed," and so forth. They tend to portray themselves as fortune's plaything and, not uncommonly, as the victim of bad luck and fate. Therefore, they may consciously and unconsciously minimize the influence of their choices in shaping their lives. One patient, for example, when discussing several important life situations, including her decision to enter psychotherapy, said, "I had no choice."

Indeed, psychotherapy for adults, including the elderly, may be looked upon as a kind of laboratory for the making of choices. Psychotherapy patients learn to reconsider past situations as the result of choices unwittingly made or evaded. This change in perspective may help them to redefine the present and the future as inherently open to influence. The next step is making new choices and dealing with their consequences, both external and internal. It is for this reason that some adults make use of at least brief psychotherapy at several times during their development and view it as an invaluable aid in their efforts to negotiate more successfully adult transitions.

ACKNOWLEDGMENT

The authors thank Susan Shelton, MD, for reviewing this chapter in its original form and for many contributions to the sections on childlessness and on the single parent.

ANNOTATED BIBLIOGRAPHY

Colarusso C, Nemiroff R: Adult Development. New York, Plenum Press, 1981
> This standard work presents a problem-oriented approach to the main stages of adult development.

Colarusso CA: Child and Adult Development: A Psychoanalytic Introduction for Clinicians. New York, Plenum Press, 1992
> This is a good introduction to psychodynamic and psychoanalytic theories and concepts of development; it is written in a clear, engaging, and clinically relevant manner.

Erikson EH: Childhood and Society. New York, WW Norton, 1963
> This classic on adult development contains the "eight ages of man" schema, which has served as a foundation for much subsequent research in the field.

Gould RL: Transformations. New York, Simon & Schuster, 1978
> Gould's paradigm of adult development stresses transitional stages such as the "age 30 transition."

Levinson DJ, Darrow CM, Klein EB, et al: The Seasons of a Man's Life. New York, Alfred A Knopf, 1978
> Based on more than a decade of rigorous research on the stages of adult development, this work achieved a fresh perspective on adulthood by viewing it as a series of transitions.

Mahler MS, Pine F, Bergman A: The Psychological Birth of the Human Infant. New York, International Universities Press, 1975
> The product of many years of observational study on mothers and their infants, this classic work offered a new developmental schema for the first 3 years of life, based on the notion of separation–individuation. It originated the idea of a normative crisis—the so-called rapprochement crisis—at the age of about 21 months.

Vaillant G: Adaptation to Life. Boston, Little, Brown & Co, 1977
> This book discusses the results of a large prospective study of male college students in which psychological traits were correlated with measures of physical and psychological health over several decades.

Viorst J: Necessary Losses. New York, Ballantine Books, 1986
> Viorst elaborates the thesis that each advance to a new developmental stage is associated, to a greater or lesser extent, with the loss of an emotionally invested portion of previous stages.

Winnicott DW: The Maturational Processes and the Facilitating Environment. New York, International Universities Press, 1965
> Winnicott's concepts of the "holding environment," "primary maternal preoccupation," and "the good-enough mother" are useful in appreciating the tasks of parenting.

REFERENCES

Anzieu D: Freud's Self-Analysis. Madison, CT, International Universities Press, 1986

Ariès P: Western Attitudes toward Death: From the Middle Ages to the Present. Baltimore, Johns Hopkins University Press, 1974

Bibring GL, Dwyer TF, Huntington DS, et al: A study of the psychological processes in pregnancy and of the earliest mother-child relationship. Psychoanal Study Child 16:9–24, 1961

Blos P: The second individuation process of adolescence. Psychoanal Study Child 22:162–186, 1967

Colarusso C, Nemiroff R: Adult Development. New York, Plenum Press, 1981.

Erikson EII: Identity and the lifecycle (monograph). Psychological Issues, Vol. 1, No. 1. New York, International Universities Press, 1959

Erikson EH: Childhood and Society. New York, WW Norton, 1963

Freud A: The concept of developmental lines. Psychoanal Study Child 8:245–265, 1963

Freud S: Three essays on the theory of sexuality. 1905. In Strachey J (ed): The Standard Edition of the Complete Psychological Works, Vol. 7. London, Hogarth Press, 1958

Freud S: Mourning and melancholia. 1917. In Strachey J (ed): The Standard Edition of the Complete Psychological Works, Vol. 14. London, Hogarth Press, 1958

Gould RL: The phases of adult life: A study in developmental psychology. Am J Psychiatry 129:521–531, 1972

Greenspan S: "The second other": The role of the father in early personality formation and the dyadic-phallic phase of development. In Cath S, Gurwitt A, Ross JM (eds): Father and Child. Boston, Little, Brown & Co, 1982

Jaques E: Death and the mid-life crisis. Int J Psychoanal 46:502–514, 1965

Kernberg O: Internal World and External Reality Object Relations Theory Applied. New York, Jason Aronson, 1980

Kiley D: The Peter Pan Syndrome. New York, Dodd, Mead, 1983

Koenig HG, Cohen HJ, Blazer DG, et al: Religious coping and depression among elderly, hospitalized medically ill men. Am J Psychiatry 149:1693–1700, 1992

Kübler-Ross E: On Death and Dying. New York, Macmillan, 1969

Levenson JL, Kay R, Monteferrante J, et al: Denial predicts favorable outcome in unstable angina pectoris. Psychosom Med 46:25–32, 1984

Levinson DJ, Darrow CM, Klein EB, et al: The Seasons of a Man's Life. New York, Alfred A. Knopf, 1978

Levinson DJ, Goodeneh WE: The life cycle. In Kaplan HI, Sadock BJ (eds): Comprehensive Textbook of Psychiatry. Baltimore, Williams & Wilkins, 1985

Lifton RJ: Death in Life: Survivors of Hiroshima. New York, Simon and Schuster, 1967

Mahler MS: The rapprochement subphase of the separation–individuation process. Psychoanal Q 41:487–506, 1972

Mahler MS, Pine F, Bergman A: The Psychological Birth of the Human Infant. New York, International Universities Press, 1975

Schafer R: The psychoanalytic vision of reality. Int J Psychoanal 51:279–297, 1970

Settlage CF, Curtis J, Lozoff M, et al: Conceptualizing adult development. J Am Psychoanal Assn 36:347–369, 1988

Sheehy G: The Silent Passage. New York, Pocket Books, 1991

Sholevar P (ed): The Handbook of Marriage and Marital Therapy. Jamaica, NY, SP Medical and Scientific Books, 1981

Simons RC (ed): Understanding Human Behavior in Health and Illness. Baltimore, Williams & Wilkins, 1985

Tolstoy L: The Death of Ivan Ilych. New York, Bantam Books, 1981

Vaillant G: Adaptation to Life. Boston, Little, Brown & Co, 1977

Van Gennep A: The Rites of Passage. Chicago, University of Chicago Press, 1960

Viorst J: Necessary Losses. New York, Ballantine Books, 1986

Winnicott DW: The Maturational Processes and the Facilitation Environment. New York, International Universities Press, 1965

11 The Psychology and Psychobiology of Developmental Trauma

Bessel A. van der Kolk

Section II and the preceding chapters in this section on human development have laid the groundwork for considering the possible consequences of developmental stresses for human behavior and vulnerability to psychiatric illness. A growing body of psychiatric research has confirmed that certain types of adverse stresses, losses, and deprivations within the family system may cause abnormalities in psychological development with lifelong effects on the individual's personality, susceptibility to stressful events in later life, and vulnerability to certain types of mental illness. Moreover, the long-term *neurobiological* effects of developmental stress also have begun to be elucidated. These findings, some of which will be summarized here, provide an excellent model to integrate biological, psychological, and social theories of human behavior and mental illness. This chapter provides an overview of some of this evidence from a psychobiological perspective. This chapter also provides an entreé and transition to Section IV of this text, which considers in some detail neurobiological aspects of behavior.

INTRODUCTION

The United States Department of Health and Human Services reported that in 1993 1,530,000 children were repeatedly beaten, sexually molested, left unattended, or severely emotionally abused. Violence in the family is one of the major causes of physical and emotional injuries. Children who witness violence in the family are, in turn, at great risk of perpetuating violence when they grow up. Boys who witness violence by their fathers have a 1,000% greater likelihood of growing up to abuse their partners than men who were not exposed to marital violence when they were young.

Battering is the greatest single cause of injury to women in the U.S., more than by car accidents, rapes, and muggings combined. It is estimated that between 30 and 80% of women receiving treatment for spousal battering witnessed violence between their parents as children. It has been estimated that 21% of all emergency surgery for women is for injuries due to battering.

THE PSYCHOLOGICAL IMPACT OF VIOLENCE

Exposure to extreme stress influences how people organize their perceptions of themselves and others, as well as how their bodies will react to subsequent experience. Exposure to trauma can have particularly profound effects on how children view themselves and their world. In psychiatric settings, where histories of trauma are extremely common, the mental organization of acute or chronic exposure to trauma may be expressed in formal psychiatric diagnoses, among which posttraumatic stress disorder (PTSD) is the easiest to recognize. This diagnosis involves the involuntary repetitive reliving of the trauma in thoughts, images, or action (intrusions), an inability to calm one's body down (hyperarousal), and a loss of capacity to engage in love and work with pleasure and zest (avoidance and numbing).

Recent research has shown that PTSD is one of the most common psychiatric diagnoses, affecting almost 10% of the population during their lifetime (Kessler, 1995). However, histories of childhood trauma set the stage for developing a range of problems that go well beyond the core definition of PTSD: how to trust people after you know how much they can hurt you, how to calm yourself down when you are upset, how to pay attention while faced with emotionally arousing situations, how to deal with bodily responses to upsetting events, and how to think positively about oneself when faced with adversity. A substantial proportion of traumatized individuals engage in self-mutilation, eating disorders, or substance abuse (van der Kolk et al, 1996a). Many people with histories of severe childhood trauma meet diagnostic criteria for trauma-related psychiatric disorders such as borderline personality disorder (Herman et al, 1989), somatization disorder, and dissociative disorders.

Often, the extreme emotional distress of these patients or the bizarre or disorganized behaviors in which they engage obscure the fact that their current problems have their origins in past trauma. However, being able to recognize how people deal with traumatic life experience helps one realize that many of these patients organize much of their lives around repetitive patterns of reliving and warding off traumatic memories, reminders, and feelings.

Recognizing these symptoms as misguided attempts to regain a sense of control and safety, rather than as bizarre behaviors that need to be merely controlled, will critically determine how one approaches the treatment of these patients.

ATTACHMENT AND DEVELOPMENT IN CHILDREN

The Development of Cognition

Maturation of the brain and the development of cognitive capacities go hand-in-hand. As children mature, structural and neurochemical changes in the brain allow for ever more complex cognitive organization of experience: experience and brain combine to determine the interpretation of subsequent reality in a use-dependent manner. Existing biological and psychological structures determine how new experiences are perceived, remembered, and integrated into the totality of a person's inner world.

As long as children lack the capacity to categorize, contrast, and compare, and know that "what you see is not necessarily what you get," they have no choice but to see themselves as the center of the universe. Everything that happens is directly related to their own sensations. As they mature, they move from *being* their actions and sensations to *having* them (Kegan, 1982).

Very young infants have not yet learned to distinguish between stimuli that come from their own bodies and those that come from outside. During the first year of life, infants learn to make the first mental associations between stimulus and response. This association modifies their reflexive patterns and sets the stage for their gaining control over their physical, reflexive reactions: the critical pathway that leads from *being* one's reflexes, movements, and sensations to *having* them (Kegan, 1982).

Development consists of learning to master and "own" one's experiences. In this process of differentiation, individuals need to detach from their "embeddedness" in the experience. The Swiss psychologist Jean Piaget called this "decentration" (the loss of an old center) that needs to be replaced by the placement of sensations and perception into personal categories. In order to develop the critical capacity to imagine playing a role in what is happening, children need to learn to place what is happening to them in relative space and time. Only when they do this can they acquire an understanding that sensations have a beginning, middle, and end, and develop a sense of continuity of the self that transcends how they feel at any particular moment.

People who develop PTSD in some ways resemble immature children: confronted with a reminder of their trauma, they become victims of their reflexes. They no longer are able to distinguish between exposure to an actual trauma and sensations that remind them of it. They feel as if the event is actually happening again.

The Social Context as a Mediator of Development

All people live within a social environment that has a major influence on the way they cope with life's stresses. Early in life, children's caregivers not only play a critical role in buffering a child against the impact of stressful situations, they also help them to build the biological capacities to deal with future life stresses. No mammal has developed more varied and complex ways of maintaining attachment bonds between caregivers and their offspring than human beings. While nonhuman primates express attachment bonds mainly with physical contact, such as grooming and imitative behavior, humans have evolved to supplement this physical contact with language, which allows them to communicate about the subtleties of how they feel and what they think.

The separation cry of infants, which fulfills the function of eliciting caregiving, can be viewed as a precursor of language. Its primary function is to induce adults to provide safety, nurturance, and social (i.e., pleasurable) stimulation. MacLean (1985) considers the human capacity to maintain attachment bonds over space and time by means of verbal communication as one of the principal reasons for the human ascendancy in the animal kingdom. This capacity also has a dark side: "when mammalians opted for a family way of life, they set the stage for the most distressful forms of suffering, a condition that, for us, makes being a mammal so painful, and that is having to endure separation and isolation from loved ones, and, in the end, the utter desolation of death" (MacLean, 1985).

Early attachment relationships are critical because they help individuals construct a psychological map of the world (Bowlby, 1980). These maps determine how people see themselves, their significant others, and the ways that the world works in general. This internal representational map contains both objective (cognitive) and subjective (affective) knowledge about the world. The feelings (i.e., the subjective knowledge) that people attach to situations allow them to rapidly appraise the personal meaning of that experience by linking what is currently going on with behavioral responses that were effective in the past. The intensity of these feelings determines the intensity of the response: the more one is capable of modifying feelings with thought, the more flexibility one has to consciously figure out the appropriate response to any given challenge.

One of the primary functions of parents is to help their children learn to modulate their physiological arousal by providing them with their own acquired knowledge about the world. This transfer of knowledge takes place principally by means of modeling: displaying behavior that is effective in modifying distress. Parents model by being attuned to their children's needs and by providing them with well-timed feeding, playing, comforting, cleaning, and resting. The quality of the caregivers' response to children's needs helps them gradually to learn to modulate their arousal and to build self-soothing skills.

As children mature, there is less need for caregivers to be constantly and immediately available to help them modulate their arousal. They learn to do some self-modulating by relying on the skills they have learned and by deriving comfort from friends and other social supports. Gradually, most children learn that coping with stress involves mobilizing skills to take care of themselves and that they need to ask for help when their own resources are inadequate.

The Development of Emotional Regulation

Caregivers play a critical role in modulating children's physiological arousal by providing a balance between soothing and stimulation. This balance, in turn, regulates normal play and exploratory activity. Stern (1985) calls this "affect attunement" between caregivers and infants. When children are removed from their caregivers, they lose their capacity to calm themselves down and go through an initial period of behavioral agitation, which is accompanied by increases in heart rate and body temperature and followed by depression. Separated children tend to suffer from sleep problems (an increase in arousal and time spent awake) and by a decrease in autonomic activity. Upon reunion with their mothers, children may continue to show behavioral changes. The caregivers' response during this time seems to play a critical role in modulating the long-term effects of separation. As they mature, most children gradually become less vulnerable to overstimulation and learn to tolerate higher levels of excitement. Over time, they have less need for physical proximity of a caregiver to maintain their comfort, and they start spending more time playing with their peers and with their fathers. Securely attached children learn how to take care of themselves effectively as long as the environment is more or less predictable. Simultaneously, they know how to get help when they are distressed.

Early Attachment and the Development of Coping Styles

While adequate caregivers maintain an optimal level of physiological arousal, unresponsive or abusive parents may promote chronic hyperarousal that can have enduring effects on the child's ability to modulate strong emotions. Research has shown that as many as 80% of abused infants and children have disorganized/disoriented attachment patterns, including unpredictable alterations of approach and avoidance toward their mothers, as well as other conflict behaviors, such as prolonged freezing, stilling, or slowed "underwater" movements. Thus, early attunement combines with temperamental predispositions to "set" the capacity to regulate future arousal. This plays a major role in the long-term vulnerability to develop psychopathological problems after exposure to stressful experiences.

The ways that people cope with stress can be divided roughly into two general categories: (1) problem-focused coping (channeling resources to solve the stress-creating problem); and (2) emotion-focused coping (easing the tension aroused by threat through changing one's feelings, such as denying what is happening or changing one's attitude toward the threatening circumstances). Under most circumstances, problem-focused coping clearly is the most adaptive of these two coping styles. However, under extreme conditions, emotion-focused coping may be the only option. While being assertive can help people escape from danger, it may be useless when one is dependent on an unpredictable or irrational person and outright dangerous when one is being physically or sexually abused or is a witness to parental violence (van der Kolk et al, 1996a).

There are situations in which people simply are unable to control the outcome of events and in which active resistance is likely to provoke retaliation from the perpetrator. In such cases, spacing out and disengaging can help people survive. Unfortunately, when children are exposed to chronic abuse and neglect, emotion-focused coping may become their habitual way of dealing with stresses, which, in the long range, is likely to reinforce their sense of powerlessness and to decrease their capacity to gain satisfaction.

In her studies on infants, Mary Ainsworth has described roughly three ways in which infants organize their behavior in regard to their caregivers: secure, anxious/avoidant, and ambivalent. These patterns have been related to differences in mothers' responsiveness to infant signals and to subsequent ways of coping in social settings. These early patterns of attachment have powerful effects across the lifespan because they are thought to set the stage for different patterns of information processing (Crittenden, 1992). Secure infants tend to grow up to become individuals who are able to rely on both emotions and thinking to help them in determining their reactions to any given situation. They carry with them an overarching sense of feeling understood because they encode the responsiveness of their caregivers in their views of themselves and carry with them a sense that they are capable of making good things happen.

When caregivers are extraordinarily inconsistent, frustrating, violent, intrusive, or neglectful, children are likely to experience a sense of distress that cannot be relieved by active manipulation of their environment. Not being able to rely on their caregivers, these infants experience excessive anxiety, anger, and desire for their attachment figures. When they fail to find a way of resolving these feelings, their distress escalates and often culminates in the development of dissociative states or self-defeating aggression. These frightened, spaced out, and hyperaroused children learn to ignore aspects of their own experience or the reality of what they are seeing and perceiving. Not being able to effect the behavior of their caregivers in the direction of comfort and safety, they engage in emotion-focused coping that allows them to modulate their arousal levels by reconstructing their inner experience.

The solutions that young infants construct to deal with such experiences have been classified roughly as: (1) avoidant, (2) anxious/ambivalent, and (3) chaotic. Avoidant infants deal with the inconsistency of their attachment figures in responding to their needs by ignoring what they feel and by depending excessively upon the logic of situations. They learn to inhibit the display of distress and desire and over time, lose touch with what it is that they actually feel. Observations of maltreated children show that many display an incongruent falsely positive exterior, which does not match what is happening to them (Crittenden, 1992). Being able to inhibit their distress has many benefits for these children and protects them against the experience of further hurt. However, it also contains the basis for great confusion regarding the true nature of who they are and what they need to do to gratify themselves. As a result, they appear more independent than other individuals, but they are emotionally distant and unable to derive comfort from friendships and intimacy.

In contrast to avoidant people, individuals who were labeled anxious/ambivalent in infancy tend to grow up relying on what they are feeling but disregard thinking. Confused about perceptual reality, they tend to tune into their own feelings at the expense of being able to think about the meaning of their experiences. This tuning into their inner reality at the expense of shared social reality condemns them to remain socially isolated. However, in contrast to the avoidant group, they tend to continue to feel a need, and they ask for social support in which they tend to repeat relationships in which they feel misunderstood and mistreated and in which logical arguments have little impact on their capacity to adjust their expectations to the reality of what is being offered. Chaotic individuals tend to have very little order or apparent control over their actions and emotions.

TRAUMA AND LOSS OF SELF-REGULATION

When a child does not have enough resources to deal with states of arousal, external agents need to come to the rescue to reestablish a sense of security and predictability. When caregivers fail to quiet the child down, the child experiences a state of extreme stimulation, and the child's coping mechanisms will be overwhelmed.

Becoming overwhelmed by extreme emotional states may produce longlasting alterations in their physiological reactivity and effect brain development. While trauma at the hands of caregivers is probably the most common form of trauma for infants and young children, accidents, repeated surgical procedures, chronic medical illnesses, forced separations, witnessing violence, and other forms of uncontrollable experiences may have a similar impact on the psychology and biology of a developing child.

Loss of capacity for self-regulation is possibly the most far-reaching effect of psychological trauma because it affects the capacity to inhibit fight and flight reactions under threat (van der Kolk et al, 1996a). This interferes with the ability to think clearly about the precise nature of the presenting stimulus and to formulate the optimal behavioral response. Because they tend to experience current stressors with emotions that have an intensity that belongs to the past, traumatized and neglected individuals are vulnerable to rely on action, rather than thought, when they feel threatened.

Research about people's reactions to trauma has clearly demonstrated that the younger the age at which they are traumatized and the longer the trauma lasts, the more they are likely to have long-term problems with the regulation of anger, anxiety, and sexual impulses (van der Kolk et al, 1996b). Loss of self-regulation may be expressed on several different levels: as attentional problems (i.e., as a loss of ability to focus on appropriate stimuli) or as an inability to inhibit action when aroused (loss of impulse control, i.e., responding with uncontrollable feelings of rage, anger, or sadness). Unaware of the traumatic origins of these feelings, they are prone to experience both their own affect storms, as well as emotional reactions from others, as retraumatizing. Thus, the feelings that belong to the trauma are continually re-experienced on an interpersonal level: they often lead the person to traumatizing and traumatized lives.

Numbing and Self-destruction as Attempts at Self-regulation

Traumatized people use a variety of methods to regain control over their deficient capacity for emotional regulation. In an apparent attempt to compensate for their hyperarousal, some of them "shut down" on a behavioral level by avoiding stimuli reminiscent of the trauma and on a psychobiological level by emotional numbing, which may extend to both trauma-related stimuli and to everyday experience. Thus, people with chronic post-traumatic stress disorder (PTSD) tend to suffer from numbing of responsiveness to the environment, which gets in the way of taking pleasure in ordinary events. Other traumatized individuals may engage in particular behaviors that are geared to alter their physiological states. Often, these efforts are self-destructive and bizarre and range from self-mutilation to unusual sexual practices, from binging and purging to drug and alcohol abuse. Self-mutilation is a common reaction to social isolation and fear. Many abused children engage in head-banging, biting, burning, and cutting. Clinical studies consistently report childhood histories of extreme neglect, physical or sexual abuse, or repeated surgery in self-mutilators (van der Kolk et al, 1991).

Research has shown that the more severe people's histories of childhood neglect, the more serious were their suicide attempts, self-mutilation, and other destructive behaviors. People who could not remember feeling special or loved by anyone as children and those who, as children, had sustained prolonged separations from their primary caregivers were least able to rely on friends and others to help them feel better when they were upset and to control self-destructive impulses. Many people who habitually engage in deliberate self-harm report that self-mutilation makes them feel better and makes them feel alive.

Substance Abuse

Studies of populations with substance abuse consistently report childhood histories of abuse and neglect in much higher proportions than the general population. Ed Khantzian (1985) has proposed a self-medication theory of substance abuse, which suggests that drugs of abuse are selected according to their specific psychotropic effects. For example, heroin has powerful effects of muting feelings of rage and aggression, whereas cocaine has significant antidepressant action. Alcohol probably is the oldest medication for the treatment of posttraumatic stress and may well be an effective short-term medication for sleep disturbances, nightmares, and other intrusive posttraumatic symptoms. Self-help groups, such as Alcoholics Anonymous, often seem to intuitively have grasped the importance of these issues and have incorporated elements of effective posttraumatic treatment in their 12 steps.

Somatization: The Loss of Words and Symbols to Communicate with Self and Others

Trauma and neglect often lead to problems in developing the capacity to use words and symbols to identify what one is feeling. Research has shown that secure children spend more time describing physiological states, such as hunger, thirst, and states of consciousness, and speak more often about negative emotions, such as hate, disgust, and anger, whereas maltreated toddlers use fewer words to describe how they feel (Cicchetti and White, 1990). Not knowing how and what one feels may contribute to the impaired impulse control seen in abused children. Having problems putting feelings into words and formulating flexible response strategies makes people liable to act on their feelings. Anticipating recent neuroimaging studies (see below). Cicchetti and White (1990) hypothesized that "the special difficulties that abused toddlers have expressing feelings in words may not be simply a reflection of psychological intimidation but rather a manifestation of neuroanatomical and neurophysiological changes secondary to abusive or neglectful treatment." Being unable to create verbal constructs to identify what one is feeling in one's body puts a person at risk for developing psychosomatic reactions. Recent studies have shown that being able to talk about upsetting experiences decreases psychosomatic symptoms and enhances people's immune response.

DISSOCIATION

Splitting Off the Experience

Many traumatized children and adults who were traumatized as children have described how, under stress, they can make themselves disappear while watching what is going on from a distance. This gives them the sensation that what is happening is not really occurring to them, but to someone else. Dissociation can be an effective way to continue functioning while the trauma is going on, but if it continues to be utilized after the acute trauma has passed, it comes to interfere with everyday functioning. When children are repeatedly exposed to extreme stress, they often develop dissociative problems. Elements of the traumatic experience may be organized in separate states of mind that may be activated only under circumstances that match some emotional or sensory element of the trauma. Very complex forms of such secondary dissociations can be found in dissociative identity disorder (DID, formerly called multiple personality disorder).

Amnesia

For well over a century, psychiatrists and psychologists have noted that dissociation at the moment of the trauma may cause memory disturbances in which people may not be able remember some, or all, of the experience. For example, after the evacuation of Dunkirk at the start of the Second World War, Sargeant and Slater (1941) observed amnesia of the trauma in 144 of 1,000 consecutive admissions to a field hospital. The DSM has classified the issue of posttraumatic memory disturbances under the rubric of dissociative amnesia.

When Sigmund Freud (1914:150) observed such amnesias, he claimed that if a person does not remember a trauma, he is likely to act it out: "he reproduces it not as a memory but as an action; he repeats it, without knowing, of course, that he is repeating, and in the end, we understand that this is his way of remembering."

During the past decade, some people have called into question the validity of dissociative amnesia in adults with childhood sexual abuse histories. However, every study of adults with histories of childhood sexual abuse, whether prospective or retrospective, has consistently found that dissociative amnesia is relatively common in childhood victims of interpersonal violence (Williams, 1995), that when they return to consciousness, such memories tend to have a sensory and perceptual quality (van der Kolk and Fisler, 1995), and that they tend to be quite accurate (Williams, 1995). These sorts of amnesias also have been noted following medical and surgical procedures in children and adults. Amnesias for emotional and cognitive material seems to be age and dose related: the younger the age at the trauma and the more prolonged the trauma, the greater the likelihood of significant amnesia.

THE EFFECTS OF DEVELOPMENTAL TRAUMA ON CHARACTER FORMATION

A person's past shapes the schemes and assumptions that determine the perceptions of day-to-day experience. When a person is traumatized, this experience may come to color the traumatized person's views of himself and of the world. These schemes then serve as roadmaps for subsequent actions and expectations. Having a history of helplessness with people in power, they tend to cast most further relationships in terms of dominance and submission. When they are in a position of power, they often inspire fear and loathing, while, in a subordinate position, they often feel helpless, behave submissively, do not stand up for themselves, and tend to engage in idealization (and/or devaluation) at the expense of being able to experience their own competence. Many repeat their family patterns in interpersonal relationships, in which they may alternate between playing the role of victim or of persecutor, often justifying their behavior by their feelings of betrayal and helplessness.

Responsibility

When trauma occurs early in life, it may interfere with the capacity to properly attribute responsibility. Young children, by virtue of their cognitive level of development, attribute everything that happens to their own actions or their own magical thinking. Many traumatized people, particularly those first traumatized as children, suffer from a profound sense of responsibility for their own abuse and for subsequent problems over which they have no control. They often continue to have great difficulty in seeing various people's contributions to interpersonal problems.

Play

One of the principal tasks of childhood is to learn to negotiate collaborative relationships with other human beings. Traumatized children often have serious problems in their capacity to play (Terr, 1991). They tend to be either excessively shy and withdrawn or to bully and frighten other children (Cicchetti and White, 1990). Their inability to regulate their arousal, to articulate their feelings in words, and to attend to appropriate stimuli, and being triggered to reexperience feelings and sensations related to the trauma make it difficult to be attuned to their environments. The function of play in childhood is to try out different roles and different outcomes, to learn to appreciate how others experience the world, and to gain mastery over dreaded feelings, people, and situations.

When children do not learn to play, they have a hard time integrating the positive and negative aspects of life. Good and bad, power and helplessness, and affection and anger continue to be experienced as separate egostates. The overall result is that many traumatized children miss a critical developmental stage in which issues of competition, intimacy, and play are being negotiated. Without these skills, these children may grow up fearful or incapable of tackling the inevitable hassles that are part of all human relationships.

The Cycle of Violence:
The Compulsion to Repeat the Trauma

Many traumatized people become involved in social situations that bear a striking similarity to the context in which they were first traumatized. People engaged in these behavioral reenactments rarely are consciously aware that they are repeating earlier life experiences. In behavioral reenactments of the trauma, a person may play the role of victim, victimizer, or both.

Victimizing Others

Numerous studies of family violence have found a direct relationship between the severity of childhood abuse and later tendencies to victimize others (Widom, 1987). Reenactment of one's own victimization seems to be a major cause of the cycle of violence. Numerous studies have shown that criminals often have histories of physical and/or sexual abuse. For example, Dorothy Lewis found that of the 14 juveniles condemned to death for murder in the U.S. in 1987, 12 had been brutally physically abused and 5 had been sodomized by relatives (Lewis et al, 1988).

Revictimization

Once people have been traumatized, they are vulnerable to being victimized again on future occasions. Diane Russell's (1986) careful study on the effects of incest on the life of women found that few women made a conscious connection between their childhood victimization and their drug abuse, prostitution, and suicide attempts. Whereas 38% of a random sample of women reported incidents of rape or attempted rape after age 14, 68% of those with a childhood history of incest reported such an incident.

THE PSYCHOBIOLOGY
OF DEVELOPMENTAL TRAUMA

The task of the developing brain is to create an internal schema of the external world that can serve as a template for future adaptation. Although the fundamental neuroanatomical structure of the brain is determined by the genome, it is not fully configured by genetic factors alone (Spinelli, 1990). The particular template that is formed for the further categorization and interpretation of experience in the early years of life depends to a significant degree on the patterns, intensity, and frequency of neuronal stimulation received during critical periods of brain development (Schwartz and Goldman-Rakic, 1990). Experience thus creates the neuronal filters that determine how a person interprets the relevance of incoming information. While this plastic ability of the human brain facilitates the greatest degree of adaptability, it also makes the developing infant most vulnerable to the influences of caretakers who have a very large impact in determining the future learning predispositions and potential of the infant.

Thus, the template of the brain is, in part, a function of the sensory signals that are processed by the central nervous system (CNS). These signals are transcribed into neurochemical and cellular processes that affect brain structure and function. Particularly early in life, when the brain is still in the process of being organized, the patterns of experience affect the particular designs of dendritic branching and neuronal structures in a use-dependent fashion. This early organization has a major impact on the subsequent long-term organization of learning and cognition.

Different areas of the brain mature at different speeds, depending on the complexity of their function. For example, at birth, the brain stem areas responsible for regulating cardiovascular and respiratory function already are "on line." This allows the infant to execute these functions without outside help. The biological regulation mediated by the hypothalamus and brain stem is complemented by controls of the limbic system. The limbic system takes much longer to mature. For example, the hippocampus is not myelinated until later in childhood, which helps explain why people generally are incapable of verbal recall before the age of 3 or 4. Input from the limbic system controls activity of the pituitary gland, which, in turn, controls the production of hormones in the thyroid and adrenal glands. As we will see, irregularities of the hypothalamic–pituitary–adrenal (HPA) axis are among the major deficits produced by exposure to trauma. The limbic system also plays a role in the functions necessary for self-preservation and procreation, as well as parental care and play, all of which are known often to be disrupted in individuals with histories of trauma and neglect.

The neocortex is primarily oriented toward the external world and is involved in problem solving, learning, and complex stimulus discriminations. In addition, it plays a critical role in mediating the transcription of subjective states into communicable language to self and others. A well-functioning neocortex is necessary for deciding which sensory stimuli are relevant and which are not, for reasoning strategies to attain personal goals, for weighing a range of options for action, and for predicting the outcome of one's behavior. Traumatized individuals often have a great deal of trouble carrying out a host of these functions associated with a well-functioning prefrontal cortex. The neocortex is not fully myelinated until adolescence, and even then it continues to be flexible to further adaptation for much of a person's life. Thus, it is likely that trauma at an early age might disrupt subtle capacities for stimulus discrimination and social judgment.

The CNS of infants and children is more malleable than that of adults. Thus, they may, on the one hand, be more vulnerable to enduring damage in response to disruptive influences, and, on the other, to be more resilient if provided with proper care. As Perry states: "While experience may alter the behavior of an adult, experience literally provides the organizing framework for an infant and child" (Perry et al, 1995). While the study of the effects of environmental deprivation in humans is still in its scientific infancy, the neuro-developmental impact of extremes of sensory deprivation is very well documented in hundreds of animal studies. These studies include disruptions of visual stimuli, maternal deprivation, and social isolation (Perry et al, 1995). These studies demonstrate that there is considerable plasticity of the nervous system during the first year of life. However, mammals, including humans, require proper stimulation of certain areas of the CNS during critical periods of development in order to promote optimal functioning. If primates are exposed to potentially damaging influences *before* a critical period, the brain appears to be able to compensate for the injury. For example, one study found that non-human primates that sustained bilateral ablations of the amygdala and were returned to their mothers 6 to 12 hours later grew up no different from normal controls. However, such amygdala lesions sustained later stages of development resulted in devastating effects on social behavior. Similarly, in neonate rhesus macaques, prefrontal and temporal cortical ablation during the first 2 years of life has little effect on social affiliative bonds, provided they receive adequate mothering, but has devastating results thereafter.

If development is disrupted during critical periods, children may develop neurophysiologic sensitization and kindling. The system may become increasingly responsive to relatively minor stimuli. Sensitization could explain the behavior of many traumatized children. Minor triggers may precipitate full-blown catastrophic reactions. Over time, there may occur a generalization of responsiveness, in which these children start responding to even minor events as if they were exposed to a traumatic stimulus. As a result, many traumatized children suffer from extremes of emotional dysregulation. They may become impulsive, hyperactive, anxious, and aggressive. Lack of attention to the traumatic origins of these behaviors might lead clinicians to diagnose these children as manic–depressive (bipolar) or hyperactive, and, indeed, many of these children would meet the diagnostic criteria for these conditions.

To date, only a small number of studies have specifically addressed the biological abnormalities in abused and neglected children. Among the most noteworthy of these are the studies by Frank Putnam and his colleagues and Martin Teicher and his group. The prospective study of sexually abused girls at the National Institutes of Mental Health has shown that these girls develop major neuroendocrine disturbances, particularly in the areas of immune, corticosteroid, thyroid, and sex hormone functions (DeBellis et al, 1994a, 1994b). Martin Teicher and his colleagues have shown that childhood physical abuse is associated with limbic system abnormalities. They found a 38% increased rate of limbic system abnormalities following physical abuse, a 49% increase after sexual abuse, and a 113% increase following combined abuse. These studies confirm that early traumatic experience affects the development of the cerebral cortex and limbic system.

In a study of EEG abnormalities, Teicher and his coleagues found an association between abuse history and neurological abnormalities. Significantly, abused and nonabused patients differed only in the prevalence of left hemisphere abnormalities: left hemisphere deficits were seven times more common than right hemisphere deficits. These findings are consistent with research that has shown that abused children have significant problems in the dominant hemisphere function of language development (Cicchetti, 1991).

Hemispheric Lateralization

During the past few years, the availability of neuroimaging for documenting structural and functional abnormalities in PTSD has opened up new ways of understanding the neurobiological processes involved in trauma. While no neuroimaging studies of traumatized children have been done as yet, the brain images of traumatized adults complement the biological studies of traumatized children in providing some intriguing leads regarding the neurobiology of developmental trauma. Our recent positron emission tomography (PET) scans of adults with PTSD showed that when patients are exposed to stimuli reminiscent of their trauma, there is an increase in perfusion of the areas in the right hemisphere associated with emotional states and autonomic arousal, while there is a simultaneous decrease in oxygen utilization in Broca's area, the region in the left hemisphere responsible for generating words to attach to internal experience (Rauch et al, 1996).

These findings may account for the observation that trauma may lead to "speechless terror," which, in some individuals, interferes with the ability to put feelings into words, leaving them to be expressed mutely by dysfunction of the body. The emerging body of knowledge from these studies is stimulating a new focus on the neuronal filters concerned in the *interpretation* of sensory information, the interactions between the various parts of the CNS that process and interpret the meaning of incoming information.

The finding that there is a relative increase in right hemisphere functioning in response to stress and trauma and decreased left hemisphere functioning suggests that there is differential hemispheric involvement in the processing of traumatic experiences. Studies of split-brain patients have shown that the right hemisphere is involved in the expression and comprehension of global nonverbal emotional communication and in the regulation of autonomic and hormonal responses. People with intact right hemispheres are able to assign emotional significance to incoming stimuli and to attach physiological responses to emotional information. However, although this hemisphere may be sensitive to emotional nuances, it has, at best, a rudimentary capacity to think and to analyze the total cognitive context of incoming information (Joseph, 1989).

If, as research suggests, developmental trauma has a negative effect on left-hemisphere functioning, traumatized individuals can be expected to show deficiencies in the functions that are regulated by this hemisphere. This includes the capacity to organize problem-solving tasks into well-ordered sets of operations and to process information in a sequential fashion. The left hemisphere generates symbolic representations (words) and linguistically labels perceptions. It is in the area of categorization and labeling of internal states that traumatized individuals seem to have particular problems (van der Kolk et al, 1996a). They may be exquisitely sensitive to their environment, but they are prone to misinterpret information in the direction of threat.

Treatment Implications

Since safe attachments appear to be the primary way children learn to regulate internal emotional changes, the negotiation of interpersonal safety needs to be the first focus of treatment. Since the labeling and categorization of emotional states is one of the principal areas of functioning disrupted by developmental trauma, treatment needs to include learning how to use words to understand and interpret feelings in general and stressful events in particular. Since distrust and lack of social safety is a critical part of developmental trauma, trauma victims are at risk of becoming involved in painful misunderstandings with people who are in a position to hurt them. Learning how to identify and negotiate the fulfillment of one's emotional needs with people who are in a position to help them and to provide them satisfaction would be a critical aspect of treatment. This includes learning to interact with members of the medical profession for whom it is often very difficult to appreciate the extraordinary degree of power that their patients ascribe to them. Table 11–1 describes many of the findings related to early developmental trauma examined in this chapter.

Table 11–1 **Effects of Developmental Trauma (Complex PTSD)**

I. Alterations in regulating emotional arousal
   1. Chronic emotional dysregulation
   2. Aggression against others
   3. Self-destructive and suicidal behavior
   4. Difficulty modulating sexual involvement
   5. Impulsive and risk-taking behaviors
II. Alterations in attention and consciousness
   1. Amnesia
   2. Dissociation
III. Somatization
IV. Chronic characterological changes
   1. Alterations in self-perception: chronic guilt and shame, feelings of self-blame, ineffectiveness, and of being permanently damaged
   2. Alterations in relations with others
      A. Inability to trust or maintain relationships with others
      B. Tendency to be revictimized
      C. Tendency to victimize others
V. Neurobiology
   1. Increased right hemisphere function
   2. Decreased left hemisphere function
   3. Hypothalamic–pituitary–adrenal axis abnormalities

REFERENCES

Bowlby J: Attachment and Loss, Vol. 3. New York, Basic Books, 1980

Cicchetti D, White J: Emotion and developmental psychopathology. In Stein N, Leventhal B, Trebasso T (eds): Psychological and Biological Approaches to Emotion. Hillsdale, NJ, Erlbaum, 1990

Crittendon PM. Treatment of anxious attachment in infancy and early childhood. Dev Psychopathol 4:575–602, 1992

DeBellis MD, Chrousos GP, Dorn LD, et al: Hypothalamic-pituitary-adrenal axis dysregulation in sexually abused girls. J Clin Endocrinol Metab 78:249–255, 1994a

DeBellis MD, Lefter L, Trickett PK, et al: Urinary catecholamine excretion in sexually-abused girls. J Am Acad Child Adolesc Psychiatry 33:320–327, 1994b

Herman JL, Perry JC, van der Kolk BA: Childhood trauma in borderline personality disorder. Am J Psychiatry 146:490–495, 1989

Kegan: The Evolving Self. Cambridge, Harvard University Press, 1982

Kessler RC, Sonnega A, Bromet E, et al: Posttraumatic stress disorder in the National Comorbidity Survey. Arch Gen Psychiatry 52:1048–1060, 1995

Khantzian EJ: The self-medication hypothesis of addictive disorders: Focus on heroin and co-caine dependence. Am J Psychiatry 142:1259–1264, 1985

Lewis DO, Pincus JH, Bard B, et al: Neuropsychiatric, psychoedeucational, and family character-istics of 14 juvenile condemned to death in the US. Am J Psychiatry 145:584–589, 1988

MacLean PD: The tribune brain, emotion, and scientific bias. In Schmitt FO (ed): The Neurosciences, Second Study Program. New York, The Rockefeller University Press, 1970.

Perry BD, Pollard RA, Blakley TL, et al: Childhood trauma: The neurobiology of adaptation and use-dependent development of the brain. Infant Mental Health J 00:000–000, 1995

Reite M, Fields T (eds): The Psychobiology of Attachment and Separation. Orlando, FL, Academic Press

Russell DEH: The Secret Trauma: Incest in the Lives of Girls and Women. New York, Basic Books, 1986

Sargeant W, Slater E: Amnesic syndromes in war. Proc Royal Soc Med 34:757–764, 1941

Spinelli DN: Plasticity triggering experiences, nature, and the dual genesis of brain structure and function. Clin Perinatol 17:77–83, 1990

Stem D: The Interpersonal World of the Infant. New York, Basic Books, 1985

Terr L: Childhood traumas: An outline and overview. Am J Psychiatry 27:96–104, 1991

van der Kolk BA, Fisler R: Dissociation and the fragmentary nature of traumatic memories: Overview and exploratory study. J Trauma Stress 9:505–525, 1995

van der Kolk BA, McFarlene AC, Weisaeth L (eds): Traumatic Stress: Effects of Overwhelming Experiences on Mind, Body, and Society. New York, Guilford Press, 1996a

van der Kolk BA, Pelcovitz D, Roth S, et al: Dissociation, somatization, and affect dysregulation: The complexity of adaptation to trauma. Am J Psychiatry 153:83–93, 1996b

Widom CS: The cycle of violence. Science 244:160–165, 1987

Williams LM: Recovered memories of abuse in women with documented child sexual victimiza-tion histories. J Trauma Stress 8:649–676, 1995

IV

Biological Basis of Behavior

12 Neurobiological Aspects of Behavior

Cort A. Pedersen,
Bradley N. Gaynes,
Robert N. Golden,
Dwight L. Evans,
and John J. Haggerty, Jr.

Enormous advances in neuroscientific research in recent years have provided the basis for exciting insights into the biological basis of behavior and invigorated the search for the biochemical and genetic basis for the major psychiatric disorders. This chapter will present an overview of the major neural networks and primary neurochemical systems that underlie complex behavior. The basic neurochemical systems will be reviewed (norepinephrine, serotonin, acetylcholine, dopamine, and so forth) as well as the major neuroendocrine systems. The neurobiology of learning and memory will be reviewed, as well as basic neurobiological aspects of reproductive behavior, consumptive behavior, aggression, and stress responses. Finally, a brief overview of sleep architecture and physiology will be presented.

MAJOR COMPONENTS OF BEHAVIOR AND THEIR NEURAL CORRELATES

Behavior may be understood as the product of integrated activity of a number of interacting brain systems. Among these systems are mechanisms that monitor internal and external sensory input, focus and maintain attention to significant stimuli, and arouse other brain regions involved in behavioral response patterns. For example, if an external stimulus (e.g., food) harmonizes with an internal drive state (e.g., hunger), a specific behavioral motivational system (e.g., feeding) activates goal-directed motor sequences. If the "reward" (i.e., food) is achieved, the internal drive state is satisfied temporarily and the motivated behavior (i.e., food seeking and eating) ceases. Conversely, aversive stimuli (e.g., predator, unfamiliar object) will activate avoidant or aggressive defensive systems and initiate motor sequences, such as a fight-or-flight, freezing, or generally cautious approach. If the resulting behavioral response decreases the danger associated with the situation, avoidant or aggressive motivation usually will subside.

Activation of the brain's motivational system also is accompanied by arousal of endocrine and autonomic responses. Affective or mood-related systems also influence the intensity and quality of behavioral responses and, in higher animals and humans, generate a range of subjective experiences known as emotion.

The basic characteristics of rewarding or aversive stimuli determine the degree of emotional arousal in the organism. Frustration in achieving the goals associated with motivated or avoidant behavior also mobilizes affective responses. As discussed by Dr. Dorsett in Chapter 6, learning modifies behavior by allowing stimuli that otherwise might be neutral (conditioned stimuli) to become associated with rewarding or aversive stimuli (unconditioned stimuli). Through the learning process, conditioned stimuli become capable of activating arousal and attention mechanisms as well as motivational and affective systems. Thus, behavior is shaped by the following basic processes: arousal and attention, motivation, affect, motor performance, and learning. While much of the brain is involved to some extent in each of these components of behavior, certain brain areas and neural circuits are known to specialize in special areas. We will discuss the neuroanatomy, interconnecting pathways, and functions of brain regions that are involved in the activation and execution of behavior, specifically the reticular activating system, the hypothalamus, the limbic system, the association cortices, and the basal ganglia.

The Reticular Activating System

A diffuse network of neurons with widespread connections runs along the entire length of the midline brain stem. This system, referred to as the *reticular formation,* has long been known to influence level of consciousness (Kandel et al, 1991). We will describe later in the section on neurotransmitters ascending monoamine-containing pathways, which originate in the midbrain and ascend to forebrain structures. Neuronal cell bodies giving rise to these noradrenergic, dopaminergic, and serotonergic projections are located within the reticular formation. Reticular monoaminergic pathways influence the processing of sensory information at higher brain centers as well as at the level of the dorsal horn of the spinal cord where primary sensory neurons connect with the central nervous system (CNS). They also regulate behavioral arousal and control levels of awareness. In particular, noradrenergic pathways ascending from the locus ceruleus, a pontine nucleus, play a key role in establishing and maintaining focused attention on significant stimuli. Monoaminergic pathways ascending from the reticular formation project to many other regions of the CNS, including areas involved in initiation of motivated behaviors, affect, organization of motor output, and learning. *Thus, arousal and attention systems, originating in the midline brain stem, activate the neural substrates of other components of behavior.*

CLINICAL VIGNETTE: THE RETICULAR ACTIVATING SYSTEM AND ATTENTION

Children with attention deficit hyperactivity disorder (ADHD) have difficulty focusing their attention, are easily distracted, and appear "hyperactive." Treatment with psychostimulants such as methylphenidate have proven to be quite effective. While at first glance treating a "hyperactive" child with a stimulant appears paradoxical, the role of the noradrenergic neurons that are located in the reticular activating system explains its effectiveness. Noradrenergic projections to the cortex are thought to increase the ability to focus attention on salient stimuli. Thus, by releasing norepinephrine and stimulating noradrenergic receptors, psychostimulants counteract the attention deficit of children with ADHD.

The Hypothalamus

The hypothalamus is a midline structure at the base of the brain beneath the thalamus and attached to the pituitary gland below by the infundibulum (Fig. 12–1A). Anteriorly, it is bordered by the preoptic area, the optic chiasm, and the lamina terminalis; posteriorly, it extends to the caudal margins of the mammillary bodies. In humans, the hypothalamus is relatively small, constituting less than 1% of the entire brain. Despite its modest size, the hypothalamus contains a large number of neural circuits that regulate the internal environment and coordinate autonomic, endocrine, and behavioral systems that maintain homeostasis. Critical physiological parameters such as temperature, osmolarity, blood pressure, and glucose concentrations are monitored by specialized neurons within the hypothalamus. Other neurons are equipped with receptors that detect levels of reproductive or stress hormones.

The hypothalamus is divided by neuroanatomical convention in the anterior–posterior dimension into anterior, middle, and posterior regions and in the lateral–medial dimension into the lateral, medial, and periventricular regions (Figs. 12–1B and C). The descending column of the fornix separates the lateral and medial regions of the hypothalamus. The most well-defined nuclei of the hypothalamus are found in the medial region: the *preoptic* and *supraoptic* nuclei in the anterior region; the *paraventricular, dorsomedial,*

A

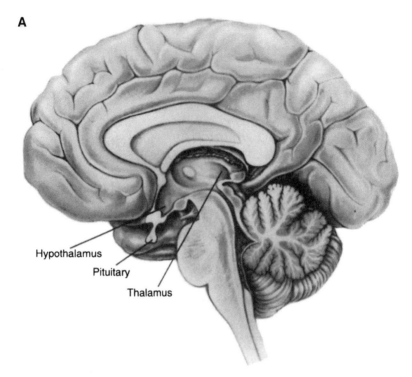

Figure 12–1. *The location and structure of the hypothalamus.* **A.** *Medial view showing the relationship of the hypothalamus to the pituitary and thalamus.*

and *ventromedial* nuclei in the middle region, and the *posterior* nucleus and *mammillary bodies* in the posterior region. The lateral region of the hypothalamus contains a number of ascending and descending pathways that connect rostrally with the forebrain. The largest of these is the *medial forebrain bundle* (MFB), which contains important fiber tracts that originate from aminergic neurons in the midbrain and project to neocortical regions. The periventricular region is composed of the portions of the hypothalamus immediately adjacent to the third ventricle. The basal parts of the medial and periventricular regions contain the *tuberal nuclei* in primates and the *arcuate nuclei* in subprimate species. The hypothalamus is interconnected with more rostral structures by fibers that course through the fornix, the mammillothalamic tract, and the stria terminalis. Connections with more caudal structures are made through the MFB, the mammillotegmental pathway, and the dorsal longitudinal fasciculus (Fig. 12–2).

Drive states originate within motivational systems located in the preoptic–hypothalamic area (Kandel et al, 1991). Some drive states (e.g., thirst, hunger, desire for warmth) result from changes in homeostasis of the internal physio-

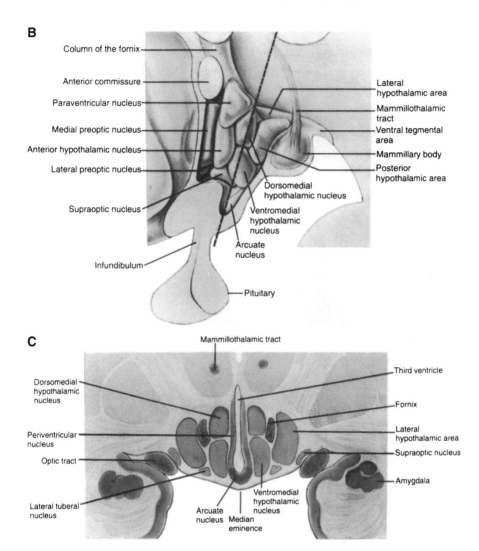

Figure 12–1. (continued). **B.** *Medial view showing positions of the main hypo-thalamic nuclei. Some nuclei are visible only in the frontal view in part C.* **C.** *Frontal view of the hypothalamus (section along plane shown in part B). (Reproduced with permission from Kandel ER, Schwartz JH, Jessell TM (eds): Principles of Neural Science. New York, Elsevier, 1991.)*

logical milieu. Indeed, specialized cells that monitor certain parameters of the internal state (osmolarity, glucose concentrations, temperature) may be directly involved in activating drive states. Sex-specific motivated behaviors (e.g. mating, parenting, social aggression) are dependent upon reproductive hormone conditions and the availability of appropriate external stimuli (e.g.,

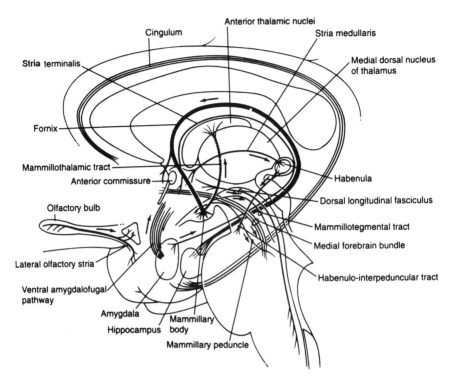

Figure 12–2. *Interconnections of the deep-lying structures included in the limbic system. The predominant direction of flow of neural activity in each tract is indicated by an arrow, but the designated tracts typically have bidirectional activity. (Reproduced with permission from Kandel ER, Schwartz JH, Jessell TM (eds): Principles of Neural Science. New York, Elsevier, 1991.)*

receptive females, newborns). As discussed earlier, threatening or painful conditions elicit avoidant, defensive, or submissive behaviors depending on the nature of the aversive situation. Output from motivational systems descends along the midline or through the MFB to the brain stem, where connections are made with pathways that control specific motor sequences. Beginning with the work of Olds and Milner in 1954, numerous investigators have found that electrical stimulation at some locations within the hypothalamus and associated structures (the limbic system and the MFB) acts as a potent reward. *Animals with electrodes in these regions stimulate themselves at very high rates for long periods of time even if they are in no drive state (i.e., not hungry, thirsty, sexually aroused, and so forth).* These findings have obvious significance for understanding the neurobiological basis of addiction. Stimulation at other hypothalamic sites elicit escape, aggressive, or submissive behavior. Dopaminergic neurons that are located in the ventral tegmental area of the midbrain and project to all parts of the limbic system are important in maintaining electrical self-stimulation and may have a more general role in the mediation of reward.

The *paraventricular* nucleus exemplifies the multifunctional role of the hypothalamus as a whole and many of its nuclei. Neurons in the paraventricular nucleus fall into three distinct groups: those projecting to the posterior pituitary, those projecting to the median eminence, and those projecting to extrahypothalamic sites in the limbic system or the brain stem. Many of the latter terminate in nuclei that regulate the autonomic nervous system. Neurons in the paraventricular nucleus, as well as throughout the mediobasal hypothalamus, synthesize and secrete into the portal hypophyseal vasculature the substances (for the most part small peptides) that promote or inhibit release of anterior pituitary hormones. Many of these hypothalamic neurons project to other brain sites where the release of peptides alter behavior. It is fascinating that the endocrine and behavioral effects of peptides are often harmonious. For example, luteinizing hormone-releasing hormone promotes both ovulation (by releasing luteinizing hormone from the anterior pituitary gland) and sexual behavior (by stimulating neurons in the ventromedial nucleus and the medial preoptic area of the hypothalamus), whereas corticotropin-releasing hormone stimulates both adrenal activation as well as various behavioral responses to stress by acting at the anterior pituitary and specific brain sites, respectively.

The Limbic System

As stated above, the hypothalamus appears to be the center of coordination of autonomic, endocrine, and behavioral aspects of affect and emotion (Kandel et al, 1991). *Ablation of the hypothalamus almost totally eliminates affective responses to stimuli.* The *parahippocampal* gyrus (including the underlying hippocampal formation), the cingulate gyrus, and the subcallosal gyrus encircle the underlying hypothalamus and midbrain (Fig. 12–3). These structures, which are considered to be phylogenetically primitive cortex, were first referred to as the limbic lobe by Paul Broca in the last century. In 1937, James Papez speculated that the limbic lobe may provide circuits through which emotional impulses arising within the hypothalamus could reach the cerebral cortex and, reciprocally, the cerebral cortex could modulate emotional states at the hypothalamic level (the Papez circuit). The limbic lobe also was thought to play a primary role in processing and integrating cognitive perceptions originating in the cerebral cortex and instinctive impulses emerging from the hypothalamus. Papez specifically proposed that information from the hypothalamus was conveyed from the mammillary bodies to the anterior thalamic nucleus along the mammillothalamic tract and then to the cingulate gyrus, where integration with information from the cerebral cortex would occur. Cortical influences then would be transmitted from the cingulate gyrus to the

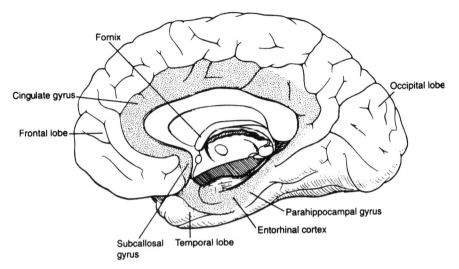

Figure 12–3. *This medial view of the brain shows the limbic lobe, which consists of primitive cortical tissue (stippled area) that encircles the upper brain stem. Also included in the limbic lobe are the underlying cortical structures (hippocampus and dentate gyrus). (Reproduced with permission from Kandel ER, Schwartz JH, Jessell TM (eds): Principles of Neural Science. New York, Elsevier, 1991.)*

hippocampal formation and from there along the fornix to the mammillary bodies (Fig. 12–4). Further processing of information would take place at each junction in this circuit.

Paul MacLean later suggested that other structures (Fig. 12–4) should be included in the limbic system first proposed by Papez. These included the *amygdala,* the *septum,* the *nucleus accumbens* (part of the striatum in the basal ganglia), portions of the *hypothalamus anterior to the mammillary bodies,* and the *orbitofrontal cortex* (part of the prefrontal and limbic association cortices).

Rostral structures within the limbic system have various modulating effects on the behavioral, autonomic, and endocrine output of the hypothalamus. For instance, in some species, lesions of the amygdala produce a placid state with muted emotional responses. On the other hand, lesions of the septum produce increased irritability and exaggerated rage responses to aversive stimuli. In primates, lesions of the orbitofrontal cortex, which connects with underlying limbic structures, *eliminate* normal levels of aggression and affective responsiveness, whereas electrical stimulation in this region has opposite effects.

Neuroanatomical studies have largely confirmed the speculations of Papez and MacLean about the organization of the limbic system and have described substantial interconnections between the hippocampal formation,

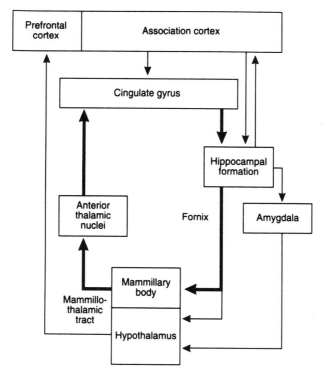

Figure 12–4. *The neural circuitry of the limbic system that probably mediates emotion. The circuit originally proposed by Papez is indicated by thick lines; additional connections later proposed by MacLean are indicated by fine lines. (Reproduced with permission from Kandel ER, Schwartz JH, Jessell TM (eds): Principles of Neural Science. New York, Elsevier, 1991.)*

amygdala, and the overlying neocortex. The association cortices project to the entorhinal cortex, which, in turn, projects along the perforant path through another area of cortex called the *subiculum* to the hippocampal formation. The subiculum, which gives rise to the efferent fibers in the fornix that innervate the hypothalamus, has extensive reciprocal connections with other brain areas, including the neocortex. The subiculum has been favored during evolution and has achieved its greatest relative size in humans. The amygdala contains a number of distinct nuclei that are reciprocally connected to the hippocampal formation, neocortex, thalamus, and hypothalamus. One of the two major projections from the amygdala, the stria terminalis, innervates the bed nucleus of the stria terminalis, the nucleus accumbens, and the hypothalamus. The other major efferent projection, the ventral amygdalofugal pathway, innervates the rostral cingulate gyrus, the dorsal medial nucleus of thalamus, and the hypothalamus (see Fig. 12–2).

CLINICAL VIGNETTE: THE LIMBIC CORTEX AND SEIZURES

Complex partial seizures, also known as "temporal lobe epilepsy," are a common form of seizure disorder. They most often originate from the limbic system area within the medial temporal lobe. Their clinical expression helps underscore the importance of the limbic system in consciousness, mood, perception, behavior, and cognition. At the beginning of a complex partial seizure, patients experience a clouding of consciousness and may seem quite confused. They may experience changes in mood, such as fear, depression, or pleasure. They may experience perceptual changes, such as auditory, visual, olfactory, or gustatory hallucinations. Their behavior may be marked by automatisms, such as lip smacking, chewing, or swallowing. After the episode has ended, patients have some degree of memory loss for the event.

The Association Cortices

During phylogeny the cerebral cortex increased enormously in size relative to other brain structures. The most impressive expansion has taken place in higher order motor and sensory cortex and association cortex (Fig. 12–5). There are three association cortices; the *prefrontal association cortex,* the *parietal–*

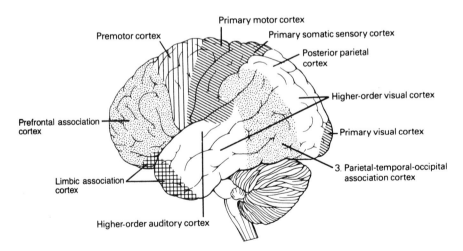

Figure 12–5. *A drawing of the lateral surface of the human brain on which are illustrated the locations of the primary sensory and motor cortices, the higher-order sensory and motor cortices, and the three association cortices. (Reproduced with permission from Kandel ER, Schwartz JH, Jessell TM (eds): Principles of Neural Science. New York, Elsevier, 1991.)*

temporal–occipital association cortex, and the *limbic association cortex.* Information from sensory organs projects initially to primary sensory cortices and then to higher-order sensory cortices where more complex analysis of sensation occurs. Each higher-order sensory cortex, in turn, projects to one, two, or all three association cortices. The association cortices integrate multimodal sensory information and initiate and execute a number of higher functions. The major functions of the association cortices are summarized in Table 12–1.

The *prefrontal association cortex,* which is quite sizeable in higher primates and humans, appears to be involved in thinking through potential future outcomes and selecting plans of action (executive functions). This cortex occupies the rostral and inferior portion of the frontal lobe just anterior to the premotor and primary motor cortex. The frontal association cortex is composed of two main subregions: the prefrontal association cortex proper, which is located on the dorsolateral surface of the frontal lobe, and the orbitofrontal cortex, which is located on the medial and ventral surface of the frontal lobe. The orbitofrontal cortex also is part of the limbic association cortex and the limbic system.

The prefrontal association cortex of the monkey is subdivided into the principal sulcus and the superior and inferior prefrontal convexities (Fig. 12–6A). *The principal sulcus* is critical to the successful performance of any task that requires retention of spatial information over time. Early studies showed that monkeys with discrete lesions of the principal sulcus were unable to remember into which of two containers a morsel of food had been placed 5 or more seconds previously. Further investigation has established that lesions of the principal sulcus do not produce a generalized deficit of short-term memory but rather a specific deficit in *working memory,* i.e., the ability to temporarily retain information that is being used to plan future action (Goldman-Rakic, 1990). Lesions of the *inferior prefrontal convexity* disrupt a monkey's ability

Table 12–1 **Major Functions of the Association Cortices**

PREFRONTAL	PARIETAL–TEMPORAL–OCCIPITAL	LIMBIC
Abstract thinking	Integration of multimodal sensory information	Emotional behavior, including aggression (orbitofrontal cortex and cingulate gyrus)
Working memory	Perception of spatial relationships	Memory storage (temporal lobe)
Planning	Understanding the meaning of words and syntax (dominant side) and nonsyntactic aspects of spoken language (nondominant side)	
Appropriate delay of responses		

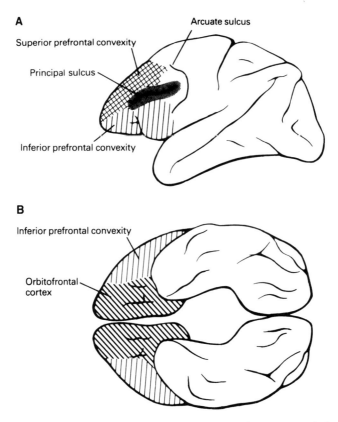

Figure 12–6. *Drawings of the basic subdivisions of the frontal association cortex of the monkey from the lateral view (**A**) and the ventral view (**B**). The orbitofrontal cortex is a subdivision of the limbic association cortex. (Reproduced with permission from Kandel ER, Schwartz JH, Jessell TM (eds): Principles of Neural Science. New York, Elsevier, 1991.)*

to perform any task involving delayed response, not just tasks that are spatial in nature. Lesions of an area of cortex adjacent to the principal sulcus, called the arcuate concavity, interfere with a monkey's ability to choose a specific motor response to a particular sensory cue. Thus, discrete portions of the prefrontal association cortex appear to subserve retention of specific sets of sensory information while the appropriate motor response is selected. The prefrontal association cortex sends projections primarily to other association cortices and to the premotor cortex.

The prefrontal cortex has been the focus of much recent speculation about the biology of schizophrenia. Neuropsychological tests reveal that schizophrenic patients have difficulty performing tasks requiring some of the delayed responses that depend upon the prefrontal association cortex.

Projections from dopaminergic neurons in the midbrain, disturbances of which are thought to occur in schizophrenia, terminate in the prefrontal cortex. Indeed, dopamine depletion in this area interferes with delayed responses. New imaging techniques show that schizophrenics do not exhibit the rise in blood flow or glucose uptake in the frontal lobes that occurs in normal subjects when they perform tasks that require prefrontal functions.

The *parietal–temporal–occipital association cortex,* which is located at the juncture between the three cerebral lobes for which it is named, is surrounded by and highly interconnected with higher-order somatic, visual, and auditory cortices. The primary function of this association cortex is to integrate multimodal sensory information to create a three-dimensional representation of the external environment. This task appears to be shared with the prefrontal association cortex because regions in both cortices, which are involved in processing spatial information, are interconnected and project to the same targets. Damage to the parietal–temporal–occipital association cortex can produce *severe distortions in body image* and *perception of spatial relationships.* Damage to the *dominant* (usually left) side of this association area often results in *aphasia,* the inability to understand spoken or written language, and *agnosia,* the inability to recognize objects. Patients with lesions of the *nondominant* (usually right) side of this association cortex frequently exhibit *deficits in understanding and utilizing nonsyntactic aspects of spoken language, such as the meaning conveyed by the tone, pitch, rhythm, and timing of words.*

The *limbic association cortex* is composed of two regions: the orbitofrontal cortex (Fig. 12–6B) and the *cingulate gyrus,* which are involved in emotional behavior and the *anterior and inferior pole of the temporal lobe,* which is primarily involved in memory *storage.* As mentioned in the description of the limbic system, ablation of the orbitofrontal cortex in monkeys was noted earlier in this century to markedly diminish aggressiveness and emotional responsivity. Because of these striking results in animals, prefrontal lobotomies or transection of pathways connecting the frontal lobes to other parts of the brain were performed in human patients who suffered from severe mental illnesses associated with high levels of agitation and dangerous aggressiveness. Although many of these patients became significantly calmer after surgery, a number of undesirable side effects, such as alterations in personality including loss of initiative and drive, disinhibition of behavior and speech, and impaired judgment, also became apparent. Neuropsychological testing revealed that patients who had undergone these types of psychosurgery had difficulty changing strategies when switching from one mental task to another.

The *temporal lobe* portion of the limbic association cortex is involved in the acquisition and retention of long-term *memory.* This will be described in more detail later in the section on Learning and Memory. There is some regional specificity within this portion of the limbic lobe concerning where memories involving specific sensory modalities are stored. For example, memories of visual stimuli tend to be stored in the inferior temporal lobe nearer higher-order visual cortex, whereas memories of auditory stimuli are stored selectively in the superior temporal lobe region of the limbic association cortex, which is adjacent to higher-order auditory cortex. The left (dominant) temporal lobe specializes in verbal and linguistic memory, whereas the right nondominant temporal lobe specializes in memory for spatial and temporal patterns of sensory input. The temporal lobe portion of the limbic association area probably plays a role in emotional responses as well. Stimulation of this area has been reported to produce a variety of emotions. Intensification of emotional feelings often is seen in patients suffering from temporal lobe epilepsy.

The Basal Ganglia

The essence of behavior is purposeful movement. Motor neurons arising in the anterior horn of the spinal cord or cranial nuclei are controlled directly or indirectly by cerebrospinal or cerebrobulbar neurons that originate in the motor cortex. The motor output of this system is regulated by the premotor and prefrontal cortex, the cerebellum, and the basal ganglia (Kandel et al, 1991). Voluntary movement requires a plan of action (motor plan), which is formulated in the premotor and prefrontal cortices. The cerebellum compares descending motor control signals with sensory signals resulting from motor action and then adjusts the motor signals at the level of the motor cortex and brain stem motor nuclei. In addition to processing motor information, the basal ganglia play a critical role in integrating information about motivational and emotional state into the motor planning process.

The basal ganglia are composed of five large subcortical nuclei: the caudate nucleus, the putamen, the globus pallidus, the subthalamic nucleus, and the substantia nigra. The globus pallidus (also called the pallidum) consists of an external and internal segment. The substantia nigra also is subdivided into the pars reticulata caudally and the more rostral, dark-stained pars compacta where dopamine-synthesizing cell bodies are located. Almost all of the input to the basal ganglia comes directly or indirectly from the cerebral cortex, and their output is routed through the thalamus back to the portions of the cerebral cortex involved in motor control (i.e., the prefrontal, premotor, supplementary motor, and primary motor cortices). Although this system plays a major role in controlling motor aspects of voluntary behavior, it also is involved in cognition and emotion.

The caudate nucleus and putamen, which together are called the neostriatum (most commonly referred to as the striatum), receive all of the input to the basal ganglia (Fig. 12–7A). These two structures develop from the same telencephalic tissue, are composed of similar neurons, and are fused anteriorly. Every region of the cerebral cortex projects to the striatum; these projections are topographically organized. The different portions of the striatum specialize in aspects of behavior controlled by the regions of cortex from which they receive projections. Thus, the *putamen* is primarily involved in motor control,

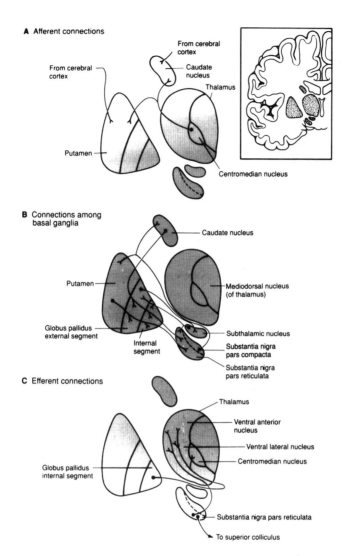

Figure 12–7. *The major connections of the basal ganglia.* **A.** *The caudate nucleus and putamen receive almost all afferent input to the basal ganglia.* **B.** *The connections between the nuclei of the basal ganglia are topographically organized.* **C.** *Efferents from the basal ganglia connect principally with the thalamus. (Reproduced with permission from Kandel ER, Schwartz JH, Jessell TM (eds): Principles of Neural Science. New York, Elsevier, 1991.)*

the *caudate* regulates eye movements and some cognitive functions, and the *ventral striatum,* which is linked to the limbic system, modulates emotion. The striatum also receives topographically organized input from the intralaminar nuclei of the thalamus. The motor cortex exerts strong control over the basal ganglia through its projection to the centromedian nucleus of the thalamus, which in turn projects to the putamen. The ventral striatum (which contains the nucleus accumbens, a portion of the limbic system) receives the important mesolimbic dopaminergic projection from the ventral tegmental area that transmits motivational and emotional information originating from the hypothalamus and limbic system to the basal ganglia. Aberrant dopaminergic neurotransmission in this pathway has been implicated in psychotic disorders such as schizophrenia (Deutch, 1992).

There are several pathways interconnecting the basal ganglia (Fig. 12–7B). The caudate and the putamen project to the external and internal segments of the globus pallidus and to the pars reticulata portion of the substantia nigra. The external segment of the pallidum projects to the subthalamic nucleus, which projects back to the external and internal segments of the globus pallidus as well as to the substantia nigra pars reticulata. The motor and premotor cortices exert additional influence on the basal ganglia through direct connections with the subthalamic nucleus. The substantia nigra pars compacta sends an important dopaminergic projection to both portions of the neostriatum.

Outputs from the basal ganglia (Fig. 12–7C) originate from the internal segment of the globus pallidus and the substantia nigra pars reticulata and project to three nuclei in the thalamus: the ventral lateral, ventral anterior, and mediodorsal nuclei. The internal segment of the globus pallidus also projects to the centromedian nucleus of the thalamus. These thalamic nuclei project to the motor cortex, supplementary motor cortex, premotor cortex, and prefrontal cortex.

Neural projections from the cerebral cortex to the striatum release the excitatory neurotransmitter *glutamate,* which activates both a direct and an indirect pathway through the basal ganglia (Fig. 12–8). The direct pathway originates in the striatum and terminates in the internal segment of the pallidum and the substantia nigra pars reticulata. Gamma-aminobutyric acid (GABA) and substance P are the neurotransmitters released by this pathway; they inhibit activity of the GABAergic projections from the output nuclei of the basal ganglia to the thalamus. Cortical activation of the striatum increases the inhibitory signals to the output nuclei of the basal ganglia, which, in turn, diminishes inhibitory transmission to the thalamic nuclei. Movement is facilitated when disinhibited thalamic projections activate premotor and supplementary motor cortex projections to the motor cortex, the brain stem, and the spinal cord.

Activation of the indirect pathway through the basal ganglia has the end result of inhibiting movement. The first link in this pathway is a projection from the striatum to the external segment of the globus pallidus mediated by GABA and enkephalin that inhibits an inhibitory GABAergic projection to the sub-

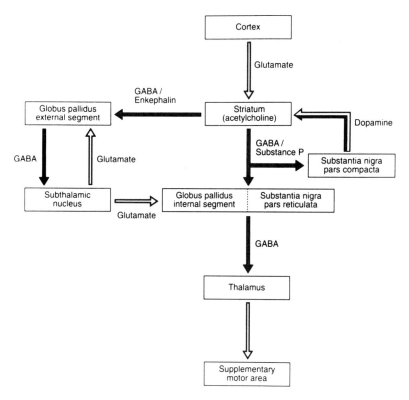

Figure 12–8. *This figure summarizes current knowledge about neurotransmitters released by afferent, efferent, and internuclear pathways of the basal ganglia. The direct and indirect routes through the basal ganglia are also illustrated. (Black arrows represent inhibitory pathways; white arrows represent excitatory pathways.) (Reproduced with permission from Kandel ER, Schwartz JH, Jessell TM (eds): Principles of Neural Science. New York, Elsevier, 1991.)*

thalamic nucleus. This produces increased activity of an excitatory glutamate-mediated link to the output nuclei of the basal ganglia, which increases inhibition of thalamic projections to motor areas of the cortex. The dopaminergic projection from the substantia nigra to the striatum excites the direct pathway but decreases activity in the indirect pathway. The result of both effects is to facilitate cortical initiation of movement.

The direct and indirect pathways through the basal ganglia appear to counterbalance each other. Deterioration, such as occurs in the nigrostriatal dopamine neurons in Parkinson's disease or trauma in the basal ganglia, may lead to imbalance between these pathways and impairment of movement (as well as cognition and emotion) of one type or another depending upon the location of the disturbance.

NEUROCHEMICAL DETERMINANTS OF BEHAVIOR

"Classic" Neurotransmitters

The Discovery of Neurotransmission

Although scientific interest and curiosity about the nervous system date back to antiquity, the concept of biochemical compounds acting as the mediators of neural transmission is less than 100 years old. In the late 19th century, a number of investigators demonstrated that adrenal extracts could produce physiological effects that were strikingly similar to those seen following stimulation of sympathetic nerves; adrenaline (epinephrine) was subsequently identified as the active compound in these extracts. In 1904, Langely demonstrated that pilocarpine could mimic the effects of parasympathetic nerve stimulation. The next year, Elliot pulled together these observations in formulating a hypothesis of chemical neurotransmission. Elliot proposed that nerve endings might release small amounts of a chemical substance, such as adrenaline, which might then act on effector sites (Elliot et al, 1977).

The initial proof of the hypothesis of neurochemical transmission focused on acetylcholine (ACH). In 1907, Dixon reexamined the physiological effects of muscarine and argued that parasympathetic nerves release a muscarinelike compound. Over the next decade, Dale and colleagues performed a series of studies that led them to conclude that ACH was involved in parasympathetic neurotransmission. Dale proposed that the parasympathetic nerve fibers should be described as "cholinergic," and that ACH and similar compounds should be called "parasympathomimetic." Then, in 1921, Loewi performed a series of elegant experiments on isolated frog hearts connected by perfusion media. He found that vagus nerve stimulation of innervated heart produced a compound, which he called "vagusstoff," which slowed the second, denervated heart. Vagusstoff was found to be acetylcholine (Elliot et al, 1977).

During the same year of Loewi's classic experiments, Cannon and Uridil isolated "sympathin," a compound that was released following stimulation of sympathetic nerves. Later studies showed that sympathin was released by all sympathetic nerves. In 1946, Von Euler identified norepinephrine as the "sympathin" neurotransmitter of the sympathetic nervous system (Elliot et al, 1977).

As interest in neurotransmission grew, a number of criteria were established for determining whether a particular substance is, in fact, a neurotransmitter (Table 12–2). It is quite difficult to demonstrate for a given substance that all of these criteria have been met. Thus, we often refer to "putative" neurotransmitters, because most, but not all, of these criteria have been met for a number of substances.

Table 12–2 **Criteria for a Neurotransmitter**

1. Neurons contain the substance.
2. Neurons synthesize the substance.
3. Neurons release the substance upon depolarization.
4. The substance is physiologically active on neurons.
5. The postsynaptic physiologic response to the substance is identical to that of the neurotransmitter released by neurons.

(Adapted from Hyman SE, Coyle JT: The neuroscientific foundations of psychiatry. In Hales RE, Yudofsky SC, Talbott JA (eds): Textbook of Psychiatry, 2nd ed. Washington, DC, American Psychiatric Press, 1994)

Further study of neurotransmission also led to the discovery of second messengers, intracellular intermediaries that are produced in response to neurotransmitters (first messengers) and create a cellular response in the target cell.

We briefly review here the physiology of some of the "classic" neurotransmitters and important second messengers. We have selected those neurotransmitters that seem to be most relevant and most extensively studied in reference to normal and pathological human behavior and those second messengers that appear prominent in the brain.

First Messengers: Representative "Classic" Neurotransmitters

How does one establish a link between a neurotransmitter and behavior? This is an exceedingly complex challenge, because the study of both neurotransmission and behavior is difficult. Nonetheless, Reis (1974) has provided useful guidelines for establishing a connection between these complex phenomena (Table 12–3).

Table 12–3 **Criteria for Linking a Neurotransmitter to a Behavior**

1. The neurotransmitter must be present in the central nervous system.
2. Precursors and enzymatic machinery for synthesis and degradation must be present in association with the transmitter.
3. A characteristic pattern of transmitter release should occur in relation to the behavior.
4. Elicitation of the characteristic transmitter release pattern should evoke the behavior.
5. Destruction of the involved neuronal system should both deplete the transmitter and abolish normal control of that behavior.
6. Increases or decreases in transmitter activity should have opposing behavioral effects.

(Reis DJ: Considerations of some specific behaviors or disease. J Psychiatr Res 11:145–148, 1974)

Representative "Classic" Neurotransmitters

Norepinephrine. Historically, the catecholamine norepinephrine (NE) has been viewed as a stress-related hormone. Hans Selye described the critical role it plays in orchestrating the physiological response to stress. Cannon identified NE and epinephrine (EPI) as key components in the mobilization of the organism for a fight-or-flight response to stimuli that are perceived as threatening.

The metabolic pathways involved in the synthesis of NE, as well as the other catecholamines dopamine (DA) and EPI, are shown in Fig. 12–9. The amino acid tyrosine is taken up into the neuronal cell body where it becomes the basic "building block" for catecholamine synthesis. The rate-limiting step involves hydroxylation by the enzyme tyrosine hydroxylase. Catabolism of the catecholamines is accomplished by several enzymes acting in an extensive pathway. Monoamine oxidase (MAO) is the enzyme that is principally involved in the intraneuronal degradation of catecholamines, where it catalyzes the oxidative deamination of NE. Catechol-O-methyltransferase (COMT) plays a similar role in the extraneuronal catabolism of NE and the other catecholamines. The O-methylated products of COMT catabolism also become substrates for further degradation by MAO. MHPG (3-methoxy-4-hydroxy-phenylglycol) is a major metabolite of NE. Figure 12–10 summarizes the metabolism of NE and DA.

In humans, noradrenergic neurons are organized into anatomically and functionally discrete nuclei in the upper brain stem. Two of the most important are the locus ceruleus, which projects extensively within the CNS (Figs. 12–11 and 12–12), and the nucleus of the tractus solitarius, which projects to the brain stem and the peripheral autonomic nervous system. Noradrenergic neurons also are organized into ganglia in the peripheral sympathetic nervous system.

Neurotransmission in noradrenergic systems is representative of synaptic transmission for the biogenic amines (NE, EPI, DA, serotonin). When NE,

Figure 12–9. *The biosynthetic pathway for catecholamines. Tyrosine hydroxylase is activated by phosphorylation by protein kinases, and the synthesis of phenylethanolamine-N-methyl transferase depends on glucocorticoids. (Reproduced with permission from Hyman SE, Coyle JT: The neuroscientific foundations of psychiatry. In Hales RE, Yudofsky SC, Talbott JA (eds): Textbook of Psychiatry, 2nd ed. Washington, DC, American Psychiatric Press, 1994.)*

Figure 12–10. *Dopamine and norepinephrine metabolism. The following abbreviations are used: DOPA, dihydroxyphenylalanine; DA, dopamine; NE, norepinephrine; DOMA, 3,4-dihydroxymandelic acid; DOPAC, 3,4-dihydroxy-phenylacetic acid; DOPEG, 3,4-dihydroxyphenylglycol; DO-PET, 3,4-dihydroxy-phenylethanol; MOPET, 3-methoxy-4-hydroxyphenylethanol; MHPG, 3-methoxy-4-hydroxy-phenylglycol; HVA, homovanillic acid; VMA, 3-methoxy-4-hydroxy-mandelic acid; NM, normetanephrine; MTA, 3-methoxytyramine; MAO, monoamine oxidase; COMT, catechol-O-methyl transferase; Dashed arrows indicate steps that have not been firmly established. (Reproduced with permission from Cooper JR, Bloom FE, Roth RH (eds): The Biochemical Basis of Neuropharmacology. New York, Oxford, 1996.)*

Figure 12–11. *The primary projections of the noradrenergic locus ceruleus. (Reproduced with permission from Hyman SE, Coyle JT: The neuroscientific foundations of psychiatry. In Hales RE, Yudofsky SC, Talbott JA (eds): Textbook of Psychiatry, 2nd ed. Washington, DC, American Psychiatric Press, 1994.)*

which is stored in presynaptic vesicles, is released, it diffuses across the synaptic cleft and interacts with postsynaptic receptors (Figs. 12–13 and 12–14). This leads to a cascade of events by a "second messenger" system (Fig. 12–15).

Noradrenergic receptors are classified, and subclassified, based on their characteristic responsivity to different agonists (Table 12–4). Thus, for *alpha₁-adrenergic* receptors, the pharmacologic potency (i.e., amount of drug required to produce a particular effect) of agonists can be "rank ordered" as EPI > NE > isoproterenol (ISO); for *alpha₂*-adrenergic *receptors,* the rank order of agonist potency is NE = EPI > ISO; the rank order of agonist potencies for *beta₁*- and *beta₂-adrenergic* receptors is ISO > EPI = NE and ISO > EPI > NE, respectively.

Alpha₁ receptors are found postsynaptically in both the sympathetic nervous system and the brain. Alpha₂ receptors are often located presynaptically in the locus ceruleus and in sympathetic terminals, where they are thought to function as autoreceptors that modulate output by serving as homeostatic regulators; they also are found postsynaptically in certain sites, such as the pituitary gland, where they play a role in regulating growth hormone release. Beta₁ receptors are found regionally in the brain, and beta₂ receptors are located on glial and neural tissues in the brain.

Electrophysiologists have advanced the concept that NE serves as an "orchestrator" or modulator of other signals in the CNS. In the cerebellum, for example, NE released following locus ceruleus stimulation decreases the spontaneous firing of Purkinje cells, thereby increasing the relative signal generated

(continued on p. 432)

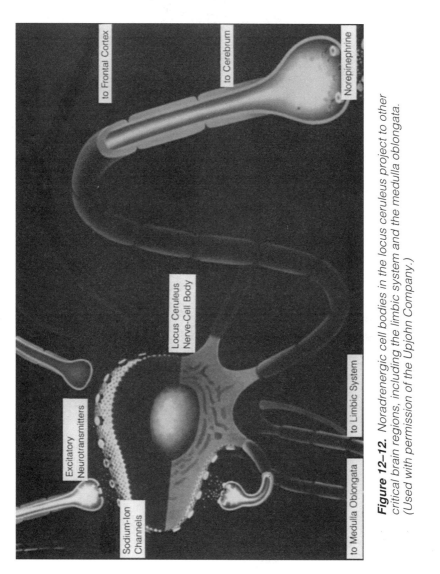

Figure 12–12. *Noradrenergic cell bodies in the locus ceruleus project to other critical brain regions, including the limbic system and the medulla oblongata. (Used with permission of the Upjohn Company.)*

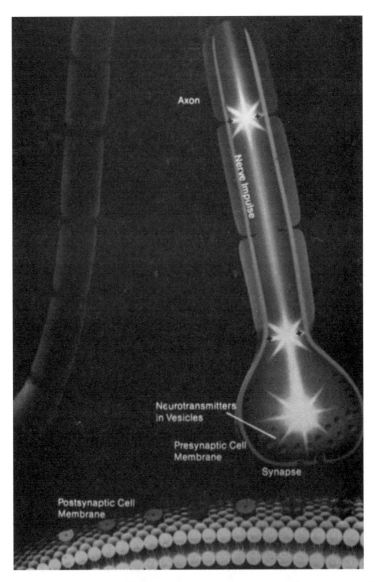

Figure 12–13. *Neurotransmitters are released from presynaptic storage vesicles and diffuse across the synaptic cleft, where they interact with the postsynaptic cell membrane. (Used with permission of the Upjohn Company.)*

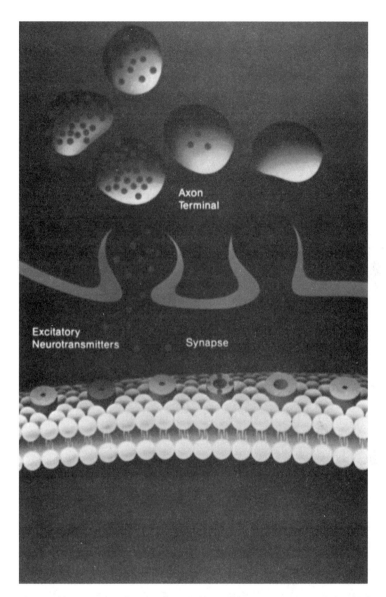

Figure 12–14. *Neurotransmitters, when released from storage vesicles in the presynaptic axon terminal, bind to those postsynaptic receptors that offer the best "fit." (Used with permission of the Upjohn Company.)*

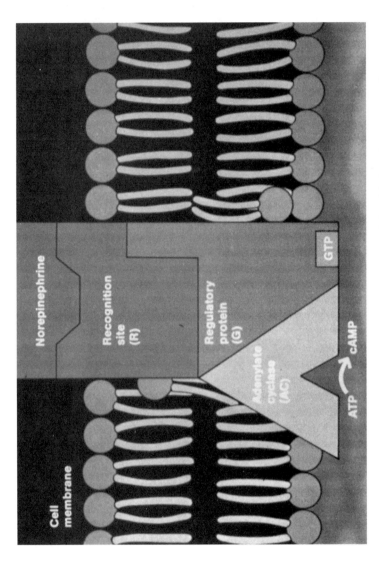

Figure 12–15. *After the neurotransmitter norepinephrine binds to its receptor site on the postsynaptic membrane, it sets into play a cascade of events, leading to the formation of cyclic AMP. (Used with permission of the Upjohn Company.)*

Table 12–4 **Drug and Neurotransmitter Receptors Relevant
to Psychopharmacology**

RECEPTOR TYPE	CHARACTERISTICS
Adrenergic	
Alpha$_1$	Located postsynaptically in both the sympathetic nervous system and brain (where it is found on both neurons and blood vessels). Produces vasoconstriction. Agonist potency: EPI > NE > ISO.
Alpha$_2$	Mostly presynaptic autoreceptor (in sympathetic terminals, locus ceruleus) but also postsynaptic (e.g., in pituitary: medicates growth hormone release). Agonist potency: NE = EPI > ISO. Clonidine is selective agonist; yohimbine is selective antagonist.
Beta$_1$	Localized in heart > lung; found regionally in brain. Stimulates heart. Agonist potency: ISO > EPI = NE. Practolol is selective antagonist.
Beta$_2$	Localized in lung > heart; found in brain, glia > neurons. Produces bronchodilation, vasodilation. Agonist potency: ISO > EPI > NE. Salbutamol, terbutaline are selective agonists.
Beta$_3$	Recently identified. Found in adipose tissue. Agonist potency: NE > ISO > EPI. Insensitive to blockade by most beta-adrenoreceptor antagonists.
Serotonin (5-HT)	Four distinct receptor classes:
5-HT$_1$	High affinity for 5-HT. Divided into subtypes that differ by nucleic acid sequencing and pharmacological profiles.
5-HT$_{1A}$	Found in gut and dorsal raphe nucleus in various species. Appears to mediate contraction in gut and neuronal inhibition in brain. Spiperone is antagonist; the anxiolytic, buspirone, is partial antagonist.
5-HT$_{1B}$	Found in cortex and sympathetic nervous system. Mediates contraction of smooth muscle and neuronal inhibition.
5-HT$_{1C}$	Found in stomach; mediates contraction.
5-HT$_{1D}$	Linked to inhibition of adenylyl cyclase.
5-HT$_{1E}$	Linked to inhibition of adenylyl cyclase.
5-HT$_{1F}$	Linked to inhibition of adenylyl cyclase.
5-HT$_2$	Found in brain, platelets, gut, and uterus. Down-regulated by antidepressant treatment. Mediates "serotonin syndrome." Methysergide, cyproheptadine, and ketanserine are antagonists.
5-HT$_3$	Linked to ligand-gated ion channels.
5-HT$_4$	Linked to stimulation of adenylyl cyclase.

(continued)

Table 12–4 *(continued)*

RECEPTOR TYPE	CHARACTERISTICS
Three potential additional receptor classes	
5-HT$_5$	Unknown effector mechanism.
5-HT$_6$	Linked to stimulation of adenylyl cyclase.
5-HT$_7$	Linked to stimulation of adenylyl cyclase.
Dopamine	All known dopamine receptors to date are members of the G-protein superfamily. They fall into two general classes based on pharmacological functional and molecular characteristics.
D$_1$-like	Two genes are known that code for two receptors: D$_1$ (or alternately D$_{1a}$) and D$_5$ (or alternately D$_{1b}$). The former exists in much higher density than the latter. Significant pharmacological and functional differences are only speculative.
	The members of this subfamily are linked to stimulatory G-protein-mediated events such as stimulation of cAMP synthesis.
	Selective antagonists include drugs chemically similar to SCH23390 (phenyltetrahydrobenzazepines). Although D$_1$-like receptors also bind many traditional antipsychotics (like haloperidol or chlorpromazine); they have low affinity for raclopride, sulpiride, and other benzamides.
D$_2$-like	At least three genes code for four different receptors: D$_{2long}$, D$_{2short}$, D$_3$, and D$_4$. Of these, the D$_{2long}$ is expressed at the highest levels. The D$_3$ and D$_4$ may occur somewhat selectively in limbic and cortical areas.
	The members of this subfamily are linked to inhibitory G-protein-mediated events such as inhibition of cAMP synthesis.
	They bind traditional antipsychotics (butyrophenones like haloperidol; phenothiazines, like chlorpromazine; etc.), but have selectivity for substituted benzamides like raclopride or sulpiride.
	Clozapine appears to have some selectivity for the D$_4$ receptor, suggesting an important role for this receptor in the unique antipsychotic action of this drug. Significant pharmacological and functional differences between these subtypes have not been conclusively resolved.
Muscarinic Cholinergic	Antagonized by atropinelike drugs, but also by tricyclic antidepressants, many antihistamines, and low-potency neuroleptics, resulting in side

(continued)

Table 12–4 *(continued)*

RECEPTOR TYPE	CHARACTERISTICS
	effects. Loss of muscarinic cholinergic transmission in Alzheimer's disease may be partly responsible for cognitive decline. Three types generally are recognized pharmacologically, but five types have been identified by cloning.
M_1	Located in sympathetic ganglia, frontal cortex, corpus striatum, and hippocampus.
M_2	Located in brain stem, cerebellum, and heart. Recently shown to open a K^+ channel by a G-protein-linked mechanism causing hyperpolarization and, therefore, bradycardia.
M_3	Major muscarinic receptor in exocrine glands; in relatively low density throughout the brain.
GABA	Two types:
GABA$_A$	Mediates classic inhibitory transmission in higher brain centers. (Glycine serves this purpose in the brain stem and spinal cord.) Thus, receptors found on majority of neurons in forebrain. The receptor also contains binding sites for benzodiazepines and barbiturates. Binding of these drugs increases the affinity of the receptor for GABA. Muscimol is a selective agonist; bicuculline (proconvulsant) is an antagonist.
GABA$_B$	Works through G proteins, not Cl⁻ channel (nonclassic effect). Baclofen is selective agonist.
Opiate	At least three types; naloxone is an antagonist at all types with affinity: $\mu > \delta > \kappa$.
mu (μ)	Localized in periaqueductal gray, thalamus, substantia gelatinosa of spinal cord, and other regions. Mediates analgesia and indifference to pain, miosis, and respiratory depression. Morphine and related opiate alkaloids are exogenous agonists; beta endorphin and the enkephalins are endogenous agonists.
delta (δ)	Highest density in limbic system. Mediates analgesia, hypotension, and miosis. Enkephalins are endogenous agonists. No selective agonists in clinical use because only peptide agonists known.
kappa (κ)	Located in deep conical layers. Mediates sedating analgesia, miosis. Benzomorphan drugs (e.g., ketamine, pentazocine) are selective agonists; dynorphins are endogenous agonists.

Abbreviations: Epi = epinephrine, ISO = isoproterenol, NE = norepinephrine.
Note: Where possible, clinically relevant agonists and antagonists are listed. The most selective agonists and antagonists often are not clinically important.

by exogenous stimuli. Thus, NE increases the "signal-to-noise" ratio in that area of the brain, thereby increasing reactivity to stimuli. In a similar way, projections from the locus ceruleus to other areas in the brain, such as the hypothalamus and cortex, may enhance responsiveness to exogenous stimuli (Golden and Potter, 1986).

Historically, NE has played a pivotal role in the development of biological theories relating to the pathogenesis of mood disorders such as depression. Two decades ago, the original formulations of the "catecholamine hypothesis of depression" identified decreased functional activity of central NE systems as an etiological mechanism in the development of depressive illness (Bunney and Davis, 1965; Schildkraut, 1965). More recently, with our growing appreciation for the complex dynamic regulatory mechanisms of neurotransmitter control, researchers have emphasized relatively subtle forms of NE systems dysregulation rather than absolute deficiencies (Golden and Potter, 1986).

More recently, the role of the locus ceruleus and the NE system has received attention as being involved in the pathogenesis of panic disorder, a severe anxiety disorder often accompanied by agoraphobia (Charney et al, 1995). Although the exact mechanisms are not clear, it is believed that some sort of disruption or dysregulation in the locus ceruleus/NE system results in a flooding of the CNS with anxiety and a plethora of secondary physiological and psychological symptoms.

Serotonin. Serotonin, or 5-hydroxytryptamine (5-HT), plays a critical role in the regulation of such diverse functions as sleep, temperature homeostasis, pain sensitivity, appetite, neuroendocrine secretions, and mood regulation. Many of these functions are felt to be regulated, in part, by 5-HT input to the hypothalamus. Cell bodies of 5-HT-containing neurons are localized in a series of nuclei in the upper pons and lower midbrain, called the raphe nuclei. Axons ascending from the raphe project to almost all brain regions (Fig. 12–16). Serotonin within these cell bodies is formed from the amino acid tryptophan, which is an "essential" amino acid in that dietary intake regulates its availability. Tryptophan is taken up into 5-HT neurons by active transport across the blood-brain barrier. The enzyme tryptophan hydroxylase catalyzes the rate-limiting step of hydroxylating tryptophan into 5-hydroxytryptophan, which is then decarboxylated to form 5-HT.

As with NE (see above), 5-HT is inactivated by reuptake into the presynaptic nerve terminal following its release and interaction with postsynaptic receptors. There it is oxidized by MAO to form 5-hydroxy-indoleacetic acid (5-HIAA), which is released into the cerebrospinal fluid (CSF) and eventually excreted in urine. Figure 12–17 summarizes the metabolic pathways involved in the synthesis and metabolism of 5-HT.

5-HT receptors also are classified based on agonist affinity; the classification is currently an area of extensive investigation and is somewhat con-

Serotonin

Figure 12–16. *The pathways of the raphe serotonergic neurons. (Reproduced with permission from Hyman SE, Coyle JT: The neuroscientific foundations of psychiatry. In Hales RE, Yudofsky SC, Talbott JA (eds): Textbook of Psychiatry, 2nd ed. Washington, DC, American Psychiatric Press, 1994.)*

troversial (see Table 12–4). 5-HT_{1A} receptors are found in the gut and in the dorsal raphe nucleus in some species. These receptors appear to mediate contraction in the gut and neuronal inhibition in the brain. The anxiolytic medication buspirone is a partial 5-HT_{1A} agonist. 5-HT_{1B} receptors are found in the cortex and in the sympathetic nervous system; they mediate smooth muscle contraction and neuronal inhibition. 5-HT_{1C} receptors mediate contraction in the stomach. 5-HT_2 receptors are localized in the brain, platelets, gut, and uterus. Several antidepressant medications have been found to down-regulate (i.e., decrease the density and responsivity of) these receptors. 5-HT_3 receptors have been described recently (Hyman, 1988), and 5-HT_3 antagonists (e.g., ondansetron) have proven extremely useful in treating the nausea and vomiting associated with cancer chemotherapy. In addition, 5-HT_D, 5-HT_{1E}, 5-HT_{1F}, 5-HT_4, 5-HT_5, 5-HT_6, and 5-HT_7 receptors now have been identified; their functional significance is currently under investigation (Mansour et al, 1995).

At about the same time that American researchers were developing the catecholamine hypothesis of depression (see above), British scientists began to emphasize the role that serotonin (5-HT) might play in depressive illness (Coppen et al, 1965). Prange and associates (1974) synthesized two bodies of data in formulating the "permissive hypothesis" of affective illness: a decrease in the functional activity of central 5-HT systems could permit the development of depressive illness when coupled with a deficiency in central NE, whereas the coexistence of decreased 5-HT and increased NE could lead to the emergence of

Figure 12–17. *The metabolic pathways available for the synthesis and metabolism of serotonin. (Reproduced with permission from Cooper JR, Bloom FE, Roth RH (eds): The Biochemical Basis of Neuropharmacology. New York, Oxford, 1996.)*

mania. Recently, a number of investigators, using various pharmacological "challenge tests" have identified 5-HT dysregulation in depressed patients as measured by altered neurohormonal response to 5-HT agonists. 5-HT also has been implicated in the pathogenesis of many other major psychiatric syndromes, including schizophrenia, personality disorders, obsessive-compulsive disorder, anxiety disorders, alcoholism, and chronic pain syndromes (Heninger, 1995).

Dopamine. Dopamine (DA), like NE, is a catecholamine neurotransmitter synthesized from the amino acid tyrosine (see Fig. 12–9) and metabolized by MAO and COMT. As shown in Table 12–4, dopamine receptors can be subdivided into two families: D_1-like and D_2-like. Such a classification originally was derived on pharmacological grounds, but it has been expanded by recent molecular biological studies. As described in Table 12–4, there are clear pharmacological and functional differences between the two subfamilies. The current trends in the field suggest that new generations of drugs (ones having binding selectivity for specific receptors forms and/or unique functional properties) are likely to appear in the immediate future. Because of the role of dopamine receptors in therapy (and etiology?) of schizophrenia (*see below*) and neurological disorders, such new drugs are likely to have important clinical impact.

There are three major DA systems in the brain: the meso-cortico-limbic midbrain-forebrain system, the nigrostriatal system, and the tuberoinfundibular system (Fig. 12–18). The meso-cortico-limbic system is felt to play an important role in regulating mood and behavior. The nigrostriatal system is involved in the control of fine movement, and disruption of DA neurotransmission in this area by neuroleptic medication can lead to the emergence of "extrapyramidal" side effects (i.e., acute dystonia, parkinsonian symptoms, and akathisia). The tuberoinfundibular system primarily contains D_2 receptors; dopamine released into the hypothalmic-pituitary portal venous system regulates prolactin and growth hormone secretion (Hyman, 1988).

Most research exploring the relationship between DA and human psychopathology has focused on psychoses (Seeman, 1995) The "dopamine hypothesis" of schizophrenia was derived, in part, from two observations: (1) clinically effective antipsychotic medications (e.g., phenothiazines,

Figure 12–18. *The three major dopaminergic pathways. These include the nigrostriatal, the mesocorticolimbic (A-10), and the tuberoinfundibular pathway from the arcuate nucleus to the infundibulum. (Modified with permission from Hyman SE, Coyle JT: The neuroscientific foundations of psychiatry. In Hales RE, Yudofsky SC, Talbott JA (eds): Textbook of Psychiatry, 2nd ed. Washington, DC, American Psychiatric Press, 1994.)*

butyrophenones, reserpine, and so forth) share a common property of diminishing central DA neurotransmission; and (2) amphetamine and other psychostimulants that enhance central dopaminergic activity have been associated with the emergence of psychotic syndromes that in some ways resemble schizophrenia. In addition, hypotheses have been developed that link alterations in central dopaminergic systems with mania and depression (Janowsky et al, 1988).

Acetylcholine. Although ACH was the first neurotransmitter to be discovered, until recently limitations in technology have slowed the pace of investigations of its role in CNS function (Janowsky et al, 1988). ACH is synthesized by choline acetyltransferase, using acetyl-coenzyme A and choline as substrates. Brain ACH formation is relatively dependent on bloodborne choline derived from dietary intake, because choline cannot be synthesized in the brain in adequate amounts.

In the brain, there are nicotinic and muscarinic, pre- and postsynaptic receptors, as well as other cholinergic receptors that do not appear to belong to either of these classic types. Muscarinic receptors (see Table 12–4) are more plentiful in the brain than nicotinic receptors and play a more vital role in behavioral regulation. Unlike the catecholamine neurotransmitters, ACH inactivation following synaptic release does not depend on reuptake, but instead takes place by hydrolysis by either neuronal acetylcholinesterase or nonneuronal (glial) pseudocholinesterases.

The limbic system and the cerebral cortex, two brain systems that are felt to play major roles in the regulation of emotion in humans, receive considerable cholinergic innervation (Fig. 12–19). Thus, there is a theoretical basis for anticipating that ACH may play a role in the regulation of mood and in the pathogenesis of mood disorders. Janowsky et al (1972) proposed a cholinergic-adrenergic balance hypothesis of mood disorders, which postulated that affect (mood) may represent a balance between cholinergic and adrenergic neurotransmitter activity in the areas of the brain that regulate mood. Depressive illness could represent a disease state of relative cholinergic predominance, whereas mania could result from relative adrenergic predominance. Numerous animal studies, clinical observations, and human studies lend support to this theory, although contradictory data also exist (Janowsky et al, 1988). Pursuit of cholinergic mechanisms as causal in mood disorders has not been fruitful.

Cholinergic projections to the cortex and hippocampus also play a critical role in cognition and its disorders (see section entitled Learning and Memory).

Gamma-Aminobutyric Acid. Gamma-aminobutyric acid (GABA) is synthesized from the amino acid glutamic acid through a decarboxylation reaction. Approximately 99% of all GABA in humans is found within the CNS, where it functions as an inhibitory neurotransmitter (Fig. 12–20).

There are at least two types of GABA receptors, $GABA_A$ and $GABA_B$ (see Table 12–4). The former is linked to the benzodiazepine receptor and chloride

Figure 12–19. *The forebrain cholinergic neurons. Cholinergic neurons in the basal forebrain (including the nucleus basalis of Meynert, the diagonal band of Broca, and the medial septal nucleus) innervate the cerebral cortex, hippocampus, and limbic structures. The striatum contains local circuit cholinergic interneurons. (Reproduced with permission from Hyman SE, Coyle JT: The neuroscientific foundations of psychiatry. In Hales RE, Yudofsky SC, Talbott JA (eds): Textbook of Psychiatry, 2nd ed. Washington, DC, American Psychiatric Press, 1994.)*

Figure 12–20. *Major GABAergic pathways. The inhibitory neurotransmitter GABA (gamma-aminobutyric acid) is synthesized by local circuit stellate cells within the cerebral cortex, by the cerebellar Purkinje cells, and by striatonigral neurons. (Reproduced with permission from Hyman SE, Coyle JT: The neuroscientific foundations of psychiatry. In Hales RE, Yudofsky SC, Talbott JA (eds): Textbook of Psychiatry, 2nd ed. Washington, DC, American Psychiatric Press, 1994.)*

ion channel and thus has been linked to the development and treatment of anxiety disorders. The benzodiazepine receptor is believed to act synergistically with the GABA receptor to increase the affinity for the neurotransmitter. In addition to its association with anxiety disorders, GABA has been implicated in the pathogenesis of affective illness, such as depression, although the data related to GABAergic theories of affective disease are quite preliminary (Janowsky et al, 1988).

Second Messengers

Five types of second messengers, cyclic adenosine monophosphate (cAMP), cyclic guanosine monophosphate (cGMP), calcium, arachidonic acid metabolites, and phosphatidylinositol (PI) metabolites, have been identified as key intermediaries in the brain (Wilcox and Gonzales, 1995). Their effects can be either stimulating or inhibiting. Most second messengers are influenced through a mechanism involving postsynaptic receptors. Neurotransmitters bind to these receptors, thereby activating G-proteins (located in the cell membrane) that regulate the activity of intracellular enzymes that produce the second messengers. These second messengers subsequently activate specific types of protein kinases, which produce immediate, short-term, and/or long-term physiological responses in the cell. Each second messenger can follow this pathway. An example of a stimulating system is the beta$_2$-adrenergic receptor. Norepinephrine binds to a postsynaptic receptor activating a G-protein in the cell membrane. This protein then activates adenylate cyclase, which catalyzes the synthesis of the second messenger, cAMP, which in turn activates a protein kinase that phosphorylates an ion channel protein, resulting in a change in ion permeability.

CLINICAL VIGNETTE: LITHIUM AND THE SECOND MESSENGERS

Although the exact mechanism and molecular site of lithium's actions are not known, effects on signal transduction involving second messenger systems may be important (Lenox and Manji, 1995). Lithium inhibits G-protein activation of enzymes that synthesize cAMP or phosphatidylinositol and the activity of some of these enzymes as well as altering protein kinase C activity. These effects slow transduction of signals initiated by transmitter occupation of membrane receptors. Neurophysiological studies indicate a damping of synaptic activity following lithium treatment, with a decrease in excessive excitation and excessive inhibition, a response consistent with the clinical effects of lithium. These actions occur at therapeutic lithium concentrations. Therefore, lithium may stabilize mood by altering second messenger-mediated signal transduction and, thereby, normalizing neuronal activity.

Neuropeptides

Neuropeptides are small proteins containing two to several dozen amino acids. They are, therefore, much larger than the "classic" small molecule neurotransmitters described above. The diversity of structure of neuropeptides is great. At least 50 are known and certainly many more will be found (Table 12–5). They occur in the CNS at concentrations far lower than classic small molecule neurotransmitters. Neuropeptides have a broad range of physiological and behavioral effects, which are exerted at concentrations three or more orders of magnitude lower than small molecule neurotransmitters. Neuropeptides also tend to have durations of effect considerably longer than classic neurotransmitters. These effects often persist well after proteolytic degradation of the neuropeptide.

Synthesis of neuropeptides is similar to that of other proteins (i.e., it involves translation of messenger RNA sequences on ribosomes [Hyman and Coyle, 1994]). This process occurs exclusively within the cell bodies and possibly dendrites of neurons. Translation usually produces a relatively large pre-proprotein or precusor of the neuropeptide. Initial proteolytic cleavage of the precursor protein occurs in the endoplasmic reticulum and the Golgi apparatus. The final stages of posttranslational processing occur after the precursor and proteolytic enzymes are packaged into neurosecretory granules, which then are transported to neuron terminals for storage or release. Processing may include further proteolytic cleavage to produce shorter peptides as well as C-terminal amidation, N-terminal acetylation, cyclization of glutamate to form pyroglutamate, disulphide bond formation, glycosylation, phosphorylation, or sulfation. Precursor molecules in some neuropeptide-synthesizing neurons contain several amino acid sequences of the same neuropeptide. This allows

Table 12–5 **Some Putative Neuropeptide Neurotransmitters**

ACTH	Interleukin-1
Angiotensin II	Leu-enkephalin
Atriopeptin	Luteinizing-hormone-releasing factor
Beta endorphin	Met-enkephalin
Bombesin	N-acetyl aspartyl glutamate (NAAG)
Bradykinin	Neurotensin
Calcitonin gene-related peptide (CGRP)	Neuropeptide Y
Carnosine	Oxytocin
Cholecystokinin	Pancreostatin
Corticotropin-releasing factor (CRF)	Somatostatin
Dynorphin	Substance P
Galinin	Thyrotropin-releasing hormone (TRH)
Gastrin	Vasoactive intestinal peptide (VIP)
Glucagon	Vasopressin
Insulin	

the neurons to produce multiple copies of a particular neuropeptide and thereby multiply the signal produced by translation of the precursor molecule. Precursor molecules in neuropeptide-synthesizing neurons also may contain amino acid sequences of several different neuropeptides. Changes in the cleavage pattern in the precursor can produce different clusters of neuropeptides, each of which may have quite different effects.

Release of neuropeptides from presynaptic sites depends on Ca^{2+} influx. Many neuropeptides act at receptors that are structurally like classic neurotransmitter receptors and exert their effects on the postsynaptic neuron through common second messenger systems such as cAMP and phosphatidylinositol (Burbach and Meijer, 1992). Thus, mechanisms of release and receptor activation within synapses are very similar in neuropeptides and small molecule neurotransmitters. Inactivation of neuropeptides appears to depend entirely on extracellular proteolysis. Unlike many small molecule neurotransmitters, presynaptic reuptake and recycling of neuropeptide molecules does not occur. Extracellular proteolysis may produce fragments that have physiological effects similar or quite different from the parent neuropeptide.

There has been much speculation about whether neuropeptides are true neurotransmitters or play a less specific neuromodulatory role. Although no neuropeptide to date has been demonstrated to meet all of the exacting criteria required for neurotransmitter status (see Table 12–2), very likely many neuropeptides function as neurotransmitters. Neuromodulators are substances that also are released presynaptically but which act both locally and at more distant postsynaptic sites to diminish or amplify the effects of neurotransmitters. Neuromodulators also may influence the rate of release of neurotransmitters from presynaptic sites. Many neuropeptides have been localized within neurons containing small molecule neurotransmitters or other neuropeptides (Hyman and Coyle, 1994). These observations suggest that neuropeptides may be coreleased with and serve as neuromodulators of small molecule or neuropeptide neurotransmitters. By diffusion through extracellular fluid and even CSF, neuropeptides may exert effects on neural activity at some distance from where they are released (Herbert, 1993). Neuropeptide receptors often are located some distance from the terminal fields of neurons synthesizing those neuropeptides. Although neuropeptides are found throughout the central and peripheral nervous systems, a large body of experimental evidence suggests that particular patterns of neuropeptide activity within limbic brain sites regulate appropriate behavioral responses to specific environmental and physiological demands (Herbert, 1993; Strand et al, 1994).

Endogenous opioids have received more investigative attention than any other family of neuropeptides. Approximately 18 separate opioid molecules have been described so far, among which beta endorphin, leu-enkephalin, met-enkephalin, and dynorphin are of primary interest. All opioids arise from three major precursor molecules, proopiomelanocortin, preproenkephalin, and preprodynorphin, each of which is synthesized in a different population of neurons.

The proteolytic cleavage products of proopiomelanocortin are summarized in Fig. 12–21. Processing of opioid precursors varies with brain region. Enkephalin and dynorphin-containing neurons form discrete pathways in many regions of the CNS. Enkephalins are found in high concentration in the basal ganglia and are often colocalized in neurons with monoamines or other neuropeptides such as substance P. Beta endorphin is synthesized primarily in neuron cell bodies in the arcuate nucleus from which project long ascending and descending pathways. A number of separate opate receptor types have been described (see Table 12–4), and several classification schemes have been suggested. Individual opioid molecules have different affinities for each of these receptor types.

Many other families of neuropeptides are found within the CNS. Neuronal processes containing the posterior pituitary hormones, vasopressin and oxytocin, project from the paraventricular nucleus of the hypothalamus to many sites in the limbic system, brain stem, and spinal cord. In addition, nests of vasopressinergic neurons are located at a number of sites outside the hypothalamus. Many hypothalamic neuropeptides that regulate release of anterior pituitary hormones also are synthesized and released in other regions of the brain. Among these are corticotropin-releasing factor, thyrotropin-releasing hormone, luteinizing hormone-releasing hormone, and somatostatin. Some peptides that were localized first in the gastrointestinal tract, such as cholecystokinin and vasoactive intestinal peptide, also have been identified in the brain. Neurotensin, first isolated from brain tissue, was subsequently found to be widely distributed in the gut. Summaries of physiological effects and brain

Figure 12–21. *Processing of proopiomelanocortin (POMC). The precursor protein, POMC, which contains 165 amino acids, is enzymatically cleaved to yield the physiologically active peptides indicated. Depending on the cellular localization (anterior pituitary, hypothalamus, midbrain nerve terminals), certain of these neuropeptides are expressed and others are not. (Reproduced with permission from Hyman SE, Coyle JT: The neuroscientific foundations of psychiatry. In Hales RE, Yudofsky SC, Talbott JA (eds): Textbook of Psychiatry, 2nd ed. Washington, DC, American Psychiatric Press, 1994.)*

localization of these and other neuropeptides can be found in Herbert (1993) and Strand et al (1994).

Steroid Hormones

Although steroid hormones have profound effects on behavior and other brain functions, they are all synthesized in peripheral tissues. Gonadal steroids are synthesized primarily in the ovaries (estrogens and progestins) or the testes (androgens), although the adrenal cortex also synthesizes significant amounts of sex steroids. The adrenal cortex is the primary site of glucocorticoid and mineralcorticoid synthesis. After secretion into the blood, steroid molecules are either tightly bound to specific steroid-binding globulins or less tightly bound to albumin. Steroids bind to albumin, much more so than steroids bind to specific binding globulins, readily dissociate, diffuse across the blood–brain barrier, and gain access to all regions of the CNS. Steroids also diffuse readily into the neuronal cytoplasm where they may undergo a variety of metabolic transformations.

Mechanisms of Effect

Steroids affect brain function by acting at both the genome and at outer membrane receptors of neurons (McEwen, 1995). In the neuronal cytoplasm, steroids form noncovalent high-affinity attachments to macromolecules called cytoplasmic steroid receptors. Binding of these receptors is quite specific in individual neurons, allowing genomic regulation of a target cell only by a particular type of steroid molecule even though other types of steroid molecules enter that cell. Once activated by hormone binding, steroid receptors are translocated into the cell nucleus where they attach to steroid-specific response elements composed of DNA sequences within genes. Binding of the hormone-steroid receptor complex to the response element then increases or decreases transcription of the target gene. Other steroid effects are exerted at receptors on the external surface of neurons that are linked to second messenger systems and gated ion channels. Genomic effects of steroids are slower in onset and persist much longer than nongenomic effects.

Location of Steroid Binding in the Brain

Neuronal cell bodies that contain receptors for specific steroids are located in discrete regions of the brain. Estrogen and androgen binding is located in the anterior and medial portions of the hypothalamus, the preoptic and septal areas, the amygdala, as well as midbrain sites such as the mesencephalic central gray. Implantation of gonadal steroids into these sites, but not into other brain sites, elicits hormonal and behavioral effects that are dependent on these steroids. Brain areas that bind gonadal steroids have been implicated in the regulation of reproductive as well as other sexually differentiated behaviors, and gonadotropin release.

Progesterone binding is localized in the same areas as estrogen binding, with the exception of the amygdala. Synthesis of some progesterone receptors requires estrogen stimulation. Progesterone receptor concentration peaks between 24 and 48 hours after estrogen treatment. If progesterone levels rise simultaneously with estrogen levels, progesterone receptor proliferation does not occur.

The pattern of glucocorticoid binding within the brain is markedly different from the pattern of gonadal steroid binding. Glucocorticoid binding is most prominent in the hippocampus (in the pyramidal cells in the CA_1 and CA_2 fields of the horn of Ammon and the granule neurons of the dentate gyrus) and, to a lesser degree, in the septal area, the amygdala, and some areas of the cerebral cortex. Behavioral effects of glucocorticoids are exerted in these limbic brain areas.

Regulatory Effects of Steroids

Estrogens and androgens have profound effects on the sexual differentiation of brain structure during early development and activate, respectively, female and male typical behaviors in adult animals. Glucocorticoids also affect some aspects of brain development and adult behavior. Progestins do not appear to influence brain development but do regulate female typical adult behaviors, especially reproductive behaviors. Steroids exert these effects by altering synthesis, release, turnover, reuptake, catabolism, and receptor concentration of small molecule neurotransmitters. These effects differ with type of steroid and vary with brain region.

Enzymatic conversion is sometimes necessary for the brain organizational and activational effects of steroids on behavior. Changes in the brain during early development that masculinize later sexual and social behavior require 5-alpha reduction of testosterone to dihydrotestosterone as well as aromatization of testosterone to estradiol. Also, brain regions differ in the activity of enzymes that convert steroids. In some species, 5-alpha reductase activity is highest in the hypothalamus whereas aromatase activity is found primarily in limbic brain sites. These regional differences may be important in the gonadal steroid activation of sexually differentiated behaviors.

Thyroid Hormone

The thyroid gland and its hormones constitute but one part of a larger regulatory system, the hypothalamic–pituitary–thyroid (HPT) axis. Key hormonal components of this system include the thyroid hormones thyroxine (T_4) and triiodothyronine (T_3), thyroid-stimulating hormone (TSH), and thyrotropin-releasing hormone (TRH). The thyroid hormones T_4 and T_3 are iodinated bi-mers of the amino acid, tyrosine. TSH, a glycoprotein synthesized in the pituitary gland, regulates the production of T_3 and T_4. TSH, in turn, is regulated by TRH, a tripeptide (pro-his-pro), which is synthesized by neurons in the hypothalamus, released in the median eminence, and delivered to the pituitary by the hypophyseal portal venous system. The activity of this system also is partially regulated by other extrathyroidal factors, such as thyroid-binding globulin, which serves as the main serum reservoir for thyroid hormone, and peripheral enzymes that convert T_4 to either T_3 or its metabolically inactive form, reverse T_3.

Some hormonal components of the thyroidal system are found in virtually all animal species, suggesting that it developed early in evolution and serves fairly basic biological ends. By interacting with membrane as well as nuclear receptors, thyroid hormone affects a variety of cellular functions including energy utilization, enzymatic rates, and cell growth and division. Although evolution appears to have adapted the HPT axis for multiple functions, its main job may be to modulate and coordinate overall metabolic activity. The ability to adjust cellular energy utilization to different circumstances such as growth, procreation, and seasonal change would provide obvious adaptational advantage. Thyroid hormone concentrations are more actively regulated in the brain than in other organ systems, suggesting that thyroid hormones may play additional specific roles in the coordination of behavior.

CLINICAL VIGNETTE: HYPOTHYROIDISM AND DEPRESSION

A 40-year-old attorney with no prior psychiatric history presents to her physician with complaints of 3 to 4 weeks of depressed mood, fatigue, weight gain, and difficulty concentrating at work. On observation, her speech and motor movements are markedly slowed, her face looks puffy, and her affect appears depressed. Her pulse and blood pressure are toward the lower range of normal. The remainder of her physical examination is normal. Her performance on a cognitive examination, despite good effort, is poor and inconsistent with her current line of work.

Laboratory evaluation shows an elevated TSH, consistent with hypothyroidism. Within 6 weeks of beginning thyroid hormone replacement, her depressive symptoms and cognitive dysfunction have resolved.

Since the turn of the century it has been known that deficiency or excess of thyroid hormone is associated with psychopathology. Severely hypothyroid adults are often depressed, demented, or psychotic. Even very mild (subclinical) thyroid hormone deficiency appears to increase the lifetime risk for mood disorder (Haggerty and Prange, 1995). Hyperthyroid persons are typically anxious or appear to have agitated depressions. The components of the HPT axis are probably partially involved in a variety of behavior responses. Based on available data, we can identify three key areas in which HPT axis activity influences behavioral adaptation: regulation of nervous system development, augmentation of catecholaminergic stress response, and modulation of biological rhythms.

Nervous System Development

Thyroid hormone has a nerve growth factorlike effect on neurons in the CNS. Dendritic and axonal growth is enhanced by thyroid hormone and is impaired in thyroid deficiency states. There appears to be a developmental window, occurring perinatally in most species, during which thyroid hormone availability is absolutely essential for brain maturation (McEwen, 1995). In humans, deprivation of thyroid hormone prenatally or in early infancy leads to the severe and irreversible form of retardation known as cretinism. The HPT axis probably also facilitates neuronal maintenance and repair in the mature organism. Administration of TRH appears to stimulate cell growth and enhance recovery of function following brain and spinal cord trauma. Although the adult CNS is more tolerant of thyroid deficiency than that of the infant, prolonged thyroid deficiency states may cause irreversible cognitive decline in adult humans.

Stress Responses

Thyroid hormone augments the firing of beta-adrenergic neurons. This is mediated by a facilitating interaction at postsynaptic beta-adrenergic receptors (Whybrow and Prange, 1981). Thus, the HPT axis may help mediate the increase in catecholaminergic neurotransmission that is an essential component of the general stress response (see section entitled Stress and Behavior), perhaps by way of a centrally induced neurohormone cascade involving TRH, TSH, and thyroid hormone. The HPT axis, in turn, can be directly tuned up or down by the sympathetic nervous system, which innervates the HPT axis at several levels. The ability of the HPT axis to enhance beta-adrenergic neurotransmission may be an important factor in recovery from clinical depression, which appears to be associated with deficient or inefficient catecholaminergic neurotransmission. A slight increase in the tone of the thyroid axis may be able to compensate, at least partially, for such a deficiency (Whybrow and Prange, 1981). This concept is strongly supported by the observation that T_3 administration has been reported to augment response to antidepressant medication in some patients. Conversely, one of the earliest and most consistent neuroendocrine findings is that 20 to 30% of depressed patients exhibit a diminished TSH response to exogenously administered TRH. Prange has postulated these findings to be the consequence of prolonged reliance in depressed persons on the ability of the HPT axis to compensate for deficient catecholaminergic neurotransmission; tachyphylaxis develops at the pituitary level to chronic TRH overdrive.

Modulation of Biological Rhythms

As with other hormonal systems, HPT axis activity fluctuates diurnally and possibly seasonally. However, there also is evidence that HPT axis activity itself regulates the length of biological rhythms (Schull et al, 1988). TRH mediates the change from hibernation to the active state in some species. In mice, the thyroid changes the length of motor activity cycles. The extent to which the HPT axis affects normal biological rhythms in humans is unknown. However, there is evidence for HPT axis abnormalities in bipolar disorder (manic-depression), a mental disorder in which mood and activity cycle at an abnormal rate and to an excessive degree. In particular, an association has been observed between hypothyroidism and rapid cycling bipolar disorder. Administration of thyroid hormone will stabilize cycling in a portion of these patients.

It can be seen from the preceding overview that there has been a dramatic and rapid expansion in our understanding of the neurobiology of behavior and an emerging body of data elucidating the biochemical basis for not only normal behavior but several of the major mental disorders as well. In the next section, the neurochemical basis of certain specific behaviors, such as learning, memory, reproductive activity, feeding, and aggression, are discussed.

THE NEUROBIOLOGY OF SPECIFIC BEHAVIORS

Learning and Memory

An impressive array of cognitive abilities enables humans to analyze situations, review past experiences, consider options, anticipate developments, and rehearse future actions. Therefore, human behavior depends on, and is the result of, a great deal of cognitive activity within the brain before overt, observable behavior occurs. Despite the critical nature of cognitive function in the shaping of human behavior, exploration of the biological basis of most cognitive functions is in its infancy. Many cognitive abilities do not appear to be localized. In brain-damaged persons impairment of cognitive functions, such as attention, concentration, calculation and inductive and deductive logic, has been related to the total amount of cortical damage but has not been associated with damage in specific areas. Some brain regions, however, have been implicated in particular cognitive tasks. As discussed earlier, the frontal lobes, for instance, play a key role in abstract thinking and planning. The neurobiological basis of most cognitive functions is unknown. However, progress has been achieved in our understanding of the mechanism of learning and memory.

The Components and Dimensions of Learning and Memory

Learning is the capacity to change behavior in response to experience. Memory is the retained record of experience and is composed of a short-term and a long-term phase. (See Table 12–6 for a summary of the phases of memory formation and the types of memory that are discussed

Table 12–6 **Types of Memory and Phases of Long-Term Memory**

TYPES OF MEMORY	CHARACTERISTICS
Short term	Seconds to minutes in duration, probably mediated by sustained neural electrical activity.
Long term	
Procedural	Involves retention of information about motor or cognitive sequences; does not depend upon the hippocampus.
Declarative	Depends upon the hippocampus; impaired in amnesiacs.
Semantic	Involves retention of information about abstract concepts or events.
Episodic	Involves retention of information about personal experiences.
PHASES OF LONG-TERM MEMORY	
Acquisition	Protein synthesis is necessary.
Consolidation	
Retrieval	Protein synthesis is not necessary.

later.) Short-term memory, lasting seconds to minutes, is probably based on a sustained pattern of activity of the primary sensory neural substrate stimulated by the new experience. Distraction by other stimuli, which disrupts the pattern of activity of the primary sensory neural substrate, results in loss of the new information stored in short-term memory. Acquisition of long-term memory requires persistent physical change either in the primary sensory neural substrate activated by the new information or physical change in cerebral cortex where information is stored after processing in the hippocampus (Squire, 1994). Changes in neural structures underlying acquisition of long-term memory depend on protein synthesis. After initial acquisition, long-term memories require a period of *consolidation* before they can no longer be abolished by pharmacological or electroconvulsive means. Consolidation of long-term memory requires a few hours to a few days in animals. Electroconvulsive therapy in psychiatric patients produces partial loss of some memories acquired as much as 3 years prior to treatment. This observation suggests that complete consolidation of memory in humans can require long periods of time. *Retrieval* of memories from long-term storage operates by mechanisms that differ from those mediating acquisition of memory. Retrieval does not involve information processing in the hippocampus nor does it depend on protein synthesis.

Recent investigations of the amnestic syndrome in humans, which results from a variety of neurological insults, have provided new insights into the complexities of long-term memory. The amnestic syndrome is characterized by impaired acquisition of new memories without accompanying sensory, motor, or other neurological deficits. Amnesics have intact short-term memory and have no problem retrieving information stored in long-term memory prior to the neurological insult. Moreover, cognitive functions other than acquisition of memories (e.g., concentration, calculation, logic, and so forth) remain intact.

Detailed investigation of which types of information can and cannot be learned by amnesics suggests the existence of different types of long-term memory mechanisms (Kandel and Hawkins, 1992). *Procedural memory* involves acquiring knowledge of motor or cognitive sequences (e.g., tying knots, solving puzzles, and so forth). *Semantic memory* is the retention of abstract knowledge or events in time (e.g., the chemical composition of water or the assassination of President Kennedy). *Episodic memory* is the recollection of personal experiences (e.g., one's last visit to the doctor). *Semantic and episodic memory together are termed declarative memory.* It is generally agreed that amnesics can acquire procedural memory but are impaired in acquiring declarative memory. This produces the interesting situation in which amnesiacs can increase their retention of procedural information with training but have no memory of having learned and, in fact, have no awareness of their increased knowledge. There is debate about the extent of the deficit in acquiring declarative memory in amnesiacs. Some argue that episodic memory is specifically eliminated in the amnestic syndrome while semantic memory capability persists. Others argue that acquisition of both episodic and semantic memory is impaired. Careful neuropsychological studies should resolve this controversy. Because amnesiacs have discrete impairment of declarative but not procedural memory, these separate types of memory are probably acquired by different mechanisms.

Studies of the effects of priming on memory retrieval in amnesics also suggest that different mechanisms underlie procedural and declarative memory. Amnesiacs are very poor at free recall of lists of words. However, when given the first three letters of words they have previously seen, amnesiacs are able to complete accurately the spelling of many words. If normal subjects are given a list of words and instructed to focus on features of the words other than their meaning (such as counting vowels), subsequent recall is also poor. However, when given the first three letters of those words, recall is much improved, demonstrating a learning effect very similar to that seen in amnesiacs. These results suggest that amnesiacs can learn but cannot store information based on meaning or category. Declarative memory, which is impaired in amnesiacs, may, therefore, involve processing and storage of information based on meaning and category, while procedural memory, which is intact in amnesiacs, involves processing and storage based on the more concrete and literal aspects of information.

Localization of Learning and Memory

Where does acquisition of memory occur? Where is memory stored? The answers to these questions depend on the complexity of learning that occurs.

Habituation, the decline and extinction of a response with repeated presentations of a particular stimulus, is the simplest type of learning. *Sensitization* is another simple learning process involving the enhancement of responses following a strong noxious stimulus. *Classical conditioning* is a more complex learning task involving the association of a conditioned and unconditioned stimulus. Classical conditioning always requires that the conditioned stimulus precede the unconditioned stimulus in time, and that only a brief period of time elapse between the conditioned and unconditioned stimulus (see Chapter 6 by Dr. Dorsett). The neurobiological basis of simple learning has been investigated in a number of animal models.

The marine snail *Aplysia californica* has a respiratory organ, the gill, and a spoutlike organ, the siphon, which is used to discharge sea water and body waste. Light tactile stimulation of the siphon causes a reflexive withdrawal of the gill and siphon. With repeated moderate tactile stimulation of the siphon, the withdrawal reflex habituates. On the other hand, strong noxious stimulation, such as electroshock of the tail of *Aplysia*, produces a subsequent increase, or sensitization, of the gill and siphon withdrawal reflex. A single aversive stimulus produces short-term sensitization whereas repeated aversive stimuli produce long-term sensitization. The gill and siphon withdrawal reflex also can be classically conditioned.

The mechanisms underlying habituation, short-term and long-term sensitization, and classic conditioning of the gill and siphon withdrawal reflex in *Aplysia* have been studied in great detail (Kandel et al, 1991). The nervous system of *Aplysia* is relatively uncomplicated. The neural circuit mediating the gill and siphon withdrawal reflex consists of sensory neurons synapsing directly on motor neurons that effect the response. Although action potentials are generated in sensory neurons by each stimulation, release of neurotransmitter from the presynaptic processes of sensory neurons decreases with repeated tactile stimulation. As a result, synaptic transmission declines until the motor neuron is no longer activated. Electroshock of the tail of *Aplysia* activates pathways that converge on and stimulate the presynaptic processes of sensory neurons involved in the gill and siphon withdrawal reflex. Subsequently, more neurotransmitter is released from the sensory neuron in response to tactile stimulation of the gill, resulting in increased activation of motor neurons. Intracellular mechanisms underlying sensitization of the gill and siphon withdrawal reflex are summarized in Fig. 12–22. The processes of short-term and long-term sensitization differ in two important ways (Bailey et al, 1994). First, short-term sensitization is based upon covalent modification of preexisting proteins, whereas long-term sensitization involves synthesis of new proteins as illustrated in Fig. 12–23. Second, the long-term process also is associated with a structural change: the growth of new synaptic connections by the sensory neurons onto their follower cells. This change can be induced by the intracellular injection of cAMP, a second messenger activated by serotonin. If light tactile stimulation is given consistently just prior to tail shock, *Aplysia* becomes conditioned to withdraw the gill and siphon vigorously in response to tactile stimulation alone. Pairing of the conditioned and unconditioned stimuli in this manner selectively increases neurotransmitter release from the presynaptic processes of sensory neurons by a mechanism that is explained in Fig.12–24, p. 454.

Figure 12–22. *Presynaptic facilitation is a factor in sensitization of the gill-withdrawal reflex in* Aplysia.
A. *Sensitization is produced by applying a noxious stimulus to another part of the body, such as the tail. Stimuli to the tail activate sensory neurons that excite facilitating interneurons. The facilitating cells, some of which use serotonin (5-hydroxy-tryptamine, or 5-HT) as their transmitter (indicated by dense core vesicles in the terminal of the facilitating neuron) in turn end on the synaptic terminals of the sensory neurons from the siphon skin, where they enhance transmitter release by means of presynaptic facilitation.*
B. *Postulated biochemical steps of presynaptic facilitation in the sensory neuron. The action of serotonin and other facilitating transmitters leads to enhanced transmitter release by modulating a number of steps in the release process; one of these is the closure of a special class of K^+ channels, which causes a consequent increase in Ca^{2+} influx through a (N-type) Ca^{2+} channel. Serotonin produces these*

Brain mechanisms underlying classic conditioning also have been studied in other animal models. In the rabbit, a brief puff of air directed at the cornea reliably produces an eyeblink response. This reflex can be conditioned by pairing a brief tone just before the puff of air. In pigeons, foot shock reliably produces an increase in heart rate. When bright illumination of the visual field is presented repeatedly prior to foot shock, heart rate acceleration becomes conditioned to the light stimulus. Classic conditioning in both of these cases does not depend on the cerebral cortex or other forebrain structures, but does appear to involve higher-order processing within the lower brain. Changes in a neural circuit within the cerebellum are necessary for eyelid conditioning to occur, whereas no changes occur in the basic reflex circuit in the brain stem during training (Rosenzweig, 1996).

Complex learning occurs by mechanisms that differ from those subserving simple learning. Midtemporal brain structures, especially the hippocampus, are essential for acquisition of complex memory (Squire, 1994). Lesions in this area eliminate the ability of animals to learn complex conditioning and operant tasks successfully. Examination of the brain of deceased amnesiacs invariably reveals damage to the midline temporal lobe area. Connections between the hippocampus and the cerebral cortex may be essential for processing and storing complex information. For instance, in the human and primate brain, the frontal association cortex (which connects with the hippocampus), the sulcus principalis, and the inferior prefrontal convexity play a critical role in sorting information in time. After processing, complex information is probably stored within the cortical areas that were involved in the processing. The importance of the cerebral cortex in the storage of complex memories is suggested by two lines of evidence. First, lesions that are restricted to the cortex interfere with

---

actions by binding to a receptor that engages a G-protein, which increases the activity of adenylyl cyclase. The adenylyl cyclase converts ATP to cyclic AMP, thereby increasing the level of cyclic AMP in the terminal of the sensory neuron. The cAMP activates the cAMP-dependent protein kinase by attaching to its regulatory subunit, which releases its active catalytic subunit. The catalytic subunit then phosphorylates the K^+ channel (either directly or by acting on a regulatory protein associated with it), thereby changing the conformation of the channel and decreasing the K^+ current (pathway 1). This prolongs the action potential, increases the influx of Ca^{2+}, and thus augments transmitter release.

In addition to broadening the action potential (pathway 1), serotonin also leads to an increase in the availability of transmitter by mobilizing vesicles from a transmitter pool to the releasable pool at the active zone (pathway 2). This second pathway concerned with mobilization of transmitter vesicles reflects the joint action of the cAMP-dependent protein kinase and protein kinase C, a second kinase activated by 5-HT (dotted line and pathway 2a). Protein kinase C (PKC) is activated by 5-HT acting through another G-protein that activates a phospholipase that in turn stimulates diacylglycerol in the membrane. Diacylglycerol activates protein kinase C. (Reproduced with permission from Kandel ER, Schwartz JH, Jessell TM (eds): Principles of Neural Science. New York, Elsevier, 1991.)

Motor neuron

Figure 12–23. *Schematic outline of the two major sets of changes in the sensory neurons of the gill-withdrawal reflex that accompany long-term memory for sensitization in* Aplysia: *persistent phosphorylation and structural changes. Serotonin (5-HT), a transmitter released by facililatory neurons, acts on a sensory neuron to initiate both the short-term and the long-term facilitation that contribute to the memory processes.*

Short-term facilitation *(lasting minutes to hours), involve covalent modification of preexisting proteins (pathways 1 and 2). Serotonin acts on a transmembrane serotonin receptor to activate a GTP-binding protein that stimulates the amplifier, the enzyme adenylyl cyclase, to convert ATP to the second messenger cAMP. In turn, cAMP activates protein kinase A, which phosphorylates and covalently modifies a number of target proteins. These include closing a K⁺ channel* the acquisition of complex learning. The size of the lesion, more so than the location, appears to be related to the degree of impairment. Second, repeated learning trials have been observed to produce hypertrophy within cortical regions that are known to process the types of sensory and motor information involved in the execution of the learned response (Rosenzweig, 1996).

In a manner analogous to simple and complex learning in animals, procedural and declarative memory in humans may depend on different neural substrates whose role changes with time. Procedural memory may be acquired and stored within subcortical connections between neurons conveying sensory information and neurons activating responses. However, acquisition and consolidation of declarative memory appear to require an intact medial temporal lobe memory system (including the hippocampus) initially (Squire, 1994). This system's role is only temporary. Over time, cortical areas become the ultimate site for declarative memory to the point where the medial temporal lobe is no longer necessary for either storage or retrieval of a specific memory. Empiric evidence supports such a localization of declarative memory; when this apparatus is damaged, as in the amnestic syndrome, impairment or complete loss of the ability to acquire declarative memory occurs while the ability to retrieve remote declarative memory remains intact. Preliminary functional brain imaging studies in humans, however, have so far provided equivocal support for this role (Ungerleider, 1995).

The Neurochemical Basis of Learning and Memory

Cholinergic pathways in the brain play a role in the acquisition and retrieval of memories (Rosenzweig, 1996). Muscarinic neurotransmission facil-

---

(pathway 1) as well as steps involved in transmitter availability and release (pathway 2). The duration of these modifications represents the retention or storage of a component of the short-term memory.

Long-term facilitation (lasting one or more days) involves the synthesis of new proteins. The switch for this inductive mechanism is initiated by the protein kinase A, which is thought to translocate to the nucleus where it is thought to phosphorylate one or more transcriptional activators that bind to cyclic AMP regulatory elements (CRE) located in the upstream region of cAMP-inducible genes (pathway 3). The transcriptional activators, thought to belong to the protein family of cyclic AMP response element binding (CREB) proteins, activate two classes of effector genes that encode two classes of proteins (β and v). Inhibiting protein synthesis during learning blocks the expression of these sets of induced proteins. These two sets of proteins have distinct functions. One set of proteins (β), one of which perhaps is a specific protease, leads to a down-regulation of the regulatory subunit. This results in persistent activity of kinase A, leading to persistent phosphorylation of the substrate proteins of pathways 1 and 2. The second set of proteins (v) is important for the growth of new synaptic connections. (Reproduced with permission from Kandel ER, Schwartz JH, Jessell TM (eds): Principles of Neural Science. New York, Elsevier, 1991).

Figure 12–24. *A molecular model of the synaptic action underlying classical conditioning. The model is based on the hypothesis that activity in the sensory neurons of the conditioned stimulus (CS) pathway prior to the presentation of the unconditional stimulus (US) permits an influx of Ca^{2+} that enhances the activity of Ca^{2+}- dependent adenylyl cyclase.*
A. *In the unpaired pathway (CS) the sensory neuron is not active prior to presentation of the CS, so its Ca^{2+} channels are closed at the time the US input arrives.*
B. *In the paired pathway (CS^+) the sensory neuron is active prior to the CS and thus its Ca^{2+} channels are open when the US input arrives. Increased intracellular Ca^{2+} binds to calmodulin, which in turn binds to adenylyl cyclase, which undergoes a conformational change as a result. This change enhances the ability of the adenylyl cyclase to synthesize cAMP in response to serotonin released by the US. The greater amount of cAMP activates more cAMP-dependent protein kinase and leads to a substantially greater amount of transmitter release than would occur normally (without paired activity). (Reproduced with permission from Kandel ER, Schwartz JH, Jessell TM (eds): Principles of Neural Science. New York, Elsevier, 1991.)*

itates initial acquisition of learning tasks but inhibits retrieval of memories from about 5 to 14 days after training. However, around 28 days after training, muscarinic neurotransmission facilitates memory retrieval. These observations suggest that memory consolidation is composed of a number of successive phases, each mediated by differing cholinergic mechanisms. Brain regions involved in learning, such as the hippocampus and the frontal cortex, are heavily innervated by cholinergic pathways.

Dementia of the Alzheimer's type has been associated with loss of cholinergic neurons in the nucleus basalis of Meynert, the major source of cholinergic projections to the cortex. The excitatory neurotransmitter glutamate also plays a role in the initial stage of memory formation. Noradrenergic neurotransmission enhances learning primarily by increasing attention. Several neuropeptides affect learning and memory. Adrenocorticotropin hormone (ACTH) or vasopressin administration after a learning trial facilitates retention of learned avoidance behavior. Oxytocin, on the other hand, inhibits retention of learned avoidance behavior.

Reproductive Behaviors: Sex and Parenting

Sexual interest is obviously a major influence on behavior in animals and humans. Perhaps less appreciated as a behavioral motivator is the drive of parents, especially mothers, to nurture and protect their offspring. Maternal behavior, along with female and male sexual behavior, are classified as reproductive behaviors because they result in propagation of species and they are under the control of reproductive hormones.

Reproductive Behavior in Subprimate Mammals

Sexual activity in subprimate mammals depends on both the early brain organizational effects and the postpubertal activational effects of gonadal steroids (McEwen, 1995). The postpubertal rise in testosterone concentrations is necessary for male copulatory behavior. Females are sexually active only when they are fertile. The sequence of changes in estrogen and progesterone concentrations that stimulate ovulation also trigger female sexual behavior. Sensitivity of the brain to gonadal steroid activation of sexual behavior during adulthood depends upon the gonadal steroid environment during fetal or neonatal life. Exposure to elevated concentrations of testosterone (and conversion to dihydrotestosterone or estradiol) during a "critical period" of brain development (this varies among species from midgestation to shortly after birth) alters the structure of the brain and ensures that gonadal steroids will activate male sexual behavior in adulthood. Male sexual behavior requires enzymatic conversion of testosterone to one or several other steroids such as androstenedione, dihydrotestosterone, other androgens, or estradiol (this varies among species). If testosterone concentrations do not rise during early development, the brain becomes sensitive to estrogen and progesterone stimulation of female sexual behavior in the adult (this also may depend upon early exposure to estrogen). Gonadal steroids stimulate sexual behavior by altering the activity of a number of neuropeptides (e.g., increasing oxytocin and decreasing opioid activity) and neurotransmitters (Pfaus and Everitt, 1995).

Female sexual behavior includes proceptive behaviors that signal the female's availability and entice the male to approach and receptive behaviors that enhance successful copulation (e.g., a receptive female rat assumes a lordotic posture and moves her tail to the side so her vagina is exposed to the penile thrusts of the male). Male sexual behavior includes penile erection, mounting, thrusting, and ejaculation. Estrogen and progesterone stimulate proceptive and receptive sexual behavior by acting on neurons in the preoptic area, mediobasal hypothalamus, and midbrain, which contain receptors for these steroids. Androgens stimulate male sexual behavior by acting on neurons in the preoptic area and anterior hypothalamus. Neural projections arising from areas in which steroids exert their activating effects on sexual behavior connect with other pathways that regulate the sensory input and motor output necessary for coordinated behavioral control. The neural circuitry underlying female sexual receptivity (lordosis) has been examined in the most detail (see Fig.12–25).

Active and sustained parental care of offspring from their birth until they are able to fend for themselves is a critical part of reproduction in mammals (Numan, 1994). Specific parental behaviors vary among species but all involve

Figure 12–25. *Schematic representation of the minimal neural circuit for lordosis behavior in the female rat. Estradiol effects are mediated at estrogen-binding neurons in the hypothalamus and the central gray. Ascending spinal fibers conveying sensory information necessary for induction of lordosis travel in the anterolateral columns of the spinal cord. mmgb, medial division of the medial geniculate body; mrf, dorsal mesencephalic reticular formation. (Reproduced with permission from Pfaff D, Modianos D: Neural mechanisms of female reproductive behavior. In Adler N., Pfaff D, Goy RW (eds): Handbook of Behavioral Neurobiology, Vol. 7: Reproduction. New York, Plenum Press, 1985, pp 423–493.)*

nursing and protecting newborns as well as keeping them warm. In most species, the mother does all of the parenting. In subprimate mammals, mothering behavior is activated by the changes in estrogen and progesterone concentrations at the end of pregnancy that stimulate parturition. Gonadal steroids exert these effects by increasing the activity of oxytocin systems as well as altering the activity of other neuropeptides and neurotransmitters in the brain. Estrogen and oxytocin activity in the medial preoptic area are particularly important for the postpartum onset of mothering behavior. In primates, parental caretaking of offspring is not as rigidly controlled by gonadal steroids and depends much more on skills learned early in life. Psychobiological investigation of parenting in animals may increase our understanding of the emotional attachments that underlie important human relationships (Carter et al, 1997).

Primate and Human Sexual Behavior

Human sexual interest and activity are influenced by reproductive hormones but to a considerably lesser degree than in animals. The human brain undergoes sexually dimorphic organization that is regulated by the testosterone concentrations that prevail during the second trimester of gestation. Testosterone concentrations are typically eight to nine times higher in male fetuses during this developmental period. The hormonal events that stimulate ovulation do not exert absolute control over the sexual behavior of female primates or women. Female sexual activity in primates is less restricted to the fertile period of the ovarian cycle than in subprimate species. Women can become sexually aroused and responsive throughout their menstrual cycles. Nonetheless, estrogen is necessary for optimal sexual interest and enjoyment in most, but not all, women. Similarily, in men, androgens enhance sexual desire and fantasy as well as penile erections. However, sexual desire and erections can be aroused by erotic stimuli in the absence of androgens. Above a threshold range, there is no relationship in men between testosterone concentration and magnitude of sexual interest or arousal (Rubinow and Schmidt, 1996). Human sexuality and sexual activity are important components in a broad range of social interactions that are not primarily reproductive in nature.

Heterosexual orientation appears to be strongly influenced by the organizational effects of gonadal steroids during early brain development. Humans are the only species in which some individuals develop exclusive sexual preference for and committed sexual relationships with members of the same sex. Evidence is accumulating that homosexual orientation is influenced by genetic and biological factors. Recent neuroanatomical studies indicate that there may be some differences in brain structure between homosexual and heterosexual men. Twin studies have found a strong genetic component for both male and female homosexuality. However, a considerably body of evidence demonstrates that human sexual identity also is powerfully determined by early experience, social expectations, and cultural factors (Collaer and Hines, 1995; Friedman and Downey, 1993).

Consumptive Behavior

Feeding behavior can be broken down into several discrete functions: initiation of feeding, food selection and maintenance of eating, and satiety. The first two are coordinated by neural structures located with the hypothalamus, especially the paraventricular nucleus. Satiety is mediated by a combination of central and peripheral mechanisms. The manner in which specific neurotransmitter systems interact varies with function, as indicated in Table 12–7. Other subcortical structures, such as brain stem motor nuclei, the nigrostriatal tract, and sympathetic pathways, play a role in carrying out the eating impulse by mediating stereotyped ingestive behaviors such as chewing and swallowing. In humans, it is clear that cortical structures can exert considerable influence over appetitive behavior, to the point of completely overriding hunger. The mechanisms by which this occurs are not yet well understood (Halmi, 1995).

The initiation of feeding is evoked in part by decreases in serum glucose concentration. Noradrenergic neurons have a strong facilitating influence on the initiation of feeding, perhaps mediated through inhibition of corticotropin-releasing factor, which has a powerful anorexic effect. Neuropeptide Y and opioids also initiate eating. Glucocorticoids facilitate eating and may regulate feeding.

Maintenance of homeostasis requires that an organism be able to select those nutrients that best fit current metabolic needs. The mechanisms involved in food choice are closely linked with reward centers in the hypothalamus. Dopaminergic neurons play a prominent role in the pleasurable reinforcement of food choice and in the maintenance of eating. Endorphins also influence food choice and, in particular, increase the consumption of fat. Noradrenergic stimulation increases fat and carbohydrate intake, whereas serotonergic stimulation decreases carbohydrate choice.

Satiety is initiated in the gut in part by food-triggered secretion of the gastrointestinal peptides cholecystokinin (CCK), satietin, and bombesin. Gut peptides exert their effects on feeding through afferent neuronal connections

Table 12–7 **Neurohormonal Regulation of Eating Behavior**

	NE	5-HT	DA	END	CCK	NPY	INS	SAT	CRF
Initiation of feeding	I	–	–	D (P,I)	D	I	I	D	D
Food choice									
CHO	I	D	–	–	–	I	–	–	–
Fat	I	–	–	I	–	–	–	–	–
Pleasure	–	–	I	–	–	–	–	–	–
Satiety	–	I	–	–	I	–	–	I	–

Abbreviations: END = endorphin, INS = insulin, SAT = satietin, D = decrease, I = increase, – = no difference, P = peripheral administration.

between the gastrointestinal tract and the CNS. For example, CCK satiety signals are transmitted to the brain through the vagus nerve. However, injection of CCK into the paraventicular nucleus also induces satiety, suggesting that direct peptide regulation of central ingestive systems also may occur.

Aggression

Aggression occurs in a number of distinct behavioral contexts. In animals and humans, aggression is one component of a larger repertoire of social behaviors, the goals of which are reproductive success as well as acquisition and protection of resources, territory, and status. Aggression also is one of a number of behavioral responses to aversive situations other than social conflict. Unfortunately, excessive, maladaptive violence directed toward others or self occurs in the form of assault, murder, or suicide. This section will focus primarily on the neurobiology of social aggression but also will review our limited understanding of pathological violence. The neurobiology of behavioral responses to stress is reviewed in the next section of this chapter.

Aggression in Subprimate Mammals
Offensive and defensive aggression in rodents and other subprimate mammals differ in a number of ways (Albert et al, 1993). The behaviors engaged in during offensive and defensive attacks are quite distinct. Offensive aggression primarily is exhibited by males toward unfamiliar members of their species, especially unfamiliar males. Competition for sexually receptive females increases offensive aggression in males. Lactating females also offensively attack animals that threaten their offspring. Male offensive aggression depends upon both the early organizational and later activational effects of testosterone. Males begin to show offensive aggression at puberty when testosterone levels increase. In contrast, defensive aggression does not require sex steroids and is exhibited by adult males and females as well as prepubertal juveniles. The brain mechanisms of offensive and defensive aggression are quite different. The medial hypothalamus and lateral septum facilitate offensive aggression but inhibit defensive aggression; the amygdala is involved in mobilizing defensive aggression but does not appear to play a role in offensive aggression. Virtually all of the classical neurotransmitter systems, including 5-HT, NE, DA, ACH, and GABA, as well as some neuropeptides (e.g., corticotropin-releasing factor, opioids) regulate aggressive behavior (Eichelman, 1992; Mann, 1995).

Aggression in Primates and Humans
Considerable evidence indicates that nonpathological aggression in primates and humans bears more resemblance to defensive than offensive aggression in subprimate mammals (Albert et al, 1993). Qualitatively similar aggression is exhibited toward familiar and unfamiliar individuals, toward

members of the same and opposite sex, and toward juveniles. Aggression is linked less predictably to particular activating situations or experiences. Testosterone does not appear to be necessary for aggression in primates and humans. Early brain organizational effects of testosterone contribute to the greater tendency of juvenile males to engage in rough and tumble play and, probably, to the greater amount of aggression exhibited by adult males. However, there is no relationship between testosterone concentrations and aggression levels. With the rise in testosterone concentrations at puberty, male aggression does not increase. Castration of adult males does not necessarily diminish aggressive behavior. Testosterone concentrations are greater in higher-rank male monkeys, but do not rise until after they have achieved their position in the dominance hierarchy. The limited clinical evidence on the behavioral effects of localized brain tumors or epileptic foci indicates that human aggression (male and female) is activated by the amygdala and inhibited by the medial hypothalamus and the lateral septum.

Human Aggression: Assault, Homicide, and Suicide

Aggressive acts of violence, directed at others or at one's self, are a major public health problem in this country. Initially, violence and suicide were studied from sociological and psychological perspectives, but beginning in the 1960s, researchers have applied increasingly sophisticated technologies to the study of the neurobiological bases of these behaviors.

Clinical Neurobiology of Aggression

Several neurotransmitters have been studied in clinical investigations exploring the neurobiological correlates of pathological human aggression. The most compelling data implicate serotonin in the pathophysiology of impulsive aggression. Low levels of the serotonin metabolite, 5-hydroxyindoleacetic acid (5-HIAA), have been found in the CSF of diverse groups of subjects with histories of violent aggression. Other peripheral measures of serotonergic function, including studies of platelet serotonin content, platelet serotonin reuptake, and whole blood serotonin content, also have supported the hypothesis that dysregulation in serotonin function is correlated with aggressive behavior. A significant positive correlation also has been found between CSF concentrations of the norepinephrine metabolite 3-methoxy-4- hydroxyphenylglycol (3, 4, MHPG) and a life history of violent aggression.

Numerous pharmacological interventions have been used in efforts to control violent, aggressive behavior. Benzodiazepines have been reported to be effective in treating aggressive outbursts. Dopamine receptor antagonists also have been applied extensively to the control of aggressive behavior in psychotic and nonpsychotic patients with aggressive behaviors, including demented patients, and children with mental retardation or conduct disorder.

Drugs that block beta-adrenergic receptors, including propranolol and nadolol, may ameliorate aggressive behavior in children with brain disease and adults with rage outbursts (Mann, 1995).

Criminal violence has been linked strongly to paranoid thinking, low intelligence, a history of head injury, physical abuse in childhood, and habitual use of cocaine, other stimulants, or alcohol (Albert et al, 1993). Most incarcerated criminals with a history of violence have abnormal electroencephalograms. These associations underscore the probable relationship between brain damage or abnormal brain development and pathological human violence.

Serotonin and Suicide

Suicide attempts are associated strongly with clinical depression. As with aggression, abnormalities in serotonergic function have been linked to suicide. Postmortem studies of suicide victims have found abnormalities in various aspects of serotonergic systems, including decreased concentrations of serotonin and 5-HIAA in the CSF and some brain sites and increased $5\text{-}HT_2$ receptor binding in the frontal cortex. These findings are related more strongly to planned, successful suicides than impulsive attempts (Mann, 1995). Increased beta-adrenergic receptor binding also has been found in the cerebral cortex of suicide victims.

CLINICAL CORRELATION: ATYPICAL ANTIPSYCHOTIC AGENTS AND AGGRESSION

The various available pharmacological regimens, including standard neuroleptics, benzodiazepines, anticonvulsants, and beta blockers, have only been partially successful in treating patients with aggressive and self-abusive behaviors. Newly available atypical antipsychotic agents, such as clozapine and olanzapine, appear especially promising in reducing aggressive behavior in patients with psychotic disorders (Mann, 1995). This antiaggressive effect may result from their actions on two neurotransmitters that play a key role in aggressive behavior: dopamine and serotonin. Unlike standard neuroleptics, which primarily antagonize the D_2 receptor and have no serotonergic effects, clozapine and olanzapine have relatively greater activity at the dopamine D_1 receptor antagonist and also function as a serotonergic agonist by blocking $5\text{-}HT_2$ receptors.

Stress and Behavior

Certain theoretical and practical aspects of stress as it affects vulnerability to physical illness (particularly the immune system) were introduced in Chapter 3 by Drs. Walker and Katon. The neurobiological mechanisms involved in stress responses are discussed here in more detail, particularly the neuroendocrine system.

The environment often subjects animals and humans to aversive stimuli and situations (stressors). Stress is the internal response to aversive conditions and includes situationally specific patterns of hormone release, central neuroendocrine change, and autonomic activation. Stressors also elicit behavioral responses, which vary widely with the type and magnitude of aversive stimulus. Hormonal and neuroendocrine components of the stress response act within the brain to stimulate appropriate behavioral responses to specific stressors.

Behavioral Responses to Stressors

Stressful conditions can be grouped into three general categories (Field et al, 1985). Specific behavioral responses as well as endocrine and autonomic responses differ with type of stressful condition. The first category is composed of *stressors for which the organism has readily available effective coping responses,* which may include escape, offensive or defensive attack, or other proactive behaviors that allow the organism to diminish or master the aversive situation. Under these conditions, cardiac output, heart rate, blood pressure, and vasodilation in skeletal muscle all increase. The second category is composed of *stressors for which the organism has no active coping option.* Under these conditions, organisms become hypervigilant but immobile, adopting either a frozen or submissive posture. Peripheral resistance and blood pressure rise while heart rate and blood flow through skeletal muscle decrease. The third category of stressors includes *unfamiliar, novel, or uncertain stimuli or situations.* Reactions to such conditions include initial hypervigilance and immobility followed by cautious exploration interspersed with behaviors that are thought to be manifestations of anxiety (e.g., self-grooming in animals; tapping, clearing the throat, pacing, and so forth in humans). Cardiovascular responses to novelty are initially (during the immobile hypervigilant phase) similar to those occurring when active coping strategies are not available, but, as the organism begins to explore and emote, the cardiovascular response shifts to that associated with active coping. The sudden onset of high-intensity aversive stimulation often elicits an initial immobile, hypervigilant response with attendant cardiovascular changes even if active coping strategies are readily available. *Repeated exposure to aversive conditions that cannot be controlled produces a state of "learned helplessness" in which the organism will passively endure stressors even when coping options become available.* Aversive stimuli also inhibit reproductive, eating, drinking, and other motivated behaviors.

Exposure to stressors early in development profoundly affects behavior and stress responses in adulthood. Male offspring of rodent mothers that were stressed during pregnancy are both demasculinized and feminized; female offspring are little affected. For instance, as adults, these males display much reduced mounting and increased lordosis behavior. Prenatal stress alters catecholamine levels in a number of brain sites. In humans, prenatal stress has been associated with behavioral, psychiatric, and sexual identity problems. Separation of infants from their mothers also has lifelong effects on behavioral, endocrine, and autonomic responses to stressors (Reite and Field, 1985) (see Chapter 11 by Dr. van der Kolk). Repeated brief periods of separation and handling of rat pups result in improved modulation of stress responses in adulthood. However, prolonged isolation of infant rhesus monkeys produces exaggerated stress responses in adulthood that resemble clinical depression in humans. Thus, stability in the face of stressors in adulthood may be enhanced by short periods of early maternal separation but impaired by excessive parental deprivation. Approximately 15% of human infants display exaggerated fear of unfamiliar objects and situations. Fearful infants had higher levels of cortisol and norepinephrine as well as elevated heart rates compared with other infants (Kagan et al, 1987). Early differences in individual temperament also may influence adult patterns of stress response.

Neuroendocrine Components of the Stress Response and Their Behavioral Effects

The hypothalamic–pituitary–adrenal (HPA) axis is particularly responsive to stressors. As established by the pioneering work of Selye, vigorous release of adrenal glucocorticoids and pituitary ACTH is a prominent feature of the stress response. Levels of beta endorphin, which is coreleased with ACTH from the anterior pituitary, also rise in response to stressors. Norepinephrine and epinephrine release from the adrenal medulla is the other component of the classic stress response (Chrousos et al, 1995).

Early stress researchers conceptualized HPA axis activation and catecholamine release as a general, nonspecific response to all types of stressors. However, more recent studies demonstrate that the pattern of release of peripheral neuroendocrine components of the stress response varies under differing stressful conditions (Field et al, 1985). Release of ACTH and adrenal glucocorticoids are most dramatic when organisms are confronted with aversive stimuli that are unfamiliar or for which they have no readily available coping mechanism. Epinephrine release also is relatively greater than norepinephrine release under these more psychologically stressful conditions.

Hypothalamic neuropeptides that are secreted into the hypophyseal portal system regulate the activity of the HPA axis by modulating the release of ACTH from the anterior pituitary. The most potent of these is corticotropin-releasing factor (CRF). However, vasopressin and oxytocin amplify CRF stimulation of ACTH release. The degree to which vasopressin and oxytocin are released into portal blood varies under different stressful conditions. Neural pathways containing CRF, vasopressin, and oxytocin, as well as beta-endorphin, enkephalins, and ACTH fragments, are widely distributed within the brain. Stressors very likely stimulate central release of these neuropeptides. Indeed, various kinds of stressors decrease concentrations of opioids and CRF and increase opioid binding in some brain regions. Turnover and synthesis of norepinephrine, epinephrine, and serotonin all increase in a number of brain regions in response to acute stressors.

Neuroendocrine components of the HPA axis influence behavioral responses to stressors. Glucocorticoids increase immobility and submissive behavior. ACTH, on the other hand, increases attack, as will exploratory behavior (Svare, 1983). Self-grooming behavior is activated by ACTH, vasopressin, oxytocin, beta endorphin, and CRF. ACTH, vasopressin, and oxytocin all influence acquisition of avoidance behavior (see section entitled Learning and Memory), suggesting that they may be crucial in gaining familiarity with novel stimuli, remembering aversive aspects of situations, and learning coping strategies. Stress inhibition of some behaviors also may be mediated by central neuroendocrine components of the HPA axis. Glucocorticoids, CRF, vasopressin, and beta endorphin all inhibit sexual behavior, whereas CRF and beta endorphin also antagonize food consumption. Central noradrenergic pathways play a key role in focusing attention and arousing appropriate behavioral responses to acute stressors. Depletion of brain norepinephrine resulting from exposure to repeated uncontrollable stress may contribute to the behavioral suppression associated with learned helplessness (Field et al, 1985).

Sleep

Sleep is a fundamental, complex, and essential behavior. Sleep was regarded as a homogeneous, passive experience until 1935, when Loomis and colleagues described distinct states of sleep that could be identified by specific electroencephalogram (EEG) patterns. By the mid-1950s, scientists had observed that bursts of conjugate rapid eye movements (REM) appear periodically during sleep; these REM sleep periods were subsequently linked to dreaming. In the past 3 decades, increasingly sophisticated technology has allowed us to decipher more of the mysteries of the experience we call "sleep." Yet even today, many medical school physiology courses virtually ignore the biology of sleep, when, in fact, the cardiovascular, respiratory, and neurochemical physiology of sleeping humans differs in many ways from the waking physiology that is usually taught.

Sleep Architecture

As Hauri (1982) has pointed out, sleep is an active, complex state, similar to a building with various components; thus, the expression "sleep architecture" is used to describe the stages and cycles of sleep and their interrelationships. The different stages of sleep are defined by distinct patterns of brain electrical activity and by distinct behavioral and physiological states.

Sleep Stages. Sleep can be divided into two broad categories: REM and non-REM (NREM) sleep. NREM sleep can be subcategorized further into four stages. NREM stages 1, 2, 3, and 4 can be conceptualized as representing a progression from very light to very deep sleep, with concurrent EEG changes from fast (high-frequency) low-amplitude waves to slow (low- frequency) high-amplitude patterns (Fig. 12–26).

Stage 1 consists of the transition from wakefulness to sleep. In normal sleepers, it lasts from 30 seconds to 7 minutes. During this stage, reactivity to

Awake - low voltage – random fast

Drowsy – 8 to 12 cps – alpha waves

Stage 1 – 3 to 7 cps – theta waves

Theta Waves

Stage 2 – 12 to 14 cps – sleep spindles and K complexes

Sleep Spindle   K Complex –

Delta Sleep – ½ to 2 cps – delta waves >75 μV

REM Sleep – low voltage – random, fast with sawtooth waves

Sawtooth Waves   Sawtooth Waves

Figure 12–26. Stages of human sleep. (Reproduced with permission from Hauri P: The Sleep Disorders. Kalamazoo, The Upjohn Co., 1982.)

external stimuli is blunted, thinking becomes less "reality oriented," and short dreams may develop as thoughts begin to drift. Many people will report that they felt that they were awake during this stage.

Stage 2 sleep is heralded by the onset of "sleep spindles" on the EEG (i.e., bursts of 12- to 14-Hz activity lasting 0.5 to 2 seconds) and "K-complexes" (i.e., sudden, high-amplitude bipolar spikes; see Fig. 12–26). By convention, sleep researchers define the onset of sleep by the appearance of the first sleep spindle or K-complex. Mentation during stage 2 consists of short, fragmented, mundane thoughts, and most people who are awakened during stage 2 will acknowledge that they were asleep and will not remember any dreams, although they may recall fragments of thoughts.

Stage 3 and Stage 4 sleep, collectively referred to as delta sleep, is characterized by slow, 0.5- to 2-Hz, high-amplitude waves on the EEG (see Fig. 12–26). Delta sleep can be thought of as "deep," or "heavy," sleep.

REM sleep derives its label from the periodic vertical and horizontal darting eye movements that are observed in this stage. The EEG during REM sleep presents a picture of low-voltage, mixed-frequency waves that resemble the pattern of Stage 1 sleep except for the additional presence of sawtooth waves (see Fig. 12–26). When people are awakened during REM sleep, they will recall dreams about 80% of the time, whereas only 5% of NREM awakenings are associated with complete dream recollection.

Sleep Cycles. During normal sleep, sleep stages do not occur at random; a pattern of progression can be described for a normal *sleep cycle* (Fig. 12–27). A healthy young adult typically moves from an awake state into a period of NREM sleep. After a brief period (e.g., 5 to 10 minutes) of relaxed, drowsy wakefulness, the sleeper passes through a brief 1- to 5-minute period of Stage

Figure 12–27. *Sequence of sleep stages in a healthy young adult. (Reproduced with permission from Mendelson WB: Human Sleep: Research and Clinical Care. New York. Plenum Press, 1987.)*

1 sleep, then descends into deeper Stage 2 sleep. Approximately thirty minutes into the sleep process, the sleeper enters delta (Stage 3 to Stage 4) sleep, which then lasts about 30 to 60 minutes. Typically, the sleeper then "ascends" back to Stage 2, during which a brief, first REM period is experienced. Following this initial REM period, the sleeper returns to Stage 2, and the second "sleep cycle" is begun. Thus, the first sleep cycle lasts about 90 minutes, with a brief REM period occurring 70 to 90 minutes after the initiation of sleep.

The typical healthy young adult sleeper will pass through four to six sleep cycles over the course of the night, and as Fig. 12–27 shows, these cycles are not identical. Following the first cycle described above, subsequent cycles show progressively less delta sleep. REM periods become progressively longer over the course of the night.

Sleep and the Lifecycle
The normal process of aging is accompanied by changes in the sleep cycle. In fact, age is the single most powerful determinant of a person's sleep physiology. Total sleep time and the total nightly amount of time spent in each of the sleep stages are age dependent. In general, total sleep time is greatest in infancy, decreases during childhood, and remains relatively stable during the adult years until a late-life decline is seen. Sleep becomes more "fragmented" over the course of a lifetime; the amount of waking time and the number of awakenings after sleep onset increase (Hauri, 1982).

In addition to these general parameters, the proportion of the various sleep stages also changes with aging. The percentage of REM sleep is highest in infancy and childhood, decreases and levels off in adulthood, and then declines in the geriatric years. Stage 4 sleep is also highest in infancy, then progressively declines with age.

The incidence and types of sleep disturbances change over the lifecycle. In childhood, sleep problems tend to include principally night terrors, enuresis, and bedtime fears and anxiety. Adolescents often are chronically sleep deprived and have difficulty getting up in the morning. In the elderly, there is a marked increase in the occurrence of insomnia, as well as in the specific sleep disorders of sleep apnea and nocturnal myoclonus. The quality of insomnia itself seems to vary with age. The elderly are inclined to experience more frequent and longer nighttime awakenings or early awakenings, whereas young insomniacs more often complain of difficulty falling asleep. In general, these changes occur earlier in women than in men (Lacks, 1987).

Circadian Rhythms
The sleep-wake cycle requires about 24 hours to complete in most humans. Thus, it is an example of a *circadian* rhythm. Other important biological functions also follow a circadian rhythm in humans, including body temperature (which reaches a nadir during nighttime sleep and peaks during the day), certain endocrine systems, and some metabolic processes. There is con-

siderable variation among people regarding the exact shape of some of these 24-hour oscillations. Scientists have suggested that people who seem to be "early birds" in terms of their preferred time of day for maximal performance may have different points of maximal efficiency for some of their circadian biological systems compared to "night owls."

When humans are placed in environments where there are no external time cues (e.g., a constantly lit, soundproof room with plenty of food but no clock), they still maintain a circadian rhythm. However, under these constant conditions, their sleep-wake cycles usually do not last exactly 24 hours. Most people settle into rhythms lasting between 24 and 28 hours, although sleep-wake cycles lasting as long as 50 hours have been observed under these conditions.

Neurobiology of Sleep

Nearly 100 years ago, Mauthner suggested that sleep induction was regulated by the area of the brain surrounding the third cranial nerve nuclei. A half century later, Bremer concluded that the junction between the diencephalon and the brain stem was crucial to sleep and wakefulness, based on his encephale isole and cerveau isole experiments (Hauri, 1982). Both Mauthner and Bremer viewed sleep as a "passive" process in which decreased cortical activation leads to a loss of wakefulness. It was later proposed that the reticular activating system plays a key role in maintaining arousal.

Other sleep researchers began to argue that sleep is a function of an active sleep-inducing center. Both stimulation and lesion experiments in animals, performed in the 1940s and 1950s, lent support to this view. Today, most sleep scientists have reconciled the "active" versus "passive" debate into an integrated theory.

Following transection at the midbrain, the forebrain above and the midbrain below both show wake-NREM sleep cycling, suggesting that there is no single center for NREM sleep. However, there are regions that do facilitate waking, including the ascending reticular activating system and the posterior hypothalamus, and regions that facilitate sleep (i.e., the basal forebrain, the area surrounding the solitary tract of the medulla, and possibly the dorsal raphe). Also, the superchiasmatic nucleus seems to serve as the major biological "clock" for most circadian rhythms and, thus, is also involved in the sleep-wake cycle.

Thus, it appears that there are two systems that regulate the sleep-wake cycle: a sleep-promoting system and a wakefulness-promoting system. For sleep onset to occur, activity in the more powerful arousal system must first passively decrease; following this, the less powerful sleep-promoting system can actively begin to play a role. Earlier, it had been suggested that serotonin controls NREM sleep, but currently it is recognized that the neurochemical control is much more complex. It appears that serotonin, acetylcholine, and norepinephrine, as well as other neurotransmitters, modulate the sleep-wake cycle in a complex, interactive manner.

In addition to the sleep-wake cycle, the REM-NREM cycle has been the subject of considerable study and debate. In the early 1960s, Jouvet (1965) reported the discovery of a REM-inducing system in the higher pons. More recently, Hobson et al (1975) have developed a model in which two classes of neural systems control the REM-NREM cycle. An aminergic system, which includes serotonergic neurons in the dorsal raphe and noradrenergic neurons in the locus ceruleus and nucleus peribrachialis lateralis, discharges at its highest rate during wakefulness, progressively decreases its discharge rate during NREM sleep, and produces very low discharge rates during REM sleep. A cholinergic reticular system, located primarily in the mesencephalic, medullary, and pontine gigantocellular tegmental fields, demonstrates the opposite pattern of activity. Thus, according to the Hobson-McCarley model, these two opposing systems continuously interact to produce the cycling between REM and NREM sleep. This model is not universally accepted, and this area remains an important focus of ongoing research.

SUMMARY

After 2 decades of breathtaking discovery, it is clear that we are now in the golden age of neuroscience. Much progress has been made in our understanding of the brain mechanisms involved in behavior. Most of this knowledge has been obtained through investigation of animal behavior. The challenge for the future is to achieve as much insight into the biological basis of human behavior. Fortunately we are on the brink of a new era in which technical advances are opening the way for safe, noninvasive study of human brain function. For instance, the availability of an increasing number of radio-emitting substances allows quantification and precise localization of blood flow, glucose utilization, and binding of specific molecules in the living brain. These methods will permit identification of brain regions and neurochemical systems involved in human behavior, cognition, and emotion. New capabilities of this sort may revolutionize our ability to diagnose and treat behavioral and psychological disorders in humans.

ANNOTATED BIBLIOGRAPHY

Bloom FE, Kupfer DJ (eds): Psychopharmacology: The Fourth Generation of Progress. New York, Raven Press, 1995

>A compendium of the field of psychopharmacology and biochemical treatments for mental illnesses; excellent reference for research and in-depth reading.

Cooper JR, Bloom FE, Roth RH (eds): The Biochemical Basis of Neuropharmacology, 7th ed. New York, Oxford University Press, 1996

>A concise but superb review of neuropharmacology; a classic small text that is "must" reading for all medical students.

Hyman SE, Coyle JT: The neuroscientific foundations of psychiatry. In Hales RE, Yudofsky SC, Talbott JA (eds): Textbook of Psychiatry, 2nd ed. Washington, DC, American Psychiatric Press, 1994

> Basic concepts in neuroscience as they relate to clinical psychiatric disorders are reviewed in this well-written chapter.

Kandel ER, Schwartz JH, Jessell TM (eds): Principles of Neural Science. New York, Elsevier, 1991

> A masterful text that is remarkable for its clarity and depth; an extremely valuable resource for students interested in recent advances in the neurosciences.

REFERENCES

Albert DJ, Walsh ML, Jonik RH: Aggression in humans: What is its biological foundation? Neurosci Biobehav Rev 17:405–425, 1993

Bailey CH, Alberini C, Ghirardi M, et al: Molecular and structural changes underlying long-term memory storage in aplysia. In Stjarne L, Greengard P, Grillner S, et al (eds): Molecular and Cellular Mechanisms of Neurotransmitter Release. New York, Raven Press, Ltd., 1994

Bunney WE Jr, Davis JM: Norepinephrine in depressive reactions: A review. Arch Gen Psychiatry 13:483–494, 1965

Burbach JPH, Meijer OC: The structure of neuropeptide receptors. Eur J Pharmacol Mol Pharmacol 227:1–18, 1992

Carter CS, Lederhendler II, Kirkpatrick B (eds): The Integrative Neurobiology of Affiliation. Ann N Y Acad Sci 807, 1997

Charney DS, Bremner JD, Redmond DE Jr (eds): Noradrenergic neural substrates for anxiety and fear: Clinical associations based on preclinical research. In Bloom FE, Kupfer DJ (eds): Psychopharmacology: The Fourth Generation of Progress. New York, Raven Press, 1995

Chrousos GP, McCarty R, Pacak K, et al (eds): Stress—Basic Mechanisms and Clinical Implications. Ann N Y Acad Sci 771, 1995

Collaer ML, Hines M: Human behavioral sex differences: A role for gonadal hormones during early development? Psychol Bull 118:55–107, 1995

Coppen A, Shaw D, Malleson A, et al: Changes in 5-hydroxytryptophan metabolism in depression. Br J Psychiatry 3:993–998, 1965

Deutch AY: The regulation of subcortical dopamine systems by the prefrontal cortex: Interactions of central dopamine systems and the pathogenesis of schizophrenia. J Neur Transmission (Suppl) 36:61–89, 1992

Eichelman B: Aggressive behavior: From laboratory to clinic. Quo vadit? Arch Gen Psychiatry 49:488–492, 1992

Elliot GR, Holman RB, Barchas JD: Neuroregulators and behavior. In Barchas JD, Berger PA, Ciaranello RD, et al (eds): Psychopharmacology: From Theory to Practice. New York, Oxford University Press, 1977

Field TM, McCabe PM, Schneiderman N (eds): Stress and Coping. Hillsdale, NJ, Lawrence Erlbaum Associates, 1985

Friedman RC, Downey J: Neurobiology and sexual orientation: Current relationships. J Neuropsychiatry Clin Neurosci 5:131–153, 1993

Golden RN, Potter WZ: Neurochemical and neuroendocrine dysregulation in affective disorders. Psychiatr Clin North Am 9:313–327, 1986

Goldman-Rakic PS: Cellular and circuit basis of working memory in prefrontal cortex of nonhuman primates. Prog Brain Res 85:325–336, 1990

Haggerty JJ Jr, Prange AJ Jr: Borderline hypothyroidism and depression. Annu Rev Med 46:37–46, 1995

Halmi KA: Basic biological overview of eating disorders. In Bloom FE, Kupfer DJ (eds): Psychopharmacology: The Fourth Generation of Progress. New York, Raven Press, 1995

Hauri P: The Sleep Disorders. Kalamazoo, The Upjohn Co., 1982

Heninger GR: Indoleamines: The role of serotonin in clinical disorders. In Bloom FE, Kupfer DJ (eds): Psychopharmacology: The Fourth Generation of Progress. New York, Raven Press, 1995

Herbert J: Peptides in the limbic system: Neurochemical codes for co-ordinated adaptive responses to behavioural and physiological demand. Prog Neurobiol 41:723–791, 1993

Hobson JA, McCarley RW, Wyzinski PW: Sleep cycle oscillations: Reciprocal discharge by two brainstem neuronal groups. Science 18:55–58, 1975

Hyman SE: Recent developments in neurobiology. Psychosomatics 29:157–165, 254–263, 373–378, 1988

Hyman SE, Coyle JT: The neuroscientific foundations of psychiatry. In Hales RE, Yudofsky SC, Talbott JA (eds): Textbook of Psychiatry, 2nd ed. Washington, DC, American Psychiatric Press, 1994

Janowsky DS, El-Yousef MF, Davis JM, et al: A cholinergic-adrenergic hypothesis of mania and depression. Lancet 2:6732–6735, 1972

Janowsky DS, Golden RN, Rapaport M, et al: Neurochemistry of depression and mania. In Georgotas A, Cancro R (eds): Depression and Mania. New York, Elsevier, 1988

Jouvet M: Paradoxical sleep: A study of its nature and mechanisms. In Himwich WA, Schade JP (eds): Sleep Mechanisms: Progress in Brain Research. Amsterdam, Elsevier, 1965

Kagan J, Reznick JS, Snidman N: Temperamental variation in response to the unfamiliar. In Krasnegor NA, Blass EM, Hofer MA, et al (eds): Perinatal Development: A Psychobiological Perspective. Orlando, Academic Press, 1987

Kandel ER, Hawkins RD: The biological basis of learning and individuality. Sci Am 267 (3) 79–86, 1992

Kandel ER, Schwartz JH, Jessell TM (eds): Principles of Neural Science. New York, Elsevier, 1991

Lacks P: Behavioral Treatment for Persistent Insomnia. New York, Pergamon Press, 1987

Lenox RH, Manji HK: Lithium. In Schatzberg AF, Nemeroff CB (eds): Textbook of Psychopharmacology. Washington, DC, American Psychiatric Press, 1995

Mann JJ: Violence and aggression. In Bloom FE, Kupfer DJ (eds): Psychopharmacology: The Fourth Generation of Progress. New York, Raven Press, 1995

Mansour A, Chalmers DT, Fox CA, et al: Biochemical anatomy: Insights into the cell biology and pharmacology of neurotransmitter systems in the brain. In Schatzberg AF, Nemeroff CB (eds): Textbook of Psychopharmacology. Washington, DC, American Psychiatric Press, 1995

McEwen BS: Neuroendocrine interactions. In Bloom FE, Kupfer DJ (eds): Psychopharmacology: The Fourth Generation of Progress. New York, Raven Press, 1995

Mendelson WB: Human Sleep: Research and Clinical Care. New York, Plenum Press, 1987

Numan M: Maternal behavior. In Knobil E, Neill JD (eds): The Physiology of Reproduction, 2nd ed. New York, Raven Press, 1994

Pfaus JG, Everitt BJ: The psychopharmacology of sexual behavior. In Bloom FE, Kupfer DJ (eds): Psychopharmacology: The Fourth Generation of Progress New York, Raven Press, 1995

Prange AJ Jr, Wilson IC, Lynn CW, et al: L-tryptophan in mania: Contribution to a permissive hypothesis of affective disorders. Arch Gen Psychiatry 30:56–62, 1974

Reis DJ: Considerations of some specific behaviors or disease. J Psychiatr Res 11:145–148, 1974

Reite M, Field T (eds): The Psychobiology of Attachment and Separation. Orlando, Academic Press, 1985

Rosenzweig MR: Aspects of the search for neural mechanisms of memory. Annu Rev Psychol 47:1–32, 1996

Rubinow DR, Schmidt PJ: Androgens, brain, and behavior. Am J Psychiatry 153:974–984, 1996

Schildkraut J: The catecholamine hypothesis of affective disorders: A review of the supporting evidence. Am J Psychiatry 122:509–522, 1965

Schull J, McEachron L, Adler NT, et al: Effects of thyroidectomy, parathyroidectomy and lithium on circadian wheelrunning in rats. Physiol Behav 42:33–39, 1988

Seeman P: Dopamine receptors: clinical correlates. In Bloom FE, Kupfer DJ (eds): Psychopharmacology: The Fourth Generation of Progress. New York, Raven Press, 1995

Squire LR: Memory and forgetting: Long-term and gradual changes in memory storage. Int Rev Neurobiol 37:243–269, 1994

Strand FL, Beckwith B, Chronwall B, et al (eds): Models of Neuropeptide Action. Ann N Y Acad
Sci 739, 1994

Svare BB (ed): Hormones and Aggressive Behavior. New York, Plenum Press, 1983

Ungerleider LG: Functional brain imaging studies of cortical mechanisms for memory. Science
270:769–775, 1995

Whybrow PC, Prange AJ Jr: A hypothesis of thyroid-catecholamine-receptor interaction. Arch
Gen Psychiatry 38:106–113, 1981

Wilcox RE, Gonzales RA: Introduction to neurotransmitters, receptors, signal transduction, and
second messengers. In Schatzberg AF, Nemeroff CB (eds): Textbook of
Psychopharmacology. Washington, DC, American Psychiatric Press, 1995

13 *Behavioral Genetics*

Miron Baron

Major advances in population genetics, cytogenetics, biochemistry, and molecular biology have heightened the awareness that much of the variation in human behavior may be attributed to complex interactions among hereditary, social, developmental, and environmental factors. These observations are in keeping with the biopsychosocial model of understanding disease and illness. Attempts to quantify the relative contributions of genetic and environmental factors in behavior have led, by necessity, to an interdisciplinary framework of scientific thought, which has replaced previously held artificial dichotomies between biological and psychological or "nature *versus* nurture." In actuality, both interact to determine behavior and vulnerability to illness.

This interdisciplinary framework is consistent with the thesis that has been repeated throughout this text—that human behavior should be understood from multiple perspectives: psychological, biological, and sociological. This chapter reviews methods of genetic investigation as they bear on studies of human behavior and mental illness. Areas to be discussed include the classic methods of family, twin, and adoption studies; pedigree analysis; the study of biological susceptibility traits and chromosomal markers; and the basic techniques of molecular biology. The implications of recent research for current trends in behavioral and psychiatric genetics also are discussed.

Supported by a Research Scientist Award MH00176 from the National Institute of Mental Health.

METHODS OF GENETIC INVESTIGATION

Family, Twin, and Adoption Studies

The following strategies constitute the most traditional approach to behavioral genetics. *Family risk studies* attempt to determine the rate of a disorder or trait among the relatives of identified index cases who are themselves affected with the condition. For the most part, family risk studies focus on first-degree relatives, but more distant relatives also can be considered. Because many behavioral disorders have variable age at onset, the observed familial rates must be adjusted by age. The *age correction procedure* yields expectancy rates or morbidity risks. The risk figures for the various groups of relatives can be compared with the expectancy rates for normal controls or the general population to determine the degree to which the condition being studied has a familial component.

Prediction studies are a variant of the family risk study. Prediction studies are concerned with the identification of behavioral or biological precursors of the disorder in subjects who are at high risk for the disorder in question by virtue of their being related to specific family constellations, for example, the children of one or two affected parents. These studies are prospective by nature and require a longitudinal approach.

Family risk studies can provide empirical risks for given conditions but are inconclusive with respect to the genetic versus environmental contribution to the observed familial patterns. By contrast, twin and adoption studies offer a way of separating genetic and environmental influences. The use of twins in genetic research commonly is based on comparing the *concordance rate* (when both twins of a pair are affected, they are said to be concordant) in monozygotic (or identical) and dizygotic (fraternal) twins. Whereas dizygotic twins share only 50% of their genetic endowment, monozygotic twins share all their genes; therefore, a higher concordance rate in monozygotic twins is taken as evidence that genetic factors are important in etiology. From the concordance rates it is possible to derive the *heritability,* which is a measure of the proportion of the genetic component in the overall familial resemblance. The concordance rate is somewhat dependent on the method of computation. Higher concordances result from the use of the proband method, whereby pairs are counted twice if each twin has an ill proband ascertained independently. In contrast, the pair method considers every pair only once. The probandwise concordance (using the proband method) is more widely used, because it can be compared with the population risk.

Adoption studies are based on three principal designs: (1) The *adoptees family method* determines the risk for a given condition to the biological and adoptive parents of index cases versus controls. A higher risk among the biological relatives of the index cases as compared with the control group points to the importance of genetic factors in the development of the disorder. A higher risk to the adoptive relatives of index cases indicates that rearing influences contribute to etiology. (2) The *adoptees study method* is concerned with the adopted-away children of affected parents. A higher risk for the disorder in this group of adoptees as compared with a matched control group indicates that heredity plays an important role in the development of the disorder. (3) The *crossfostering method* compares adoptees who have an affected biological parent (but whose adoptive parents are normal) with adoptees whose biological parents are normal but who are reared by an adoptive parent who is affected with the condition under study. Knowledge of the risk for the disorder in the two groups of adoptees is useful in evaluating the relative contributions of heredity and rearing influences. These three designs are summarized in Table 13–1.

Questions of ascertainment (case selection), adequate controls, phenotypic classification (e.g., diagnosis), and zygosity (twin studies) require careful consideration in these research strategies. These and related issues are discussed in greater detail by Rosenthal (1970) and Emery (1976).

Table 13–1 **Adoption Studies**

TYPE	DESIGN	INTERPRETATION
Adoptees family method	Compares the risk for a given condition among the biological and adoptive parents of index cases (groups I and II, respectively) and matched controls.	A higher risk to group I compared with the control group indicates that heredity contributes significantly to the condition studied. An increased risk to group II points to the importance of rearing influences.
Adoptees study method	Determines the risk for a given condition in the adopted-away children of affected parents (group III) versus matched controls.	An increased risk to group III points to the importance of genetic factors.
Crossfostering method	Compares adoptees whose adoptive parents are normal, but who have an affected biological parent (group IV) with adoptees whose adoptive parents are affected, but whose biological parents are normal (group V).	A higher risk to group IV compared with group V supports the role of heredity and minimizes the role of environment. An increased risk to group V indicates that the environment plays an important role in the disorder studied.

Pedigree Analysis

The studies described in the preceding section can point to the presence of genetic factors in etiology; however, they do not address the question of the underlying genetic mechanisms. Specifically, the mode of genetic transmission remains unknown. Discerning the mode of inheritance can strengthen the genetic evidence and can be useful both in the design and interpretation of genetic investigations (e.g., genetic linkage studies, see later) and in genetic counseling.

The search for mode of inheritance can be conducted through the use of statistical models that test the fit of specific genetic hypotheses to observed familial patterns. The method most commonly used for hypothesis testing is based on maximum likelihood, with "likelihood" referring to the probability of observing a given data set under a specific hypothesis (Thompson, 1986).

Most behavioral disorders do not have a clear single gene inheritance that conforms to Mendelian laws. The deviation from classic Mendelian inheritance has led to the introduction of concepts such as *reduced or incomplete penetrance, phenocopies or sporadic cases,* and *multifactorial–polygenic effects. Reduced penetrance* refers to the incomplete manifestation of the trait in persons who have the genotype and is usually ascribed to an interaction with other genes or to nongenetic factors. *Phenocopies* are persons who do not carry the genotype, but who nevertheless manifest the trait, a phenomenon commonly attributed to other genetic or nongenetic causes. *Multifactorial–polygenic* effects result from a large number of underlying genes and other factors that contribute to the person's liability to a given trait.

The most commonly used genetic formulations are the single major locus (or gene) (SML) and multifactorial–polygenic (MFP) models. The SML model stipulates that the transmission of a trait or disorder can be explained entirely by a single gene with two alleles resulting in three genotypes, two homozygous states and a heterozygous condition. Several subhypotheses can be tested under the SML model, such as dominant (where one dose of the abnormal allele may bring about the disorder) and recessive (where a double dose of the allele is required) modes of inheritance, as well as contributions from the environment. The parameters of the model are the frequency of the allele, the genotypic means of the three genotypes, the threshold (a point on a liability scale beyond which the penetrance is 100%), and a measure of environmental variance.

The MFP model invokes multiple genes and random environmental factors (each of small and additive effects) that contribute to phenotypic expression. The model incorporates such features as the liability of the general population and that of affected persons, and a threshold (a point on a liability scale above which all persons are affected and below which all are normal); the threshold corresponds to the genetic–environmental load that is sufficient to bring about the phenotype. Nongenetic factors, such as cultural influences that are transmitted between generations and environmental factors that are not transmissible, also can be incorporated in the models.

Other models that are thought to address more fully the complex transmission pattern of some behavioral disorders have been devised. These include: (1) the "mixed" model that combines single gene transmission, a polygenic background, and environmental effects; (2) the oligogenic model that postulates several separate genes with varying degrees of interaction; and (3) a polygenic model with graduated effects across the different loci.

One should note that the results of pedigree analysis must always be interpreted with due attention to methodological issues such as etiological heterogeneity, epistasis (the interaction between genes), reduced fertility, and assortative mating (the tendency of persons with like behavioral dispositions to marry and to reproduce).

Susceptibility Traits and Gene Markers

Pedigree analysis aims to examine the fit of a given data set to a particular genetic model; however, in the absence of additional information on inherited biological traits or chromosomal markers, statistical formulations cannot uncover the underlying genetic abnormality.

Biological susceptibility traits derive from etiological or pathophysiological hypotheses. They span diverse fields such as biochemistry, neurophysiology, and neuroanatomy, and are thought to be part of the pathway from genotype to phenotype.

Potential susceptibility traits include neurotransmitter enzymes, receptor proteins, and metabolites; attentional and electroencephalographic measures; and indices on brain scanning, such as those with positron emission tomography (PET). To qualify as a genetic susceptibility trait, the biological characteristic must be *heritable and state independent* (stable over time, regardless of clinical state); in addition, it should *segregate* with the disorder in families of affected probands (Rieder and Gershon, 1978). Although the specific mode of inheritance need not be known, traits of interest can be incorporated in genetic models that examine the underlying genetics of both the behavioral disorder and the biological trait.

Gene markers refer to chromosomal loci with known genomic position. They can be assigned to two general categories: (1) classic or conventional markers such as leukocyte antigens (HLA system), red blood cells antigens (i.e., blood groups), serum proteins, and observable traits such as color blindness; and (2) the new generation of DNA markers, namely, inherited variations that are detectable by molecular genetic techniques (see below).

The relation of gene markers to a trait or disorder can be determined by linkage analysis (Ott, 1991). Genetic linkage refers to the tendency of chromosomal loci to be coinherited. The distance between loci can be inferred from the recombination frequency (recombination is an exchange of material between homologous chromosomes during meiosis leading to a rearrangement of alleles in the offspring generation). The closer the loci are to each other, the less likely is recombination to occur between them. The odds ratio (the ratio between the probability of there being linkage at a given recombination frequency and that of there being no linkage), more commonly known as the lod score (the logarithm of odds), serves as the principal statistical measure of linkage.

By definition, gene markers have a Mendelian mode of inheritance. Unlike susceptibility traits, they need not stem from etiological or pathophysiological hypotheses of the disorder being studied. By virtue of their coinheritance with the gene for the disorder, they point to its presence and approximate chromosomal location. The most efficient approach to the study of linkage markers requires extended pedigrees with large sibships and high density of illness. An alternative approach, known as the *sibpair method,* is concerned with pairs of affected siblings and does not require multigeneration family pedigrees. An extended version of this approach, known as the affected pedigree member method, includes other relative pairs as well. Gene markers also can be studied for association with a given trait using a case-control design (a comparison between unrelated affected individuals and a general population sample). Such an association, which usually involves markers at genes believed to play a role in pathogenesis (so-called candidate genes), can imply a causal link between the marker locus and the trait.

The demonstration of linkage (or association) with gene markers is interpreted as proof of a susceptibility gene and also can provide external validation for behavioral assessments. In addition, the study of inherited biological traits and chromosomal markers can offer a means of addressing the important question of etiological heterogeneity. For example, linkage or association of a trait with different gene markers in different family pedigrees or populations would suggest the presence of several independent genetic forms.

Molecular Biology

Perhaps the single most important development in human genetics in recent years involves the application of molecular biology techniques. The insights gleaned by these methods can be summarized briefly, as follows. First, the new technology can reveal numerous DNA variations that span the entire human genome. In conjunction with linkage analysis, these DNA markers can lead to the chromosomal localization of the genes responsible for many inherited conditions. DNA markers have already been used to map the abnormal genes in numerous human disorders, including the neuropsychiatric disorders Huntington's disease, X-linked mental retardation, and familial forms of Alzheimer's disease. Second, the structure and function of the abnormal genes can be determined. This, in turn, can shed light on the underlying molecular mechanisms. A case in point is Duchenne muscular dystrophy, where the gene has been characterized and its protein product identified. Third, the molecular

Table 13–2 **Genetic Mapping of Neurobehavioral Disorders**

DISORDER	CHROMOSOMAL LOCATION	GENE DEFECT	REFERENCE
Tay–Sachs	15q22–25	Hexosaminidase (alpha chain)	Gilbert et al, 1975
Duchenne	Xp21	Dystrophin	Murray et al, 1982 Hoffman et al, 1987
Huntington's	4p16	IT15	Gusella et al, 1983 MacDonald et al, 1993
Lesch–Nyhan	Xq27	HPRT	Nussbaum et al, 1983
Wilson's	13q14	Copper binding ATPase	Tanzi et al, 1993
Neurofibromatosis	17q11	NF1LT	Wallace et al, 1990
Bipolar disorder	Xq24–28?	Unknown	Baron et al, 1993 Pekkarinen et al, 1995
	21q22?	Unknown	Straub et al, 1994
	18cen–q23?	Unknown	Berrettini et al, 1994 Stine et al, 1995 Freimer et al, 1996
	4p16?	Unknown	Blackwood et al, 1996
Schizophrenia	6p24–22?	Unknown	Straub et al, 1995
	15q13–14?	Unknown	Freedman et al, 1997
Alzheimer's	21q21	Beta APP	St. George-Hyslop et al, 1987
	19q13	ApoE4	Pericak-Vance et al, 1991
	14q24	Presenilin 1	Schellenberg et al, 1992
	1q31–42	Presenilin 2	Levy-Lahad et al, 1995

Note: q,p. the long and the short arms of the chromosome, respectively; cen. the centromere; preceding these notations are the chromosome numbers; following the q,p notations are the numbers of the chromosomal bands.

biology approach can increase the precision of genetic diagnosis and might lead to improved preventive and treatment measures. The chromosomal mapping and the gene defects for some selected neurobehavioral disorders are summarized in Table 13–2.

DNA markers have evolved in stages. The first-generation markers, also known as restriction-fragment-length polymorphisms (RFLPs), are detected by a method known as Southern hybridization, whereby a DNA molecule digested by restriction enzymes (endonucleases) is hybridized to a genetic probe specific for the DNA segment suspected to be variant. The resultant pattern of DNA fragments that contain complementary genetic information then can be displayed by autoradiography and tested for linkage with presumed genes for a given disorder. Localization of the gene to a specific chromosomal region can be inferred from prior evidence that the marker is on a particular chromosome, or by physical methods such as somatic cell hybridization.

RFLPs are being supplanted by the more abundant and more polymorphic microsatellite markers. These markers, which already span the entire length of the genome, are detected by a molecular method known as polymerase chain reaction (PCR).

As noted earlier, a linked marker merely points to the approximate chromosomal location of the gene of interest, but is not likely to contain it. Several molecular genetic methods have been developed to bridge the distance between the marker and the putative disease gene. These include saturation mapping, physical mapping, DNA sequencing, and cDNA (complementary DNA) cloning. Once the DNA segment containing the gene has been identified and its structure (nucleotide sequence) has been determined, both the messenger RNA and the associated protein product can be characterized according to the principles of transcription and translation. Conversely, knowledge of the gene product can lead to identification of the gene itself. Namely, the DNA sequence corresponding to the nucleotide code of the protein can be synthesized, cloned, and used as a probe to screen for the DNA segment that includes the relevant gene. This method has been used successfully to identify the genes for the hormones insulin and erythropoietin, coagulation factor VIII, and the globin chains, among other protein-encoding genes. In behavioral disorders, such genes, also known as candidate genes, include genomic regions that code for neurotransmitter receptors and enzymes. The Human Genome Project, which is well on its way to completion, will alter dramatically the landscape of molecular biology: with precise knowledge of all DNA sequences (and oftentimes their function) in any region of interest, candidate genes for any genetic condition could be readily identified once linkage has been established.

The availability of tightly linked DNA markers or gene-specific probes can provide powerful and accurate tools for genetic diagnosis of a given trait or disorder. These tools also can be used for risk prediction (and thereby genetic counseling) by the detection of carriers of abnormal alleles. Inherited disorders where these methods are being applied include sickle cell disease,

Table 13–3 **Clinical Applications of Molecular Biology Techniques**

	APPLICATION	
DISORDER	**Risk Prediction**	**Treatment***
Sickle cell anemia	+	
Thalassemia	+	
Phenylketonuria	+	
Lesch–Nyhan	+	
Cystic fibrosis	+	
Diabetes mellitus		+ (Insulin)
Hemophilia	+	+ (Coagulation factor VIII)

* Therapeutic products produced by molecular biology techniques.

thalassemia, phenylketonuria, and Lesch–Nyhan syndrome. The characterization of genes and their products can lead to specific drugs of a therapeutic or preventive nature; in some instances (e.g., insulin, erythropoietin, and the antihemophilic factor VIII), the product itself can be used for treatment purposes. Eventually, the replacement of defective genes with normal clones could be contemplated. The clinical applications of molecular biology techniques to some medical disorders are listed in Table 13–3.

The principles that underlie the new DNA technology and its implications for psychiatry are reviewed in detail elsewhere (Martin, 1987; Baron and Rainer, 1988; Owen and Craddock, 1996).

Phenotypic Classification

An accurate definition of the phenotype is crucial in behavioral genetics. The current emphasis on structured, criterion-based approaches to the assessment of behavior has improved reliability and consensus between investigators and practitioners. "Ill" versus "well" dichotomies largely depend on descriptive diagnostic practices in the absence of external validating measures. The question of external validity pertains to the likely heterogeneity both within and among diagnostic categories. Additional information, such as biochemical measures, can aid in refining behavioral and psychiatric nosology and lead to the demarcation of homogeneous subgroups, which, in turn, may enhance the prospects of genetic studies. Conversely, data on biological vulnerability traits, linked genetic markers, and differential familial loading can aid in the classification of behavioral conditions by circumventing the uncertainties inherent in descriptive diagnostic phenomenology, which is largely based on behavioral signs and symptoms.

Genes and Environment

Although the main emphasis in this review is on the genotypic determination of inherited conditions, *the environment can play an important role in the pathway from genotype to phenotype.* The environment shapes and modifies the transmission and expression of the genetic makeup at all levels, from the cellular to the behavioral. This regulation may be in the form of activation or suppression of the underlying genetic mechanisms.

The contribution of the environment to phenotypic expression in most behavioral disorders can be evidenced readily by the incomplete concordance in identical monozygotic twins. To some extent, this contribution can be quantified by statistical measures, such as heritability, and the incorporation of reduced penetrance, sporadic cases or phenocopies, multifactorial influences, and other types of environmental variance in the genetic analysis of pedigrees. The study of biological inherited traits may provide a more definitive approach to the elucidation of gene–environment interaction. For example, if a specific environmental factor operates in conjunction with the underlying genotypic makeup, this factor will more likely be present in the affected than in the unaffected relatives when the illness in both groups of subjects is linked to a particular genetic marker. A complementary approach, which falls under the rubric of high-risk paradigms, would be to study prospectively putative environmental factors in persons who carry the genetic marker and are therefore at risk for developing the disorder.

PSYCHIATRIC GENETICS

Major Disorders

Family, Twin, and Adoption Studies

The major mental disorders, schizophrenia and bipolar disorder (manic–depressive illness), occupy center stage in psychiatric genetics because both conditions run in families. In recent well-designed studies, the morbidity risk for schizophrenia in first-degree relatives schizophrenic patients is 3 to 6%, as compared with 0.2 to 0.7% in the general population. The corresponding rates for bipolar disorder in the general population are 4 to 9% and 0.2 to 0.5%, respectively. (When major depression, also known as unipolar major depressive disorder and thought to be a milder manifestation of the bipolar genotype in families of bipolar patients, is included in the bipolar "spectrum," the risk to first-degree relatives of bipolar probands is 13 to 35% versus 5 to 8% in the general population.) The variable rates among studies are attributable in part to different diagnostic practices and other methodological issues, such as sampling scheme. For example, the rate at which schizophrenia is diagnosed can vary severalfold, depending on how narrow or how broad the criteria are (Baron et al, 1985a). Similarly, the familial rate of major depressive disorder can be reduced considerably by requiring "impairment incapacitation" as an essential inclusion criterion (Gershon et al, 1982). It is of interest, however, that despite the varied methodology, the relative risk (the ratio of the risk to patients' relatives to the risk to relatives of normal controls) is high (approximately 10 to 20% for schizophrenia, 17 to 20% for bipolar disorder), indicating significant familial aggregation. When major depression is considered independently of bipolar disorder, the risk to first-degree relatives of patients with major depression is 11 to 18%, compared with 5 to 6% in controls; the relative risk is 2 to 3%. Thus, the evidence for familial clustering is not as impressive as that for schizophrenia and bipolar disorder, but is nevertheless significant. The results overall support earlier family studies dating to the beginning of the century. Morbidity risk data on schizophrenia and mood disorders are presented in Table 13–4.

Consistent with a genetic hypothesis, twin studies have consistently shown higher concordance in both mood disorders and schizophrenia rates in monozygotic than in dizygotic twins. The ratio of monozygotic versus dizygotic

Table 13–4 **Morbidity Risk for Schizophrenia and Mood Disorders**

DISORDER	MORBIDITY RISK IN FIRST-DEGREE RELATIVES (%)	MORBIDITY RISK IN RELATIVE OF CONTROLS (%)	RELATIVE RISK	REFERENCE*
Schizophrenia	5.8	0.6	9.7	Baron et al, 1985b
	4.6	0.7	6.6	Kendler et al, 1993
Bipolar disorder[†]	3.9	0.2	19.5	Tsuang et al, 1980
	4.5 (8.6)	0.0 (0.5)	(17.2)	Gershon et al, 1982
	3.9 (8.1)	No data		Andreasen et al, 1987
Major depression	11.0	4.8	2.3	Tsuang et al, 1980
	17.5	5.9	3.0	Weissman et al, 1984
	22.8	No data		Andreasen et al, 1987

* The studies cited fulfill modern criteria for genetic-family investigations. They represent six large-scale research efforts: the Iowa 500 (Tsuang et al, 1980); the New York-Columbia University Study (Baron et al, 1985a and b); the NIMH Study (Gershon et al, 1982); the New Haven–Yale University Study (Weissman et al, 1984); the NIMH Collaborative Study (Andreasen et al, 1987); and the Roscommon Irish Family Study (Kendler et al, 1993).
† Bipolar disorder has two variants: bipolar I, the more severe illness form (depressive and manic episodes), and bipolar II (depression and hypomania). The figures in parentheses are the combined morbid risks for bipolar I and bipolar II disorders; the other risk figures are for bipolar I disorder.

concordance rates is approximately 4 to 1 for schizophrenia and bipolar disorder, although the absolute rates vary among studies. The heritability estimates based on these data are 30 to 50% and 60 to 80% for schizophrenia and bipolar disorder, respectively. As with the family risk data, the evidence for a genetic component in major depression is not as strong; the monozygotic to dizygotic ratio in concordance rates is only 2 to 1. It is noteworthy that an appreciable proportion of the monozygotic twin pairs are discordant for schizophrenia and bipolar disorder (approximately 50% and 20%, respectively), pointing to the important role of environmental factors in the pathogenesis of these disorders.

Using both the adoptees family method and the adoptees study method, adoption studies have reinforced the notion that genetic factors play an important role in schizophrenia and major mood disorders. In addition, a cross-fostering study has shown that the adopted-away offspring of schizophrenic parents are at increased risk for the illness as compared with the adopted-away offspring of nonschizophrenic parents. The adopted-away offspring of normal biological parents reared by schizophrenic parents showed no increase in the risk for schizophrenia. This study has been interpreted as evidence against a strong environmental component in the etiology of schizophrenia.

Taken together, family, twin, and adoption studies support the role of heredity in the major psychoses. A spectrum of conditions thought to be related to the "core" disorders also has been considered in the genetic framework. For example, some forms of schizoaffective illness (a mixed pattern of schizophrenic and affective symptoms), schizotypal, and paranoid personality disorders are believed to belong in the schizophrenia spectrum, whereas other subtypes of schizoaffective disorder and some forms of alcoholism, sociopathy, anxiety, eating disorders, and minor disorders with affective coloring such as cyclothymia may be related to the affective spectrum. These studies are reviewed in detail elsewhere (Andreasen et al, 1987; Baron et al, 1985a and b; Gershon et al, 1982; Gottesman and Shields, 1982; Kendler et al, 1993; Weissman et al, 1984).

Pedigree Analysis

Numerous applications of genetic models to family data, including the SML and MFP models and variations thereof, have been reported. Despite the advances in statistical genetics, the analysis of clinical genetic data has not led to consistent results. Based on these studies, the mode of inheritance of either schizophrenia or major mood disorders remains elusive. The inconsistency among studies has been attributed to variations in the methods for data collection (sampling scheme, diagnosis) and analysis (mathematical formulations) and to the likely heterogeneous nature of these disorders. The prevailing wisdom is that the analysis of familial patterns using statistical genetic techniques is not likely to unravel the underlying genetic mechanism without the added benefit of biological susceptibility traits and chromosomal markers. Detailed reviews of this topic are provided by Baron (1986a) and by Goldin and Gershon (1983).

Biological Susceptibility Traits and Gene Markers

A large array of biological variables, including biogenic amine enzymes and metabolites, neuroreceptor sensitivity, neuromuscular function, immune response, attentional and electrophysiological measures, and brain morphology, have been examined as potential vulnerability traits for schizophrenia and mood disorders. As has been noted in recent reviews of this area (Baron, 1986b), some of these traits, such as attentional (Continuous Performance Test and eye tracking), neurophysiological (auditory evoked response), and brain morphology measures (brain ventricular size) appear promising, but the data are as yet not adequate to arrive at firm conclusions. In bipolar affective disorder (manic depression), alterations of the GABA (cerebrospinal fluid GABA and GABA-transaminase) and cholinergic (muscarinic receptor sensitivity) systems show promise as elaborate potential susceptibility traits. For example, induction of rapid eye movement sleep by the muscarinic agonist arecoline has been claimed to distinguish euthymic bipolar patients from controls, and is concordant in monozygotic twins. These findings suggest a genetic control of this trait. The information available to support this theory fully is incomplete (Goldin and Gershon, 1983). Based on the available evidence, none of the proposed biological traits qualifies as a major factor in the genetic susceptibility to the major psychoses.

Potential breakthroughs in this area may come about by means of linkage studies with chromosomal markers. Baron et al (1987) reported close linkage of bipolar affective illness to the X chromosome markers for color blindness and glucose-6-phosphate dehydrogenase (G6PD) activity and thus supported earlier suggestions that a gene on the distal long arm of the X chromosome plays a role in a subset of bipolar disorder (Baron et al, 1981; Risch and Baron, 1982). Subsequently, Mendlewicz et al (1987) provided further supportive evidence for the X-linkage hypothesis by demonstrating linkage between bipolar illness and a DNA marker associated with the factor IX (F9) locus on the long arm of the X chromosome. Another group of investigators (Egeland et al, 1987) reported linkage between two DNA markers on chromosome 11, the Harvey-ras (HRAS1) and insulin loci, and bipolar illness in an Old Order Amish pedigree. A similar strategy was applied to schizophrenia where linkage was reported between the illness and DNA markers on chromosome 5 (Sherrington et al, 1988); this linkage study used as an indicator an earlier report on a cytogenetic abnormality, a balanced translocation between chromosomes 5 and 1 in a family segregating schizophrenia (Bassett et al, 1988). Unfortunately, subsequent studies have failed to replicate these findings (see Baron et al, 1990 for review). Moreover, the addition of new genetic and clinical information has led to diminished evidence of linkage in these pedigrees (Baron et al, 1993; Kelsoe et al, 1989; Mankoo et al, 1991). These apparent false starts (especially the chromosomes 11 and 5 findings; some of the X-linkage data remain intriguing pending further investigation) can be traced to methodological uncertainties and other limitations in studying complex diseases (Baron, 1996 and 1997; Baron et al, 1990). Recent studies, using more extensive genome-wide searches and improved methodology, reported linkage between bipolar disorder and DNA markers on chromosome 21 (Straub et al, 1994), different segments of chromosome 18 (Berrettini et al, 1994; Freimer et al, 1996; Stine et al, 1995), the X chromosome (Pekkarinen et al, 1995), chromosome 4 (Blackwood et al, 1996), and chromosomes 6, 13, and 15 (Ginns et al, 1996), and between schizophrenia and DNA markers on chromosome 6 (Straub et al, 1995) and chromosome 15 (Freedman et al, 1997).

Subsequent studies have replicated some of these findings, but conflicting results by other investigators, as well as other methodological uncertainties, mandate caution, pending further investigation (Baron, 1996, 1997). Linkage or association studies with other genetic loci, including potential candidate genes expressed in the brain (and therefore thought to modulate behavior), yielded negative or equivocal results, but large segments of the genome in sufficiently large clinical samples have yet to be studied. Using improved molecular biology techniques and analytical paradigms, the search for genetic mechanisms that underlie the major psychoses continues.

Other Mental Conditions

Other psychiatric disorders with possible genetic components include alcoholism, behavioral conditions associated with chromosome anomalies, and nonpsychotic states such as panic disorder, eating disorders (bulimia nervosa and anorexia nervosa), agoraphobia, somatization disorder (Briquet's syndrome) and some of the personality disorders, and several neuropsychiatric disorders. The genetics of the disorders reviewed in this section are discussed further by Rainer (1989). Selected morbidity risk data are presented in Table 13–5.

Alcoholism appears to have a genetic component, evidenced by family, twin, and adoption studies, but the mode of inheritance has not been established. The role of genetic factors seems clearer in males than in females. Environmental factors also have been invoked. In some instances, alcoholism is thought to be related to affective disorder and antisocial personality, but the precise relation is unclear. It is of interest that familial alcoholics are distinguishable from the nonfamilial cases with respect to the severity of alcohol-related problems (more severe), onset of physical dependence (earlier), and treatment outcome (poorer). The two groups of alcoholics also differ on some physiological and endocrine measures. These findings point to the heterogeneous nature of this condition. A recent study reported an association of the D_2 dopamine receptor gene and alcoholism (Blum et al, 1990), but conflicting results and methodological uncertainties have rendered this finding controversial (Conneally, 1991).

Chromosome anomalies marked by behavioral features chiefly involve the sex chromosomes. These are Klinefelter's syndrome (XXY karyotype) and

Table 13–5 **Morbidity Risk for Some Psychiatric Disorders**

DISORDER	MORBIDITY RISK IN FIRST-DEGREE RELATIVES (%)	MORBIDITY RISK IN RELATIVES OF CONTROLS (%)	RELATIVE RISK	REFERENCE
Alcoholism	16.1	1.6	10.1	Pitts and Winokur, 1966
Panic disorder	17.3	1.8	9.6	Crowe, 1985
Anorexia nervosa	2.3	0.5	4.6	Strober et al, 1985
Agoraphobia	11.6	4.2	2.8	Crowe, 1985
Briquet's syndrome (somatization disorder)	7.7	2.5	3.1	Cloninger et al, 1986

the XYY aberration. The behavioral manifestations in Klinefelter's syndrome can range from mild personality changes to delinquency to psychosislike behavior. The XYY anomaly seems to occur more often than expected among delinquent and criminally inclined persons who show episodic violence and other forms of aggression and impulsive behavior. The interaction between the extra sex chromosome and other factors in the development of these behavioral conditions is not well understood.

Genetic contributions to panic disorder, eating disorders, agoraphobia, obsessive–compulsive disorder, somatization disorder, and schizotypal, borderline, and antisocial personality disorders have been surmised from family, twin, and adoption studies, although these studies are not as comprehensive as those carried out on the major psychoses. In some studies, the familial pattern of panic disorder is consistent with single gene inheritance. Panic disorder, eating disorders, agoraphobia, borderline personality disorder, and antisocial personality disorder appear to share a comorbidity with mood disorders, whereas schizotypal personality disorder is thought to be part of the schizophrenia spectrum. Obsessive–compulsive disorder may have a genetic link to Tourette's syndrome. The biological and genetic basis of these conditions and their possible relation to the major psychiatric disorders require further elucidation.

Linkage studies with DNA markers have shown the chromosomal sites for three neuropsychiatric conditions with neurological and behavioral features: Huntington's disease (chromosome 4), Lesch–Nyhan disorder (the X chromosome), and familial forms of Alzheimer's disease (chromosomes 21, 19, 14, and 1). Huntington's and familial Alzheimer's disease follow a dominant mode of inheritance, whereas Lesch–Nyhan syndrome is inherited as an X-linked recessive trait.

Particularly noteworthy is the dramatic progress on Alzheimer's disease. Following on earlier studies that mapped putative genes for this disorder at four chromosomal sites (Table 13–2), the actual genetic alterations have been identified: beta amyloid precursor protein (APP) on chromosome 21, apolipoprotein E (apoE) on chromosome 19, Presenilin 1 on chromosome 14, and Presenilin 2 on chromosome 1 (Selkoe, 1997). Of special importance is the emergence of a clarifying pattern: all four gene defects increase the production or deposition (or both) of the amyloid beta protein in the brain, a major culprit in the pathogenesis of Alzheimer's disease. Animal models, specifically transgenic mice (a new mouse strain produced by introducing into the animals a mutant version of the human gene encoding APP) that also exhibit abundant amyloid plaques, as well as memory deficits, complement this picture and suggest that molecular approaches to the development of effective treatments for this disorder may be in the offing in the not-to-distant future. This may augur well for similar prospects in psychiatric disorders proper (especially the major psychoses), which have been likened to Alzheimer's disease by way of genotypic and phenotypic complexity.

The Genetics of Personality

Although the focus of interest in behavior genetics, especially within the framework of psychiatry, has been on psychopathology, personality is an increasingly important area of inquiry. Most of the evidence on the role of heredity in shaping personality stems from twin studies. In Loehlin and Nichols's (1976) pioneering study, a wide array of personality traits measured in identical versus fraternal twins was shown to have substantial heritabilities of about 50%. No effect of shared environment was detected. In a study of identical twins reared apart, Bouchard and McGue (1981) confirmed the high heritability rates for personality traits and showed that the correlations for identical twins reared apart and those reared together were very much alike. The results indicated that the contribution of common environment to the similarity between twins reared together is fairly small as compared with genetic influences. Of interest are the findings that genes also seem to influence social attitudes and that some environmental influences are genetically mediated.

Taken together, these studies suggest that genes play a major role in determining personality traits. Compared with the person's genetic endowment, the common environment appears to exert a negligible influence on personality. The results are somewhat reminiscent of the substantial heritability shown for various cognitive abilities as measured in IQ tests. The similarity carries over to the controversy that such findings evoke, partly owing to potential social and political implications. In the absence of a clear biological substrate, questions of the nature and interpretation of personality measurement scales, prenatal and perinatal factors, and gene–environment interaction will continue to arouse debate and stimulate further investigation in this complex area. This subject matter is discussed in greater detail by Loehlin and Nichols (1976) and by Plomin and Daniels (1987). Recently, molecular biology techniques have yielded potential clues to the genetic underpinnings of personality. Linkage or association was reported between specific genomic loci and male sexual orientation (Hamer et al, 1993), novelty-seeking behavior (Benjamin et al, 1996), and anxiety-related traits (Lesch et al, 1996). Further study is needed to firm up the evidence and, in any event, the contribution of the implicated genes to the development of these traits is fairly small.

Genetic Testing

Genetic testing for diagnosis and risk prediction is available for a wide array of diseases, primarily monogenic disorders such as cystic fibrosis, phenylketonuria, thalassemia, and Huntington's disease. The specific forms of genetic testing include carrier testing, newborn screening, prenatal testing, and risk-oriented testing. Because gene-specific probes for some psychiatric disorders may become a reality in the not-too-distant future, important questions must be addressed to assess the validity and utility of such testing. These questions include, but are not limited to, the following: *First,* as noted earlier, psychiatric disorders are complex diseases where several (in some instances numerous) genes play a role, but nongenetic (environmental) effects also are essential. This poses special challenges for genetic testing. When multiple factors combine to produce a disorder, genetic testing may not be particularly helpful. Even if all genes (including those of minor effect) are identified, some effects can be caused by many different (and not readily tractable) nongenetic influences. *Second,* in complex diseases there is no simple and direct correspondence between genotype and phenotype. Owing to reduced penetrance or variable expressivity, people can vary greatly in the manner genes affect them. *Third,* even if a single gene is the primary cause of the disease in a small proportion of families, there is still room for considerable genetic variability. For example, a given disease can be caused by many mutations occurring in the *same* gene. Unless all such mutations are detected, the results of genetic testing will be ambiguous. A case in point is cystic fibrosis, a single-gene disorder, with at least 80 different mutations and less-than-perfect carrier detection. Of course, it is possible that with further advances in knowledge, some of these scientific hurdles will be overcome and a "probabilistic risk profile" could be constructed for many individuals. Other vexing problems will then come into play, in particular legal, social, and ethical issues concerning privacy and confidentiality of sensitive information. It will be critical to ensure that individuals at high risk will not be subjected to discrimination, to establish safeguards for informed consent prior to genetic testing, and to educate health professionals, patients, family members, and the public at large about the complexities of genotyping and risk prediction. Finally, because genetic counseling is concerned with human behavior, the psychological meanings of issues relating to health versus illness, procreation, parenthood, interpersonal functioning, the respective roles of counselors and counselees, and the process of counseling in general must be well understood. Substantial discussions concerning these issues are already underway among scientists, clinicians, genetic counselors, ethicists, policy makers, lawyers, and patient advocates, with the aim of jointly identifying and examining critical topics and formulating guidelines for the proper and meaningful use of genetic testing.

IMPLICATIONS

The burgeoning field of human genetics has yielded important insights into several conditions affecting behavior. Applications of the classic genetic methodologies involving family, twin, and adoption studies underscore the role of heredity in various behavioral manifestations ranging from personality traits to severe psychopathology. Studies with biological susceptibility traits and genetic linkage markers, in conjunction with molecular biology techniques, hold great promise for elucidation of etiology and pathophysiology, identification and characterization of abnormal genes, refinement of phenotypic classification, disentangling gene–environment interaction, risk prediction, and, eventually, improved prevention and treatment measures.

ANNOTATED BIBLIOGRAPHY

Baron M, Endicott J, Ott J: Genetic linkage in mental illness: Limitations and prospects. Br J Psychiatry 157:645–655, 1990

> Reviews methodological issues in genetic linkage strategies, with special reference to psychiatric disorders.

Baron M, Rainer JD: Molecular genetics and human disease: Implications for modern psychiatric research and practice. Br J Psychiatry 152:741–753, 1988

> Reviews the principles and potential applications of molecular biology techniques in medicine and psychiatry.

Emery EH: Methodology in Medical Genetics, 2nd ed. New York, Churchill Livingstone, 1986

> Reviews statistical methods and research designs in medical genetics.

Lander E, Kruglyak L: Genetic dissection of complex traits: Guidelines for interpreting and reporting linkage results. Nature Genet 11:241–247, 1995

> Provides guidelines for the analysis and interpretation of genetic linkage data in complex disorders.

Rainer JD: Genetics and psychiatry. In Kaplan HI, Sadock BJ (eds): Comprehensive Textbook of Psychiatry, 5th ed. Baltimore, Williams & Wilkins, 1989

> Overall review of genetic theories and findings in psychiatry.

Rosenthal D: Genetic Theory and Abnormal Behavior. New York, McGraw-Hill, 1970

> Reviews classic research designs and methodologies in psychiatric genetics.

REFERENCES

Andreasen NC, Rice J, Endicott J, et al: Familial rates of affective disorder: A report from the National Institute of Mental Health Collaborative Study. Arch Gen Psychiatry 44:461–469, 1987

Baron M: Genetics of schizophrenia. I. Familial patterns and mode of inheritance. Biol Psychiatry 21:1051–1066, 1986a

Baron M: Genetics of schizophrenia. II. Vulnerability traits and gene markers. Biol Psychiatry 21:1189–1211, 1986b

Baron M: Linkage results in schizophrenia. Am J Med Genet 67:121–123, 1996

Baron M: Genetic linkage and bipolar affective disorder: Progress and pitfalls. Mol Psychiat. 2:200–210, 1997

Baron M, Endicott J, Ott J: Genetic linkage in mental illness: Limitations and prospects. Br J Psychiatry 157:645–655, 1990

Baron M, Freimer NF, Risch N, et al: Diminished support for linkage between manic depressive illness and X-chromosomes markers in Israeli pedigrees. Nat Genet 3:49–55, 1993

Baron M, Gruen R, Kane J, et al: Modern genetic criteria and the genetics of schizophrenia. Am J Psychiatry 142:697–701, 1985a

Baron M, Gruen R, Rainer JD, et al: A family study of schizophrenia and normal control probands: Implications for the spectrum concept of schizophrenia. Am J Psychiatry 142:447–454, 1985b

Baron M, Rainer JD: Molecular genetics and human disease: Implications for modern psychiatric research and practice. Br J Psychiatry 152:741–753, 1988

Baron M, Rainer JD, Risch N: X-linkage in bipolar affective illness: Perspectives on genetic heterogeneity, pedigree analysis and the X-chromosome map. J Affect Disord 3:141–157, 1981

Baron M, Risch N, Hamburger R, et al: Genetic linkage between X-chromosome markers and bipolar affective illness. Nature 326:289–292, 1987

Bassett AS, McGillivray BC, Jones BD, et al: Partial trisomy chromosome 5 cosegregating with schizophrenia. Lancet 8589:799–801, 1988

Benjamin J, Li L, Patterson C, et al: Population and familial association between the D4 dopamine receptor gene and measures of novelty seeking. Nature Genet 12:81–84, 1996

Berrettini WH, Ferraro TN, Goldin LR, et al: Chromosome 18 DNA markers and manic-depressive illness: evidence for a susceptibility gene. Proc Natl Acad Sci USA 91:5918–5921, 1996

Blackwood DHR, He L, Morris SW, et al: A locus for bipolar affective disorder on chromosome 4p. Nature Genet 12:427–430, 1996

Blum K, Noble EP, Sheridan PJ, et al: Allelic association of human dopamine D_2 receptor gene in alcoholism. JAMA 263:2055–2060, 1990

Bouchard TJ Jr, McGue M: Familial studies of intelligence: A review. Science 212:1055–1059, 1981

Cloninger CR, Martin RL, Guze SB, et al: A prospective follow-up and family study of somatization in men and women. Am J Psychiatry 143:873–878, 1986

Conneally PM: Association between the D_2 dopamine receptor gene and alcoholism: A continuing controversy. Arch Gen Psychiatry 48:664–666, 1991

Crowe RR: The genetics of panic disorder and agoraphobia. Psychiatry Dev 2:171–186, 1985

Egeland JA, Gerhard DS, Pauls DL, et al: Bipolar affective disorder linked to DNA markers on chromosome 11. Nature 325:783–787, 1987

Emery EH: Methodology in Medical Genetics. New York, Churchill Livingstone, 1976

Freedman R, Coon H, Myles-Worsley M, et al: Linkage of a neurophysiological deficit in schizophrenia to a chromosome 15 locus. Proc Natl Acad Sci USA 94:587–592, 1997

Freimer NB, Reus VI, Escamilla MA, et al: Genetic mapping using haplotype, association and linkage methods suggests a locus for severe bipolar disorder at 18q22-q23. Nature Genet 12:436–441, 1996

Gershon ES, Hamovit J, Guroff JJ, et al: A family study of schizoaffective, bipolar I, bipolar II, unipolar, and normal control probands. Arch Gen Psychiatry 39:1157–1167, 1982

Gilbert F, Kucherlapati R, Creagan RP, et al: Tay–Sachs and Sandhoff's diseases: The assignment of genes for hexosaminidases A and B to individual human chromosomes. Proc Natl Acad Sci USA 72:263–267, 1975

Ginns EI, Ott J, Egeland JA, et al: A genome-wide search for chromosomal loci linked to bipolar affective disorder in the Old Order Amish. Nature Genet 12:431–435, 1996

Goldin LR, Gershon ES: Association and linkage studies of genetics marker loci in major psychiatric disorders. Psychiatric Dev 4:387–418, 1983

Gottesman II, Shields J: Schizophrenia: The Epigenetic Puzzle. Cambridge, Cambridge University Press, 1982

Gusella JF, Wexler NS, Conneally PM, et al: A polymorphic DNA marker genetically linked to Huntington's disease. Nature 306:234–238, 1983

Hamer DH, Hu S, Magnuson VI, et al: A linkage between DNA markers on the X chromosome and male sexual orientation. Science 261:321–327, 1993

Hoffman EP, Brown RH, Kunkel LM: Dystrophia: The protein product of the Duchenne muscular dystrophy locus. Cell 51:919–928, 1987

Kelsoe JR, Gings EI, Egeland JA, et al: Reevaluation of the linkage relationship between chromosome 11_p loci and the gene for bipolar affective disorder in the Old Order Amish. Nature 342:238–243, 1989

Kendler KS, McGuire M Gruenberg AM, et al: The Roscommon Family Study. Arch Gen Psychiatry 50:527–540, 1993

Lesch K-P, Bengel D, Heils A, et al: Association of anxiety-related traits with a polymorphism in the serotonin transporter gene regulatory region. Science 274:1527–1530, 1996

Levy-Lahad E, Wijsman EM, Nemens E, et al: A familial Alzheimer's disease locus on chromosome 1. Science 269:970–973, 1995

Loehlin JC, Nichols RC: Heredity, Environment and Personality. Austin, University of Texas Press, 1976

MacDonald ME, Ambrose CM, Duyao MP, et al: A novel gene containing a trinucleotide repeat that is expanded and unstable on Huntington's disease chromosomes. Cell 72:971–983, 1993

Mankoo B, Sherrington R, Brynjoltsson J, et al: New microsatellite polymorphisms provide a highly polymorphic map of chromosome 5 bands 911.2–913.3 for linkage analysis of Icelandic and English families affected by schizophrenia. Psychiat Genet 2:17, 1991

Martin JB: Molecular genetics: Applications to the clinical neurosciences. Science 238:765–772, 1987

Mendlewicz J, Simon P, Sevy S, et al: Polymorphic DNA marker on X-chromosome and manic depression. Lancet 8544:1230–1232, 1987

Murray JM, Davies KE, Harper PS, et al: Linkage relationship of a cloned DNA sequence on the short arm of the X chromosome to Duchenne muscular dystrophy. Nature 300:69–71, 1982

Nussbaum R, Brennand J, Chinault C, et al: Molecular analysis of the hypoxanthine phosphoribosyltransferase locus. In Caskey CT, White RL (eds): Recombinant DNA Application to Human Disease. New York, Cold Spring Harbor Laboratory, 1983

Ott J: Analysis of Human Genetic Linkage. Revised edition. Baltimore, The Johns Hopkins University Press, 1991

Owen MJ, Craddock N: Modern molecular genetic approaches to complex traits: Implications for psychiatric disorders. Mol Psychiatry 1:21–26, 1996

Pekkarinan P, Terwilliger J, Bredbacka P-E, et al: Evidence of a predisposing locus to bipolar disorder on Xq24-q27.1 in an extended Finnish pedigree. Genome Res 5:105–115, 1995

Pericak-Vance MA, Bebout JL, Gaskell PC Jr, et al: Linkage studies in familial Alzheimer's disease: Evidence for chromosome 19 linkage. Am J Hum Genet 48:1034–1050, 1991

Pitts FN, Winokur G: Affective disorder. VII. Alcoholism and affective disorder. J Psychiat Res 4:37–50, 1966

Plomin R, Daniels D: Why are children in the same family so different from one another? Behav Brain Sci 10:1–60, 1987

Rainer JD: Genetics and psychiatry. In Kaplan HI, Sadock BJ (eds): Comprehensive Textbook of Psychiatry, 5th ed. Baltimore, Williams & Wilkins, 1989

Rieder RO, Gershon ES: Genetic strategies in biological psychiatry. Arch Gen Psychiatry 35:866–873, 1978

Risch N, Baron M: X-linkage and genetic heterogeneity in bipolar-related major affective illness: Reanalysis of linkage data. Ann Hum Genet 46:153–166, 1982

Rosenthal D: Genetic Theory and Abnormal Behavior. New York, McGraw-Hill, 1970

Schellenberg GD, Bird TD, Wijsman EM, et al: Genetic linkage evidence for a familial Alzheimer's disease locus on chromosome 14. Science 258:668–671, 1992

Selkoe DJ: Alzheimer's disease: Genotypes, phenotype, and treatments. Science 275:630–631, 1997

Sherrington R, Brynjolfsson J, Petursson H, et al: Localization of a susceptibility locus for schizophrenia on chromosome 5. Nature 336:164–167, 1988

St. George-Hyslop PH, Tanzi RE, Polinsky RJ, et al: The genetic defect causing familial Alzheimer's disease maps on chromosomal 21. Science 235:885–889, 1987

Stine OC, Xu J, Koskela R, et al: Evidence for linkage of bipolar disorder to chromosome 18 with a parent-of-origin effect. Am J Hum Genet 57:1384–1394, 1995

Straub RE, Lehner T, Luo Y, et al: A possible vulnerability locus for bipolar affective disorder on chromosome 21q22.3. Nature Genet 8:291–296, 1994

Straub RE, MacLean CJ, O'Neill FA, et al: A potential vulnerability locus for schizophrenia on chromosome 6p24-22: Evidence for genetic heterogeneity. Nature Genet 11:287–293, 1995

Strober M, Morell W, Burroughs J, et al: A controlled family study of anorexia nervosa. J Psychiatr Res 19:239–246, 1985

Tanzi RE, Petrukhin K, Chernov I, et al: The Wilson disease gene is a copper transporting ATPase with homology to the Menkes disease gene. Nature Genet 5:344–350, 1993

Thompson EA: Pedigree Analysis in Human Genetics. Baltimore, John Hopkins University Press, 1986

Tsuang MT, Winokur G, Crowe R: Morbidity risks of schizophrenia and affective disorders among first degree relatives of patients with schizophrenia, mania, depression and surgical conditions. Br J Psychiatry 137:497–504, 1980

Wallace MR, Marchuk DA, Andersen LB, et al: Type 1 neurofibromatosis gene: Identification of a large transcript disrupted in three NF1 patients. Science 249:181–186, 1990

Weissman MM, Gershon ES, Kidd KK, et al: Psychiatric disorders in the relatives of probands with affective disorders: The Yale University-National Institute of Mental Health Collaborative Study. Arch Gen Psychiatry 41:13–21, 1984

V Clinical Applications

14 Supportive Psychological Care of the Medically Ill: A Synthesis of the Biopsychosocial Approach in Medical Care

Stephen A. Green

This entire text has been a prodrome to this concluding chapter, which addresses how a knowledge of human behavior contributes to the compassionate psychological and emotional care of patients again, focusing on the critical importance of the doctor–patient relationship. In addition, the basic themes of the biopsychosocial model introduced by Drs. Cole and Levinson are discussed again in light of the multiple perspectives that have been presented in previous chapters as well as the model's practical application in patient care.

THE DOCTOR–PATIENT RELATIONSHIP AND THE BIOPSYCHOSOCIAL MODEL

The interaction between physician and patient is too often an impersonal, mechanistic encounter due to their shared cause-and-effect mindset concerning the diagnosis and treatment of specific symptoms. Medical practice has long been considered an exercise of determining etiology, prescribing the indicated therapeutic regimen, and monitoring the patient's response, a perspective that highlights intellectual problem solving while neglecting central emotional factors that influence the course of an illness. This approach is based on the biomedical model, discussed in Chapters 1 and 2, which is a parochial viewpoint rooted in the oversimplification and misinterpretation of the theories of René Descartes involving mind–body duality.

A strictly biomedical model compromises patient care by supporting the inaccurate belief in a mind–body dichotomy and perpetuating the simplistic notion that complex pathophysiological phenomena are ultimately explained by a single principle (Engel, 1977). For example, it defines peptic ulcer disease as the anatomical end product of gastric hypersecretion, implying that definitive treatment consists solely of appropriate medication and dietary restrictions. These are necessary measures; however, they may be no more than palliative if medical interventions fail to address specific psychosocial issues affecting and affected by the patient's ulcer. The biomedical model promotes "the physician's preoccupation with the body and disease and the corresponding neglect of the patient as a person," and it fails to consider "how the patient behaves and what he reports about himself and his life [because] it does not include the patient and his attributes as a person, a human being" (Engel, 1980). In sum, the biomedical model suggests that treating one's specific physical pathology is synonymous with treating the patient, which ignores the fundamental truth that all illness simultaneously affects the mind and the body.

Every patient must be seen as a singular human being if medical care is to be appropriate and effective. This requires application of the biopsychosocial model, a theoretical construct that assesses a person within the distinctive context of supports and stressors affecting his or her daily functioning. As discussed in Chapters 1, 2, and 3, an understanding of the interplay among each patient's medical disorder, intrapsychic life, and the positive and negative impact of his or her external environment is important for several reasons.

First, the genesis and exacerbation of an illness (Rahe, 1973), even mechanisms of sudden death (Engel, 1968; Reich et al, 1981), are affected by numerous psychosocial factors. Second, as discussed in Chapters 3, 11, and 12, extensive scientific research has demonstrated mind–body interactions in specific physiological, endocrinological, and immunological processes, as well as in generalized stress reactions. Third, one's willingness and ability to cooperate in prescribed care is often affected by myriad nonphysical factors, including intrapsychic issues (Lipowski, 1975) and sociocultural norms (Zola, 1963). Finally, physical illness itself can precipitate a variety of abnormal psychological states that adversely influence the disease process, or reach a degree of severity so intense that they become more threatening to patients than their original medical disorder (Green, 1985).

The preceding discussion demonstrates that optimal medical treatment requires the biopsychosocial treatment approach, which Engel (1980) conceptualizes by interposing the patient between two hierarchies that combine to form an overall hierarchy of natural systems (Fig. 14–1). The person is at the same time at the highest level of an organismic hierarchy, which ranges from subatomic particles through the nervous system, and the lowest stratum of a social hierarchy, which ranges from a two-person system to the biosphere. These two hierarchies are in a dynamic equilibrium, because every system (e.g., cells or two-person) within each hierarchy is a distinctive whole that is simultaneously interrelated with every other system. Consequently, disturbances at any system level can alter any other system level; through feedback controls, they may modify or aggravate the system originally affected. Engel presents a clinical case to illustrate the workings of this medical model, which as discussed next, is ultimately based on the clinician's appreciation of the meaning of illness to an individual patient.

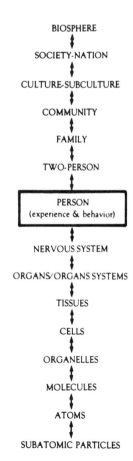

Figure 14–1. *Hierarchy of natural systems. (Reprinted with permission from Engel G: The clinical application of the biopsychosocial model. Am J Psychiatr 137:535–544, 1980.)*

ILLNESS DYNAMICS

The biopsychosocial model demonstrates that nonphysical issues are part and parcel of the disease process and can transform the same organic pathology into vastly different illnesses in different patients. Consider that premise in terms of the following two men who suffered similar myocardial damage from a heart attack. Their histories highlight the many psychosocial factors that influenced when and to what degree they became ill, as well as their response to treatment and ultimate prognosis.

TWO CASE STUDIES

Mr. A., a 40-year-old widower, is a midlevel manager diligently working his way up the corporate ladder while supporting three young children. In addition to family responsibilities and professional obligations, he devotes considerable time to a flourishing relationship with a coworker he hopes to marry. His past history is significant for the unexpected death of his mother from a cerebrovascular accident when he was 13 years old.

In contrast, Mr. B. is a 63-year-old executive vice-president on the threshold of retirement, a husband of 40 years eagerly anticipating more leisure time with his wife and grown family. He has consistently enjoyed good health; his only major medical event, a cholecystectomy, was a scheduled procedure that caused minimal disruption to his life. Although Mr. B.'s father died of metastatic carcinoma at the age of 70, his mother, siblings, wife, and children are all in good health.

After surviving the immediate threat of death from a myocardial infarction, each man exhibited a unique reaction to his damaged myocardium. Mr. A.'s initial anxiety was progressively supplanted by a growing sense of helplessness. The death of his mother at his early age had generally sensitized him to loss and specifically affected his psychological development by enhancing dependent yearnings. Moreover, because she died of a cardiovascular illness, he more closely associated his heart disease with her sudden demise. He also identified with his children's concerns, as he had experienced the same anxiety that comes from recognizing that one's future is largely dependent on the welfare of a single parent. Significant feelings of anger and depression arose when he considered the impact of his illness on the course of his career and the developing relationship with his girlfriend. All these factors contributed to a heightened affective response to his heart attack, making it more difficult to resolve those intense feelings that fostered an increasing helplessness and dependency on those around him.

>   *Mr. B., on the other hand, was also angered and depressed by his bad luck but basically because it occurred at a stage of life primarily reserved for relaxation. However, the intensity of his feelings was tempered by the knowledge that his family was grown, that his loving spouse had consistently provided reassurance and support when needed, that he had already realized his professional ambitions, and that he was financially secure. For these reasons, Mr. B. more easily worked through the emotions stirred by his physical impairment and quickly returned to his premorbid level of functioning.*

Although these patients suffered the exact same anatomical and physiological pathology, each reacted to the period of ill health in a highly distinctive fashion due to the impact of idiosyncratic psychological and social issues. Mr. A.'s heart attack precipitated a considerable emotional upheaval, marked by anxiety, depression, and helplessness, because it reawakened traumatic memories and painful feelings related to his mother's death, and he experienced it as a significant threat to many important aspects of his current life. Although some concerns were more imagined than real, they interfered with his ability to assess accurately and, consequently, to accept the effect of an uncomplicated heart attack on his daily existence.

The relationship among one's biological status (e.g., genetic constitution and physical pathology), emotional makeup, and the supports and stresses of a social matrix constitutes that person's *illness dynamics* (Green, 1985). This idiosyncratic standard, which represents the patient's understanding of a specific disease during a particular period of life, is portrayed schematically in Fig. 14–2. The shaded area defines the distinctive interrelationship between the conscious and unconscious psychosocial factors affecting and affected by a patient's biological status (Table 14–1), which predisposes to certain diseases and pro-

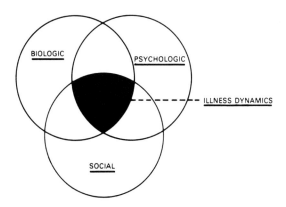

Figure 14–2. *Illness dynamics. (Reprinted with permission from Green S: Mind and Body: The Psychology of Physical Illness. Washington, DC, American Psychiatric Press, 1985.)*

Table 14–1 **Major Components of Illness Dynamics**

Biological
Nature, severity, and time course of disease
Affected organ system, body part, or body function
Baseline physiological functioning and physical resilience
Genetic endowment

Psychological
Maturity of ego functioning and object relationships
Personality type
Stage in the lifecycle
Interpersonal aspects of the therapeutic relationship
  (e.g., countertransference of healthcare providers)
Previous psychiatric history
Effect of past history on attitudes toward treatment
  (e.g., postoperative complications)

Social
Dynamics of family relationships
Family attitudes toward illness
Level of interpersonal functioning (e.g., educational and occupa-
  tional achievements; ability to form and maintain friendships)
Cultural attitudes

tects against others. Illness dynamics incline one to assess all illness-related information in light of singular values, wishes, needs, and fears, *ultimately causing the patient to perceive, assess, and defend against the loss of health in a highly subjective manner.* As demonstrated by the preceding case histories, this may significantly affect the patient's ability to cope with disease.

Both Mr. A. and Mr. B. shared the common pathology of an uncomplicated myocardial infarction; however, the most significant biological component of Mr. A.'s illness dynamics was his mother's genetic endowment. The affected organ system also bore special meaning, raising doubts that he would have sufficient strength and stamina to devote to a rising career or to meet the emotional—and sexual—demands of a second marriage. Mr. A.'s excessive dependency was an important psychological component of his illness response, a probable legacy of the early loss of his mother that was intensified by the death of his wife. His stage in the lifecycle contributed to his significant depression because the heart attack occurred at a time when persons are more focused on the challenges and joys of life than on the fear of death. The predominant social determinants of Mr. A.'s illness dynamics concerned family relationships. His heart disease had considerable effect on his young children, whose welfare depended on his wage-earning ability. This lack of flexibility in the family system placed greater stress on him to recuperate rapidly and completely. All of these issues were in contrast to the impact of a heart attack on Mr. B.'s life. His physical resilience, psychological strength, and the supports of his social network combined to help him readily negotiate this period of ill health.

These patients' distinctive illness dynamics, illustrated in Fig. 14–3, greatly influenced their ability to cope with heart disease *by affecting a grief process that normally accompanies loss of health.* Emotionally processing an episode of illness, reaching an accommodation with the diverse and powerful feelings that accompany it, is a prerequisite for return to healthy functioning. As discussed next, the working through of these emotions, in order to prevent them from intruding on one's daily responsibilities and interpersonal relationships, is analogous to grieving for a loved one.

THE GRIEF PROCESS AND ILLNESS

Illness is universally experienced as a loss, namely the loss of health, because it decreases one's degree of autonomy. Illness imposes restrictions on people that may be transient and mild (e.g., immobilization of a sprained joint) or chronic and severe (e.g., hemiparesis following a cerebrovascular accident). Although feelings of loss are most intense when a serious health problem permanently and profoundly alters one's physical status, they also occur with minor ailments. The bedridden patient suffering a febrile viral syndrome often feels anxious, frustrated, and depressed about the inability to pursue his or her

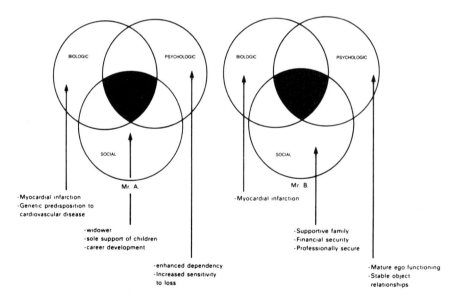

Figure 14-3. *Comparative illness dynamics. (Reprinted with permission from Green S: Mind and Body: The Psychology of Physical Illness. Washington, DC, American Psychiatric Press, 1985.)*

daily activities and responsibilities. Illness also precipitates a sense of loss due to its various symbolic meanings. The concrete demonstration of physical vulnerability deprives one of infantile invulnerability, while idiosyncratic reactions to disease cause patients to experience more specific losses, such as Mr. A.'s conviction (founded on his mother's medical history) that his heart attack inevitably signaled an early death.

Whether illness has a predominantly symbolic or concrete effect, it precipitates a predictable psychological reaction—namely, a grief reaction during which patients mourn the loss of their previous healthier functioning. The process is identical to bereavement, causing an outpouring of varied and shifting emotions as patients acknowledge their current state of health and contrast it with a premorbid level. Grieving entails recognition of the good and bad associated with a particular loss, which prompts a series of feeling states— *denial, anxiety, anger,* and *depression*—that a person must progress through before resolving those emotions and coming to terms with a temporary or permanent health impairment. The emotional response to a myocardial infarction illustrates this process.

Although well aware that severe precordial pain may signal an evolving heart attack, patients often attempt to deny that reality by minimizing the symptom or explaining it away as indigestion, myalgia, or bronchitis. That denial recedes as persisting angina underscores the medical reality and precipitates a host of intense feelings. There is immediate anxiety about the prospect of dying, the discomfort of acute treatment, and the need to abdicate considerable responsibility and autonomy to anonymous caretakers.

Anxiety persists into the recuperative period due to concern about long-range effects of the illness (e.g., dietary and physical limitations), although anger becomes the predominant feeling once patients feel secure that they will survive the medical emergency. During this phase of illness, patients direct their resentments globally, as well as toward specific targets. They curse the gods for their bad luck, while blaming specific family members, friends, and medical personnel for real and imagined transgressions and omissions that promoted ill health. As the anger abates, patients may experience a growing depression, characterized by emotional, behavioral, and cognitive changes that reflect their extreme preoccupation with real and potential losses brought on by the heart attack. In the short-term, all aspects of their lives (e.g., family, professional, and social commitments) must assume secondary importance to health concerns. Patients also mourn longer-term losses caused by their diseased myocardium, such as restricted physical activities because of persistent angina.

The grief process proceeds toward closure as patients begin to achieve a realistic perspective concerning the consequences of illness. This entails acknowledgment of all limitations imposed by the disease and of one's physical vulnerabilities and ultimate mortality. "Working through," or attempting to resolve those issues, is a dynamic process that allows reestablishment of the emotional equilibrium that characterized premorbid functioning, illustrated by Mr. B. Patients unable to resolve feelings precipitated by loss may develop one of several syndromes that characterize pathological grief reactions (Brown and Stoudemire, 1983). These may take the form of a mood disturbance (e.g., the heightened anxiety and depression that complicated Mr. A.'s recuperation and persisted even after his physical recovery), a behavioral disturbance (e.g., compulsive eating or substance dependence), or impaired interpersonal relationships. As discussed in preceding chapters, there also may be neurobiological correlates to the inability to work through feelings precipitated by ill health. Severe stress, such as physical illness and other circumstances involving loss of control, influences the neurochemistry by endogenous opiods, catecholamines, indoleamines, and pituitary functioning. Dr. van der Kolk in Chapter 11 suggests that these changes promote heightened anxiety, difficulties modulating aggression, and depression—affective disturbances characteristic of unresolved grief—that may represent adult responses to the effects of earlier trauma and stress. Similarly, immunological and neuroendocrinological data highlight the correlation between grief and discrete physiological changes (Irwin et al, 1987). Consequently, a patient's ability to come to terms with the loss of health is a comprehensive psychobiological response. One's illness dynamics facilitate or impede this grief process; in the latter circumstance, the person is likely to develop one of the following pathological reactions.

ABNORMAL ILLNESS RESPONSES

Persons unable to acknowledge and put into perspective the disturbing feelings brought on by disease are prone to abnormal illness responses, which significantly detract from physical and/or mental health. In these circumstances, individuals may deny their feelings or, more often, strongly experience one emotion while significantly minimizing all others. In essence, the patient becomes mired in one stage of the grief process, promoting a preoccupation with feelings characteristic of that phase, thereby preventing resolution of the varied emotions precipitated by loss of health; the situation is analogous to pathological grief. Because of the interdependence between emotional and somatic functioning, abnormal illness responses can aggravate medical conditions (e.g., increased cardiac irritability due to heightened anxiety following a heart attack), often promoting psychological and biological distress more disabling than the initial illness. The most common abnormal illness responses include the following.

The Denial Response

Denial is a common defense mechanism that enables one to reject cognitive and emotional aspects of anxiety-provoking unpleasant external reality. Despite this function, denial usually serves an adaptive role (Vailliant, 1977), such as facilitating continued functioning by moderating the impact of an overwhelming stressor that might otherwise threaten one's psychological health (e.g., the massive anxiety that precedes battle or other potentially life-threatening situations). Denial becomes maladaptive only when it is exclusively defensive, causing significant distortions in the assessment and acceptance of life's realities. For example, persons who never recognize their contribution to their recurrent failed relationships will probably perpetuate the pattern and increasingly become isolated as life progresses.

Pathological denial may be present throughout the course of a medical or surgical illness. A common example of denial during an acute medical emergency is seen in cardiac patients who dismiss severe precordial pain as heartburn. Persistent denial is often reflected in noncompliance with a therapeutic regimen, which may commence immediately after a medical crisis (e.g., refusal to maintain bedrest while recuperating from a myocardial infarction) and continue throughout a chronic illness (e.g., continued smoking in a patient with chronic obstructive pulmonary disease). Denial is seen in terminal patients who refuse to acknowledge impending death. In sum, denial, if extreme, may interfere with accurate diagnosis, impede definitive treatment, and, consequently, perpetuate the disease state.

The Anxiety Response

Anxiety is an adaptive feeling that signals danger, prompting one toward purposeful action. The fight–flight behavior of animals confronted by a predator illustrates how this affect spurs self-protective behavior. In relation to illness, anxiety promotes preventive behaviors (e.g., scheduled immunizations, healthy diet) and timely medical attention following the onset of symptoms. Its persistence during an episode of ill health, secondary to patients' concern about a multitude of diverse issues (e.g., the discomfort of diagnostic and therapeutic procedures, long-term limitations to daily functioning), further motivates compliance with treatment. However, anxiety can become excessive, prompting an irrational preoccupation with health issues that evolves into a pathological illness response.

Anxiety is maladaptive when the concern it causes the person exceeds its protective function. In this circumstance, patients may become hypersensitive to all aspects of an illness (e.g., ruminating about casual remarks passed by caretakers, obsessing to the point of indecision about therapeutic options). Such absorption with one's physical status greatly detracts from all other aspects of life, progressively displacing former pleasures with a debilitating angst. Paradoxically, this also interferes with medical care. Heightened anxiety compromises objectivity and, consequently, one's ability to provide an accurate history, tolerate diagnostic procedures (e.g., colonoscopy, an MRI scan), or even cooperate in a routine physical examination. Should such pervasive apprehension progress into a chronic anxiety, the patient is then burdened with an unpleasant, counterproductive affective state, in addition to the limitations caused by his or her physical pathology. Finally, continued demands for reassurance from friends, family, and healthcare personnel may progressively alienate those support systems. The anxiety response compromises diverse aspects of medical treatment and, consequently, diminishes the patient's potential for returning to premorbid or optimal functioning.

The Anger Response

All medical and surgical patients become frustrated, resentful, or overtly hostile about their plight, and vent those feelings in several directions. The anger is directed globally and specifically. Patients may curse the fates, God, the unfairness of life, or, alternatively, castigate themselves for being ill whether or not such self-criticism is warranted (e.g., cirrhosis secondary to alcohol abuse) or unreasonable (e.g., the result of an uncontrollable infectious disease). They may lash out at family members and friends for varied reasons—condemning ancestors for passing on a defective gene, blaming friends or family for causing exacerbations of an illness (e.g., the impact of marital discord on labile hypertension), or basically resenting the reality of heightened dependency on people in their social network who enjoy continued good health. Medical personnel are often primary and direct targets for patients' hostility because of the restrictions they impose (e.g., constraints on diet and physical activity), the discomfort they may cause (e.g., performing painful diagnostic procedures, prescribing medications with unpleasant side effects), the limitations of the profession (e.g., inability to cure many diseases), and their role as bearers of grim news about patients' welfare and mortality.

Patients who fail to work through these angry feelings may develop an illness response that is often characterized by severe interpersonal conflicts. They engage in overt and covert struggles with the people in their lives, which fosters a progressive isolation from necessary support and undermines their medical care. Patients may angrily refuse to submit to important diagnostic tests, comply with rehabilitative programs, or take prescribed medications; these behaviors frustrate family members, control caretakers, and also reflect a self-directed anger because all these actions are ultimately detrimental to the patient. Struggles may also occur in subtle, unstated ways, by passive–aggressive behaviors (e.g., failing to adhere to a prescribed diet or medication regimen), which afford the pleasure of secret control over persons. In this manner, the anger response progressively transforms the patient's supportive alliances into adversarial relationships, with widespread negative effects on treatment and day-to-day life.

The Depression Response

This illness response is characterized by the common cognitive, mood, and behavioral signs and symptoms that constitute a clinical depression. These include changes in mood, most commonly a sustained sadness with tearfulness and anhedonia (loss of pleasure and interest in life), although irritability and agitation may be present as well. The patient also manifests physiological sequelae of depression, which span the spectrum from the usual neurovegetative complaints (e.g., insomnia, anorexia, fatigue, decreased sexual drive) to somatic disturbances of any organ system (Lindemann, 1944). The most prominent behavioral manifestation of this illness response is a change in established daily patterns, which most often takes the form of generalized withdrawal from one's environment. Patients can manifest more specific behaviors, such as neglecting professional responsibilities or avoiding family interactions, reactions influenced by the particular illness and/or its treatment (e.g., one may be inclined to retreat from social commitments and to rely more on family support following a disfiguring surgical procedure). Behavioral changes also include radical departures from usual routines of life, such as quitting a satisfying job, precipitously moving, or ending a long-term marriage. Finally, diminished self-esteem is a prominent feature of this illness response. Already stressed by the effects of a physical impairment that may prevent one from returning to a healthy premorbid level of functioning, the psychological reaction to that reality can provoke a negativistic spiral of self-criticism and self-reproach that ultimately leaves the patient feeling helpless and worthless. Each of these four areas of objective and subjective signs and symptoms can vary in intensity, with the result that the depression response may range from a relatively mild adjustment disorder to a major depression.

The depression response detracts from medical care by direct effects on patients and its impact on their relationships with healthcare personnel. Diverse psychophysiological symptoms are often mistaken as primary manifestations of serious underlying medical illness, which complicates accurate diagnosis and, consequently, treatment. The differentiation becomes even more difficult when depression causes such withdrawal that the patient is unwilling or unable to provide an adequate medical history or report objective and subjective responses to a therapeutic regimen. Depression also interferes with normative healing processes by debilitating neurovegetative symptoms (e.g., anorexia), a diminished immunological response (Stein et al, 1985), the passive abandonment of a will to live (Engel, 1968), or even purposeful self-destructive behaviors (Slaby and Glicksman, 1985). In sum, depression may become so severe that it becomes a greater threat to one's welfare and survival than the original underlying physical pathology.

The Dependency Response

As discussed in Chapter 5, behavioral regression is common to all illness, the result of factors endemic to patients (e.g., general preoccupation with one's illness, restrictions caused by specific symptoms) and external issues (e.g., limitations of a structured hospital routine, constraints of the treatment regimen, like a controlled diet). Such adaptive regression forms the basis of effective medical care. Reversion to more passive behaviors, characteristic of early developmental stages, allows a patient the comfort and familiarity of diminished responsibility while simultaneously enabling caretakers to assume a necessary degree of control over the treatment. Diminished autonomy also serves the defensive purpose of helping a patient deal with distressing emotions by assigning accountability for one's welfare to others and readily accepting their concern and support.

As previously mentioned in Chapter 2, Parsons (1951) discusses these aspects of regression in his description of the dynamics of the *sick role,* emphasizing the *collaborative* nature of medical treatment. He outlines the usual course of enhanced dependence on healthcare personnel during the early stages of illness, but he emphasizes the importance of patients assuming increased responsibility for their welfare as they progress toward wellness. For example, the stable postmyocardial infarction patient is expected to adhere to a prescribed diet and exercise regimen, important steps toward recovery and maintenance of healthy, independent functioning. Some persons, however, are so gratified by the ministrations of others they refuse to cooperate in their treatment. Warmed by the concern and constant attention of healthcare providers and, consequently, disinclined to strive for the autonomy of premorbid life, they abdicate increasing responsibility to family, friends, and caretakers. This can lead to an increasing dependency that may ultimately culminate in a semihelplessness that endangers one's physical and emotional well-being.

Treatment noncompliance is a common manifestation of excessive dependency, as patients haphazardly adhere to prescribed therapies (e.g., a medication regimen, physical rehabilitation following a traumatic injury). Although the motivation for such behavior may be purposeful or unconscious, it yields the same endpoint: prolonged dependence on healthcare personnel, who must then compensate for the patient's self-neglect by providing an even greater degree of care. At a minimum, this slows one's return to optimal functioning; at worst, it aggravates the illness by intensifying its pathophysiological effects.

Individuals' interpersonal relationships also suffer when illness spawns excessive dependency. Established family patterns must adapt to the patient's prolonged regression, sometimes causing considerable disruption to relatives, who now tend to matters usually managed by the patient. Growing resentments may, in turn, detract from their supportive efforts. A parallel situation occurs when healthcare providers develop a negative reaction to so-called hateful patients (Groves, 1978), fostering conscious or unconscious neglect of their care. The dependency response signals the evolution of an individual into a professional patient who is more concerned with being cared for than with achieving an optimal level of coping. When physicians fail to recognize this illness response, which may be hidden by a patient's stated desire to get well quickly, there is greater risk that the collaborative doctor–patient relationship will steadily degenerate into an adversarial association harmful to both parties.

THE DOCTOR–PATIENT RELATIONSHIP IN THE PSYCHOLOGICAL CARE OF THE MEDICALLY ILL

Psychotherapy, in general, can be broadly classified as *supportive* (anxiety-suppressing) or *introspective* (anxiety-provoking). The former seeks to preserve the patient's psychological status quo; the latter attempts to heighten insight by obliging the patient to explore painful memories and emotional experiences.

Introspective therapy is usually required with medically ill patients if they manifest symptoms of a *pathological* illness response. Treatment is then administered by a psychiatrist or other mental health professional specifically trained to help patients work through abnormal affective states (Green, 1985). More often, however, psychotherapeutic care of the medically ill patient is initially *supportive.* Usually effected by primary caretakers (e.g., nonpsychiatrist physicians, nursing staff, rehabilitation therapists), it is designed to help patients identify and ventilate the intense feelings precipitated by ill health, thereby enabling them to contain emotional distress within limits that were acceptable premorbidly. As discussed by Frank (1961) in his classic study concerning the process of healing, this type of treatment is highly dependent on the personal influence exerted by caretakers. For example, a positive relationship can yield favorable effects even with *symbolic* interventions, such as the administration of an inert medication. Alexander and French (1946) specifically exploit the doctor–patient interaction in this manner by the technique of manipulating the transference during psychotherapy (see Chapter 5).

Whether supportive or introspective psychotherapeutic treatment is indicated, patients' comprehensive medical care derives from an accurate appreciation of their emotional condition caused by their ill health in addition to a thorough knowledge of their underlying physical disease. The biopsychosocial approach, which acknowledges the inextricable link between mind and body, requires an understanding of patients' illness dynamics and the application of standard psychotherapeutic principles to medical management (Kahana and Bibring, 1964; Reichard, 1964). A necessary requirement for this treatment approach is *empathic* communication between patients and their caretakers.

As mentioned by Dr. Shelton in Chapter 1, the concept of *empathy* involves a process that enables clinicians to appreciate the conscious and unconscious internal experiences of patients, that is, the capacity "to think and feel oneself into the inner life of another person" (Kohut, 1984). A somewhat intuitive capacity, empathy is a response to emotional signals from patients, such as their facial expressions, level of motor activity, speech patterns, and content of mental productions (Greenson, 1960). These emotional signs from the patient evoke intrapsychic responses in their caretakers, which, in turn, are influenced by their own emotional makeup (Buie, 1981), autonomic reactions (Basch, 1983), and associated memories and overall personality style. In this manner a physician can experience the patient's emotional states by "oscillating" between the role of observer and participant (Book, 1988), which Jaffe (1986) describes as alternately "thinking *with* the patient and then *about* the patient." This process involves transiently identifying with the patient; that is, imagining what it would be like to be in his or her situation, then "pulling back" as an understanding, more objective yet empathic observer.

A CASE STUDY

Dr. L. entered Mr. M.'s hospital room and saw a young teenager lying on top of the bedsheets, his right leg supported by a series of pillows and heavily bandaged around the knee. Dr. L. immediately felt a sinking feeling in his stomach, then found himself recalling a serious childhood accident of his own that had required an extended hospitalization. Mr. M. trembled slightly as he greeted Dr. L., attributing it to the air conditioning that had given him a chill, then grimaced in pain as he propped himself up in bed. When asked how he was feeling, Mr. M. reported that he was being "treated like a rock star" by "a hundred people taking care of me." Although Dr. L. did not have the patient's obvious physical pain, he felt he understood Mr. L.'s anxiety and helplessness and could also understand his wish that a multitude of caretakers minister to all his needs.

The physician's emotional reaction to this patient derived primarily from the young man's signals of emotional and physical distress, data that afforded an accurate appreciation of Mr. M.'s affective and cognitive condition. He felt empathy for the frightened young man, but this empathy nevertheless did not necessarily benefit the patient until it was used positively. Empathy does not lead to an empathic interaction until observations by clinicians are communicated in a genuine manner to the patient (Bachrach, 1976). This requires conveying to the patient an understanding of his or her internal emotional states in a manner that causes the patient to feel that the physician is emotionally "with them" (Book, 1988).

Mr. M's ability to maintain a facade of artificial cheerfulness quickly faltered as he began describing the details of his injury. The victim of a hit-and-run driver, he had suffered considerable trauma to his knee that required extensive reconstruction and a regimen of rehabilitative therapy, the extent of which would be determined by the success of his surgery. His agitation steadily increased during the interview, until he abruptly stopped speaking "because I'm tired and want to crash for a while." Dr. L. agreed that rest was a good idea and suggested that he return later. Shortly before leaving, Dr. L. recalled how the conversation brought back memories of his own hospitalization for a concussion when he was 15. He remembered feeling frightened by the strangeness of the hospital and the uncertainty of his prognosis, and guessed that Mr. M. might have similar feelings. As Dr. L. reflected to the patient how he might be feeling in this situation, the young man sensed the physician's empathy and invited Dr. L. to stay "a little longer," then ventilated myriad thoughts and feelings about his injury. He concluded with the prediction that he'd be "jogging again by Christmas."

As the case illustrates, empathy is only therapeutic when "accurate reception [is] complemented by accurate feedback" (Keefe, 1976). This results in "empathic communication" (Miller, 1989), an affective experience similar to the good feeling that follows discussion of a problem with a close friend and leaves one feeling better due to the sense of being heard and understood. A measure of the existence and benefit of this type of interaction between Dr. L. and his patient was Mr. M.'s emotional catharsis, which greatly diminished his anxiety and concluded with a positive and probably realistic hope of running again.

Cohen-Cole and Bird's (1986) discussion of common supportive technical interventions used with the medically ill (briefly referred to in Chapter 2 in this text) and Buckley's (1986) exploration of their theoretical basis highlight the role of empathy in psychotherapy. In general, physicians should present themselves as available and concerned, which requires "giving of self" as a real person as opposed to being neutral, objective, and analytic. They should use a personable, conversational tone to offer advice and reassurance (e.g., commenting on the patient's response to a treatment regimen), praise when warranted (e.g., when the patient progresses in a rehabilitative program), and didactic instruction about the illness (e.g., identifying normal emotional and behavioral aspects of the sick role). They should consistently attempt to involve patients in the treatment (e.g., inviting input into decisions concerning therapeutic options) in order to strengthen the working alliance. This overall posture helps limit patients' behavioral regression by retaining focus on the here-and-now, improves their compromised ego functioning by supporting usual defense mechanisms, and enhances self-esteem by acknowledging inherent strengths and therapeutic gains.

Hollis's (1964) description of the supportive approach also underscores the importance of empathic communication. He discusses four categories of intervention: (1) sustaining procedures (e.g., demonstration of a desire to help); (2) procedures of direct influence (e.g., offering suggestions and advice); (3) facilitation of catharsis (e.g., sanctioning the expression of emotions); and (4) guidance concerning the day-to-day implications of illness (e.g., urging the return to work or a change in one's living situation). The physician's ability to pursue these tasks, to sense when patients require an empathic response and then respond in an appropriate manner, is what makes the practice of medicine an art as well as a science. The shifting back and forth from the more objective, technical, and analytic clinical functions to those of an empathic therapist is difficult to achieve and to maintain. Nevertheless, it is *the* essential quality of being a physician, one that fundamentally rests on the practitioner's ability for self-scrutiny regarding two personal attributes, namely his or her emotional makeup and ethical beliefs.

First, effective psychological care of medical patients is exquisitely dependent on the ability of physicians to maintain perspective on their *own* emotions. Frequent exposure to severely ill individuals may cause considerable distress to physicians frustrated by patients' marginal improvement or continued decline. Clinicians' heightened anxiety or mounting depression may cause them to deny unconsciously their own physical and emotional needs, grow increasingly emotionally distant by becoming increasingly aloof and/or spending less time with the patient, or generally neglect a patient's psychological needs by simply ignoring signs and symptoms of affective distress. Reacting to patients' emotional needs in these ways is antithetical to empathic concern and detrimental to patient welfare.

Effective psychological care of medical patients additionally requires that physicians refrain from imposing their own ethical beliefs on patients whose dependence on caretakers makes them potentially more vulnerable to the values those caretakers might bring to the medical setting. As Strupp (1974) notes in his discussion of the psychotherapeutic process, clinicians are constantly at risk of promoting their values over those of their patients, whether wittingly or unconsciously, because all physicians incorporate idiosyncratic moral beliefs into their work. It is therefore essential that they commit themselves to placing the values and interests of patients first, then acting as their agents. Lacking that perspective, the patients' well-being may suffer. The mechanism for protecting patients' autonomous wishes in the medical environment is the maintenance of an ongoing collaborative relationship between physician and patient in which therapeutic goals, and the means to achieve those goals, are continually considered. This rests on informed consent, the process of ensuring that patients participate in medical decision-making in a manner that maximizes their ability to advance their own autonomy. Informed consent rests on four basic elements: (1) the provision of information to patients concerning recommended actions, benefits, risks, and alternatives of medical treatments; (2) assurance that patients understand the information provided concerning various medical treatments; (3) assurance that the patients' decisions concerning medical treatment are made voluntarily, in the absence of coercion; and, (4) eliciting patients' consent via active authorization, as opposed to passive assent.

Although informed consent is often conceptualized as applying to a single instance of medical decision-making (e.g., consent to a surgical procedure), it is actually a dynamic process inherent in the ongoing relationship between physician and patient. For example, a patient suffering from insulin-dependent diabetes over many years should continually be discussing with his or her physician the course and treatment implications of the illness, in addition to any therapeutic determination that must be made in acute situations. The physician should not be allowed to disclose medical information selectively in order to advance a therapeutic regimen that he or she considers to be the best option, as that approach unfairly promotes values that may conflict with the patient's longstanding autonomous wishes. Although supportive psychotherapeutic techniques require the clinician to indulge in a certain degree of guidance and influence, to interpret those maneuvers as a *caveat* for allowing physicians to unilaterally impose their own values on patients is to undermine any attempt at empathic communication with the medically ill. The current era of medicine increasingly requires physicians to make treatment decisions that balance commitment to individual patients against a broader societal commitment to allocate medical resources over growing populations of patients. This atmosphere may foster a desire to advocate for policies whose values are contrary to those of individual patients, a temptation that clinicians must guard against vigilantly.

An empathic approach in the context of a biopsychosocial frame of reference is ". . . to treat the whole patient and not merely characterize the nature of an illness and impede biologic deterioration" (Slaby and Glicksman, 1985). Excellent, integrated, and compassionate treatment of each patient as a unique individual is the ultimate goal of the complete physician—and the goal of this text.

ANNOTATED BIBLIOGRAPHY

Bloch S, Chodoff P (eds): Psychiatric Ethics, 2nd ed. Oxford, Oxford University Press, 1991

> This text offers a comprehensive overview of the ethical dilemmas facing mental health professions. The individual chapters present material that is highly relevant to all practitioners, including issues concerned with the philosophical basis of psychiatric ethics, the concept of disease, and ethical aspects of psychotherapy.

Engel G: The need for a new medical model: A challenge for biomedicine. Science 196:129–136, 1977

> In this article, Engel carefully articulates the shortcomings of the biomedical model, which he feels leaves no room within its framework for the social, psychological, and behavioral dimensions of illness. He demonstrates a need for the biopsychosocial approach as a "blueprint for research, a framework for teaching, and a design for action in the real world of health care."

Engel G: The clinical application of the biopsychosocial model. Am J Psychiatry 137:535–544, 1980

> An excellent complement to the above, this article uses the biopsychosocial model to describe the impact of an acute myocardial infarction on a middle-aged man. It explores the effect of relevant psychosocial issues (e.g., the role of family mem-

bers, healthcare providers, and coworkers) on the onset, treatment, and course of his illness.

Frank J: Persuasion and Healing. Baltimore, Johns Hopkins University Press, 1961

> In this classic study of psychotherapy, the author explores the relationship between healer and sufferer, stressing the fundamental importance of the clinician's personal influence. Frank's observations concerning general attitudes and specific procedures that facilitate communication with patients constitute the basis of all forms of psychotherapy, including the supportive care of the medically ill.

Green S: Mind and Body: The Psychology of Physical Illness. Washington, DC, American Psychiatric Press, 1985

> This text expands on the basic principles discussed in this chapter, including the clinical applications of the biopsychosocial model and psychodynamic factors in the doctor–patient relationship.

Lipowski Z: Psychiatry of somatic disease: Epidemiology, pathogenesis, classification. Compr Psychiatry 16:105–124, 1975

> In this comprehensive article, the author presents a wealth of information concerning the linkage between psychiatric and physical illness. It is particularly notable for discussion of psychological responses to disease and injury, and the psychosocial determinants influencing those responses.

Lindemann E: Symptomatology and management of acute grief. Am J Psychiatry 101:141–146, 1944

> This landmark paper discusses the psychological and widespread psychophysiological manifestations of acute grief. Although subsequent investigations of bereavement modify Lindemann's initial conclusions (e.g., Rynearson E: Psychotherapy of pathologic grief: Revisions and limitations. Psychiatr Clin North Am 10:487–500, 1987), the work remains a standard in the field.

Parsons T: The Social System. Glencoe, IL, The Free Press, 1951

> Part of this lengthy sociological text is devoted to study of medical practice, including a sophisticated discussion of the dynamics of the sick role. Emphasizing the collaborative nature of medical care, Parsons details distinctive roles for patient and clinician during the various stages of illness. Of particular importance is his description of the changing levels of dependency and autonomy required of the patient by different aspects of the treatment.

REFERENCES

Alexander F, French T: Psychoanalytic Therapy. New York, Ronald Press, 1946

Bachrach H: Empathy: We know what we mean, but what do we measure? Arch Gen Psychiatry 33:35–38, 1976

Basch M: Empathic understanding: A review of the concept and some theoretical considerations. J Am Psychoanal Assoc 31:101–125, 1983

Book H: Empathy: Misconceptions and misuses in psychotherapy. Am J Psychiatry 145:420–424, 1988

Brown J, Stoudemire GA: Normal and pathological grief. JAMA 250:378–382, 1983

Buckley P: A neglected treatment. Psych Ann 16:515–521, 1986

Buie D: Empathy: Its nature and limitations. J Am Psychoanal Assoc 29:281–307, 1981

Cohen-Cole S, Bird J: Interviewing the cardiac patient II: A practical guide for helping patients cope with their emotions. Qual Life Cardiovasc Care 3:53–65, 1986

Engel G: A life-setting conducive to illness: The giving-up–given-up complex. Ann Intern Med 69:293–298, 1968

Engel G: The need for a new medical model. A challenge for biomedicine. Science 196:129–136, 1977

Engel G: The clinical application of the biopsychosocial model. Am J Psychiatry 137:535–544, 1980

Frank J: Persuasion and Healing. Baltimore, Johns Hopkins University Press, 1961

Green S: Mind and Body: The Psychology of Physical Illness. Washington, DC, American Psychiatric Press, 1985

Greenson R: Empathy and its vicissitudes. Int J Psychiatry 41:418–424, 1960

Groves J: Taking care of the hateful patient. N Engl J Med 298:883–887, 1978

Hollis F: Casework: A Psychosocial Therapy. New York, Random House, 1964

Irwin M, Daniels M, Weiner H: Immune and neorendocrine changes during bereavement. Psychiatr Clin North Am 10:449–466, 1987

Jaffe D: Empathy, counteridentification, countertransference: A review, with some personal perspectives on the "analytic instrument." Psychoanal Q 55:215–243, 1986

Kehana R, Bibring G: Personality types in medical management. In Zinberg N (ed) Psychiatry and Medical Practice in a General Hospital. New York, International Universities Press, 1964

Keefe T: Empathy: The critical skill. Social Work 21:10–14, 1976

Kohut H: How Does Analysis Cure? Chicago, University of Chicago Press, 1984, p 82

Lindemann E: Symptomatology and management of acute grief. Am J Psychiatry 101:141–146, 1944

Lipowski Z: Psychiatry of somatic disease: Epidemiology, pathogenesis, classification. Compr Psychiatry 16:105–124, 1975

Miller I: The therapeutic empathic communication (TEC) process. Am J Psychother 43:531–545, 1989

Parsons T: The Social System. Glencoe, IL, The Free Press, 1951

Rahe R: Subjects' recent life changes and their near-future illness reports. Ann Clin Res 4:1–16, 1973

Reich P, DeSilva R, Lown B, et al: Acute psychological disturbances preceding life-threatening ventricular arrhythmias. JAMA 246:233–235, 1981

Reichard J: Teaching principles of medical psychology to medical house officers: Methods and problems. In Zinberg N (ed): Psychiatry and Medical Practice in a General Hospital. New York, International Universities Press, 1964

Slaby A, Glicksman A: Adapting to Life-Threatening Illness. New York, Praeger, 1985

Stein M, Keller S, Schleifer S: Stress and immunomodulation: The role of depression and neuroendocrine function. J Immunol 135(Suppl 2):827–833, 1985

Strupp H: Some observations on the fallacy of value-free psychotherapy and the empty organism: Comments on a case study. J Abnorm Psychol 83:199–201, 1974

Vailliant G: Adaptation to Life. Boston, Little, Brown, & Co, 1977

Winston A, Pinsker H, McCullough L: A review of supportive psychotherapy. Hosp Comm Psychiatry 37:1105–1114, 1986

Zola I: Socio-cultural factors in the seeking of medical aid: A progress report. Transcult Psychiatr Res 14:62–65, 1963

Subject Index

A

Acetylcholine (ACH), and behavior, 420, 436, 437
ACH *See* Acetylcholine
ACTH *See* Adrenocorticotrophic hormone
Acting out, as defense mechanism, 162
Adaptive Behavior Scale, 270
Adaptive point of view, psychoanalytic theory, 142, 149
Adolescence, development, 298–302
  affective development, 299–302
    critical developmental issues, 300
    defense mechanisms, 300
    family relationships, 302
    risk-taking behavior, 300–301
    sexuality, 301–302
    turmoil, 299
  cognitive development, 298–299
    Piaget's stages, 298–299
  physical development, 298
    endocrine, 298
    neurological, 298
  response to physical illness, 312–313
  social development, 302
Adoption studies, 475
Adrenocorticotropic hormone (ACTH), 53
  as regulator in stress response, 97
Adulthood
  developmental concepts, 342–348
    Erikson's eight stages of man, 346–348
    identity and lifecycle, 347–348

    psychological concepts, 343
    stage, transition, and normative crisis, 342–346
      lines, 344
      normative crisis, 344
      normative crisis in health and illness, 344
      regression, 345–346
      repetition, 346
      stages, 342
      timing, 345
      transitions, 342–343
  lifecycle, 340–342
  psychological stages of lifecycle, 341, 350
  sexuality in, 244–245
  stages, 349–381
    bereavement, 368–371
      case study, 370–371
    choices, 379–381
    consolidation of adulthood, 353–355
      case study, 355
    courtship, marriage, and marital crisis, 355–361
      alternatives, 359–360
      childlessness, 360–361
      counseling and psychotherapy, 358–359
      courtship, 355–356
      marital crisis, 357–358
      marriage, 356–357
    death and dying, 374–379
      case study, 377

Adulthood, stages (*continued*)
    late life transition, 371–374
        case study, 372–373
        integrity during, 373–374
    midlife, 366–368
    pregnancy, childbirth, and
        parenting, 361–366
        childbirth and early postpartum
            period, 362–363
        parenting, 363–365
        pregnancy, 361–362
        separation and divorce, 366
        single parent, 365–366
    transition to adulthood, 349–353
        failures in early adult
            development, 351–352
        precocious adult, 353
        "pseudo-adult," 352–353
            case study, 352–353
Affective development *See* Emotional
    development
African-American culture, 124–126
Age
  and decision time, 73
  and mental disorders, 62
  and physical disorders, 61–62
  selected lifetime prevalence, 57
Aggression, neurobiological aspects,
    459–460
  clinical neurobiology, 460–461
  in primates and humans, 459–460
  in subprimate mammals, 459
AIDS, 244, 248
Alcoholism, 486
Altruism, as defense mechanism, 163
Alzheimer's disease, 487
Amnesia, 392
Anal stage, 142
Androgen insensitivity syndrome, 237, 238
Anger, 505
Antecedents, in behavioral psychology,
    201–203
Anticipation, as defense mechanism, 163
Anxiety
  psychoanalytic view, 160–161
  response to illness, 504–505
  therapy techniques, 214, 215
Asian-American culture, 129–130

Assault, neurobiological aspects, 460
Attachment, in children, 385–389
  affect regulation development, 387
  cognitive development, 385
  coping styles, 387–389
  social context as a mediator of
    development, 386–387
Autocratic style, and doctor–patient
    relationship, 10
Autonomic nervous system, and sexual
    development and physiology,
    254

B
Bandura, Albert, 184
Bayley Scales of Infant Development-
    Revised, 270
Bechterev, Vladimir, 183, 184
Behavior
  Type A
    as risk factor for coronary artery
      disease, 90
Behavioral genetics, 473–492
  implications, 489–490
  methods of genetic investigation,
    474–482
    family, twin, and adoption studies,
      474–475
    genes and the environment, 481–482
    molecular biology, 478–481
    pedigree analysis, 476–477
    phenotypic classification, 481
    susceptibility traits and gene
      markers, 477–478
  overview, 473
  psychiatric genetics, 482–489
    alcoholism, 486
    Alzheimer's disease, 487
    biological susceptibility traits and
      gene markers, 484–485
    Klinefelter's syndrome, 486–487
    major disorders, 482–484
    morbidity risk, 483
    pedigree analysis, 484
    personality genetics, 488
    testing, genetic, 488–489
Behavioral model, criticisms, 224–226
Behavior modification, cognitive, 211

Behavior, neurobiological components, 403–419
  association cortices, 412–416
  basal ganglia, 416–419
  hypothalamus, 405–409
  limbic system, 409–412
  reticular activating system, 404–405
Behavioral psychology
  antecedents, 201–203
  behavioral medicine, 221–222
    case study, 221–222
  behavioral model, criticisms, 224–226
  behavioral and psychoanalytic models compared, 223–224
    clinical applications of behavior therapy to health-related problems, 221
  classical conditioning, 183–187
  clinical applications, 210–213
    Beck's cognitive therapy, 212–213
    cognitive behavior modification, 211
    rational-emotive therapy (RET), 211–212
  contributions of behavioral approach, 226–227
  emotional development, 186–187
  extinction, 185, 192–193
  illness and disease prevention, 222–223
  imitation, 192
  negative consequences, 199–201
  operant conditioning, 187–203
    antecedents, 201–203
    consequences, 189
    new behavior development, 191–192
      case study, 191–192
    reinforcement, 188–190
  overview, 182–183
  punishment, 194–199
    case study, 196–199
    negative effects, 200
  reciprocal inhibition, 203–204
  schedules of reinforcement, 193–194
  social learning theory, 204–210
    modeling, 204–207
      component processes, 206
      functions, 205
    self-efficacy, 209–210

    self-regulation, 207–208
      case study, 208
      self-direction, 207
      self-evaluation, 207–208
      self-observation, 207
      self-reaction, 208
  therapy techniques, 213–221
    for anxiety disorders, 214, 215
    biofeedback, 217, 219
    case study, 218–221
    cognitive restructuring, 217, 219
    contingency contract, 213, 219
    contingency management, 213, 219
    exposure to fear-provoking stimuli, 214
    flooding *in vivo*, 216, 219
    imaginal flooding, 215–216, 219
    parent training, 213, 219
    problem-solving skills training, 217, 219
    relaxation techniques, 216–217, 219
      diaphragmatic breathing, 217
      progressive muscle relaxation (PMR), 216–217
      visualization techniques, 217
    response prevention, 216, 219
    social skills training, 213, 219
    stress-management training, 217–218, 219
    systematic desensitization, 214–215, 219
Bereavement, 368–371
  case study, 370–371
Biofeedback, 217, 219
Biomedical model
  definition, 5
Biomedicine, 130–133
Biopsychosocial model, 5–6, 36–84
  areas of study, 37–40
  case formulation, 40–46
    biological variables, 40
    biopsychosocial formulation, 42
    biopsychosocial management, 42–45
      biological management, 43
      psychological interventions, 43–45
      social interventions, 45
    psychological variables, 41
    social variables, 41–42
      case studies, 5–6, 39–40

Biopsychosocial model (*continued*)
  epidemiology of psychiatric disorders
       in general medical practice,
       55–61
    in the community, 55–59
    in primary care, 59–61
  in medical practice, 46–55
    influence of psychosocial variables
       on course and outcome of
       illness, 51–52
    interviewing skills, 54–55
    onset of illness, 48–50
    psychobiological mechanisms, 53–54
    psychological and behavioral
       predisposition to physical
       illness, 46–48
    psychosocial intervention in
       outcome of physical illness,
       52–53
    use of medical services, 51–52
  overview, 36–37
  for psychiatric patients, 77–78
  social epidemiology and illness
       behavior, 61–70
    age factors, 61–62
      mental disorders, 62
      physical disorders, 61–62
    gender factors, 62–67
      mental disorders, 66–67
      physical disorders, 62–66
    racial factors, 67–68
      mental disorders, 68
      physical disorders, 67–68
    social class, 68–70
      mental disorders, 69–70
      physical disorders, 68–69
  utilization and related illness
       behaviors, 70–77
    decision time, 71–76
      age, 73
      background factors, 71
      ethnicity, 73–75
      gender, 73
      psychological processes, 71–72
      social class, 73–75
      social networks, 75
      social-psychological factors, 75–76

      social variables, 72–73
      definitions, 70–71
      sick role, 76–77
Birth control counseling, 247

C
Cardiovascular disease
  and stress, 101–102
Case studies
  behavioral medicine, 221–222
  bereavement, 370–371
  biopsychosocial model, 5–6, 39–40
  consolidation of adulthood, 355
  countertransference, 175
  death and dying, 377
  doctor–patient relationship, 31–33
  dreams, 147–148
  dynamic-motivational point-of-view,
      149–150
  ego, and structural model, 159–160
  family medicine, 318, 321, 335
  "hateful" patient, 24
  in-hospital patient, 27–28
  illness dynamics, 498–499
  late-life transition, 372–373
  mentally disturbed patient, 28–29
  object relations, 169–170
  operant conditioning, 191–192
  patient with multiple complaints,
      25–26
  professional boundaries, 14
  psychoanalytic view, 140–141, 147–148
  psychological care of the mentally ill,
      509–510
  psychological factors affecting medical
      condition, 87, 509–510
  psychosexual development, 151,
      152–153, 157
  punishment, 196–199
  seductive patient, 22–23
  self-psychology, 171–172, 172–173
  self-regulation, 208
  stress, 87
  therapy techniques, 218–221
  transition to adulthood, 352–353
Character disorder, psychoanalytic
      theory, 142

Character formation, 392–394
  play, 393
  responsibility, 393
  revictimization, 394
  victimizing others, 394
Childhood, early
  development, 287–293
    affective development, 290–291
      dreams, 291
      family relationships, 292
      fears, 290
      gender-related issues, 290
      imaginary companions, 291
      object relations, 290
      sexuality, 290–291
    cognitive development, 288–289
      milestones, 289
      Piaget's stages, 288–289
    physical development, 287–288
      fine motor-adaptive skills, 287
      gross motor skills, 287
      sleep, 287
      toilet training, 288
    response to physical illness, 312
    school, 292
    social development, 291–292
    speech and language, 289–290
    television, 292
Childhood, middle, 293–298
  affective development, 295–296
    conscience, 295–296
    fears, 296
    sexuality, 296
    superego, 295–296
  cognitive development, 294–295
    milestones, 294–295
    Piaget's stages, 294
  physical development, 293–294
    fine motor-adaptive skills, 293
    gross motor skills, 293
    growth and pubertal changes, 294
    neurological, 293
    sleep, 293
  response to physical illness, 312
  social development, 296–298
Childlessness, 360–361
Chromosomes, abnormalities in sex
    differentiation, 237

Cigarette smoking
  fetal development risk, 274
Cognitive behavior modification, 211
Cognitive development
  adolescent, 298–299
  in early childhood, 288–289
  infancy, 276
  in middle childhood, 294–295
  in toddlers, 283
Cognitive restructuring, 217, 219
Communication
  cross-cultural, 120–122
  infancy, 276–277
Compliance, 17–21
  factors affecting, 18
  factors enhancing, 20–21
  factors related to noncompliance,
    19–20
  fostering, 21
Compromise formation, 142
Conditioning, classical, 183–187
Conscience
  in middle childhood, 295–296
Conscious stage, 142
Consumer-based style, and doctor–patient
    relationship, 11
Consumptive behavior, neuorobiological
    basis, 458–459
Contingency contract, 213, 219
Contingency management, 213, 219
Corticotropin-releasing factor (CRF), 53
  as regulator in stress response, 97
Countertransference
  in doctor—patient relationship, 16–17
  medicine and the family, 334–335
  psychoanalytic theory, 142
Courtship, 355–356
Couvade syndrome, 362
CRF *See* Corticotropin-releasing factor
Culture, and the practice of medicine,
    109–136
  African-American, 124–126
  Asian-American, 129–130
  biomedical, 130–133
  concept, 111–112
  "culture-bound syndromes," 113–114
  ethnocentrism, 110, 113

Culture, and the practice of medicine
    (*continued*)
  ethnomedical systems, typology,
    117–118
  and health 112–122
    cross-cultural communication,
      120–122
    epidemiological risk, 112
    models of illness, 117–119
    normality, disease, and health,
      112–115
    and personality development,
      115–117
  Hispanic-American, 126–129
  influence of family, 302–303
  LEARN model, 120–122
  materialistic model, 111
  medical care, 122–124
  overview, 109–110

D

Death and dying
  in adult development, 374–379
    case study, 377
  age-adjusted death rates according to
    sex and rate, 64
  and doctor–patient relationship, 29–33
    case study, 31–33
  leading causes of death for adults, 65
Decision-making process, and
    doctor–patient relationship,
    9, 11
Decision time, 71–76
  and age, 73
  and background factors, 71
  and ethnicity, 73–75
  and gender, 73
  and psychological processes, 71–72
  and social class, 73–75
  and social networks, 75
  and social-psychological factors, 75–76
  and social variables, 72–73
Defense mechanisms, 161–163
  in adolescent development, 300
  as developed by Freud, 158–160
  psychoanalytic theory, 142
  in toddlers, 285
Delusional projection, as defense
    mechanism, 162

Denial
  as defense mechanism, 162
  response to illness, 503–504
Denver II, 266–267
Dependency, 506–507
Depression, 505–506
Development
  adolescent, 298–302
    affective development, 299–302
      critical developmental issues, 300
      defense mechanisms, 300
      family relationships, 302
      risk-taking behavior, 300–301
      sexuality, 301–302
      turmoil, 299
    cognitive development, 298–299
      Piaget's stages, 298–299
    physical development, 298
      endocrine, 298
      neurological, 298
    response to physical illness, 312–313
    social development, 302
  children at risk, 307–310
    children of alcoholic parents, 308
    children of mentally ill parents, 309
    divorce, 308
    prevention and early intervention,
      309–310
    resilient children and adolescents,
      309
  early childhood, 287–293
    affective development, 290–291
      dreams, 291
      family relationships, 292
      fears, 290
      gender-related issues, 290
      imaginary companions, 291
      object relations, 290
      sexuality, 290–291
    cognitive development, 288–289
      milestones, 289
      Piaget's stages, 288–289
    physical development, 287–288
      fine motor-adaptive skills, 287
      gross motor skills, 287
      sleep, 287
      toilet training, 288
    response to physical illness, 312

school, 292
social development, 291–292
speech and language, 289–290
television, 292
family's role, 302–307
cultural influences, 302–303
nontraditional families, 307
parenting styles, 303–304
response to physical illness, 313
stages of development, 304–305
adolescent, 305
child aged 3 to 6 years, 304–305
first baby, 304
school-age child, 305
sibling rivalry, 305
toddler, 304
tasks, 303
working parents, 306–307
infancy, 275–281
affective development, 277–281
early attachment, 277–279
maternal deprivation, 279–281
separation-individuation, 281
transitional object, 281
cognitive development, 276
communication, 276–277
physical development, 275–276
gross motor skills, 275
growth, 276
neurological, 275
sleep, 276
response to physical illness or
handicap, 310–311
intelligence, 269–272
evaluation, 269
mental retardation, 269–272
causes, 271
tests, 270
in medically ill children, adolescents,
and families, 310–313
family response to physical illness,
313
parental response to physical illness
or handicap in a newborn,
310–311
response to illness and hospitalization during the toddler phase,
311–312

response to physical illness in
adolescence, 312–313
response to physical illness in early
childhood, 312
response to physical illness in middle
childhood, 312
middle childhood, 293–298
affective development, 295–296
conscience, 295–296
fears, 296
sexuality, 296
superego, 295–296
cognitive development, 294–295
milestones, 294–295
Piaget's stages, 294
physical development, 293–294
fine motor-adaptive skills, 293
gross motor skills, 293
growth and pubertal changes, 294
neurological, 293
sleep, 293
response to physical illness, 312
social development, 296–298
models, 262–269
milestones, 264
Piagetian cognitive development,
265–269
temperament, 263–264
clusters, 264
dimensions, 263
normal, 262
overview, 261–272
prenatal, 272–274
communication, 274
fetal risks, 272–274
adolescent pregnancy, 273
and cigarette smoking, 274
complications in the newborn
period, 274
emotional factors, 274
fetal alcohol syndrome (FAS), 273
genetic abnormality, 273
low birth weight, 272–273
maternal disease, 273
maternal substance abuse, 273–274
outcome, 274
toddler, 281–287
affective development, 284–286
defense mechanisms, 285

Development, toddler (*continued*)
    emotions, 285
    fears, 285
    gender-related issues, 285–286
    object relations, 284–285
    cognitive development, 283
    milestones, 283
    Piaget's stages, 283
    physical development, 281–283
    fine motor-adaptive skills, 282
    gross motor skills, 281
    growth and feeding, 282
    sleep, 282
    toilet training, 282–283
    response to illness and
        hospitalization, 311–312
    social development, 287
    speech and language development,
        283–284
    views, 262
Developmental point of view, in
        psychoanalytic theory, 142,
        149
Diagnostic and Statistical Manual of
        Mental Disorders (DSM-IV),
        86, 117
Disease, prevention, 222–223
Displacement, as defense mechanism,
    162
Dissociation, as defense mechanism, 162
Distortion, as defense mechanism, 162
Divorce, 308
Doctor–patient relationship, 3–35
    biomedical model
        definition, 5
    biopsychosocial model, 5–6, 495–497
        case study, 5–6
    compliance, 17–21
        factors affecting, 18
        factors enhancing, 20–21
        factors related to noncompliance,
            19–20
        fostering, 21
    difficult relationships, 21–33
    and dying patient, 29–33
        case study, 31–33
    empathy, 6–9
    ethics, 13

    and "hateful" patient, 23–24
        case study, 24
    in-hospital patient, 26–28
        case study, 27–28
    mentally disturbed patient, 28–29
        case study, 28–29
    overview, 3–5
    patient with multiple complaints, 24–26
        case study, 25–26
    professional boundaries, 12–16
        case study, 14
    psychoanalytic view, 173–176
    and the psychological care of the
        medically ill, 508–512
        case study, 509–510
    and seductive patient, 22–23
        case study, 22–23
    styles of relating, 9–11
        consumer-based, 11
        decision-making process, 9
        paternalistic or autocratic, 10
        quality of interaction, 9
        shared decision-making, 11
    transference and countertransference,
        16–17
    trust, 12
Dopamine, and behavior, 422–424, 430,
    432, 434–436
Dreams
    early childhood, 291
    psychoanalytic view, 146–148
        case study, 147–148
DSM-IV *See Diagnostic and Statistical*
        Manual of Mental Disorders
Dynamic-motivational point-of-view,
        psychoanalytic theory, 142,
        148–150
    case study, 149–150
Dynamic unconscious, 143

E
ECA *See* Epidemiologic Catchment Area
        study
Ego
    psychoanalytic theory, 143
    and the structural model, 157–160
        case study, 159–160
Ego-ideal, psychoanalytic theory, 143

Elderly, sexuality in, 245–246
Emotional development, 186–187
  adolescent, 299–302
  early childhood, 290–291
  infancy, 277–281
  in middle childhood, 295–296
  in toddlers, 284–286
Empathy
  and doctor–patient relationship, 6–9
  psychoanalytic theory, 143
Endocrine system
  adolescent, 298
  and sexual development and
      physiology, 255
Epidemiologic Catchment Area (ECA)
      study, 56
Epidemiology
  cultural risk, 112
Ergotropic system, 99–100
  characteristics, 100
Erikson's eight stages of man, 346–348
Ethics
  and doctor–patient relationship, 13
Ethnicity *See also* Race
  and decision time, 73–75
Ethnocentrism, 110, 113
Ethnomedical systems, typology, 117–118
Extinction, 185, 192–193

F
Family
  developmental role, 302–307
    cultural influences, 302–303
    nontraditional families, 307
    parenting styles, 303–304
    response to physical illness, 313
    stages of development, 304–305
      adolescent, 305
      child aged 3 to 6 years, 304–305
      first baby, 304
      school-age child, 305
      sibling rivalry, 305
      toddler, 304
    tasks, 303
    working parents, 306–307
  and doctor–patient relationship, 21
  and medicine, 318–339
    case studies, 318, 321, 335
    consultation and referrals, 335–336

countertransference to the family,
      334–335
    family definition, 320–321
    family therapies, 326–331
      integrative model for families and
          illness, 329–331
      multigenerational family, 328–329
      structural family, 326–327
    historical perspective, 319–320
    overview, 319
    physician involvement, 331–334
      family therapy, 333–334
      feelings and support, 332
      minimal family emphasis, 331
      ongoing medical information and
          advice, 331
      systematic assessment and
          planned intervention, 333
    theory, 322–326
      case study, 323–324
  response to physical illness, 313
  social support during illness, 96
FAS *See* Fetal alcohol syndrome
Fears
  early childhood, 290
  middle childhood, 296
  in toddlers, 285
Females
  adrenogenital syndrome, 237
  cyclic changes, 253
  genital anatomy, 252–254
  hormone changes during menstrual
      cycle, 241
Fetal alcohol syndrome (FAS), 273
Fixation, psychoanalytic theory, 150
Flooding
  imaginal flooding, 215–216, 219
  in vivo, 216, 219
Follicular stimulating hormone (FSH),
      238, 255
Free association, psychoanalytic theory,
      143
Freud, Sigmund, 89–90, 146, 148–149
  and development of defense
      mechanisms, 158–160,
      161–163
  and development of the ego, 157–160

Freud, Sigmund (*continued*)
  and role of anxiety, 160–161
  and psychosexual development, 150–157
FSH *See* Follicular stimulating hormone

G

GABA *See* Gamma-Aminobutyric acid
Gamma-Aminobutyric acid (GABA), and
      behavior, 436–438
Gender
  and age-adjusted death rates, 64
  and decision time, 73
  identity, 239
  and life expectancy, 63
  and mental disorders, 66–67
  and physical disorders, 62–66
  selected lifetime prevalence, 57
Genetics, behavioral, 473–492
  implications, 489–490
  methods of genetic investigation,
      474–482
    family, twin, and adoption studies,
      474–475
    genes and the environment, 481–482
    molecular biology, 478–481
    pedigree analysis, 476–477
    phenotypic classification, 481
    susceptibility traits and gene
      markers, 477–478
  overview, 473
  psychiatric genetics, 482–489
    alcoholism, 486
    Alzheimer's disease, 487
    biological susceptibility traits and
      gene markers, 484–485
    Klinefelter's syndrome, 486–487
    major disorders, 482–484
    morbidity risk, 483
    pedigree analysis, 484
    personality genetics, 488
    testing, genetic, 488–489
Genogram, 329, 330
Grief process, 501–503

H

Habituation, 448–449
"Hateful" patient, and doctor–patient
      relationship, 23–24
  case study, 24

Hemispheric lateralization, 397–398
Hispanic-American culture, 126–129
HIV-positive patients, sexuality in,
      248–249
Homeostatic equilibrium, 91
Homosexuality, 247–248
Hormones
  changes during menstrual cycle, 241
  steroid hormones, 442–443
    location of steroid binding in the
      brain, 442–443
    mechanisms of effect, 442
    regulatory effects, 443
  thyroid hormones, 443–446
    biological rhythms modulation,
      445–446
    nervous system development, 445
    stress responses, 445
Hospital patient, and doctor–patient
      relationship, 26–28
  case study, 27–28
Humor, as defense mechanism, 163
Hypochondriasis, as defense mechanism,
      162

I

ICD *See International Classification of
      Disease*
Id, psychoanalytic theory, 143
Illness
  influence of psychosocial variables on
      course and outcome, 51–52
  prevention, 222–223
Imitation, 192
Infancy, 275–281
  affective development, 277–281
    early attachment, 277–279
    maternal deprivation, 279–281
    separation-individuation, 281
    transitional object, 281
  cognitive development, 276
  communication, 276–277
  physical development, 275–276
    gross motor skills, 275
    growth, 276
    neurological, 275
    sleep, 276

response to physical illness or
handicap, 310–311
sexual development and physiology,
238–240
Insight, psychoanalytic theory, 143
Instinctual drives, psychoanalytic theory,
143
Intellectualization, as defense
mechanism, 162
Intelligence, development, 269–272
evaluation, 269
mental retardation, 269–272
causes, 271
tests, 270
Interaction, quality of, in doctor–patient
relationship, 9
Intercourse, 243
International Classification of Disease
(ICD), 117
Interpretation, psychoanalytic theory,
143, 177
Interviewing skills, 54–55
IQ tests, 270

K
K-ABC *See* Kaufman Assessment Battery
for Children
Kaufman Assessment Battery for
Children (K-ABC), 270
Klinefelter's syndrome, 237

L
Latency, psychoanalytic theory, 143
Latino philosophical premises about
health and curing, 128
"Lay referral system," 75
LCU *See* Life-change unit
LEARN model, 120–122
Learning and memory, 446–455
components and dimensions, 446–448
localization, 448–453
neurochemical basis, 453–455
phases, 447
types, 447
Leiter International Performance Scale,
270
LH *See* Luteinizing hormone
Life-change unit (LCU), 92–93, 94

Lifecycle, 340–342
psychological stages, 341, 350
Luteinizing hormone (LH), 238, 255

M
Males
cyclic changes, 251
genital anatomy, 250
reproductive system, 250
Marriage, 356–357
Masturbation, 242
Medical condition, psychological factors
affecting (PFAMC), 85–108
cardiovascular disease and stress,
101–102
case study, 87
diagnostic criteria, 86
historical development of mind-body
relationship, 89–91
model of illness onset, 88
neuroendocrine and neuroimmune
response, 99–101
ergotropic system, 99–100
characteristics, 100
trophotropic system, 100–101
characteristics, 100
overview, 85–89
psychoneuroimmunology, 102–104
T-cell regulation, 103
psychophysiological pathways, 97–99
stress, influence on disease, 91–97
biological predisposition to stress-
induced illness, 96–97
cognitive appraisal of life-change
events, 94
coping and defense mechanisms,
94–95
social support, 95–96
treatment strategies, 104–106
Medical illness, biopsychosocial approach
in medical care, 495–514
doctor–patient relationship
and the biopsychosocial model,
495–497
and the psychological care of the
medically ill, 508–512
case study, 509–510
grief process, 501–503

Medical illness, biopsychosocial approach
        in medical care (*continued*)
    illness dynamics, 498–501
        case studies, 498–499
        components, 500
    illness response, abnormal, 503–507
        anger, 505
        anxiety, 504–505
        denial, 503–504
        dependency, 506–507
        depression, 505–506
Medical practice, and biopsychosocial
        model, 46–55
    influence of psychosocial variables on
            course and outcome of
            illness, 51–52
    interviewing skills, 54–55
    onset of illness, 48–50
    psychobiological mechanisms, 53–54
    psychological and behavioral
            predisposition to physical
            illness, 46–48
    psychosocial intervention in outcome
            of physical illness, 52–53
    use of medical services, 51–52
Medical regimen
    and doctor–patient relationship, 21
Medical services, use of, 51–52
Medicine, behavioral, 221–222
    case study, 221–222
Medicine, and the family, 318–339
    case studies, 318, 321, 335
    consultation and referrals, 335–336
    countertransference to the family,
            334–335
    family definition, 320–321
    family therapies, 326–331
        integrative model for families and
            illness, 329–331
        multigenerational family, 328–329
        structural family, 326–327
    historical perspective, 319–320
    overview, 319
    physician involvement, 331–334
        family therapy, 333–334
        feelings and support, 332
        minimal family emphasis, 331

ongoing medical information and
        advice, 331
    systematic assessment and planned
            intervention, 333
    theory, 322–326
        case study, 323–324
Menstrual cycle, hormone changes
        during, 241
Mental illness
    mentally disturbed patient, and doctor-
            patient relationship, 28–29
    case study, 28–29
Mental retardation, 269–272
    causes, 271
Metapsychology, psychoanalytic theory,
        144
Midlife, 366–368
Mind–body relationship
    historical development, 89–91
Modeling, 204–207
    component processes, 206
    functions, 205
Molecular biology, and behavioral
        genetics, 478–481
Mortality
    life expectancy by race and sex, 63

N
Narcissism, 170–171
Nervous system, and sexual development
        and physiology, 254
Neurobehavioral disorders, genetic
        mapping, 479
Neurobiology, 403–472
    behavior components, 403–419
        association cortices, 412–416
        basal ganglia, 416–419
        hypothalamus, 405–409
        limbic system, 409–412
        reticular activating system, 404–405
    neurobiology of specific behaviors,
            446–469
        aggression, 459–460
            clinical neurobiology, 460–461
            in primates and humans, 459–460
            in subprimate mammals, 459
        assault, 460

consumptive behavior, 458–459
learning and memory, 446–455
    components and dimensions,
        446–448
    localization, 448–453
    neurochemical basis, 453–455
    phases, 447
    types, 447
neurohormonal regulation of eating
    behavior, 458
reproductive behavior, 455–457
    in primates and human sexual
        behavior, 457
    in subprimate mammals, 455–457
sleep, 464–468
    architecture, 464–467
        cycles, 466–467
        stages, 464–466
    circadian rhythms, 467–468
    and lifecycle, 467
    neurobiology, 468–469
stress, 461–464
    behavioral responses to stressors,
        462–463
    neuroendocrine components of
        stress response and
        behavioral effects, 463–464
suicide, 461
neurochemical determinants of
    behavior, 420–446
neuropeptides, 439–442
neurotransmitters, classic,
    420–438
    criteria, 421
    drug and neurotransmitter
        receptors relevant to
        psychopharmacology,
        429–431
    linking neurotransmitter to
        behavior, 421
    neurotransmission, discovery,
        420–421
steroid hormones, 442–443
    location of steroid binding in the
        brain, 442–443
    mechanisms of effect, 442
    regulatory effects, 443

thyroid hormones, 443–446
    biological rhythms modulation,
        445–446
    nervous system development, 445
    stress responses, 445
Neuroendocrine and neuroimmune
        response, 99–101
    ergotropic system, 99–100
        characteristics, 100
    trophotropic system, 100–101
        characteristics, 100
Neurological system
    adolescence, 298
    infancy, 275
    middle childhood, 293
Neurosis, psychoanalytic theory, 144,
        163–164
Norepinephrine, and behavior, 422–424,
        432

O

Object, psychoanalytic theory, 144
Object relations, theory of development,
        164–170
    case studies, 169–170
    parallel lines of human development,
        168
    separation-individuation process,
        166–167
Operant conditioning, 187–203
    antecedents, 201–203
    consequences, 189
    new behavior development, 191–192
        case study, 191–192
    reinforcement, 188–190
Oral stage, psychoanalytic theory, 144

P

Palliation, 95
Paraphilias, 239
Parents, 363–365
    children of alcoholic, 308
    children of mentally ill, 309
    response to physical illness or
        handicap in a newborn,
        310–311
    single, 365–366

Parents (*continued*)
  styles, 303–304
  training, 213, 219
Passive-aggressive behavior, as defense
      mechanism, 162
Paternalistic style, and doctor–patient
      relationship, 10
Patient care
  styles of relating, 9–11
    consumer-based, 11
    decision-making process, 9
    paternalistic or autocratic, 10
    quality of interaction, 9
    shared decision-making, 11
Pavlov, Ivan, 183, 184
Peabody Picture Vocabulary Test
      (PPVT-R), 270
Personality
  and the biopsychosocial model, 47
  development, and culture, 115–117
PFAMC *See* Medical condition, psy-
      chological factors affecting
Phallic-oedipal stage, psychoanalytic
      theory, 144
Phenylketonuria (PKU), 272
Physical development
  early childhood, 287–288
Physician *See also* Doctor–patient
      relationship
  styles of relating, 9–11
    consumer-based, 11
    decision-making process, 9
    paternalistic or autocratic, 10
    quality of interaction, 9
    shared decision-making, 11
Piaget, Jean, 265–269
PKU *See* Phenylketonuria
Pleasure-unpleasure principle,
      psychoanalytic theory, 144
PMR *See* Progressive muscle relaxation
POMC *See* Proopiomelanocortin
PPVT-R *See* Peabody Picture Vocabulary
      Test
Preconscious, psychoanalytic theory, 144
Pregnancy, childbirth, and parenting
  adolescent, 273
  childbirth and early postpartum period,
      362–363

parenting, 363–365
pregnancy, 361–362
separation and divorce, 366
single parent, 365–366
teenage, 247
Prenatal development, 272–274
  communication, 274
  fetal risks, 272–274
    adolescent pregnancy, 273
    and cigarette smoking, 274
    complications in the newborn
        period, 274
    emotional factors, 274
    fetal alcohol syndrome (FAS), 273
    genetic abnormality, 273
    low birth weight, 272–273
    maternal disease, 273
    maternal substance abuse, 273–274
    outcome, 274
Primary conscious, psychoanalytic
      theory, 144
Progressive muscle relaxation (PMR),
      216–217
Projection, as defense mechanism, 162
Prolactin, 255
Proopiomelanocortin (POMC), 441
Psychiatric disorders, in general medical
      practice, 55–61
  in the community, 55–59
  epidemiology, 55–61
  in primary care, 59–61
Psychiatric genetics, 482–489
  alcoholism, 486
  Alzheimer's disease, 487
  biological susceptibility traits and gene
        markers, 484–485
  Klinefelter's syndrome, 486–487
  major disorders, 482–484
  morbidity risk, 483
  pedigree analysis, 484
  personality genetics, 488
  testing, genetic, 488–489
Psychic determinism, psychoanalytic
      theory, 145
Psychoanalytic and behavioral models
      compared, 223–224
  clinical applications of behavior
        therapy to health-related
        problems, 221

Psychoanalytic theory, 139–181
  anxiety, 160–161
  aspects, 140–141
  case study, 140–141
  concepts, 141–150
    dreams, 146–148
      case study, 147–148
    dynamic-motivational point-of-view,
      148–150
      case study, 149–150
  defense mechanisms, 161–163
  and the doctor–patient relationship,
    173–176
    countertransference, 174–175
      case study, 175
    transference, 173–174
    treatment alliance, 175–176
  ego, and the structural model,
    157–160
    case study, 159–160
  neurosis, 163–164
  object-relations theory of development,
    164–170
    case studies, 169–170
    parallel lines of human development,
      168
    separation-individuation process,
      166–167
  overview, 139–140
  parallel lines of human development,
    168
  psychoanalytic psychotherapy,
    176–178
  psychosexual development, 150–157
    anal stage, 152–153
      case study 152–153
    oral stage, 151–152
      case study, 151
    phallic-oedipal stage, 153–157
      case study, 157
  self-psychology, 170–173
    case studies, 171–172, 172–173
  separation-individuation process,
    166–167
Psychobiology, 394–398
Psychoneuroimmunology, 102–104
Psychophysiological pathways, 97–99

Psychosexual development, stages,
    psychoanalytic theory, 145,
    150–157 *See also* anal stage,
    oral stage, phallic-oedipal
    stage
Psychotherapy
  psychoanalytic, 176–178
  as treatment for physical illness, 53
Puberty, sexuality during, 240–244
Punishment, 194–199
  case study, 196–199
  negative effects, 200

R

Race *See also* Ethnicity
  and age-adjusted death rates, 64
  and life expectancy, 63
  and mental disorders, 68
  and physical disorders, 67–68
Rational-emotive therapy (RET),
    211–212
Reaction formation, as defense
    mechanism, 162
Reciprocal inhibition, 203–204
Regression, psychoanalytic theory,
    149–150
Reinforcement, 188–190
  schedules, 193–194
Relationships
  difficult, doctor–patient, 21–33
Relaxation techniques, 216–217, 219
  diaphragmatic breathing, 217
  progressive muscle relaxation (PMR),
    216–217
  visualization techniques, 217
Repetition compulsion, psychoanalytic
    theory, 145
Repression, as defense mechanism, 162
Resilience, 97
Resistance, psychoanalytic theory, 145
Response prevention, 216, 219
RET *See* rational-emotive therapy

S

Schedule of Recent Life Events (SRE),
    92–93
Schizoid fantasy, as defense mechanism,
    162

Schizophrenia, 414
School
  in early childhood, 292
Sechenov, Ivan, 183, 184
Secondary process, psychoanalytic
      theory, 145
Seductive patient, and doctor–patient
      relationship, 22–23
  case study, 22–23
Self-direction, 207
Self-efficacy, 209–210
Self-observation, 207
Self-psychology, 170–173
  case studies, 171–172, 172–173
Self-reaction, 208
Self-regulation, 207–208
  loss, 389–391
  numbing and self-destruction, 390
  somatization, 391
  substance abuse, 391
Separation-individuation process,
      166–167
Serotonin
  and behavior, 429–430, 432–434
  and suicide, 461
Sexual development and physiology,
      233–260
  in adolescence, 301–302
  adulthood, 244–245
  birth control counseling, 247
  chromosomal abnormalities in sex
      differentiation, 237
  in early childhood, 290–291
  elderly, 245–246
  in HIV-positive patients, 248–249
  homosexuality, 247–248
  hormone changes during menstrual
      cycle, 241
  impact of life events on, 249
  infant and young child development,
      238–240
  intercourse, 243
  masturbation, 242
  in middle childhood, 296
  overview, 233–234
  pregnancy, teenage, 247
  prenatal development, 236–238
  puberty, 240–244

sexual history interview, 234–236
sexual physiology, 254–255
sexual response, 249–257
  cycle, 255–257
  females
    cyclic changes, 253
    genital anatomy, 252–254
    hormone changes during
      menstrual cycle, 241
  males
    cyclic changes, 251
    genital anatomy, 250
    reproductive system, 250
    sexual physiology, 254–255
Skinner, B. F., 184, 187
Sleep
  in early childhood, 287
  during infancy, 276
  in middle childhood, 293
  neurobiological aspects, 464–468
    architecture, 464–467
      cycles, 466–467
      stages, 464–466
    circadian rhythms, 467–468
    and lifecycle, 467
    neurobiology, 468–469
  in toddlers, 282
Social class
  and decision time, 73–75
  and mental disorders, 69–70
  and physical disorders, 68–69
Social development
  adolescent, 302
  early childhood, 291–292
  in middle childhood, 296–298
  in toddlers, 287
Social learning theory, 204–210
  modeling, 204–207
    component processes, 206
    functions, 205
  self-efficacy, 209–210
  self-regulation, 207–208
    case study, 208
    self-direction, 207
    self-evaluation, 207–208
    self-observation, 207
    self-reaction, 208
Social readjustment rating scale, 49

Social skills training, 213, 219
Speech and language development
early childhood, 289–290
in toddlers, 283–284
Spouse
and doctor–patient relationship, 21
SRE *See* Schedule of Recent Life Events
Stanford-Binet Intelligence Scale, 270
Stress, 48–50
neurobiological aspects, 461–464
behavioral responses to stressors,
462–463
neuroendocrine components of
stress response and
behavioral effects, 463–464
psychological factors affecting,
85–108
and cardiovascular disease, 101–102
case study, 87
diagnostic criteria, 86
historical development of mind-body
relationship, 89–91
influence on disease, 91–97
biological predisposition to stress-
induced illness, 96–97
cognitive appraisal of life-change
events, 94
coping and defense mechanisms,
94–95
social support, 95–96
model of illness onset, 88
neuroendocrine and neuroimmune
response, 99–101
ergotropic system, 99–100
characteristics, 100
trophotropic system, 100–101
characteristics, 100
overview, 85–89
psychoneuroimmunology, 102–104
T-cell regulation, 103
psychophysiological pathways,
97–99
treatment strategies, 104–106
Stress-management training, 217–218,
219
Structural model, psychoanalytic theory,
145
Sublimation, as defense mechanism, 163

Superego
in middle childhood, 295–296
psychoanalytic theory, 145
Suppression, as defense mechanism, 163
Systematic desensitization, 214–215, 219

T
T-cell regulation, 103
Teenagers, pregnancy, 247 *See also*
Adolescence
Television
and early childhood development, 292
Testosterone, 238
Therapeutic alliance, psychoanalytic
theory, 145
Therapy, techniques in behavioral
psychology, 213–221
for anxiety disorders, 214, 215
biofeedback, 217, 219
case study, 218–221
cognitive restructuring, 217, 219
contingency contract, 213, 219
contingency management, 213, 219
exposure to fear-provoking stimuli, 214
flooding *in vivo*, 216, 219
imaginal flooding, 215–216, 219
parent training, 213, 219
problem-solving skills training, 217, 219
relaxation techniques, 216–217, 219
diaphragmatic breathing, 217
progressive muscle relaxation
(PMR), 216–217
visualization techniques, 217
response prevention, 216, 219
social skills training, 213, 219
stress-management training, 217–218,
219
systematic desensitization, 214–215, 219
Thorndike, Edward L., 184
Toddler, development, 281–287
affective development, 284–286
defense mechanisms, 285
emotions, 285
fears, 285
gender-related issues, 285–286
object relations, 284–285
cognitive development, 283
milestones, 283
Piaget's stages, 283

Toddler, development (*continued*)
  physical development, 281–283
    fine motor-adaptive skills, 282
    gross motor skills, 281
    growth and feeding, 282
    sleep, 282
    toilet training, 282–283
  response to illness and hospitalization,
    311–312
  social development, 287
  speech and language development,
    283–284
Toilet training
  in early childhood, 288
  in toddlers, 282–283
Tolman, Edward C., 184
Topographic model, psychoanalytic
    theory, 145
Training
  parent, 213, 219
  problem-solving skills, 217, 219
  social skills, 213, 219
  stress-management, 217–218, 219
Transference
  in doctor–patient relationship, 16–17
  psychoanalytic theory, 145
Trauma, developmental, 383–399
  attachment, in children, 385–389
    affect regulation development, 387
    cognitive development, 385
    coping styles, 387–389
    social context as a mediator of
      development, 386–387
  character formation, 392–394
    play, 393
    responsibility, 393
    revictimization, 394
    victimizing others, 394
  dissociation, 391–392
    amnesia, 392
    splitting-off the experience, 391–392
  effects, 398
  hemispheric lateralization, 397–398
  overview, 383–384
  psychobiology, 394–398
  self-regulation, loss, 389–391
    numbing and self-destruction, 390
    somatization, 391

  substance abuse, 391
  treatment, 398
  violence, psychological impact,
    384–385
Trophotropic system, 100–101
  characteristics, 100
Trust, in doctor–patient relationship, 12
Turner's syndrome, 237

U
Unconscious stage, psychoanalytic
    theory, 145

V
Vascular system, and sexual development
    and physiology, 255
Vineland Adaptive Behavior Scales, 270
Violence, psychological impact,
    384–385

W
WAIS-R *See* Wechsler Adult Intelligence
    Scale-Revised
Watson, John B., 184, 186
Wechsler Adult Intelligence Scale-
    Revised (WAIS-R), 270
Wechsler Individual Achievement Test
    (WIAT), 270
Wechsler Intelligence Scale for Children,
    3rd Edition (WISC-III), 270
Wechsler Preschool and Primary Scale
    of Intelligence Revised
    (WPPSI-R), 270
WIAT *See* Wechsler Individual
    Achievement Test
Wide Range Assessment of Memory and
    Learning (WRAML), 270
WISC-III *See* Wechsler Intelligence Scale
    for Children, 3rd Edition
Wolpe, Joseph, 184
WPPSI-R *See* Wechsler Preschool and
    Primary Scale of Intelligence
    Revised
WRAML *See* Wide Range Assessment of
    Memory and Learning

X
XYY chromosome syndrome, 237